Statistics for Biology and Health

For other titles published in this series, go to
http://www.springer.com/series/2848

Alexander Krämer · Mirjam Kretzschmar ·
Klaus Krickeberg
Editors

Modern Infectious Disease Epidemiology

Concepts, Methods, Mathematical Models, and Public Health

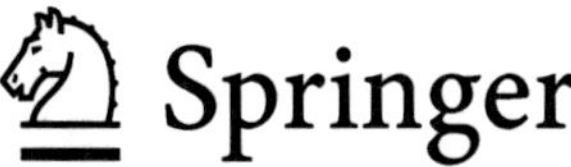

Editors

Alexander Krämer
Universität Bielefeld Fak.
Gesundheitswissenschaften
Universitätsstr. 25
33615 Bielefeld
Germany
alexander.kraemer@uni-bielefeld.de

Mirjam Kretzschmar
University Medical Center Utrecht
Julius Center for Health
Sciences & Primary Care
Heidelberglaan 100
3584 CX Utrecht
The Netherlands
m.e.e.kretzschmar@umcutrecht.nl

Klaus Krickeberg
Le Châtelet
F-63270 Manglieu
France
krik@ideenwelt.de

Statistics for Biology and Health Series Editors

ISSN 1431-8776
ISBN 978-0-387-93834-9 e-ISBN 978-0-387-93835-6
DOI 10.1007/978-0-387-93835-6
Springer New York Dordrecht Heidelberg London

Library of Congress Control Number: 2009939504

Printed on acid-free paper

Springer is part of Springer Science+Business Media (www.springer.com)

Foreword

Infectious diseases have been, alongside cardiovascular diseases and cancer, the main threat to human health. Acute and chronic respiratory diseases, especially pulmonary tuberculosis, but also malaria, AIDS and acute infections of the digestive tract are responsible for a large portion of mortality, both in developing and developed countries. Moreover, the role of infectious agents in the genesis of various severe ailments, such as cardiovascular diseases, certain carcinomas and stomach ulcers, is more and more being brought to light.

Fighting infectious diseases has many aspects – all of them characterized by their dynamic nature. First, infections travel. The plague did so extensively already in the Middle Ages and up to the end of the nineteenth century. The Spanish flu at the end of World War I cost the lives of several million people all over the world. At present, high mobility of people through travel and migration and an ever-increasing exchange of goods are driving the rapid spread of infections around the world. The first aspect of the fight against these infections is, therefore, what is commonly called "epidemic control". This means fast information on new cases, on incidences and mortalities, on strains and transmission routes of the infectious pathogen, if possible centralized in a supranational institution such as the World Health Organization (WHO). It also means making rapid decisions on intervention and treatment strategies, for example, isolation and prophylaxis or treatment with antivirals, for example, stockpiling drugs. The efficacy of modern methods of epidemic control was demonstrated during recently emerging diseases like the bovine spongiform encephalopathy (mad cow disease), the severe acute respiratory syndrome (SARS) and avian influenza ($A|H_5N_1$), which finally did not reach large proportions of the population, especially compared to the diseases mentioned in the beginning. It is to be hoped that $A|H_1N_1$ can also be contained by rigorous control.

A second aspect of the fight against infectious diseases is the changing environment in which disease transmission is taking place. The transmission of an infection in a community or between communities is influenced by many characteristics of modern societies such as growing urbanization accompanied by changing structures of cities as well as of the country side, different housing conditions, growing social inequalities that imply growing health inequalities, pollution and malnutrition that may weaken the immune system, and consequences of climate change. Classical hygiene, both public and personal, still plays a pivotal role in environmental prevention, but needs to be complemented by measures that respond to the aforementioned factors.

A third aspect of dealing with infectious diseases is large-scale primary prevention, of which immunization is by far the most important tool. Starting with vaccination against smallpox, this public health measure has helped to reduce the burden of vaccine-preventable infections enormously. In many scientific studies, both the effectiveness and possible adverse effects of large-scale immunizations have been investigated.

However, fighting infectious diseases is like shooting at a moving target. Pathogens are continuously evolving, among others under the pressure of large-scale infection control measures like antibiotic treatment and vaccination. This aspect generates renewed challenges to infectious disease control and creates the need for continued efforts in the development of monitoring and control. While antibiotic and antiviral resistance have emerged and led to increasing problems in the control of infections like tuberculosis and hospital infections around the world, molecular biology and bioinformatics have, on the other hand, provided us with tools that allow increasingly detailed insight into the transmission patterns and dynamics of pathogens. Molecular sequencing in combination with epidemiological studies has elucidated transmission routes among individuals, risk groups and populations.

The successful implementation of infectious disease control depends critically, if not predominantly, on thorough knowledge of epidemiologic facts. Epidemic control is based on surveillance and detailed knowledge of the paths of transmission in a population. Environmental prevention rests on epidemiological studies of environmental risk factors. The planning and monitoring of immunization measures requires a deep understanding of their mechanisms and effects on transmission dynamics in a given community. Mathematical modelling is employed to compute and estimate parameters that are important for understanding the transmission dynamics. Mathematical modelling can be used to simulate outbreaks and to assess the effectiveness of different prevention and intervention strategies. Results from modelling studies help with interpreting epidemiological data and support evidence-based decisions for targeting interventions for effective disease control.

The aim of our book is to present the reader with a general picture and the main ideas of the subject. We do not aim at covering the complete field of infectious disease epidemiology, but more to introduce the reader to different methodological aspects of epidemiology that are specific for infectious diseases. Furthermore, we give insight into the epidemiology of some classes of infectious diseases characterized by their main modes of transmission. With this choice of topics we hope to bridge the gap between scientific research on the clinical, biological, mathematical, social and economic aspects of infectious diseases and their applications in public health. We would like the reader to understand the impact of infectious diseases on modern society and the instruments that policy makers have at their disposal to deal with these challenges. Hardly a day goes by without news headlines concerning infectious disease control. At the time of writing these lines, the spectre of a pandemic of influenza $A|H_1N_1$ is raising its head and containment seems a lost cause. At the same time, heated debates are taking place in many societies about the pros and cons of vaccinating young girls against human papillomavirus, while in the Netherlands one of the largest outbreaks of Q fever ever observed in humans is unfolding. It seems as if the momentum of the challenges posed by infectious diseases to our ability to control them is increasing rather than decreasing, maybe due to the increasing pace of changes in human societies and their natural environments. In order to meet these challenges we need solid scientific knowledge and an understanding of all aspects of infectious diseases and their controls. With this book we hope to provide the reader with the basic groundwork for this knowledge and understanding. We hope that it will contribute to an evidence-based and responsible communication of infectious disease topics to avoid misunderstandings and overreaction of the public.

The book is written for students of the health sciences, both of curative medicine and public health, and for experts that are active in these and related domains. It may also be of interest for the educated layman since the technical level is kept relatively low. It has evolved from a rich experience of continuous teaching and research in many places, but particularly at the School of Public Health of Bielefeld University, Germany, where an international summer school in our field has been held every year since 1999. We hope that it will fill a gap and prove useful by "infecting" the reader with fascination for the features and the dynamics of infectious disease epidemiology.

The first two parts of the text are general, treating the background and general methods for studying infectious diseases, while the third part deals with specific transmission routes and related infectious diseases.

Acknowledgements

We would like to thank the doctoral student Arina Zanuzdana from the Department of Public Health Medicine of the School of Public Health, Bielefeld University for her great engagement as technical editor, Mrs. Regine Myska for her secretarial assistance, and Erich Wehmeyer for his help in improving the English language of the chapters. In addition, we are indebted to the many critical comments of our students and colleagues that will hopefully continue to improve the quality of our book in future editions.

Bielefeld, Germany — Alexander Krämer
Utrecht, The Netherlands — Mirjam Kretzschmar
Le Châtelet (Manglieu), France — Klaus Krickeberg

Contents

Contributors

Manas Akmatov Department of Experimental Mouse Genetics, Helmholtz Centre for Infection Research, Inhoffenstraße 7, 38124 Braunschweig, Germany, manas.akmatov@helmholtz-hzi.de

Charlotte van den Berg Cluster Infectious Diseases, Public Health Service of Amsterdam, Amsterdam, The Netherlands, cvdBerg@ggd.amsterdam.nl

Stuart M. Berman Centers for Disease Control and Prevention, Atlanta, GA, USA, smb1@cdc.gov

M.J.M. Bonten Department of Medical Microbiology and the Julius Center for Health Sciences and Primary Care; University Medical Center Utrecht, Utrecht, The Netherlands, mbonten@umcutrecht.nl

M.C.J. Bootsma Faculty of Science, Department of Mathematics, Utrecht University, Utrecht, The Netherlands; Julius Center for Health Sciences and Primary Care University Medical Center Utrecht, Utrecht, The Netherlands, m.c.j.bootsma@uu.nl

Sylvia M. Bruisten Cluster Infectious Diseases, Public Health Service of Amsterdam, Amsterdam, The Netherlands, sbruisten@ggd.amsterdam.nl

Roel Coutinho Center for Infectious Disease Control, RIVM, Bilthoven, The Netherlands, roel.coutinho@rivm.nl

A.S.G. Faruque International Centre for Diarrhea Disease Research, Bangladesh (ICDDR,B), Dhaka, Bangladesh, gfaruque@icddrb.org

Eduardo L. Franco Division of Cancer Epidemiology, Departments of Oncology and Epidemiology and Biostatistics, McGill University, Montreal, Canada, eduardo.franco@mcgill.ca

Wolfgang Greiner Bielefeld School of Public Health, Health Care Management (AG5), University of Bielefeld, Postfach 10 01 31, D-33501 Bielefeld, Germany, wolfgang.greiner@uni-bielefeld.de

Oliver Gruebner Geography Department, Geomatics Lab, Humboldt-Universität zu Berlin, Berlin, Germany, oliver.gruebner@geo.hu-berlin.de

Susan Hahné Center for Infectious Disease Control, RIVM, Bilthoven, Netherlands, susan.hahne@rivm.nl

Lars Henning International Centre for Diarrhea Disease Research, Bangladesh (ICDDR,B), Dhaka, Bangladesh; Swiss Tropical Institute, Basel, Switzerland, lars.henning@unibas.ch

Md. Mobarak Hossain Khan Department of Public Health Medicine, School of Public Health, University of Bielefeld, Bielefeld, Germany, mobarak.khan@uni-bielefeld.de

Patrick Hostert Geography Department, Geomatics Lab, Humboldt-Universität zu Berlin, Berlin, Germany, patrick.hostert@geo.hu-berlin.de

Tomas Jelinek Berlin Center for Travel and Tropical Medicine, Jägerstrasse 67–69, 10117 Berlin, Germany, jelinek@bctropen.de

Robert E. Johnson Centers for Disease Control and Prevention, Atlanta, GA, USA, rej1@cdc.gov

David Klemperer School of Social Sciences, University of Applied Sciences, Regensburg, Germany, david.klemperer@soz.fh-regensburg.de

Alexander Krämer Department of Public Health Medicine, School of Public Health, University of Bielefeld, Bielefeld, Germany, alexander.kraemer@uni-bielefeld.de

Gérard Krause Department for Infectious Diseases Epidemiology, Robert Koch Institute, Nordufer 20, 13353 Berlin, Germany, krauseg@rki.de

Mirjam Kretzschmar Julius Centre for Health Sciences and Primary Care, University Medical Centre Utrecht, Utrecht, The Netherlands; Center for Infectious Disease Control, RIVM, Bilthoven, The Netherlands, mirjam.kretzschmar@rivm.nl

Klaus Krickeberg Formerly, Universitè de Paris V, France; Bielefeld, Germany, krik@ideenwelt.de

Thijs van de Laar Cluster Infectious Diseases, Public Health Service of Amsterdam, Amsterdam, Netherlands, tvdlaar@ggd.amsterdam.nl

Charles P. Larson International Centre for Diarrhea Disease Research, Bangladesh (ICDDR,B), Dhaka, Bangladesh; Centre for International Child Health, British Columbia Children's Hospital and Department of Pediatrics, University of British Columbia, Vancouver, Canada, clarson@icddrb.org

Reiner Leidl Helmholtz Zentrum München, German Research Center for Environmental Health (GmbH), Institute of Health Economics and Health Care Management (IGM), Ingolstädter Landstr. 1, 85764 Neuherberg, Germany, leidl@helmholtz-muenchen.de

Karen Lindenburg Cluster Infectious Diseases, Pubic Health Service of Amsterdam, Amsterdam, The Netherlands, klindenburg@ggd.amsterdam.nl

Thomas Löscher Department of Infectious Diseases and Tropical Medicine (DITM), University of Munich, Munich, Germany, loescher@lrz.uni-muenchen.de

Stephen Luby International Centre for Diarrhea Disease Research, Bangladesh (ICDDR,B), Dhaka, Bangladesh, sluby@icddrb.org

Colin D. Mathers Department of Measurement and Health Information Systems, World Health Organization, Geneva, Switzerland, mathersc@who.int

Rafael Mikolajczyk Department of Public Health Medicine, School of Public Health, University of Bielefeld, Germany, rafael.mikolajczyk@uni-bielefeld.de

Richard Pebody Health Protection Agency, Communicable Disease Surveillance Centre, London, England, richard.pebody@hpa.org.uk

Paulo Pinheiro Department of Public Health Medicine, School of Public Health, University of Bielefeld, Germany, paulo.pinheiro@uni-bielefeld.de

Maarten Postma Groningen Research Institute of Pharmacy (GRIP), Antonius Deusinglaan 1, University of Groningen, 9713 AV Groningen, Groningen, The Netherlands, m.j.postma@rug.nl

Maria Prins Cluster Infectious Diseases, Public Health Service of Amsterdam, Amsterdam, Netherlands, mprins@ggd.amsterdam.nl

Luise Prüfer-Krämer Travel Clinic, Bielefeld, Germany, pruefer-kraemer@gmx.de

Ralf Reintjes Department of Public Health, Hamburg University of Applied Sciences, Hamburg, Germany, ralf.reintjes@haw-hamburg.de

Leo Schouls Laboratory for Infectious Diseases and Perinatal Screening, National Institute for Public Health and the Environment, Antonie van Leeuwenhoeklaan 9, 3721 MA Bilthoven, The Netherlands, leo.schouls@rivm.nl

Helen Trottier Division of Cancer Epidemiology, Departments of Oncology and Epidemiology and Biostatistics, McGill University, Montreal, Canada, helen.trottier@mcgill.ca

Timo Ulrichs Koch-Metschnikow-Forum, Luisenstr. 59, 10117 Berlin, Germany, timo.ulrichs@bmg.bund.de

Jim van Steenbergen Center for Infectious Disease Control, RIVM, Bilthoven, The Netherlands, jim.van.steenbergen@rivm.nl

Jacco Wallinga Julius Centre for Health Sciences and Primary Care, University Medical Centre Utrecht, Utrecht, The Netherlands; Center for Infectious Disease Control, RIVM, Bilthoven, The Netherlands, jacco.wallinga@rivm.nl

Robert Welte Helmholtz Zentrum München, German Research Center for Environmental Health (GmbH), Institute of Health Economics and Health Care

Management (IGM), Ingolstädter Landstr. 1, 85764 Neuherberg, Germany, robert.welte@helmholtz-muenchen.de

Aryna Zanuzdana Department of Public Health Medicine, School of Public Health, University of Bielefeld, Bielefeld, Germany, aryna.zanuzdana@uni-bielefeld.de

Freke Zuure Cluster Infectious Diseases, Public Health Service of Amsterdam, Amsterdam, Netherlands, fzuure@ggd.amsterdam.nl

Part I
Challenges

Chapter 1
The Global Burden of Infectious Diseases

Paulo Pinheiro, Colin D. Mathers, and Alexander Krämer

1.1 Introduction

Over the last century, infectious diseases have lost a lot of their threat to individuals' health as well as to the health of populations living in industrialized countries. The continuous reduction and effective control of both mortality and morbidity from infectious diseases marks an impressive story of success in the history of public health in the developed world and has been linked to a wide range of improvements that occurred alongside the socioeconomic modernization of these societies. Although many factors (e.g., improved sanitation, development of antibiotics and vaccines, improved living conditions and food quality/availability, and improved health care and surveillance systems) that contributed significantly to the success have been identified, there are, however, still uncertainties about the underlying mechanisms and interactions that led to the decline of infectious disease mortality (Sagan 1987). The sustainable control of infectious diseases was also accompanied by an impressive rise of life expectancies which, in turn, gave chronic (non-communicable) diseases the opportunity to increase in quantity and importance for public health. This so-called epidemiological transition (Omran 1971, Olshansky and Ault 1986) may have resulted in the fact that infectious diseases have become somewhat marginalized in the public perception of the developed world.

From a global perspective, however, infectious diseases still play, and will continue to play, a significant role in public health since most of the regions of the world have not reached a level of modernization that is comparable with the industrialized world. Especially developing countries and countries in transition still face an enormous burden posed by communicable diseases on their populations' health. Changes in environment and human behavior due to the globalization of the world and the evolutionary dynamics of microbial agents may, furthermore, produce new ecological niches that enable the emergence or re-emergence of infections, thus posing a persistent threat to the developed world too.

P. Pinheiro (✉)
Department of Public Health Medicine, School of Public Health, University of Bielefeld, Germany
e-mail: paulo.pinheiro@uni-bielefeld.de

A. Krämer et al. (eds.), *Modern Infectious Disease Epidemiology*,
Statistics for Biology and Health, DOI 10.1007/978-0-387-93835-6_1,

This chapter aims to give an overview of the global and regional distribution of infectious diseases and puts its emphasis on the impact of infectious diseases on the population's health. For this purpose, the findings presented here will mainly rely

on results from the Global Burden of Disease Project (Lopez et al. 2006). Using this approach, one is able to not only make comprehensive estimates of the magnitude of the burden of infectious diseases, but also to make comparative assessments of the burden of disease posed by non-communicable diseases and injuries. This makes it possible to identify the importance of communicable diseases relatively to other diseases.

The first part of this chapter provides an introduction to the GBD study, i.e., its conceptual and methodological basis, and dwells on the GBD core measure, the
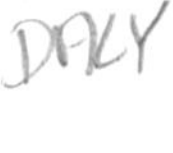
Disability-Adjusted Life Year (DALY). In the second part, main empirical findings on the current and future burden of disease that can be related directly to infectious conditions will be presented. These findings include published data from the GBD study as well as own estimates that were generated on the basis of available GBD statistics.

1.2 The Burden of Disease Approach

1.2.1 Conceptual Framework

Undisputedly, population health statistics are an important source of information for decision-makers and researchers in public health. Although there has been an increase in volume and quality of health data in the past, statistics on the health status of populations still suffer from several limitations that reduce their value for policy making and research purposes. These limitations include difficulties in comparing health indicators over time, across population groups, before and after specific health interventions, or the making of comparisons related to different health states and disease events. Furthermore, health statistics are globally unevenly distributed with many countries still lacking basic information on mortality and morbidity data.

In order to approach these difficulties, the World Bank, in collaboration with the World Health Organization (WHO) and the Harvard School of Public Health, started the Global Burden of Disease Project in the late 1980s. The main objective of the study was to generate a comprehensive and internally consistent, thus comparable set of estimates of mortality and morbidity by age, sex, and regions of the world. First estimates were made for the year 1990 (Murray and Lopez 1996). Also, the 1990 GBD study provided the public health community with a new conceptual und methodological framework, which was developed for integrating, validating, analyzing, and disseminating partial and fragmented information on the health of populations. The characteristics of this framework included the development of methods to estimate missing data and to assess the quality of available data, the incorporation of data on non-fatal health outcomes into summary measures of population health, and the development of a new metric, the Disability-Adjusted Life

Year (DALY) , to summarize the disease burden (Murray and Lopez 1996, 1997a). Since the original 1990 GBD study, WHO has undertaken some major revisions of the methodology resulting in improved updates of the global burden of disease for the years 2000–2002 (e.g., World Health Organization 2002).

The 2001 GBD study, which is the central source of information for this chapter, has quantified the burden of premature mortality and disability by age, sex, and region for 136 causes. These 136 causes are closely related to the diagnostic categories of the International Classification of Diseases (ICD) and are classified using a tree structure with four levels of disaggregation. In the GBD classification system, the first level of disaggregation defines three broad cause groups: group I causes include communicable, maternal, perinatal, and nutritional conditions; group II and group III causes comprise non-communicable diseases and injuries, respectively (Mathers et al. 2006).

Regional assessments of the burden of disease have been presented on a country level or on either the WHO (World Health Organization 2002) or the World Bank (World Bank 2002) regional grouping level. In this chapter, the estimates are presented in terms of the income and regional groupings of countries as given by the World Bank. Based on the economic and social data compilation according to the World Development Report 2003 (World Bank 2002) countries are divided into seven groups: the high-income countries constitute one group and the low- and middle-income countries comprise another group that can further be subdivided into six geographical regions.

1.2.2 The Measurement Unit Disability-Adjusted Life Year (DALY)

The measurement unit Disability-Adjusted Life Year (DALY) is a core element of the GBD study since it was exclusively designed to meet the major objectives of this study, i.e., the inclusion of non-fatal health outcomes in debates on international health policy, the decoupling of epidemiological assessments from advocacy, and the quantification of the burden of disease with a measure that could further be used for cost-effectiveness analysis. The technical basis for the DALY calculation is characterized by a high degree of complexity since a number of different features had to be incorporated into the development of the DALY formula in order to fulfil the overall aims of the GBD study. Thus, an adequate interpretation of results that are generated with this measure requires some methodological knowledge.

The DALY is a composite measure that combines time lost due to premature mortality with time of healthy life lost due to living in health states worse than ideal health (see Fig. 1.1). Thus, the DALY measure is a health gap measure that quantifies the difference between the actual health of a population and some defined ideal or goal for population health. Just like DALYs, the quality adjusted life year (QALY) measure is a way of measuring disease burden, including both the quality and the quantity of life lived. Though having several similarities in methodology and semantics with DALYs, QALYs are frequently used to measure the number of

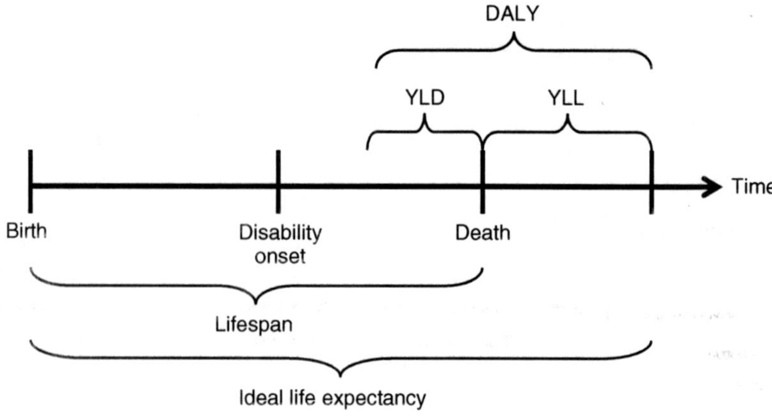

DALY = YLL + YLD
DALY: Disability Adjusted Life Years
YLL: Years of Life Lost due to premature death
YLD: Years of Life Lost due to Disability

Fig. 1.1 The GBD measure Disability-Adjusted Life Year (DALY). It sums up years of life lost due to premature death (YLL) and healthy years of life lost due to disability (YLD). Premature death refers to some ideal goal of the life expectancy. YLD estimates use disability weights in order to determine the extent of health losses in lifetime. DALYs can be calculated for disease grouping like infectious diseases or cancers or injuries, and for single disease entities like, e.g., tuberculosis, thus making all kinds of comparisons possible

additional years of healthy life that would be added by a certain intervention, be it preventive or curative, population-based, or clinical.

For the DALY development some general assumptions were made in order to achieve the goals of the GBD study (Murray 1994, 1996). First, it was demanded that any health outcome that affects social welfare should in some way be reflected in the indicator of the burden of disease. Second, individual characteristics that should be considered in estimating the burden of disease should be restricted to age and sex since these variables are general to all communities and households. For the GBD purposes, socioeconomic variables were explicitly excluded from consideration reflecting the developers' notions of social justice. Third, like-health outcomes should be treated as like. The principle of treating like events equally was articulated in order to ensure comparability of the burden of disease across different communities or in the same community over a period of time, and implies that the health status of a person does not depend on his/her neighbor's health status. Fourthly, time was chosen to be the unit of measure for the burden of disease.

Estimates of the duration of time lost due to premature death are reflected in the DALY formula by the component Years of Life Lost (YLL). There are several options to estimate time lost due to mortality. For the calculation of DALYs, the use of the standard expected years of life lost method was chosen (Murray 1994, 1996). Basically, this method calculates the time of life lost due to premature death with regard to a standard cohort life expectancy at each age. For the ideal standard, the expectations of life at each age are based on a model life table which has a life expectancy at birth for females of 82.5 years. This value was chosen since it was close to the highest national period life expectancy observed at that time. For males, a life expectancy at birth of 80 years was defined. This sex difference in life expectancies at birth of 2.5 years obviously does not reflect the average observed differences in populations which are significantly higher. It was chosen according to the developers' assumption about the biological differences in life expectancies when behavioral or contextual factors are equally distributed between the sexes.

Years of Life Lost due to Disability (YLD) are the morbidity component of the DALYs and are considered to be the most difficult estimate in a burden of disease study (Mathers et al. 2001). The assessment of the impact of non-fatal health outcomes on the burden of disease requires an in-depth understanding of the diseases specific epidemiology. Non-fatal health conditions are measured in the DALY formula in terms of disability, i.e., the functional loss of capacity. The data required to estimate the YLD component are the disability incidence and duration, the age of onset, and the distribution by severity classes, all of which must be disease specific and disaggregated by age and sex. To make the specified disabilities comparable, YLDs were combined with a disability weight ranging from 0 (full health equivalent) to 1 (health state equivalent to death). The bigger a disability weight, the more health losses are estimated. The disability weights again implied value choices since it was required to give preferences for health states in terms of a single number on an interval level scale. In the GBD framework, health state valuation was done by means of the person trade-off (PTO) technique (Murray 1996). The PTO method is a group exercise where specific descriptions of patients in different health states are presented to the participants. The participants are then asked to do an explicit trade-off between a collection of 1000 fictive, healthy people and each of the people in the presented health state, i.e., to indicate the number of disabled people equivalent to the 1000 healthy people. Disability weights are then calculated as the ratio of the number of the imaginary healthy people divided by the number of virtual people in the disabled health state. In the original 1990 GBD study, disability weights were derived for all conditions based on a set of 22 indicator conditions by expert panels from different regions of the world. Disability weights used for the updated GBD studies were based on the 1990 GBD disability weights.

Other key features of the DALY measure that affect the calculation of both YLL and YLD are social values with respect to age and time preferences (Murray 1994). An age weighting function was developed for the original GBD study based on findings indicating that there are social preferences to value years of life lived at young adult ages higher than years lived by young children or older ages. It was postulated that societies in general assign greater importance to preventing the deaths of young adults than of very young children or older adults because of different economic and social roles. Thus, according to the DALY developers, dependency of young children and elderly on young/middle-aged adults should be included in the DALY formulation. Technically, age weights are derived by the use of an exponential function. The proposal to incorporate age weights into the DALYs has led to controversial discussions (e.g., Anand and Hanson 1997) and, as a consequence, resulted in updated GBD assessments that present estimates with, as well as without, age preferences.

Time preferences have been considered in the GBD study by means of a discounting rate that was applied to the DALY calculation (Murray 1994). Discounting of future benefits is a widely accepted economic concept that reflects the fact that most individuals prefer benefits now rather than in the future. It refers to the practice that things are valued in the future as less or more valuable than in the present. This concept was transferred to the GBD study in terms of valuing future health losses in comparison with the present ones. Similar to the age weights, a number of arguments have been presented for and against discounting future health. DALY incorporates an arbitrarily chosen 3% discount rate per year.

1.3 The global and Regional Burden of Infectious Diseases

1.3.1 Infectious Diseases and the Global and Regional Causes of Death

Worldwide, slightly more than 56.2 million people out of about 6.1 billion people living globally died in 2001. About 14.7 million, or 26%, of these deaths were from infectious diseases. Maternal and perinatal conditions and nutritional deficiencies (other group I conditions) accounted for 3.5 million deaths (6%), noncommunicable diseases (group II) for about 32.9 million deaths (59%), and injuries (group III) for about 5.2 million deaths (9%) (see Fig. 1.2).

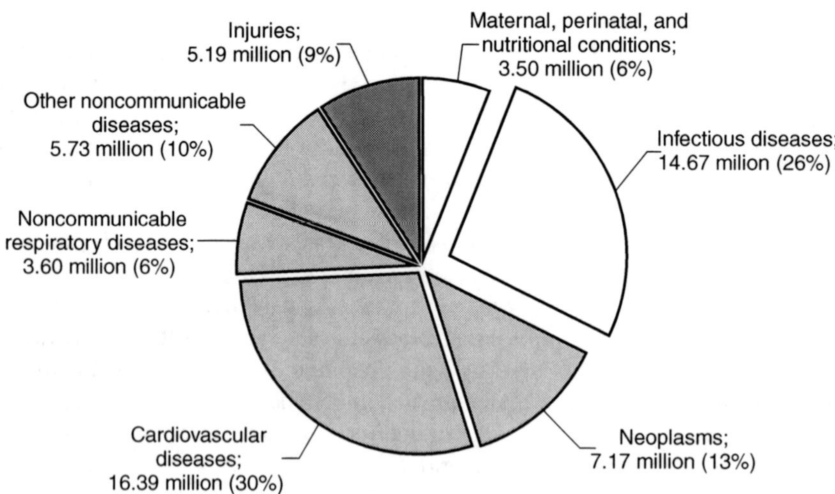

Fig. 1.2 Global causes of death, 2001 (GBD group I conditions: *white*; group II conditions: *gray*; group III conditions: *black*)

Among the infectious disease group, respiratory infectious diseases are the most common cause of death (3.8 million; 26.1% of all infectious causes of death), followed by HIV/AIDS (2.6 million; 17.5%), diarrheal diseases (1.8 million; 12.2%), tuberculosis (1.6 million; 10.9%), vaccine preventable childhood diseases (1.4 million; 9.3%), malaria (1.2 million; 8.2%), sexually transmitted diseases excluding HIV/AIDS (0.18 million; 1.2%), meningitis (0.17 million; 1.2%), hepatitis B and C (0.15 million; 1.0%), and tropical-cluster diseases (0.13 million; 0.8%). Other infectious diseases contributed to approx. 1.7 million deaths (11.4%) (see Fig. 1.3).

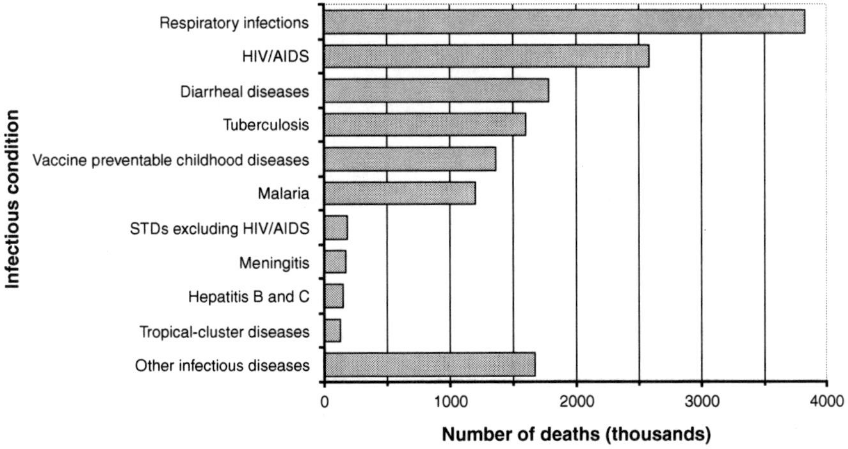

Fig. 1.3 Leading infectious causes of death worldwide, 2001

Table 1.1 shows the top 10 disease and injury causes of death in 2001 for low-and-middle-income countries and for high-income countries according to the World Bank's classification. Ischemic heart disease and cerebrovascular disease were the leading cause of death in both groups of countries, together responsible for more than one fifth of all deaths worldwide. Only 1.4 million of the total 7.1 deaths from ischemic heart disease, and 0.8 million of the total 5.4 million of deaths from cerebrovascular diseases lived in high-income countries reflecting the importance of cardio- and cerebrovascular diseases for health in low-and-middle-income countries. Lung cancer (0.5 million deaths) was the third leading cause of death in high-income countries, but was not among the ten leading causes of death in low- and middle-income countries. Here, five of the ten most common causes of death were infectious diseases, including lower respiratory infections, HIV/AIDS, diarrheal diseases, tuberculosis, and malaria. In contrast to these findings, only lower respiratory infections (0.34 million deaths) appear as an infectious condition in the top ten ranking of causes of death in high-income countries. According to the mortality data, high-income countries suffer not only a much lower burden than low- and middle-income countries but also a burden that is predominantly affected by non-communicable conditions.

When stratifying the mortality estimates by age groups, about 12.1 million deaths (21.5%) were attributable to children younger than 15 years of age in 2001. Nearly

Table 1.1 The ten leading causes of death, by broad income group, 2001

Low- and middle-income countries				High-income countries			
S.No.	Cause	Deaths (millions)	Percentage of total deaths	S.No.	Causes	Deaths (millions)	Percentage of total deaths
1	Ischemic heart disease	5.70	11.8	1	Ischemic heart disease	1.36	17.3
2	Cerebrovascular disease	4.61	9.5	2	Cerebrovascular disease	0.78	9.9
3	Lower respiratory infections	3.41	7.0	3	Trachea, bronchus, and lung cancers	0.46	5.8
4	HIV/AIDS	2.55	5.3	4	Lower respiratory infections	0.34	4.4
5	Perinatal conditions	2.49	5.1	5	Chronic obstructive pulmonary disease	0.30	3.8
6	Chronic obstructive pulmonary disease	2.38	4.9	6	Colon and rectal cancers	0.26	3.3
7	Diarrheal diseases	1.78	3.7	7	Alzheimer's and other dementias	0.21	2.6
8	Tuberculosis	1.59	3.3	8	Diabetes mellitus	0.20	2.6
9	Malaria	1.21	2.5	9	Breast cancer	0.16	2.0
10	Road traffic accidents	1.07	2.2	10	Stomach cancer	0.15	1.9

94% of these deaths occurred in low- and middle-income countries with seven of the top ten causes of death being infectious diseases and killing about 6.5 million children in 2001. Leading infectious diseases were lower respiratory infections, diarrheal diseases, and malaria.

The cause-of-death pattern distributed by age among people living in high-income countries is mainly characterized by the rise of non-communicable diseases in older age groups (see Fig. 1.4). Infectious diseases, as well as injuries play a negligible role here. Low- and middle-income countries show a different pattern when stratifying causes of death by age (see Fig. 1.4). Besides the increasing contribution of non-communicable diseases to the death numbers at higher ages that shows similarities with the pattern of high-income countries, there is also a crucial impact of infectious diseases on the mortality of the lower age groups, especially among children younger than age 5 in low- and middle-income countries. Furthermore, injuries

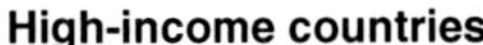

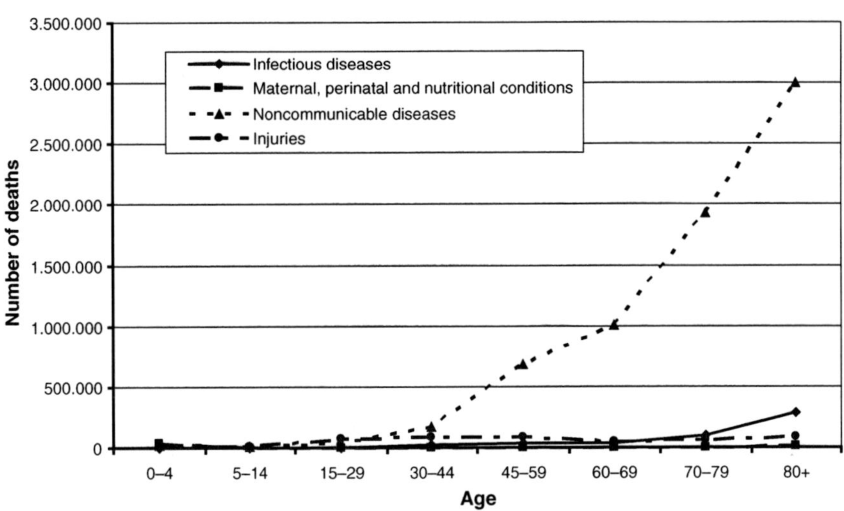

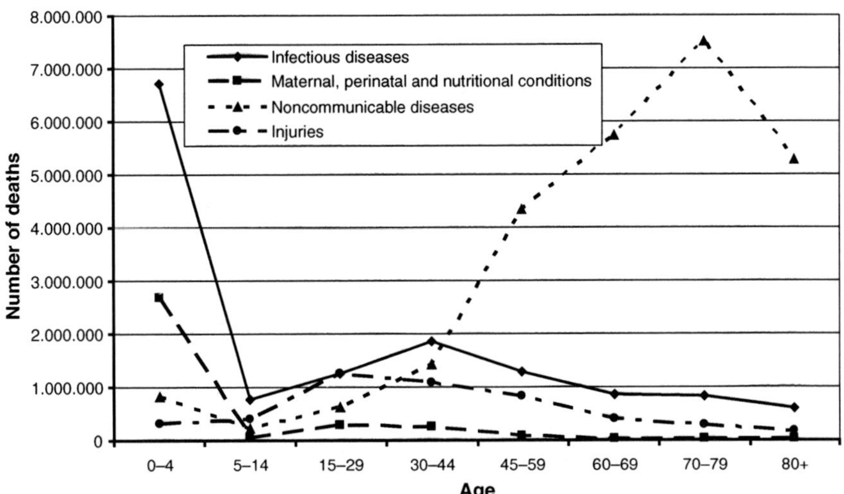

Fig. 1.4 Causes of death by age in high-income and low- and middle-income regions, 2001

can be identified in low- and middle-income countries as an important cause of death among young adults (peak values in age group 15–29 years).

According to the GBD estimates, child mortality (age 0–4 years) generally declined between 1990 and 2001 in all regions of the world mainly due to a substantial decrease of death rates from communicable diseases, especially for diarrheal and respiratory diseases. Mortality from diarrheal diseases fell from 2.4 million deaths in 1990 to about 1.6 million deaths in 2001 as a result of improvements in diarrheal case management. Death rates from acute respiratory infections declined by more than 40% in all regions of the world except in South Asia (25%) and sub-Saharan Africa (15%). On the other hand, malaria and HIV/AIDS are the two diseases for which death rates have increased from 1990 to 2001 in children younger than 5 years, primarily in sub-Saharan Africa. Here, the proportion of deaths caused by malaria in children younger than 5 years increased from 15 to 22%.

Among adults aged 15–59 years, HIV/AIDS has become the leading cause of death worldwide in 2001 being responsible for 2.1 million adult deaths (14% of all deaths in adults). Deaths rates among adults aged 15–59 years have generally declined in all WHO regions of the world from 1990 to 2001 with two exceptions: Europe and Central Asia, and sub-Saharan Africa. Europe and Central Asia were the only regions where deaths rates from cardiovascular diseases and injuries have increased within this period. In sub-Saharan Africa, the rise of mortality among adults aged 15–59 years has been attributed to HIV/AIDS. In 2001, about 80% of the 2.1 million adult deaths from HIV/AIDS occurred in sub-Saharan Africa. Among all infectious diseases, HIV/AIDS has generally become the most important contributor to the global mortality. While HIV/AIDS accounted for 2% of all deaths in 1990, the proportion increased to 14% in 2001. Other deaths due to communicable diseases (including maternal, perinatal, and nutritional conditions) fell from one third of total deaths in 1990 to less than one fifth in 2001.

1.3.2 *Infectious Diseases and the Global and Regional Burden of Disease*

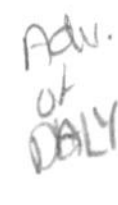

In addition to the mortality estimates presented in the section before and expressed in terms of death numbers, an assessment of the health burden caused by diseases and injuries as measured in DALYs offers several advantages: At first, the incorporation of non-fatal health outcomes into burden of disease calculations enables the assessment of the impact of chronic diseases, especially of those that are characterized by a low case-fatality, on a population's health. Then, the combination of non-fatal with fatal outcomes allows comparability between mortality with morbidity information. Finally, the presentation of results in terms of health losses gives an idea about a virtually existing preventive potential.

There have been several ways of how to report DALY estimates, depending on the fact whether or not non-uniform age weights and discount rates were applied to the DALY formula. Noteworthy is that these inconsistencies have resulted in limitations when comparing the presentations of GBD results by use of different publication sources. In the present section, DALYs will be used with uniform age weights and the standard GBD discount rate as presented by Lopez et al. (2006).

In 2001, the total global burden of disease was more than 1.536 million DALYs according to the GBD estimates. Across all regions of the world, the average burden of disease was 250 DALY per 1000 population, of which almost two thirds were due to years of life lost due to premature mortality and one third due to years of life lived with disability. The global burden of disease attributable to infectious diseases accounted for slightly more than 400 million DALYs and thus for about 26% of the total burden of disease. Maternal and perinatal conditions and nutritional deficiencies (other group I conditions) accounted for about 148 million DALYs (10%), non-communicable diseases (group II) for about 808 million DALYs (53%), and injuries (group III) for about 167 million DALYs (11%) (see Fig. 1.5). In contrast to the cause-of-death analyses, DALY estimates capture the relevance of chronic conditions with low case-fatality such as neuropsychiatric disorders and sense organ disorders.

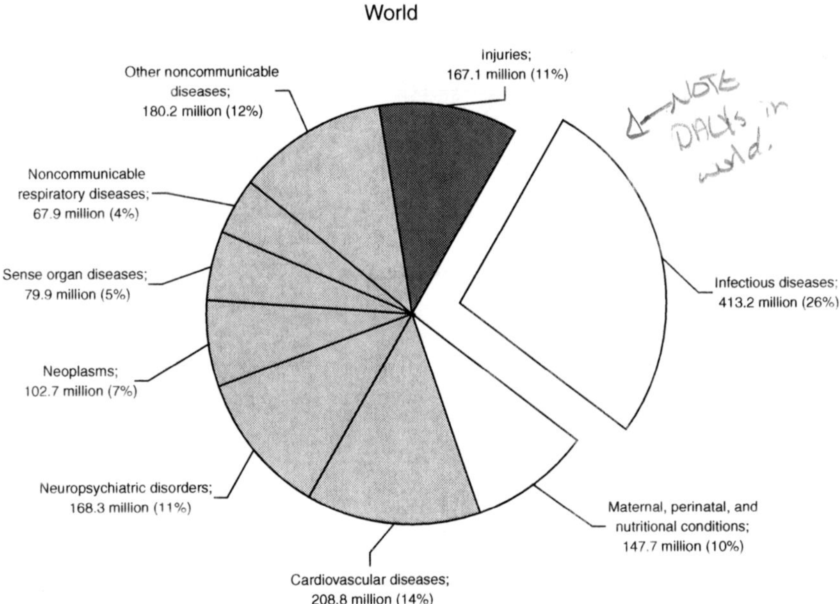

Fig. 1.5 Global burden of disease estimated by DALYs, 2001 (GBD group I conditions: *white*; group II conditions: *gray*; group III conditions: *black*)

Among all infectious diseases, respiratory infectious diseases were the most common cause of DALYs (89.2 million; 21.6% of all infectious disease DALYs), followed by HIV/AIDS (71.5 million; 17.3%), diarrheal diseases (59.1 million; 14.3%), vaccine preventable childhood diseases (43.3 million; 10.5%), malaria (40.0 million; 9.7%), tuberculosis (36.1 million; 8.7%), tropical-cluster diseases (10.3 million; 2.5%), sexually transmitted diseases excluding HIV/AIDS (9.5 million; 2.3%), meningitis (5.6 million; 1.4%), and hepatitis B and C (3.2 million; 0.8%). Other infectious diseases contributed to approx. 45.5 million DALYs (11.0%) (see Fig.1.6).

When comparing the DALY ranking with the death number ranking among the infectious condition group, respiratory infectious diseases, HIV/AIDS, and diarrheal diseases were the leading causes in both statistics. Using DALYs, a higher relevance to the burden can be attributed to vaccine preventable diseases, malaria, and tropical-cluster diseases, whereas, e.g., for tuberculosis less importance can be assigned. An

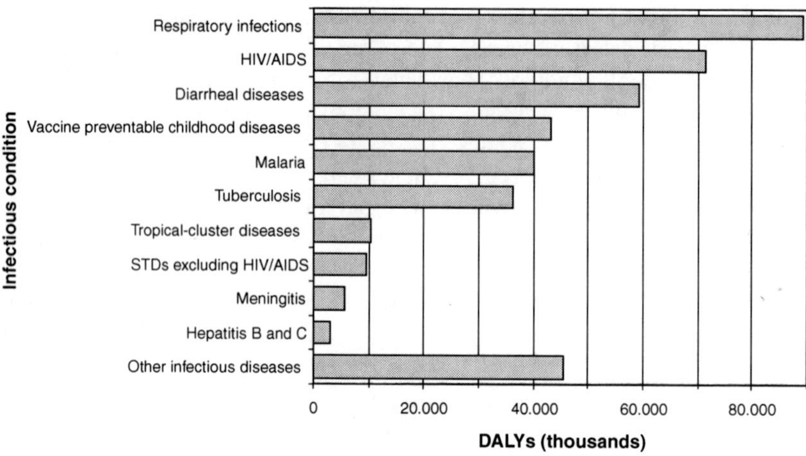

Fig. 1.6 Leading infectious conditions of the global burden of disease, 2001

important reason for the variability in the rankings is that DALYs incorporate the age at death into the calculation of years of life lost and thus assign a higher burden to diseases that cause premature death in early ages.

Table 1.2 shows the 20 leading causes of the global burden of disease. In contrast to the cause-of-death ranking, perinatal conditions and lower respiratory infectious

Table 1.2 The 20 leading causes of global burden of disease, 2001

S.No	Cause	DALYs (millions of years)	Percentage of total DALYs
1	Perinatal conditions	90.48	5.9
2	Lower respiratory infections	85.92	5.6
3	Ischemic heart disease	84.27	5.5
4	Cerebrovascular disease	72.02	4.7
5	HIV/AIDS	71.46	4.7
6	Diarrheal diseases	59.14	3.9
7	Unipolar depressive disorders	51.84	3.4
8	Malaria	39.97	2.6
9	Chronic obstructive pulmonary disease	38.74	2.5
10	Tuberculosis	36.09	2.3
11	Road traffic accidents	35.06	2.3
12	Hearing loss, adult onset	29.99	2.0
13	Cataracts	28.64	1.9
14	Congenital anomalies	24.95	1.6
15	Measles	23.11	1.5
16	Self-inflicted injuries	20.26	1.3
17	Diabetes mellitus	20.00	1.3
18	Violence	18.90	1.2
19	Osteoarthritis	17.45	1.1
20	Alzheimer's and other dementias	17.11	1.1

diseases are the two leading causes of burden followed by ischemic heart diseases and cerebrovascular diseases, these two conditions being the leading causes of death. Besides lower respiratory infections, 5 other infectious disease conditions are among the 20 leading causes of the global burden of disease: HIV/AIDS (5th rank), diarrheal diseases (6th), malaria (8th), tuberculosis (10th), and measles (15th).

Virtually, the entire global burden of disease (>98%) due to infectious diseases can be found in low- and middle-income countries. Here, infectious diseases account for 30% (407 million DALYs) of the total burden of disease. Maternal, perinatal, and nutritional conditions account for 10% (145 million DALYs), non-communicable diseases for 49% (678 million DALYs), and injuries for 11% (167 million DALYs). In high-income countries, the picture is completely different: Infectious diseases account for only 4% (5.8 million DALYs) of the total burden of disease, while other group I conditions contributed 2% (2.7 million DALYs), non-communicable diseases 86% (129 million DALYs), and injuries 8% (11.2 million DALYs) (see Fig. 1.7). The higher importance of infectious diseases for low- and middle-income countries can be confirmed by the fact that, in 2001, the leading causes of burden of disease included five communicable diseases (lower respiratory infections, HIV/AIDS, diarrheal diseases, malaria, and tuberculosis). The leading causes in high-income countries were all non-communicable conditions and included three conditions with few direct deaths but high disability (unipolar depressive disorders, adult-onset hearing loss, and alcohol use disorders).

HIV/AIDS was the fourth leading cause of burden of disease worldwide as well as in low- and middle-income countries in 2001. According to the GBD estimates it was the leading cause in the sub-Saharan Africa region, where it was followed by three other infectious diseases: malaria, lower respiratory infections, and diarrheal diseases. These four leading causes of burden of disease bore more than 42% of the total burden of disease in sub-Saharan Africa measured by DALYs.

The age-dependent distribution of the burden of disease in low- and middle-income and high-income countries shows patterns that are similar to those related to the mortality numbers with some slight modifications (see Fig. 1.8). In high-income countries, non-communicable diseases play an outstanding role in the burden of disease across all age groups. The use of DALYs not only depicts the importance of non-communicable conditions for higher age groups but also gives some hints to their relevance for younger age groups. Low- and middle-income countries face a double burden of disease: Children younger than 5 years of age are predominantly affected by infectious diseases. In addition, non-communicable conditions replace infectious diseases as the leading cause for the burden of disease in the subsequent age groups. When comparing the burden with the mortality pattern, the rise of the importance of non-communicable diseases becomes visible in earlier ages and thus enhances the relevance of non-communicable diseases for the younger age groups.

Between 1990 and 2001, there was a 20% decrease in the global per-head burden of disease due to the group I diseases (communicable, maternal, perinatal, and nutritional conditions). Without HIV/AIDS and the associated persistence of the burden attributable to tuberculosis, the reduction of group I conditions would have

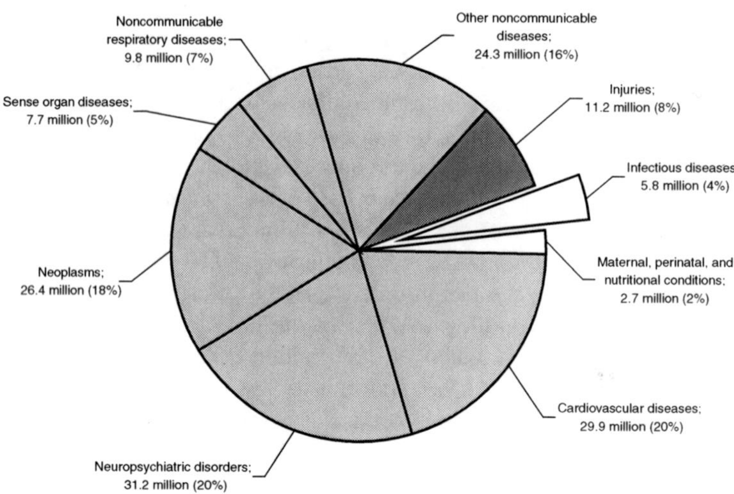

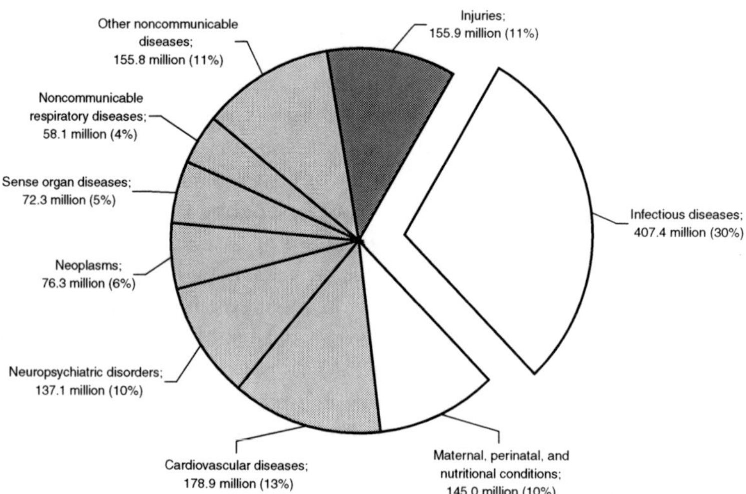

Fig. 1.7 Burden of disease in high-income and low- and middle-income countries estimated by DALYs, 2001 (GBD group I conditions: *white*; group II conditions: *gray*; group III conditions: *black*)

been almost 30% according to the GBD results. In line with the decrease of communicable diseases, the proportion of the burden of disease due to non-communicable diseases has shown a rise. In low- and middle-income countries almost half of the disease burden is from group II conditions, what marks an increase of 10% in its relative share since 1990.

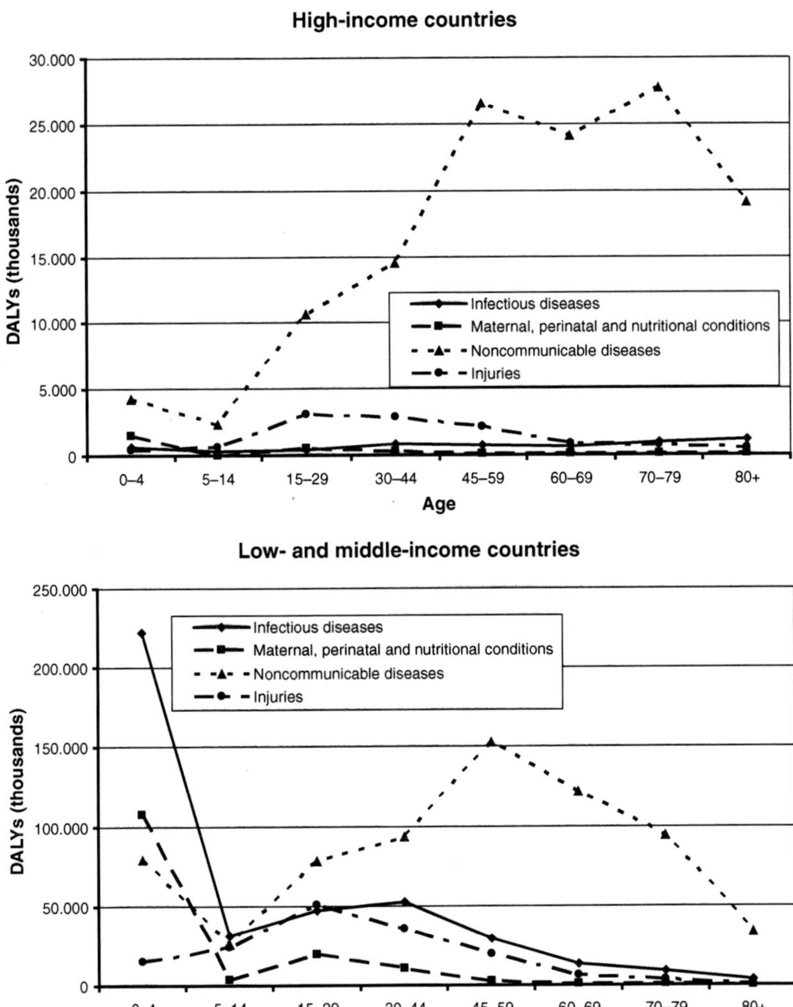

Fig. 1.8 The burden of disease by age in high-income and low- and middle-income regions, 2001

1.3.3 Projections of the Global Burden of Infectious Diseases from 2002 to 2030

The preparation of projections of mortality and burden of disease by cause represents another crucial part of the Global Burden of Disease project. On the basis of the initial estimates for 1990, first forecasts of global mortality and burden of disease trends by cause for 2000, 2010, and 2020 were presented under the assumption of three alternative scenarios (Murray and Lopez 1997b). However, it was shown that the HIV/AIDS projections based on the GBD 1990 results substantially underestimated the spread of the HIV epidemic and the level of HIV/AIDS mortality around 2000; thus, the first projections are now considered to be outdated (Mathers and Loncar 2006). As a consequence, updated projections of mortality and burden of disease from 2002 to 2030 were prepared using new input information and methods similar to those of the original GBD study (Mathers and Loncar 2006). The main results of these projections with regard to infectious conditions are presented below.

Future health trends were projected under three scenarios – baseline, pessimistic, and optimistic – that were based on economic and social development. Age- and sex-specific deaths rates at country level were projected for ten major-cause clusters comprising infectious diseases within a cluster that summarizes group I conditions excluding HIV/AIDS. For forecasts of HIV/AIDS trends, separate projections were developed under several scenarios derived from existing UNAIDS (Joint United Nations Programme on HIV/AIDS) and WHO models.

Life expectancy at birth is projected to increase in all regions of the world in 2030, with the largest increases in the Africa and South Asia regions and the highest projected life expectancy for Japanese women at 88.5 years. Projected global deaths vary from 64.9 million (optimistic scenario) to 80.7 million (pessimistic scenario). Compared with death numbers in 2002 by age, a dramatic shift in the distribution of deaths from younger to older age is forecasted for 2030.

Large declines in mortality between 2002 and 2030 are projected for all of the major infectious disease conditions, with the exception of HIV/AIDS. The average annual rate of decline in age-standardized death rates is projected to vary between about 1.4% (malaria) and 5.3% (tuberculosis) and is greater for communicable causes than for non-communicable causes. In the opposite direction, HIV/AIDS projections show an average annual rate of increase of 3% for males and 2% for females.

Under the baseline scenario, HIV/AIDS deaths increase from 2.8 million in 2002 to 6.5 million in 2030. The total number of deaths caused by other communicable, maternal, perinatal, and nutritional conditions declines from 15.5 million in 2002 to 9.0 million in 2030. By contrast and as a result of the population aging and the increasing number of road traffic accidents, total deaths due to group II (non-communicable) and group III conditions (injuries) will significantly increase until 2030.

DALYs are projected to increase worldwide from 1.48 billion in 2002 to 1.54 billion in 2030. Although this means an increase of 3% of the total burden of disease, there is a decrease of the per-capita burden since the global population increase is projected to be 27%. Another factor that contributes to a decrease of DALY rates is the postponement of the age at death to older ages that is projected to occur from 2002 to 2030 and that results in a reduction of measured years of life lost. With regard to the three major GBD cause groups, the projections show significant changes in the proportional contribution to the burden of disease. Group I diseases are projected to contribute to 30% of the burden in 2030 as compared to more than 40% in 2002. In low-income countries the decline of the group I proportion is more pronounced, from 56% in 2002 to 41% in 2030. Group II conditions are projected to increase to 57% in 2030; thus, non-communicable diseases will become the most important contributor to the global burden in 2030. According to the baseline scenario, there will be substantial changes in the global rank order of the leading causes of DALYs between 2002 and 2030. With the exception of HIV/AIDS, infectious diseases are projected to decline substantially in importance. Lower respiratory infections, tuberculosis, diarrheal diseases, and malaria are projected to move down up to 15 places in the global burden ranking. On the other hand, HIV/AIDS is projected to move up one place becoming the third most important contributor to DALYs in 2030. However, infectious diseases are projected to maintain an important role in low-income countries in 2030 where they account for four of the ten leading causes of burden of disease. These are HIV/AIDS (2nd rank), lower respiratory infections (5th), diarrheal diseases (8th), and malaria (10th).

1.4 Discussion

The estimates of the GBD study show that only a minor burden can be attributed to infectious diseases in high-income countries and, thus, this may suggest that the impact of communicable diseases on the population's health is of less importance compared with non-communicable diseases or injuries. However, in low- and middle-income countries the burden of infectious diseases will continue to remain high with implications for more efficient public health strategies. The planning of interventions should take into account the relative changes in incidence of different infectious disease entities.

According to the published projections of mortality and burden of disease, the impact of HIV/AIDS on population health is going to increase over the next decades. The estimates for HIV/AIDS, however, have recently been revised downward quite substantially. Due to better data from population-based surveys and due to new evidence on survival with HIV/AIDS, UNAIDS and WHO revised estimates for India (halving prevalence estimate from half a million to closer to quarter of a million) and for a number of African countries (UNAIDS 2007). The overall effect was a reduction of the death estimates from around 2.5 million to 2.1 million for 2007. For 2001, there would presumably be a similar, but smaller reduction in the total number of deaths and DALYs, respectively. Also, based on the new evidence, and on more optimistic assumptions that incidence will decline with increasing antiretroviral therapy (ART) coverage, the new projections of UNAIDS predict peak HIV/AIDS death numbers of around 2.3 million in 2012 and a decline to around 1.2 million by 2030. This is in strong contrast to the previous projections which predicted a continuing rise in HIV deaths to around 6 million in 2030. An update of GBD estimates which include the HIV/AIDS revisions is currently being completed, but has not yet been released.

When thinking about the relevance of infectious diseases for public health, there are other aspects specific to infectious diseases that have to be taken into account separately since they cannot be assessed with the burden of disease methodology, but add a potential and unpredictable burden to public health. They are not only important for high-income countries with effective infectious disease control mechanisms but also affect low- and middle-income countries (see Chapter 3 for emerging infections).

Another important issue that has to be considered in the context of the burden of infectious diseases is the fact that microbial agents are increasingly being recognized as triggers and thus as causative factors for a number of chronic diseases (Carbone et al. 2005). Chronic diseases for which there is a strong evidence of infectious etiology are, e.g., allergic disorders (house dust mites, respiratory syncytial virus), peptic ulcer diseases and gastric lymphoma (*Helicobacter pylori*), cervical carcinoma (human papilloma virus), hepatocellular carcinoma (hepatitis B and C viruses), or post-streptococcal glomerulonephritis and rheumatic fever (group A streptococcus). Furthermore, there is a range of other chronic diseases for which there is suspicion of an infectious disease origin, e.g., multiple sclerosis (Epstein–Barr virus), Alzheimer's diseases (*Chlamydia pneumoniae*), and diabetes mellitus (enteroviruses) (Carbone et al. 2005). Even obesity, a risk factor for several chronic diseases, has recently been discussed to have an infectious etiology (Adenovirus 36) (Atkinson et al. 2005). Therefore, the assessment of the burden of infectious diseases by means of the GBD study might underestimate the real burden since the GBD approach links the burden estimates to primary causes. In conclusion, refined estimates to identify the proportion of the burden due to non-communicable diseases that can be attributed to an infectious etiology are helpful for a comprehensive assessment of the contribution of infectious diseases to the burden of disease.

References

Anand S, Hanson K (1997) Disability-adjusted life years: a critical review. J Health Econ 16(6):685–702

Atkinson RL, Dhurandhar NV, Allison DB, Bowen RL, Israel BA, Albu JB, Augustus AS (2005) Human adenovirus-36 is associated with increased body weight and paradoxical reduction of serum lipids. Int J Obes (Lond) 29:281–286

Carbone KM, Luftig RB, Buckley MR (2005) Microbial triggers of chronic human illness. American Academy of Microbiology, Washington

Lopez AD, Mathers CD, Ezzati M, Jamison DT, Murray CJL (eds) (2006) Global burden of disease and risk factors. Oxford University Press, New York

Mathers CD, Loncar D (2006) Projections of global mortality and burden of disease from 2002 to 2030. PLoS Med 3(11): e 442

Mathers CD, Lopez AD, Murray CJL (2006) The burden of disease and mortality by condition: data, methods, and results for 2001. In : Lopez AD, Mathers CD, Ezzati M, Jamison DT, Murray CJL (eds) Global burden of disease and risk factors. Oxford University Press, New York, pp 45–93

Mathers CD, Vos T, Lopez AD, Salomon J, Ezzati M (eds) (2001) National burden of disease studies: A practical guide. Edition 2.0. World Health Organization, Geneva

Murray CJL (1994) Quantifying the burden of disease: the technical basis for disability-adjusted life years. Bull World Health Organ 72(3):429–445

Murray CJL (1996) Rethinking DALYs. In: Murray CJL, Lopez AD (eds.) The Global Burden of Disease: a comprehensive assessment of mortality and disability from diseases, injuries, and risk factors in 1990 and projected to 2020. Harvard University Press, Cambridge, pp 1–98

Murray CJL, Lopez AD (eds.) (1996) The Global Burden of Disease: a comprehensive assessment of mortality and disability from diseases, injuries, and risk factors in 1990 and projected to 2020. Harvard University Press, Cambridge

Murray CJL, Lopez AD (1997a) Mortality by cause for eight regions of the world: Global Burden of Disease Study. Lancet 349(9061):1269–1276

Murray CJ, Lopez AD (1997b) Alternative projections of mortality and disability by cause 1990-2020: Global Burden of Disease Study. Lancet 349(9064):1498–1504

Olshansky SJ, Ault AB (1986) The fourth stage of the epidemiologic transition: the age of delayed degenerative diseases. Milbank Q 64(3):355–391

Omran AR (1971) The epidemiologic transition. A theory of the epidemiology of population change. Milbank Mem Fund Q 49(4):509–538

Sagan LA (1987) The health of nations:True causes of sickness and well-being. Basic Books, New York

UNAIDS (2007) AIDS epidemic update: December 2007. World Health Organization, Geneva

World Bank (2002) World Development Report 2003: sustainable development in a dynamic world: transforming institutions, growth, and quality of life. Oxford University Press, New York

World Health Organization (2002) The world health report 2002 - reducing risks, promoting healthy life. World Health Organization, Geneva

Chapter 2
Global Challenges of Infectious Disease Epidemiology

Alexander Krämer and Md. Mobarak Hossain Khan

2.1 Introduction

As we have seen in the last chapter, infectious and parasitic diseases are major causes of morbidity and mortality worldwide, particularly in developing countries. Approximately 26% of global deaths and 26% of global burden of disease were attributed to infectious diseases in 2001 (Lopez et al. 2006; see Chapter 1). One in two deaths that are mostly preventable occurs in developing countries (Kim-Farley 2004; Folch et al. 2003). Looking to the remaining 21st century, we could imagine a decline in major infectious diseases like malaria and AIDS as a result of an adoption of effective prevention strategies and treatments or, like in the case of hepatitis B, as a consequence of worldwide vaccination programs in children. In addition, new vaccines, new treatment technologies, as well as an improvement in infrastructures can contribute to win the "battle against infectious diseases." However, for these prospects not to be doomed to fail, measures will have to be integrated much more than they are now into international health and public health policies, and there needs to be a multi- and interdisciplinary approach, a stronger facilitation of the participation of affected populations, and – above all – a committed and sustainable effort of all stakeholders. In this context, infectious disease public health plays the role of a moderator, and infectious disease epidemiology has the role of providing high-quality data and indicators for monitoring and surveillance as a basis for concerted and efficient public health actions.

2.2 Challenges

In an increasingly globalized world there are several structural aspects that determine and characterize the growing importance of infectious diseases in the modern world (Saker et al. 2004) (Table 2.1).

A. Krämer (✉)
Department of Public Health Medicine, School of Public Health, University of Bielefeld, Bielefeld, Germany
e-mail: alexander.kraemer@uni-bielefeld.de

A. Krämer et al. (eds.), *Modern Infectious Disease Epidemiology*, Statistics for Biology and Health, DOI 10.1007/978-0-387-93835-6_2,

Table 2.1 Challenges of infectious diseases

Aspects	Components
Demographic and behavioral	Demographic transition Aging and immune dysfunction Changing behaviors Intravenous drug use
Mobility, migration, and globalization	High mobility and rural–urban migration Modern transportation systems International migration and migration of refugees International travel and tourism Travel medicine
Modern medical practices	Organ or tissue transplantation Chemotherapy Drugs causing immunosuppression Widespread use of antibiotics and antibiotic resistance Microbial adaptation and change Hospital infections Use of intensive care medicine
Modern food technology	Industrialized food production Food processing and food preservation technology Antibiotics and chemicals used in food production Global trade, commerce, and distribution of foods Changing demand, consumption, and behavioral pattern
Politics, ecology, and environment	War and civil conflict Political pressure (minorities) Social inequality (vulnerable groups) Global warming and climate change Environmental disasters (e.g., floods, hurricanes)
Urbanization and megacities	Accelerating urbanization and megacities Pollutions (e.g., water) Overcrowding, poverty, and lack of resources Inadequate infrastructure and governability Changing sexual behavior (e.g., prostitution) Ecological change due to urban extension (e.g., deforestation)
Emerging diseases	See Chapter 3

2.2.1 Demographic Transition and Aging

The shift from high to low mortality and fertility is known as the demographic transition. This shift occurred throughout Europe, North America, and a number of other areas in the 19th and early 20th centuries and started in many developing countries in the middle of the 20th century. The life expectancy has increased rapidly during the last century. For instance, in 1900, life expectancy at birth was 47 years in the United States, by 1950 it was 68 years, and it reached 77 years by 2000. Life expectancy rose even higher in Japan and many European countries, and it continues to increase. Many low-fertility countries have entered what some describe as a "second demographic transition" in which fertility falls below the replacement rate (Population Reference Bureau 2004). It is estimated that by 2025, 120 countries would have reached total fertility rates below replacement level (fertility rate of 2.1 children per woman), a substantial increase as compared to 1975, when only 22 countries had a total fertility rate below or equal to the replacement level (WHO 2002). This transition has been linked with greater educational and job opportunities for women, the availability of effective contraception, a shift away from formal marriage, the acceptance of child bearing outside marriage, and the rise of individualism and materialism (Population Reference Bureau 2004).

The global population aged 65 or older is projected to increase from 8% (almost 500 million) in 2006 to 13% (about 1 billion) in 2030 (National Institutes of Health 2007). Industrialized countries have the highest percentages of older people in the world today, although 60% of the world's older population now live in less developed countries and in 2030, this proportion is projected to increase to 71% (Kinsella and Phillips 2005).

Although advances in controlling infectious diseases have contributed a lot to increasing life expectancy (mainly by reducing child mortality) and resulted in a large population of elderly people, they are, ironically, the most vulnerable groups to serious infectious diseases clinically and are at greatest risk for death and complications from infections (Yoshikawa 2000). New emerging infectious disease variants can be especially risky for older people, who are more vulnerable than younger people to acute respiratory diseases. For example, the outbreak in 2003 of severe acute respiratory syndrome (SARS) affected older people disproportionately. In Hong Kong, people aged 65 and older accounted for about one-fifth of the reported SARS cases and two-thirds of the SARS deaths in 2003 (Kinsella and Phillips 2005), while the percentage of the older population (aged 65+ years) was about 12% in 2003 (HKSAR Government 2003).

Older persons have greater susceptibility to certain infections than do younger adults because aging is associated with immune dysfunction, especially in cell-mediated immunity. Elderly persons suffer from a variety of chronic disorders, some of which affect the integrity of host resistance to infections. Urinary tract infections, lower respiratory tract infections, skin and soft tissue infections, intra-abdominal infections (cholecystitis, diverticulitis, appendicitis, and abscesses), infective endocarditis, bacterial meningitis, tuberculosis, and herpes zoster appear to have a special predilection for elderly persons. The mortality rates of most of these infections are about three times higher among elderly patients than among younger adult patients with the same disease. In addition to the above-mentioned factors, perhaps several other factors such as delays in diagnosis and therapy, poor tolerance to invasive diagnostic and therapeutic procedures, delayed or poor response to antimicrobial therapy, and greater risk and incidence of nosocomial infections contribute to this higher morbidity and mortality (Yoshikawa 2000).

2.2.2 *Mobility*

Population mobility is not a new phenomenon. Since ancient times, there have been relentless movements of people in search of food, water, wealth, and security.

Nonetheless, despite this continual migration, large-scale movement of populations across continents is a relatively recent phenomenon. Advances in transportation technology, in particular the advent of fast trains, automobiles, and jet aircrafts, have played a crucial role in facilitating dramatic increases in population mobility during the last 50 years. Global travel has grown from 25 million trips in 1950 to 341 million in 1980 and 500 million in 1993 and is estimated to reach 1 billion by 2010 (Rodriguez-Garcia 2001).

Of all travel-related illnesses, infectious diseases pose perhaps the greatest threat to global health. Since most infectious diseases have an incubation period exceeding 36 h and any part of the world can now be reached within this time frame, the potential for rapid geographical spread is obvious (Saker et al. 2004). A recent example of the worldwide spread of an infectious agent through travel is the SARS epidemic. This epidemic started in Guangzhou, province of Guangdong, China, in late 2002 and then spread to Hong Kong, Taiwan, Singapore, Vietnam, Toronto (Canada), the United States, and Europe (e.g., Germany, France and Sweden). The cumulative total of probable SARS cases surpassed 5,000 on April 28, 6,000 on May 2, 7,000 on May 8, and 8,000 on May 22, 2003 (WHO 2003a). Results from mathematical modeling and computer simulations demonstrated that important air travel routes had played a crucial role in the worldwide SARS spread (Hufnagel et al. 2004).

Furthermore, medical advice to travelers is often poor. This points to the importance of services of travel medicine through experts who are well trained in the prevention of infections caused by travel. Such advice applies not only to the consultation of clients before they start their journey but also to persons who come home from foreign countries. It is often the case that imported infections such as diarrheal diseases, hepatitis, malaria, and many others are not diagnosed at all or not diagnosed in due time and may thus cause avoidable morbidity and mortality.

Another structural element for the growing importance of infectious diseases in this context of population mobility is mass migration. According to the estimate of the United Nations, in 2005 about 191 million people – 3% of the world's population – were international migrants. Between 1995 and 2000, around 2.6 million migrants per year moved from less developed to more developed regions and mostly settled in the United States and Canada (Population Reference Bureau 2007). Various kinds of migrations can be distinguished such as labor migration and migration due to education. Another important group of migrants are refugees (rose from 8.7 million to 9.9 million globally during 2006) (Population Reference Bureau 2007), which have increased rapidly during the last 50 years due to interstate war, internal conflicts, political and economic instability, natural disasters (e.g., droughts), cultural and religious reasons (Saker et al. 2004). Such a huge migration exposes people to high health hazards including the potential acquisition of infections (vulnerable populations). An example is the high prevalence of infectious diseases such as cholera and dysentery among inhabitants in a refugee camp of Zaire who had moved there from Rwanda in 1994. Normally the refugee camps or temporary shelters in low-income countries are overcrowded, and the provision of sanitation, clean water, food, and health care is inadequate. Moreover, barriers to vectors and animals carrying infectious diseases are insufficient, and person-to-person contact is amplified (Saker et al. 2004).

2.2.3 Modern Medical Practices

One of the causes of an increasing importance of infectious diseases is unwanted effects of modern medical practices. During the 1960s and 1970s, there was a great deal of hope that humankind had tackled some of the worst infectious diseases through medical advances in antibiotics, vaccines, and other treatments (Brower and Chalk 2003). Without doubt, emergency and intensive care medicines provide life-saving services, but high-tech medicines may also cause threats to patients. Increasingly aggressive medical and therapeutic interventions, including implanted foreign bodies, organ transplantations, and xenotransplantations, have created a cohort of particularly vulnerable persons and increased the risk of infections. According to the report of Weinstein (1998), nosocomial infection rates in adults and pediatric intensive care units (ICUs) are approximately three times higher than elsewhere in hospitals. Artificial ventilation can lead to pneumonias and arterial and venous catheters can cause local or generalized infections due to insufficient hygiene. When a catheter is inserted through the patient's skin into a blood vessel, this can provide a route for bacteria living on the patient's skin to reach the patient's bloodstream and cause potentially lethal infection (Farr 2002). Patients with vascular catheters and monitoring devices have more bloodstream infections due to coagulase-negative staphylococci. Fungal urinary tract infections have also increased in ICU patients, presumably because of extensive exposure to broad-spectrum antibiotics (Weinstein 1998). In order to prevent the rejection of organ transplants in transplantation surgery, immunosuppressive therapy that may facilitate generalized infections in immunosuppressed transplant patients is required. In patients in oncology wards with tumors, chemotherapy is beneficial for the suppression of tumor growth but may facilitate the invasion of various infectious agents – potentially leading to life-threatening generalized infections. Therefore, the mortality of tumor patients is also determined by potential side effects of medical tumor therapy. Examples are generalized infections in immunosuppressed patients due to cytomegalovirus, aspergillosis, cryptococcosis, and many other agents.

Antibiotic resistance is a serious and growing public health threat in all nations around the globe. The past few decades have seen an alarming increase in the prevalence of resistant microbial pathogens in serious infections (Masterton 2005). An obvious example is penicillin. In 1942, the first US patient with streptococcal infection was miraculously cured with a small dose of penicillin. Nowadays penicillin-resistant streptococcus is widespread. Increasing travel and migration probably contributes to the growth of resistance problems (Zhang et al. 2006). Antibiotic-resistant infections are important because they result in more prolonged illness, longer hospitalization, greater risk of death, and higher costs for the health-care system than do infections with antibiotic-sensitive strains of the same species. The two most important causes of patients receiving antibiotic-resistant pathogens in hospitals have been the volume of antibiotic use and patient-to-patient transmission (Farr 2002). Resistant strains are found in various types of infectious agents, such as parasites (e.g., malaria), viruses (e.g., HIV, hepatitis B), and bacteria (e.g., methicillin-resistant *Staphylococcus aureus*, MRSA). Interestingly, the prevalence of MRSA varies greatly between different developed countries (high prevalence in the United States and low prevalence in The Netherlands), thus pointing to the challenge of reducing the burden through controlled use of antibiotics and efficient hygienic measures. Recently, multi-drug-resistant (MDR) tuberculosis is a growing problem – particularly in Russia, the Newly Independent States, and countries in Eastern Europe – that will require increasing public health intervention efforts in the future. While the WHO strategy of directly observed treatment (DOTS) proves successful in settings and regions where it is applied, at the same time the emergence of extremely multi-drug-resistant tuberculosis (XMDR), in which all known antibiotics against tuberculosis fail, poses enormous challenges for public health and necessitates the development of new anti-tuberculosis drugs (see Chapter 16).

Antibiotic resistance also contributes to the growing disease burden due to nosocomial infections. Nosocomial infections are usually linked to sophisticated medical technology and the use of invasive devices (Allegranzi and Pittet 2007). These infections make up a substantial proportion of the infectious disease burden in both developed and developing countries. For instance, at any time, over 1.4 million people worldwide suffer from infectious complications associated with health care (WHO 2005b). In developed countries, between 5 and 10% of patients acquire one or more nosocomial infections and approximately 15–40% of those admitted to intensive care are thought to be affected. Every year approximately 3 million people in the European Union contract a nosocomial infection, of which 50,000 die (ECDC 2007). In 2002, the estimated number of nosocomial infections in the United States was approximately 1.7 million and the estimated deaths associated with these infections were 98,987; of these, 35,967 were for pneumonia, 30,665 for bloodstream infections, 13,088 for urinary tract infections, 8,205 for surgical site infections, and 11,062 for infections of other sites (Klevens et al. 2007). The risk of nosocomial infection for patients is 2–20 times higher in developing countries than in industrialized countries (Allegranzi and Pittet 2007; Lazzari et al. 2004). An estimated 40% or more patients could suffer from health care-associated infections which are preventable and every day 4,384 children die due to such infections in developing countries (WHO 2005a).

A complex array of factors that promote nosocomial infections include pre-existing diseases and decreased patient immunity, invasive diagnostic and therapeutic techniques, the widespread antimicrobial resistance, lack of infection control measures and environmental hygiene, lack of resources, inappropriate use of antibiotics, use of counterfeit drugs, understaffing and lack of training of health-care professionals, and governments that are overwhelmed with larger health issues and cannot commit to infection control procedures and standards (Allegranzi and Pittet 2007; WHO 2005a; Lazzari et al. 2004). At least 50% of all medical equipments in most developing countries are unusable, or only partly usable, at any given time. Approximately 77% of all reported cases of substandard and counterfeit drugs occur in developing countries. About 4.2 billion injections are administered each year in India and two out of three injections given are unsafe, posing serious health hazards to recipients, health workers, and the community. In Brazil and Indonesia, more than half of newborn babies admitted to neonatal units acquire a nosocomial infection, and 12–52% of them die (WHO 2005a).

2.2.4 Modern Food Technology

The globalization of food increases the likelihood of pandemics of foodborne diseases. These diseases are a considerable burden for both developing and developed countries, and hence they are a growing public health concern (Elmi 2004). For instance, each year, foodborne diseases cause approximately 76 million illnesses, 325,000 hospitalizations, and 5,000 deaths in the United States (Mead et al. 1999), 5.4 million cases in Australia (OzFoodNet 2006), and 1.7 million cases, 21,997 hospitalizations, and 687 deaths in the United Kingdom (Adak et al. 2005). The causes of foodborne diseases include viruses, bacteria, parasites, toxins, metals, and prions and the symptoms of foodborne diseases range from mild gastroenteritis to life-threatening neurologic, hepatic, and renal syndromes. Foodborne disease outbreaks are now more far-reaching due to modern mass food production and widespread food distribution (Hall et al. 2002).

A number of factors such as increasing travel, international food supply and trade, changes in animal husbandry and agronomic processes, changes in food technology, production, processing, and distribution, changes in lifestyle (e.g., introduction of uncooked items into our diets) and consumer demands, and increasingly susceptible populations (e.g., growing number of elderly) can facilitate foodborne infections all over the world (Elmi 2004; Blaser 1996). Due to modern transportation systems, food grown in one country can now be transported and consumed all across the world. A person can be exposed to a foodborne illness in one country and expose others to the infection in a location thousands of kilometers from the original source of infection (ECDC 2007; Elmi 2004). Food can be contaminated in one country and cause outbreaks of foodborne diseases in another one due to globalization of food trade (Sanders 1999). International trade has three main consequences: (i) the rapid transfer of microorganisms from one country to another; (ii) the time between processing and consumption of food is increasing, leading to increased opportunity for contamination and time/temperature exposure of the products and hence the risk of foodborne illness; and (iii) people are more likely to be exposed to a higher number of different strains/types of foodborne pathogens (Elmi 2004).

Currently, prevailing food insecurity and food crisis including rising food prices may pose enormous challenges particularly in developing countries. There are over 800 million undernourished people in the world and this number could increase sharply as a result of the current food crisis. Extrapolation suggested that globally up to 105 million people could become poor due to rising food prices between 2005 and 2007 (World Bank 2008). Food insecurity and food crisis may influence the risk of acquiring infectious diseases as well as the number of deaths through poverty and malnutrition. Only in Ethiopia, about 12 million children under the age of 5 years are at risk for severe malnutrition as a result of the current food crisis

(USAID 2008). Malnutrition causes severe deficiencies – calories, zinc, and vitamin A – that facilitate infectious diseases in these populations. People weakened by diarrhea, pneumonia, malaria, and measles are becoming sicker or die if they cannot get adequate food. Globally, malnutrition is responsible for 3.5–5.5 million child deaths every year (USAID 2008).

The extensive use of chemical fertilizers and pesticides, in addition to damaging the environment, introduces toxic residues into the food chain and consequently into our bodies. The use of untreated sewage for irrigation and increased use of manure rather than chemical fertilizers contribute to an increased risk of infections through the consumption of fresh fruits and vegetables. People demand a wider variety of food than in the past and nowadays almost every type of fruit is available on the international food markets the entire year round regardless of seasonal changes in growth. Long storage of food and the increased use of refrigeration to prolong the shelf-life of food may lead to its deterioration – including the development of infectious agents. Changing lifestyles such as going to restaurants frequently, eating foreign cuisine, and consuming fresh fruits and vegetables also increase the risk of foodborne diseases (Elmi 2004). Consumption patterns may enhance unhealthy food production and distribution because the consumer desires ubiquitous availability of all foods at low prices. Additionally, hygienic measures in the processes of food production and consumption may be insufficient and thus facilitate the spread of infections.

2.2.5 Politics and Environment

Ecological factors and political and socioeconomic conditions also influence the spread of infectious diseases. As we have already seen, political pressure may result in migration movements of populations. Low socioeconomic status is often associated with a higher burden of infectious diseases (see Chapter 6). For migrants, the access to health-care services may be reduced due to cultural or language barriers. Also for poorer native inhabitants of a country, the utilization of health-care services is less efficient compared to representatives of the high socioeconomic class. Due to recently growing levels of social inequality, not only in developing countries but also in developed ones, these problems are currently increasing and will probably continue to increase in the future. Therefore, health security particularly for vulnerable groups remains an important tool of national and international politics. This also holds for the growing worldwide fear of international terrorism including the use of biological agents such as the smallpox virus, *Bacillus anthracis*, and others.

Increasingly, there is scientific evidence that most of the recent global climate changes are man-made (anthropogenic) and mainly are due to increased CO_2 levels in the atmosphere resulting from industrialization and traffic. During the 20th century, world average surface temperature increased by approximately 0.6°C and approximately two-thirds of that warming occurred since 1975. Climatologists forecast further warming along with changes in precipitation and climate variability during the coming century and beyond. Climate change influences the functioning of many ecosystems and is a major threat to human health in lower income countries, predominantly within tropical and subtropical countries (WHO 2003b). This is of major importance for the prevalence and spread of infectious diseases because the breeding sites of vector-borne diseases such as malaria, dengue, yellow fever, and many others are extended. Generally, warmer temperatures enhance vector breeding and reduce the pathogen's maturation period within the vector organism. It is estimated that if the global temperature increased by 2–3°C, the number of people who are at risk of malaria would increase by around 3–5%, i.e., several hundred million. In 2030, the estimated risk of diarrhea will be up to 10% higher in some regions than it would have been without climate change (WHO 2003b). In existing endemic areas the spread of vector-borne infections is facilitated and the endemic regions themselves may grow, with a consequence that, in the future, parasitic diseases will occur in areas not yet or not anymore endemic for these infections (see Chapter 3).

In addition, there are further manifestations of global climate changes associated with infectious diseases. Climate changes will cause greater frequency of infectious disease epidemics following floods and storms. It will also cause substantial health effects following population displacement from the sea level rise and increased storm activity (Intergovernmental Panel on Climate Change 2007; WHO 2003b). Flooding has always occurred due to seasonal variations and special weather conditions such as monsoon rains and others. What is alarming, however, is the amount of rainfall and the frequency with which it occurs not only in flooding endemic regions like India and Bangladesh but also in areas that until recently have only rarely or never been affected by heavy rains. It is obvious that waterborne infectious agents can multiply at much higher rates under such conditions. Rainfall can also influence the transportation and dissemination of infectious agents, while temperature affects their growth and survival (WHO 2003b). Environmental catastrophes and disasters such as earth quakes including massive tsunamis on December 26, 2004, in south and southeast Asia mainly in Indonesia, Sri Lanka, and India (USAID 2005), Hurricane Katrina in Louisiana on August 29, 2005 (US Department of Commerce 2006), and Cyclone Sidr in Bangladesh on November 15, 2007 (United Nations 2007), led to the spread of infections in the affected regions. Briefly, climate changes cause population displacement, crowding, inadequate shelter, poor access to safe water, inadequate hygiene and sanitation, unsafe food preparation and handling practices, malnutrition, poor access to health services along with huge logged water as a result of severe flooding/cyclones/tsunamis, all of which increase the risk of waterborne, foodborne (cholera, typhoid, *Shigella dysenteriae*), and vector-borne diseases (malaria, typhoid, dengue) among the affected people (WHO 2007; Khasnis and Nettleman 2005; Wilder-Smith 2005).

2.2.6 *Urbanization and Megacities*

Urbanization processes represent one of the most important dimensions that determine present and future public health needs. For 200 years, the proportion of the population living in cities has constantly been rising: from approximately 3% in the year 1800 to approximately 13% in 1900, 29% in 1950, 38% in 1975, 47% in 2000, and 49% in 2005 (United Nations 2006; Moore et al. 2003; Dadao and Hui 2006). While the whole world has been predominantly rural until 2005, now the world is on the verge of becoming more urban than rural for the first time. In 2008, more than half of the world population lived in urban areas (Population Reference Bureau 2007). By 2030, urban dwellers will make up roughly 60% of the world's population. Cities offer the lure of better employment, education, health care, and culture; and they contribute disproportionately to national economies (Moore et al. 2003). Whereas until World War II urbanization had primarily been a major feature of developed countries, after World War II, urbanization processes were increasingly observed in the developing world also due to intensified industrialization and migration processes.

Recently the term "megacities" was created to characterize very big cities (Hinrichsen et al. 2002; United Nations 2006). However, there is no adequate definition, as the benchmark of the population concentration that differentiates megacities from other urban areas varies. Planetearth (2005) and the German National Committee on Global Change Research (NKGCF 2005) defined megacities as the metropolitan areas with more than 5 million inhabitants. The United Nations (UN) coined the term megacities to describe cities with 8 million or more inhabitants but its present threshold for a megacity is 10 million (Hinrichsen et al. 2002; United Nations 2006). Hence we distinguish three different categories: megacities from 5 to <8 million inhabitants, megacities from 8 to <10 million inhabitants, and those with a population above 10 million citizens. The future growth is predominantly expected in developing countries, particularly in south Asia, southeast Asia and China. The overall growth of the urban population from 1970 to 2025 is expected to be much higher in developing countries than in developed countries. It is estimated that by the year 2030 approximately 4.9 billion people will live in urban areas (United Nations 2006).

According to Kraas (2003), megacities share some common characteristics such as the fact that they represent nodal points of globalization processes, in which a concentration of national, regional, and global economic activities can be observed with particularly high concentrations of industrial production. Besides their high population densities, megacities are often characterized by uncontrolled spatial expansion, increasing traffic volumes, and severe infrastructural deficits that may represent manifestations of a loss of governability. The latter can lead to unregulated and disparate land and property markets, resulting in an insufficient housing provision. In these megacities a trained and highly specialized workforce can be distinguished from a cheap labor market, and accordingly a formal economic sector can be distinguished from an informal economic sector.

Worldwide, approximately 1 billion people are estimated to live in shanty towns, favelas, or so-called marginal settlements (Riley et al. 2007). Megacities are endangered by both environmental and man-made hazards (Kraas 2007). High burdens of health risks originate from these hazards and threaten megacity populations. Higher air and surface temperatures in combination with other environmental conditions, especially in big cities, make them "urban heat islands." Higher temperature in these cities is caused by daytime heat retained by the fabric of multi-storied buildings and by a reduction in cooling vegetation (Grimm et al. 2008; Kovats and Akhtar 2008). However, low temperature levels, frost, and avalanches can also harm megacity populations. Man-made hazards, which can be distinguished from environmental hazards, may lead to pollutions of air, water, and soil, to accidents with a much higher burden in developing countries (e.g., car crashes), to large-scale fires, and to industrial explosions and releases of toxic gas (see Kraas 2003 for details and examples).

Briefly, increased health problems in megacities are associated with many dimensions such as loss of governability, lack of infrastructure, poverty, diversity of culture and ethnicity, migration, pollution, lack of health knowledge, and insufficient health-care systems. Here we want to highlight some factors that influence the occurrence of infectious diseases in megacity populations (Fig. 2.1). With respect to the climate, it is noteworthy to mention that most megacities are located in tropical and subtropical areas predisposing their inhabitants to tropical diseases. Housing conditions can be characterized by poor sanitation and sewage disposal, overcrowding, and a high prevalence of vermin, which may transmit infections. A poor infrastructure may lead to a high contact rate in, e.g., buses and trains (due to overcrowding) and to a lack of adequate water supply and health-care services (e.g., vaccinations) and therefore facilitates the occurrence of outbreaks and epidemics. The clean water supply may be insufficient, particularly in marginal settlements or slums, and available water can be heavily contaminated by infectious agents due to discharge of untreated industrial wastes, leaching from waste dumps into surface and water, inadequate treatment of sewage, and poor solid waste management. Sanitation may be poor, rivers may be contaminated, and sewage and garbage disposal may be missing. Prostitution enhances the spread of sexually transmitted infections (e.g., HIV) and immigration can lead to the import of infections. Educational deficits particularly in women and mothers facilitate unsafe practices and deficient services for their children (e.g., in the case of diarrheal diseases). Knowledge deficits also arise when important information on outbreaks or epidemics is only insufficiently distributed to the general public. Moreover, health-care system services may be characterized by scarce or lacking equipment (posing

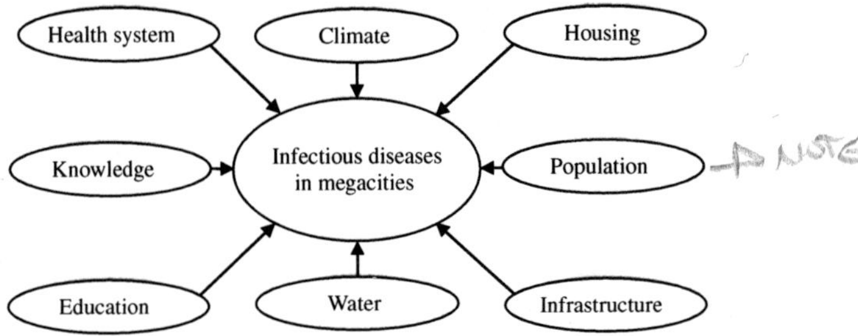

Fig. 2.1 Factors related to infectious diseases in megacities

problems with sterility), poor overall hygienic standards, the overuse and misuse of antibiotics, and low vaccination rates.

2.3 Solution Strategies to Meet These Challenges

2.3.1 Functions of Infectious Disease Epidemiology

Preventing and reducing the spread of infectious disease among humans is an essential function of public health. Epidemiology is often called the core science of public health, which studies the distribution and determinants of disease risk in human populations. Starting in the middle of the 19th century, infectious disease epidemiology applies the fundamentals of epidemiology to study infectious diseases and deals with questions about conditions for disease emergence, spread, and persistence. It describes the prevalence and incidence of infectious diseases through which the epidemiological trends can be characterized for different world regions (see Chapters 5 and 11).

A further task is to assess the expansion and transmission routes of the infectious pathogens in human population groups and, where appropriate, to investigate the nature of transmission, the infection probability per contact between the infected and the susceptible persons, the frequency and intensity of this contact and to determine the risk and protective factors of infectious and associated diseases. In collaboration with microbiologists, infectious disease epidemiology characterizes the features of the pathogen as well as its virulence, its pathogenicity, and, where appropriate, its resistance. It also specifies different molecular subtypes and strains of the pathogens (see also Chapter 7). Another vital task of infectious disease epidemiology is to investigate outbreaks. This investigation includes verifying, confirming the diagnosis, developing a case definition and case finding, describing the data in terms of time, place, and person, identifying risks, formulating and testing of a hypothesis, planning for further studies, establishing control measures, and communicating the findings to prevent larger epidemics (see Chapter 9).

Infectious disease epidemiology also identifies population groups vulnerable to specific infections for targeted prevention and intervention measures. Furthermore, it includes investigation of the immune status of the populations among others to evaluate the effectiveness and coverage of vaccination programs, thereby contributing to public health surveillance. Mathematical models help to better understand the transmission dynamics and spread of infections, to identify the factors governing the transmission process in order to develop effective control strategies, and to evaluate the effectiveness of surveillance strategies and intervention measures. Mathematical modeling in combination with health economic analyses supports public health experts and policy makers in designing effective public health policy to best protect populations from detrimental effects of infectious diseases. Model calculations also provide information about where the existing infectious disease surveillance must be replaced by new and more effective surveillance methods (for advanced reading, see Chapters 8 and 12).

2.3.2 Interdisciplinary Approaches

Infectious diseases are a leading cause of death worldwide and hence a great challenge for every nation. The present chapter shows that many structural aspects are associated with the increasing burden of both re-emerging and new infectious diseases. Taken together, these structural aspects of infectious diseases are highly interrelated and therefore the study of infectious disease clearly requires expertise from numerous fields such as public health, epidemiology, demography, social science, sociology, anthropology, economics, food science, medicine, hospital management, clinical studies, environmental science, climatology, ecology, agriculture, microbiology, geography, geomatics, urban and regional planning, meteorology, statistics, and mathematics. Coordinated collaborations among various disciplines will promote our understanding of the many possible perspectives on infectious disease problems.

As an example, the role of climate in the emergence of human infectious diseases requires interdisciplinary cooperation among physicians, climatologists, biologists, and social scientists (Patz et al. 1996). Combating emerging infectious diseases will succeed only when various disciplines work together, such as animal studies, epidemiology, immunology, ecology, environmental studies, microbiology, pharmacology, public health, medicine, nursing, cultural, political, and social studies (Lashley 2004). To control and eradicate malaria, proper physical and social planning, understanding the geography, entomology, epidemiology, behavior, and lifecycle of malarial parasites, cooperation between the policy makers, malaria specialists, neighboring countries, and international communities are important (Woube 1997). Increasing population mobility and large-scale migrations within and between countries in association with rapid urbanization have particularly profound implications for the ecology of infectious diseases, interacting in complex ways with other biological and social factors and opening multiple pathways for the emergence of new infections and the resurgence of existing ones. Therefore, collaboration between ecologists, urban planners, and epidemiologists is extremely important (Eisenberg et al. 2007). Quantifying the contributions of various factors to emergence and spread of infections requires expertise from statistics and mathematics. Dedicated efforts from many other partners such as local and state health departments, agencies, professional societies, universities, research institutes, health-care providers and organizations, domestic and international organizations are also needed to effectively organize infectious disease control and prevention.

The public health community, in particular, must take the leading responsibility to work more actively with other sectors that have important roles and interests in reducing infectious diseases. Even greater efforts will be necessary to deal with poverty, a particularly recalcitrant contributor to, and consequence of, some infectious diseases (Binder et al. 1999). At the national level, coordination among public health authorities at all levels of government needs to be substantially enhanced and developed in conjunction with mechanisms that allow for greater interaction across state borders and local boundaries. Greater involvements with private sectors are also important in relation to the research, development, and manufacture of vaccines and antibiotics and the development of microbial surveillance technology. Increased state investment is critical to develop a functional and coherent national policy for combating infectious disease. In conclusion, through the reinforced interdisciplinary collaboration in scientific research and increased knowledge transfer, we hope to be able to ultimately control infectious diseases, to reduce the burden of morbidity and mortality they cause, and to improve the quality of life of populations.

References

Adak GK, Meakins SM, Yip H, Lopman BA, O'Brien SJ (2005) Disease risks from foods, England and Wales, 1996–2000. Emerg Infect Dis 11: 365–372

Allegranzi B, Pittet D (2007) Healthcare-associated infection in developing countries: simple solutions to meet complex challenges. Infect Control Hosp Epidemiol 28: 1323–1327

Binder S, Levitt AM, Sacks JJ, Hughes JM (1999) Emerging infectious diseases: public health issues for the 21st century. Science 284: 1311–1313

Blaser MJ (1996) How safe is our food? Lessons from an outbreak of salmonellosis. N Engl J Med 334:1324–1325

Brower J, Chalk P (2003) Factors associated with the increased incidence and spread of infectious diseases. In: The global threat of new and reemerging infectious diseases: Reconciling U. S. National Security and Public Health Policy. Rand Science and Technology, McLean, VA, pp. 13–30

Dadao L, Hui L (2006) Urbanization and environmental issues in China. In: Wuyi W, Krafft T, Kraas F (eds) Global change, urbanization and health. China Meteorological Press, China, pp. 3–10

ECDC (2007) The first European communicable disease epidemiological report. European Centre for Disease Prevention and Control, Stockholm

Eisenberg JNS, Desai MA, Levy K, Bates SJ, Liang S, Naumoff K, Scott JC (2007) Environmental determinants of infectious disease: a framework for tracking causal links and guiding public health research. Environ Health Res 115: 1216–1223

Elmi M (2004) Food safety: current situation, unaddressed issues and the emerging priorities. Eastern Mediterranean Health J 10: 794–800

Farr BM (2002) Prevention and control of nosocomial infections. Business Briefing: Global Healthcare 3: 37–41

Folch E, Hernandez I, Barragan M, Franco-Paredes C (2003) Infectious diseases, non-zero-sum thinking, and the developing world. Am J Med Sci 326: 66–72

German National Committee on Global Change Research (NKGCF) (2005) Global change research in Germany. Department of Earth and Environmental Sciences, München

Grimm NB, Faeth SH, Golubiewski NE, Redman CL, Wu J, Bai X, Briggs JM (2008) Global change and the ecology of cities. Science 139:756–760

Hall GV, D'Souza RM, Kirk MD (2002) Foodborne disease in the new millennium: out of the frying pan and into the fire? Med J Australia 177: 614–618

Hinrichsen D, Salem R, Blackburn R (2002) Meeting the urban challenge. Population Reports, Series M, No. 16. The John Hopkins Bloomberg School of Public Health, Baltimore

The Hong Kong Special Administrative Region (HKSAR) Government (2003) Hong Kong: The Facts. Hong Kong 2003

Hufnagel L, Brockmann D, Geisel T (2004) Forecast and control of epidemics in a globalized world. PNAS 101: 15124–15129

Intergovernmental Panel on Climate Change (2007) Climate change 2007: Synthesis report. World Meteorological Organization, UNEP, Geneva

Khasnis AA, Nettleman MD (2005) Global warming and infectious disease. Arch Med Res 36: 689–696

Kim-Farley RJ (2004) Global strategies for control of communicable diseases. In: Detels R, McEwen J, Beaglehole R, Tanaka H (eds) Oxford textbook of public health. Oxford University Press, Oxford, pp. 1839–1859

Kinsella K, Phillips DR (2005) Global aging: The challenge of success. Population Bulletin 60, No. 1. Population Reference Bureau, Washington DC

Klevens RM, Edwards JR, Richards Jr. CL, Horan TC, Gaynes RP, Pollock DA, Cardo DM (2007) Estimating health care-associated infections and deaths in U.S. hospitals, 2002. Public Health Reports 122: 160–166

Kovats S, Akhtar R (2008) Climate, climate change and human health in Asian cities. Environ Urban 20:165–175

Kraas F (2003) Megacities as global risk areas. Petermanns Geographische Mitteilungen 147: 6–15

Kraas F (2007) Megacities and global change in East, Southeast and South Asia. Asien 103: s9–s22

Lashley FR (2004) Emerging infectious diseases: vulnerabilities, contributing factors and approaches. Expert Rev Anti Infect Ther 2: 299–316

Lazzari S, Allegranzi B, Concia E (2004) Making hospitals safer: the need for a global strategy for infection control in health care settings. World Hosp Health Serv 40: 32, 34, 36–42

Lopez AD, Mathers CD, Ezzati M, Jamison DT, Murray CJL (eds) (2006) Global burden of disease and risk factors. Oxford University Press, New York

Masterton RG (2005) A new understanding of antibiotic resistance in nosocomial infections. Br J Intensive Care Spring: 20–26

Mead PS, Slutsker L, Dietz V, McCaig LF, Bresee JS, Shapiro C, Griffin PM, Tauxe RV (1999) Food-related illness and death in the United States. Emerg Infect Dis 5: 607–625

Moore M, Gould P, Keary BS (2003) Global urbanization and impact on health. Int J Hyg Environ Health 206: 269–278

National Institutes of Health (2007) Why population aging matters: A global perspective. National Institute on Aging (Publication No. 07–6134) Washington, DC

OzFoodNet (2006) Burden and causes of foodborne disease in Australia: annual report of the OzFoodNet network, 2005. Commun Dis Intell 30: 278–300

Patz JA, Epstein PR, Burke TA, Balbus JM (1996) Global climate change and emerging infectious diseases. JAMA 275: 217–223

Planetearth (2005) Megacities-our global urban future. Earth Sciences for Society Foundation, Leiden

Population Reference Bureau (2004) Transitions in world population. Population Bulletin 59, No. 1. Population Reference Bureau, Washington DC

Population Reference Bureau (2007) World population highlights. Population Bulletin 62, No. 3. Population Reference Bureau, Washington DC

Riley LW, Ko AI, Unger A, Reis MG (2007) Slum health: diseases of neglected populations. BMC Int Health Human Rights 7: 2 (doi:10.1186/1472–698X-7-2)

Rodriguez-Garcia R (2001) The health-development link: travel as a public health issue. J Commu Health 26: 93–112

Saker L, Lee K, Cannito B, Gilmore A, Campbell-Lendrum D (2004) Globalization and infectious diseases: a review of the linkages. WHO, Geneva

Sanders TAB (1999) Food production and food safety. BMJ 318: 1689–1693

United Nations (2006) World urbanizations prospects: the 2005 revision. United Nations, New York

United Nations (2007) SIDR cyclone Bangladesh 2007. Office of the UN Resident Coordinator, Dhaka

USAID (2008) Global food insecurity and price increase update # 3. May 30, USAID

USAID (2005) Indian Ocean-Earthquake and Tsunamis. Office of US Foreign Disaster Assistance (OFDA), USAID

US Department of Commerce (2006) Hurricane Katrina August 13–31, 2005. National Oceanic and Atmospheric Administration (NOAA), Silver Spring

Weinstein RA (1998) Nosocomial infection update. Emerg Infect Dis 4: 416–420

WHO (2002) Active ageing: a policy framework. Second United Nations World Assembly on Ageing, Madrid

WHO (2003a) Update 62 – More than 8000 cases reported globally, situation in Taiwan, data on in-flight transmission, report on Henan Province, China. WHO, Geneva. Available at: http://www.who.int/csr/don/2003_05_22/en/

WHO (2003b) Climate change and human health-risks and responses: summary. WHO, Geneva

WHO (2005a) Preventable hospital infections are a major cause of death and disability for patients (SEA/PR/1407). WHO: Regional Office for South-East Asia, New Delhi

WHO (2005b) Global patient safety challenge 2005–2006: clean care is safer care. World Alliance for Patient Safety, Geneva

WHO (2007) Communicable disease risk assessment and interventions: Cyclone Sidr disaster-Bangladesh. WHO, Geneva

Wilder-Smith A (2005) Tsunami in South Asia: what is the risk of post-disaster infectious disease outbreaks? Ann Acad Med Singapore 34: 625–631

World Bank (2008) Addressing the food crisis: the need for rapid and coordinated action. A document prepared for G8 Finance Ministers Summit, June 13–14, Osaka.

Woube M (1997) Geographical distribution and dramatic increases in incidences of malaria: consequences of the resettlement scheme in Gambela, SW Ethiopia. Indian J Malariol 34: 140–163

Yoshikawa TT (2000) Epidemiology and unique aspects of aging and infectious diseases. Clin Infect Dis 30: 931–933

Zhang R, Eggleston K, Rotimi V, Zeckhauser R (2006) Antibiotic resistance as a global threat: evidence from China, Kuwait and the United States. Globalization Health 2: 6 (doi: 10.1186/1744-8603-2-6)

Chapter 3
Emerging and Re-emerging Infectious Diseases

Thomas Löscher and Luise Prüfer-Krämer

3.1 Definition

Emerging infectious diseases (EIDs) are characterized by a new or an increased occurrence within the last few decades. They include the following categories:

1. Emerging diagnosis of infectious diseases: old diseases that are newly classified as infectious diseases because of the discovery of a responsible infectious agent,
2. Newly emerging infectious diseases,
3. Re-emerging infectious diseases: reoccurrence or new outbreaks of old infectious diseases with important public health relevance, and
4. Emerging resistance: increasing resistance of infectious agents to antimicrobial substances.

3.2 Factors Contributing to Emergence

Human activities that change the ecology of the microbial world are important factors for the emergence of infectious diseases on a macro- and microlevel, which was noted in the Institute of Medicine (IOM) report in 1992. The main factors that were listed are deforestation, change in air quality, and climate. The report was updated in 2003 when additional factors were included: human susceptibility to infection (HIV, aging population), changing ecosystems, poverty and social inequality, war, famine, lack of political will (e.g., breakdown of public health), and the intent of harm (bioterrorism). The convergence model of the various factors shows that environmental factors interact with genetic and biological factors, social and political, as well as economic factors. Figures 3.1 and 3.2 demonstrate examples of different categories of EIDs and the influencing factors on the macro-, meso- and microlevel.

T. Löscher (✉)
Department of Infectious Diseases and Tropical Medicine (DITM), University of Munich, Munich, Germany
e-mail: loescher@lrz.uni-muenchen.de

A. Krämer et al. (eds.), *Modern Infectious Disease Epidemiology*,
Statistics for Biology and Health, DOI 10.1007/978-0-387-93835-6_3,

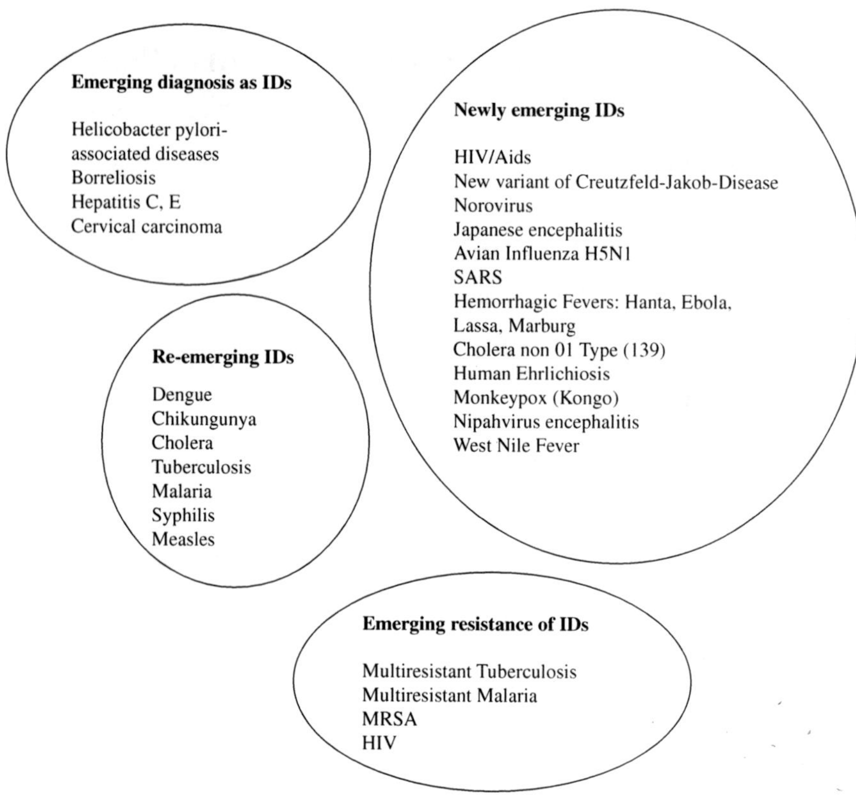

Fig. 3.1 Categories of emerging infectious diseases (EIDs) with examples

An interdisciplinary consortium recently analyzed 335 EID events between 1940 and 2004 (Jones et al. 2008) and demonstrated nonrandom global patterns. It gave analytical support that EID events rose significantly over time with a peak incidence in the 1980s concomitant with the HIV pandemic. EID events are dominated by zoonoses (over 60%), originating mostly in wildlife (almost 72% of zoonoses, e.g., hantavirus infections). The authors showed that 54% of EID events were caused by bacteria or *Rickettsia*, including a large number of drug-resistant microbes. They proved that new EID events are significantly associated with socioeconomic, environmental, and ecological factors, which can provide a basis for identifying regions where new EIDs are most likely to originate (emerging disease "hot spots"). They showed that the risk of wildlife zoonotic and vector-borne EIDs is high in lower latitudes where reporting effort is low. Population density is the most important driver for EID events in zoonotic wildlife and non-wildlife transmission, drug resistance, and the vector-borne transmission mode. The trends in the last decade were the following:

a. The proportion of viral diseases compared to other infectious agents,
b. The zoonotic wildlife transmission type,

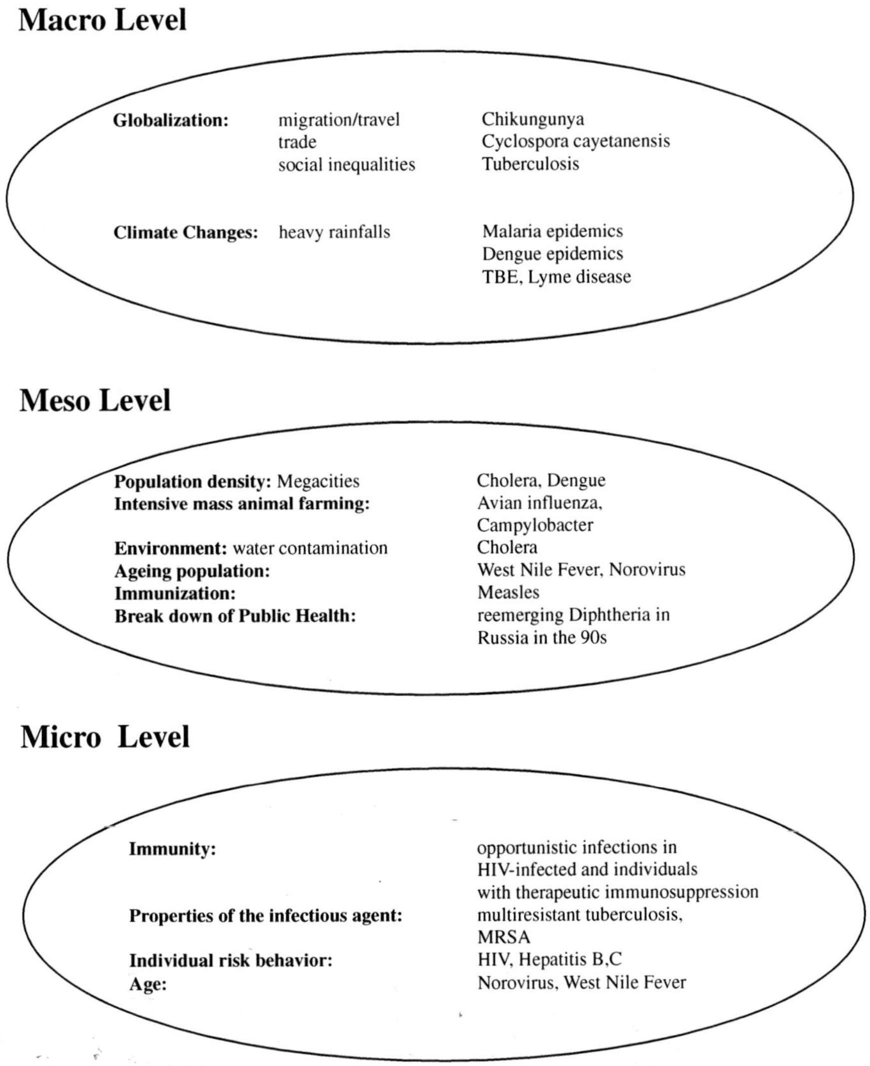

Macro Level

Globalization:	migration/travel trade social inequalities	Chikungunya Cyclospora cayetanensis Tuberculosis
Climate Changes:	heavy rainfalls	Malaria epidemics Dengue epidemics TBE, Lyme disease

Meso Level

Population density: Megacities	Cholera, Dengue
Intensive mass animal farming:	Avian influenza, Campylobacter
Environment: water contamination	Cholera
Ageing population:	West Nile Fever, Norovirus
Immunization:	Measles
Break down of Public Health:	reemerging Diphtheria in Russia in the 90s

Micro Level

Immunity:	opportunistic infections in HIV-infected and individuals with therapeutic immunosuppression
Properties of the infectious agent:	multiresistant tuberculosis, MRSA
Individual risk behavior:	HIV, Hepatitis B,C
Age:	Norovirus, West Nile Fever

Fig. 3.2 Factors contributing to the emergence of infectious diseases with examples

c. The vector-borne transmission mode, and
d. The non-drug-resistant pathogens increased their proportion of EID events compared to the previous decade.

The "hot spots" for EID events were located in India for all four categories (zoonotic wildlife, zoonotic non-wildlife, drug resistance, and vector borne), clustered in densely populated areas throughout the world for zoonotic pathogens from wildlife, and were found for non-wildlife zoonotic diseases mainly in western

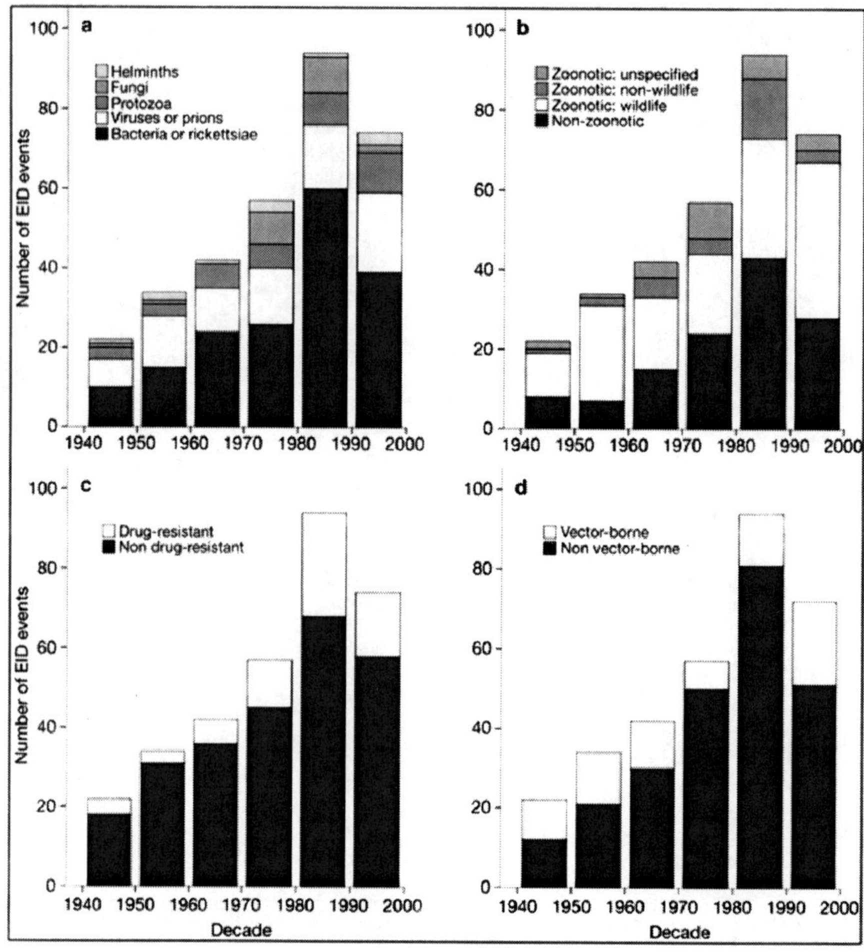

Fig. 3.3 Number of EID events per decade. Adapted from Nature 451, 990–993 (2008)

Europe including Great Britain as well as in India, China, and Japan. Emerging vector-borne disease events concentrated in densely populated subtropical and tropical regions mostly in India, Indonesia, China, sub-Saharan Africa, and Central America (see Figs. 3.3, 3.4, and 3.5).

3.3 New Infectious Agents in Old Diseases

The identification of new infectious agents in old diseases with unknown etiology is still the basis in many epidemiological studies. Such newly detected bacteria and viruses in the last few decades are listed in Table 3.1.

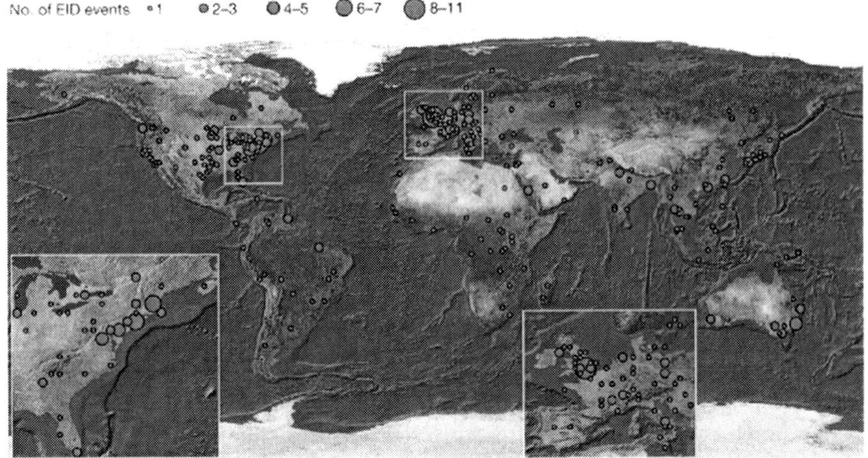

Fig. 3.4 Global richness map of the geographic origins of EID events from 1940 to 2004. Adapted from Nature 451, 990–993 (2008)

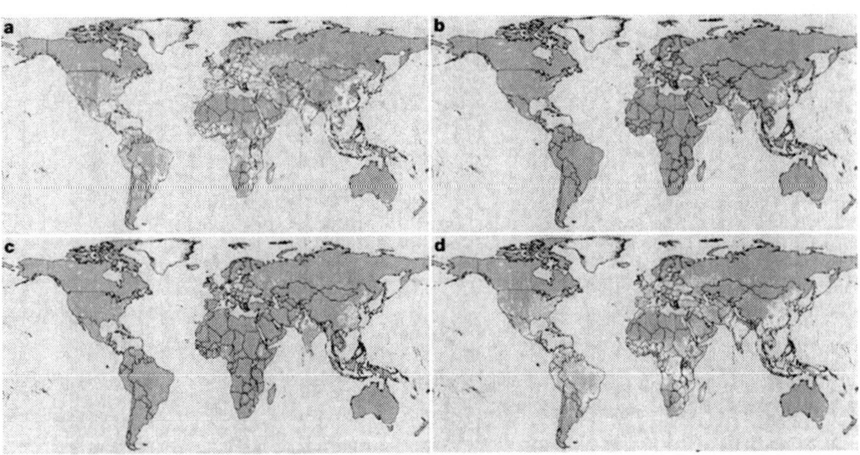

a. zoonotic pathogens from wildlife
b. zoonotic pathogens from non-wildlife
c. drug-resistant pathogens
d. vector-borne pathogens

Fig. 3.5 Global distribution of relative risk of an EID event; (**a**) zoonotic pathogens from wildlife, (**b**) zoonotic pathogens from non-wildlife, (**c**) drug-resistant pathogens, (**d**) vector-borne pathogens. Adapted from Nature 451, 990–993 (2008)

Table 3.1 New infectious agents of old diseases that had been classified as infectious diseases in the last decades

Infectious agent	Discovery year	Disease
H. pylori	1983	H.p.-gastritis
		Peptic ulcer
		Stomach cancer
		MALT lymphoma
B. burgdorferi	1982	Lyme disease (borreliosis)
		Erythema chronicum migrans
		Arthritis
		Neuroborreliosis
Hepatitis C virus (HCV)	1989	Hepatitis C
Hepatitis E virus (HEV)	1983/1990	Hepatitis E
Chlamydia pneumoniae	1986	Community-acquired pneumonia
		Coronary heart disease
Tropheryma whipplei	1992	Morbus whipple
Bartonella henselae	1994	Cat scratch disease
		Bacillary angiomatosis
Human papillomavirus (HPV)	1983	Cervix carcinoma

3.3.1 Emerging Diagnosis of Infectious Diseases

3.3.1.1 *Helicobacter pylori*-Associated Diseases

Since the detection of *Helicobacter pylori* in 1983, this infection has been identified as the causative agent in 90% of B-gastritis cases. The risk of duodenal ulcer is increased by 4–25-fold in patients with *Helicobacter*-associated gastritis. WHO declared *H. pylori* as a carcinogen of first order because of its potential to enhance the risk of stomach carcinoma and MALT lymphoma in long-term infection. In high-prevalence regions for *H. pylori*, the frequency of stomach carcinoma is significantly higher compared to low-endemic areas (Correa et al. 1990). The identification of *H. pylori* facilitates curative treatment of most associated diseases in individuals. But the most important epidemiological effect on associated diseases is attributed to increased hygienic standards in industrialized countries with a substantial reduction of *H. pylori* prevalences in younger age cohorts.

Transmission of *H. pylori* occurs mainly in childhood. In western developed countries the overall prevalence is around 30%, higher in older age groups due to a cohort effect, and this increases with low socioeconomic status (Rothenbacher et al. 1989). In countries with low hygienic standards the prevalences are still high in younger age groups and reach 90% in developing countries. In developed countries, migrant subpopulations from less-developed regions show significantly higher prevalences in comparison to the nonmigrant population (Mégraud 1993).

3.3.1.2 Lyme Disease, Tick-Borne Encephalitis

Since the early 20th century, a characteristic expanding skin lesion, erythema migrans (EM), and an arthritis associated with previous tick bites were known.

Molecular investigations in conserved ticks showed that ticks had been infected with *Borrelia* for many decades. Increased outdoor activities facilitated contacts between humans and ticks in the 1970s and the 1980s and increased transmission of *Borrelia* to humans at the northeastern coast of North America, leading to the discovery of *Borrelia burgdorferi* in 1981 by Willy Burgdorfer. Three different stages of the disease that describe the stage of infection and the involvement of different organ systems are known: stage 1, early localized infection; stage 2, early but disseminated infection; and stage 3, late stage with persistent infection.

Lyme disease is endemic at the east coast and in Minnesota in the United States, in eastern and central Europe, and Russia. Seroprevalence rates that reflect about 50% of nonclinical infections vary between 2 and 18% in the general population in Germany (Hassler et al. 1992; Weiland et al. 1992). In high-risk groups like forest workers in Germany the prevalences reach 25–29% (Robert Koch Institute 2001a). In ticks (*Ixodes*) the prevalences are between 2 and 30% depending on the geographical area and the testing method used [immunofluorescence test, IFT and polymerase chain reaction (PCR)]. In most studies the main risk factors of infection are age (children: 4–9 years, adults 35–60 years), outdoor activities, skin contacts with bushes and grass, and the presence of ticks in domestic animals (Robert Koch Institute 2001b). The probability of infection (seroconversion) after a tick bite in Germany is 3–6% and the probability of a clinical disease is 0.3–1.4%. The probability that the bite of an infectious tick leads to infection in the host is 20–30%. This depends on the time duration that the tick is feeding on the human body. Since the detection of the etiologic infectious agent and the subsequent development of laboratory diagnostic tests in the 1980s, the number of reported cases of Lyme disease has increased from 0 to 16,000 per year, indicating that it is an "emerging diagnosis." The reported numbers vary depending on the reproduction of the hosting rodents for ticks as well as the contacts between humans and nature (Spach et al. 1993).

Ticks may live for several years and their survival, reproduction rate, and activity are directly affected by changes in seasonal climate through induced changes in vegetation zones and biodiversity, hence causing local alterations of the tick's habitat and in the occurrence of animals that are carriers of different pathogens (like small rodents). Several studies in Europe have shown that in recent decades the tick *Ixodes ricinus*, transmitting Lyme borreliosis and tick-borne encephalitis (TBE), has spread into higher latitudes (e.g., Sweden) and altitudes (e.g., Czech Republic, Austria), and has become more abundant in many places. Such variations have been shown to be associated with recent variations in climate. As a result, new risk areas of both diseases have recently been reported from the Czech Republic. Climate change in Europe seems likely to facilitate the spread of Lyme borreliosis and TBE into higher latitudes and altitudes, and to contribute to extended and more intense transmission seasons. Currently, the most effective adaptive strategies available are TBE vaccination of risk populations and preventive information to the general public (Danielova et al. 2004; Lindgren et al. 2006; Materna et al. 2005).

An effective vaccine was licensed for *B. burgdorferi* in 1999. In Europe, where different variants of *Borrelia* are present (mostly *B. afzelii* and *B. garinii*), this vaccine is not protective. Trivalent vaccines for Europe are in clinical trials.

3.3.1.3 Norovirus

In recent years, norovirus infections are increasingly recognized as the cause of large outbreaks of diarrheal diseases in the general population, school classes, nursing homes, hospitals, and cruise ships in western countries with peaks in colder seasons (winter epidemics) (Centers of disease control 2006; Verhoef et al. 2008; Robert Koch Institute 2008a). This is a typical example for emerging diagnosis due to increasing availability of routine PCR testing for these viruses in stool samples. Noroviruses (family *Caliciviridae*) are a group of related, single-stranded RNA viruses first described in an outbreak of gastroenteritis in a school at Norwalk, Ohio, in 1968. Five genogroups are known. Immunity seems to be strain specific and lasts only for limited periods, so individuals are likely to get the infection repeatedly throughout their life. It is estimated that noroviruses are the cause of about 50% of all food-borne outbreaks of gastroenteritis. For several years there has been an ongoing epidemic in several European countries due to drift variants of a new genotype (GG II.4jamboree) previously unknown to this nonimmune population (Robert Koch Institute 2008a).

As a result of an analysis of 232 outbreaks in the United States between 1997 and 2000, direct contamination of food by a food handler was the most common cause (57%), person-to-person transmission was less prevalent (16%), and even less frequently waterborne transmission could be proved (3%) (Centers for Disease Control 2006). Vomiting is a frequent symptom of norovirus enteritis and may result in infectious droplets or aerosols causing airborne or contact transmission. This may explain the difficulty to stop outbreaks in hospitals, nursing homes, and similar settings despite precautions to prevent fecal–oral transmission. Also on cruise ships, person-to-person transmission is most likely in those closed settings, and drinking tap water is a risk factor as well (Verhoef et al. 2008).

3.3.1.4 Hepatitis E

Searching for an agent which causes large outbreaks of enterically transmitted non-A hepatitis in Asia and other parts of the world, the hepatitis E virus (HEV) was first described in 1983 and cloned and sequenced in 1990 (Reyes et al. 1990). Meanwhile, HEV has been shown to be a zoonotic virus circulating in pigs and other animals. It is implicated in about 50% of sporadic cases of acute hepatitis in developing countries and associated with a high case fatality rate in the third trimester of pregnancy (10–25%). HEV is a major cause of large epidemics in Asia, and to a lesser extent in Africa and Latin America, typically promoted through postmonsoon flooding with contamination of drinking water by human and animal feces.

Recent data show HEV also to circulate in European countries and to be associated with severe and fatal disease not only during pregnancy but also in the elderly and in patients with chronic liver conditions. In patients with solid organ transplants, HEV may even cause chronic hepatitis and liver cirrhosis (Kamar et al. 2008). A recombinant HEV vaccine candidate has demonstrated a high protection rate of approximately 95% during clinical trials in Nepal (Shrestha et al. 2007).

3.3.1.5 Cervix Carcinoma and Human Papillomavirus Infection

For 30 years, specific human papillomaviruses have been linked to certain human cancers and have been identified as causative agents of malignant proliferations. In the 1980s the detection of papillomavirus DNA from cervical carcinoma biopsies were published, showing that HPV types 16 and 18 are the most frequent (Dürst et al. 1983; Boshart et al. 1984). The relation of HPV infections and cancer is further discussed in Chapter 23.

3.4 Newly Emerging Infections

Definition: only infections that are newly discovered in humans are listed in this chapter: HIV, new variant of Creutzfeldt–Jakob disease (vCJD), hemorrhagic uremic syndrome (HUS) caused by enterohemorrhagic *Escherichia coli*, viral hemorrhagic fevers like Hanta, Lassa, Ebola, and Marburg fever, Nipah virus encephalitis, monkeypox, human ehrlichiosis, severe acute respiratory syndrome (coronavirus infection, SARS), and avian influenza (H5N1) (see Fig. 3.1 and Table 3.2).

Table 3.2 Newly emerging infectious diseases

Infectious agent	Discovery year	Disease	Important outbreak; prevalence
Hantaan virus	1976	Hemorrhagic fever with renal syndrome (HFRS)	More than 3,000 cases in 1951 in US soldiers in the war of Korea, case fatality rate 5%
Puumala virus		HFRS	Central and northern Europe (seroprevalence up to 3%), outbreak in Germany 2007
Dobrava (central and southeast European variant)		HFRS	Central and southeast Europe (seroprevalence 2.4% in lumbermen in Brandenburg, Germany)
Various types of hantaviruses Muerto Canyon, Sin Nombre, Louisiana et al.	1993	Hantavirus pulmonary syndrome (HPS)	First outbreak in the United States through favorable climatic conditions for the chronically infected deer mice population, 465 cases until 2007, case fatality rate 35%
Nipah virus (related to Hendra virus)	1999	Encephalitis	1997/1998 in Malaysia among butchery workers, 265 cases, case fatality rate 40%, disease transmission by infected pigs, in India 66 cases in 2001 Outbreaks in Bangladesh since 2001
West Nile virus	1999	Encephalitis	Since 1999 at the east coast of the United States, spread in the whole country within 4 years

Table 3.2 (continued)

Infectious agent	Discovery year	Disease	Important outbreak; prevalence
V. cholerae 0139 Bengal	1992	Cholera	Originated from India and Bangladesh, epidemic with 200,000 cases in seven Asian countries
Cyclospora cayetanensis	1993	Long-lasting diarrhea	1996/1997 outbreaks in the United States with 1465 diseases through contamination of imported strawberries
Presumably PrPSc (Prion), presumably identical to BSE virus	1996	New variant of Creutzfeldt–Jakob Disease (vCJD)	First cases in 1994/1995 in the United Kingdom, 163 deaths in the United Kingdom until June 2008
Ehrlichia chaffeensis, *E. ewingii*, etc.	1986, 1994, 1999	Human monocytogenic and granulocytogenic ehrlichiosis	Several clinical cases, seroprevalence in lumbermen in Brandenburg, Germany, in 2000 6.2%
Coronavirus	2002	Severe acute respiratory syndrome (SARS)	8097 cases between 11-2002 and 2004 (China, Hong Kong, Taiwan, Singapore, Canada), case fatality rate 9.6%
Influenza virus H5N1	1996 in a farmed goose in China, 2003 first human confirmed cases from China	Avian influenza	Since 2003 until June 2008, 385 confirmed human cases with 243 deaths in China, Vietnam, Thailand, Indonesia, Cambodia, Azerbaijan, Djibouti, Egypt, Iraq, Turkey, Laos, Myanmar, Nigeria, Pakistan, Bangladesh
Influenza virus A H1N1	2009 in children and mostly young adults in Mexico	New influenza A H1N1	Since 2009, outbreak in Mexico with further spread to neighborhood countries, North and South America, Europe, Asia, and Africa (56,000 cases worldwide by the end of June 2009)

These infections mostly have their origin in zoonotic wildlife (e.g., avian influenza, monkeypox, hantavirus, Nipah virus, and filoviruses) or livestock (e.g., vCJD). Factors promoting the spread of these infections in humans are contacts with wildlife, mass food production of animal origin, and globalization (migration, transportation of goods and vectors) (see Fig. 3.2).

In addition, new strains or variants of well-known pathogens have emerged showing increased or altered virulence such as *Clostridium difficile* ribotype 027 or *Staphylococcus aureus* strains expressing the Panton–Valentine leukocidin (see also Chapter 22).

The epidemiology of HIV is treated in Chapter 18 and that of avian influenza and new influenza H1N1 in Chapter 16.

3.4.1 New Variant of Creutzfeldt–Jakob Disease

In the year 1995, 3 years after the peak of the BSE epidemic in the United Kingdom, with an annual incidence rate in cows of 6.636 per million bovines aged over 24 months, the first mortalities in humans with a new variant of Creutzfeldt–Jakob disease were observed in the United Kingdom. Until 2007, smaller incidence rates of BSE cases had been reported by 21 other European countries in indigenous bovines and up to more than 43,000 per million in 2004 in Ireland. From 1999, BSE started to increase in Switzerland and Portugal, from 2004 in Spain and in recent years has spread to eastern European countries (Organisation Mondiale de la Santé Animale 2008). The infectious agent is a self-replicating protein, a "prion." The source of infection for cows is infectious animal flour. The transmission to humans occurs through oral intake of cow products, most likely undercooked meat and nerval tissues as well as transplants of cornea, dura mater, contaminated surgical instruments, or the treatment with hypophyseal hormones extracted from animal tissues. After a statuary ban on the feeding of protein derived from ruminants to any ruminant and the export ban of all cow products from England, the epidemic of BSE in cows and the occurrence of human infections decreased in the United Kingdom since 2004. By June 2008 the total number of deaths in definite/probable cases of vCJD in the United Kingdom was 163 (The National Creutzfeldt–Jakob Disease Surveillance Unit 2008). Only a few numbers of vCJD were reported from other European countries and the United States (WHO 2008).

3.4.2 Nipah Virus Encephalitis

Nipah virus encephalitis was first observed in 1997/98 in Malaysia. The disease was transmitted by pigs to laborers in slaughterhouses and showed a lethality of 40%. The infectious agent was detected in 1999 (Chua et al. 2000; Lam and Chua 2002). Since then, several outbreaks of Nipah virus infections have been observed in Asian countries: Singapore in 1999, India 2001, and Bangladesh since 2003 (WHO 2004a; Harit et al. 2006). The virus has been isolated repeatedly from various species of fruit bats, which seem to be the natural reservoir (Yob et al. 2001).

3.4.3 West Nile Encephalitis

West Nile is a mosquito-borne flavivirus that was first isolated from a woman with a febrile illness in Uganda in 1937. From the 1950s, West Nile fever endemicity and epidemics started being reported from Africa and the Middle East. Severe neurological symptoms were thought to be rare. More recent epidemics in northern Africa, eastern Europe, and Russia suggested a higher prevalence of meningoencephalitis with case fatality rates of 4–13%. In 1999, West Nile virus was identified as the cause of an epidemic of encephalitis at the east coast of the United States (Nash et al. 1999). A seroepidemiological household-based survey showed that the first outbreak consisted of about 8,000 infections of which about 1,700 developed fever and less than 1% experienced neurological disease (Mostashari et al. 2001). Since then, epidemics occur during summer months in North America each year, with an estimated 35,000 febrile illnesses and over 1,200 encephalitis or meningitis cases in the United States in 2007 (Centers for Disease Control 2008). Age above 50 years is the main risk factor for developing severe disease. The virus is transmitted mainly by *Culex* mosquitoes, but also by sandflies, ceratopogonids, and ticks, with birds as reservoir hosts and incidental hosts such as cats, dogs, and horses. Efforts are made to reduce the transmitting mosquito population and to prevent mosquito bites through personal protection as well as to prevent transmission through blood donations by screening (Centers of Disease Control 2008).

3.4.4 Severe Acute Respiratory Syndrome (SARS)

The first case of SARS occurred in Guangdong (China) in November of 2002, leading to an outbreak with 7082 cases in China and Hong Kong (8096 cases worldwide) until July 2003. The case fatality rate was 9.6%. A new coronavirus (SARS-CoV) was identified as the causative agent (Drosten et al. 2003), being transmitted first by infected semidomesticated animals such as the palm civet and subsequently from human to human. Some cases were exported to other countries, causing smaller outbreaks there, Canada being the most affected country outside Asia with 251 cases, before control of transmission was effective. Eight thousand and ninety-six cases were reported worldwide, until July 2003, then further transmission stopped (besides one more case of laboratory transmission in 2004), indicating an efficient international cooperation in disease control (WHO 2004b). Recently, SARS-CoV has been found in horseshoe bats, which seem to be the natural reservoir of the virus.

3.4.5 Hantavirus

About 150,000–200,000 cases of hemorrhagic fever with renal syndrome (HFRS) caused by hantaviruses are reported annually worldwide, with more than half in China, many from Russia and Korea, and numerous cases from Japan, Finland, Sweden, Bulgaria, Greece, Hungary, France, and the Balkan with different death rates depending on the responsible virus, ranging from 0.1% in Puumala to 5–10% in Hantaan infections (Schmaljohn and Hjelle 1997).

Hantaviruses are transmitted from rodent to rodent through body fluids and excreta. Only occasionally do humans get infected. Different types of hantaviruses are circulating in Europe and the eastern hemisphere, predominantly Puumala virus, Dobrava virus, and Tula virus, adapted to different mouse species. Depending on the virus type the case fatality rate is between 1 and 50%. As an example, the annual rate of reported cases in Germany was about 100 cases per year from 2001 onward. This started to change in 2005 with 448 reported cases and rose dramatically to 1687 cases in 2007. That year, hantavirus infections were among the five most reported viral infections in Germany. Reasons for the rise in human infections were an increase in the hosting rodent population due to a very mild winter 2006/2007 and an early start of warm temperatures in spring which led to favorable nutritional situations for the mice influencing their population dynamics. In addition, favorable climatic conditions enhanced the outdoor behaviors of humans facilitating transmission in rural areas (Robert Koch Institute 2008b; Hofmann et al. 2008).

Since 1993, a previously unknown group of hantaviruses (Sin Nombre, New York, Black Creek Canal, Bayou—in the United States and Canada; Andes, in South America) emerged in the Americas as a cause of hantavirus pulmonary syndrome (HPS), an acute respiratory disease with high case fatality rates (approx. 35%), causing a new, significant public health concern. A total of 465 cases had been reported until March 2007 in 32 states, most of them in the western part of the United States (Centers for Disease Control 2007).

3.4.6 Filoviruses and Lassa Virus

Lassa virus was detected for the first time in 1969 during an outbreak affecting nurses in a missionary hospital in Lassa, Nigeria. However, the disease had previously been described in the 1950s. Lassa virus is enzootic in a common peridomestic rodent in West Africa, the multimammate rat *Mastomys natalensis*, which is chronically infected and sheds the virus in urine and saliva. Human infection through direct or indirect contact with rats or their excretions is rather common in some West African countries and estimates from seroepidemiological and clinical studies suggest that there are several hundred thousand cases annually. However, only a minority of infections seems to progress to severe hemorrhagic disease with a case fatality rate of 5–30% in hospitalized cases. The virus can be transmitted by close person-to-person contact and nosocomial spread has been observed under poor hygienic conditions.

Marburg and Ebola viruses, which were first detected during outbreaks in 1967 and 1975, respectively, have so far been observed only during several limited outbreaks and a few isolated cases in certain countries of sub-Saharan Africa. However, very high case fatality rates (25–90%), the occurrence of outbreaks that were difficult to control in resource-poor settings, and the obscure origin of these viruses have attracted considerable public interest worldwide. Recently, evidence was found for both Marburg and Ebola viruses to occur in certain species of bats that probably constitute the natural reservoir of these filoviruses (Towner et al. 2007).

Although the disease burden of these viral hemorrhagic fevers is low, they gained considerable international attention due to

- their high case fatality rates,
- the risk of person-to-person transmission,
- several imported cases to industrialized countries, and
- fears of abuse of these agents for bioterrorism.

As a consequence, considerable resources have been invested, even in non-endemic countries, in the setting up of task forces and high containment facilities for both laboratory diagnostic services and treatment of patients using barrier nursing.

3.4.7 C. difficile Ribotype 027

This highly virulent strain of *C. difficile* expresses both cytotoxins A and B and, in addition, the binary toxin CDT, an ADP-ribosyltransferase. Due to a deletion in the regulatory *tcdC* gene, the synthesis rates of toxin A and B are increased by 16- and 23-fold, respectively. This strain was detected in 2000 for the first time in Pittsburgh, USA. Since then it has spread to Canada, and in 2003 it reached Europe causing multiple outbreaks in hospitals and nursing homes (Warny et al. 2005). *C. difficile* 027-associated colitis has shown high case fatality rates (10–22%) and an increased relapse rate. Containment of outbreaks in hospitals and other institutions necessitates isolation of patients or cohorts and strict hygienic measures.

3.5 Re-emerging Infectious Diseases

During recent decades, a large variety of well known infectious diseases has shown regional or global re-emergence with considerable public health relevance (Table 3.3). Globally, tuberculosis is probably the most important re-emerging infectious disease. In developing countries, TB infection still is extremely common and, in the wake of the HIV pandemic, the percentage of those developing overt disease has increased dramatically. Worldwide, TB is the most common opportunistic infection in patients with AIDS. The significance of TB and HIV/TB coinfection is reviewed in Chapters 16 and 18.

The re-emergence of some infectious diseases is closely related to the lack or the breakdown of basic infrastructures as seen in periurban slums and in refugee camps in developing countries, or as a consequence of war, breakdown of the civil society, or natural or man-made disasters. Cholera is a formidable example for both re-emergence and epidemic spread under those conditions.

Another important group of re-emerging infectious diseases is caused by various vector-borne infections, such as malaria, dengue fever, and yellow fever. These major vector-borne diseases are treated in more detail in Chapter 21. In addition,

Table 3.3 Re-emerging infections of public health relevance

Disease	Current epidemiology
Tuberculosis, malaria, cholera, dengue fever	See Chapters 16, 17, and 21
Yellow fever	See Chapter 21
	Numerous outbreaks in Africa and South America; in 2008 new outbreaks in southern Brazil, Argentina, and Paraguay
	Single cases in uprooting workers and gold miners in the Amazon area; in 2007–2008 new outbreak in southern Brazil, Paraguay and Argentina; single imported cases in industrialized countries (Germany, United States, and others)
Japanese encephalitis	Increasing in rural areas of Southeast Asia, spreading to the West (epidemics in northern India, Nepal, Sri Lanka); since 1995 some cases in Torres Islands (Australia)
Crimean-Congo hemorrhagic fever	Small tick-borne or human-to-human transmission-borne epidemics in 2001 (Kosovo, Albania, Iran, Pakistan, South Africa), small outbreaks in Turkey since 2002, 438 cases (27 deaths) reported in 2006
Meningococcal meningitis	Pandemic since 1996 in West Africa; epidemic with serogroup W135 in pilgrims to Mecca 2000 and 2001 with imports and contact infections in several European countries
Plague	Several epidemics in the 1990s in India, Tanzania, Madagascar (deriving from known zoonotic infections, facilitated by increased rat population and slums and poor hygiene)
Rift Valley fever	Epidemics in humans and productive livestock in North Africa and sub-Saharan Africa; in 1997–1998, outbreaks in Kenya and Somalia (heavy rainfalls, El Niño); in 2000, first occurrence outside Africa in Saudi Arabia and Yemen; in 2006–2007, outbreaks in Kenya and Tanzania
Ross River fever	Spread in Australia and to Oceania, some epidemics
Sleeping sickness	Re-emergence in areas with political destabilization, high mortality (Angola, Congo, south Sudan)
Visceral leishmaniasis	Increasing numbers in south Sudan, northeast India, west China; increasing occurrence as opportunistic infection in HIV-infected persons mainly in southwest Europe (i.v. drug user) and northeastern Brazil
Rabies	India, Nepal, China (outbreaks in dog farms)
Cholera	Tanzania, Zanzibar
Chikungunya fever	Large outbreaks in La Réunion and other Indian Ocean islands with further spread to Sri Lanka, India in 2007–2008, autochthonous outbreak in Italy in 2007

there are a variety of re-emerging infections transmitted by arthropod vectors such as various arboviral diseases and some protozoal diseases other than malaria (i.e., leishmaniasis, human African trypanosomiasis). The reasons for the emergence of several vector-borne diseases are rather variable and may range from climatic factors (e.g., global warming, rainfall), lack or breakdown of control, to changes in agriculture and farming and in human behavior (e.g., outdoor activities). These factors are usually quite specific for each of these diseases and largely depend on the specific ecology of the agent, its vectors, and reservoirs.

3.5.1 Cholera

Cholera, an acute diarrheal infection transmitted by fecally contaminated water and food, had been endemic for centuries in the Ganges and Brahmaputra deltas in the 19th century before it started to spread to the rest of the world. Since 1817, six pandemics caused by the classical biotype of *Vibrio cholerae* were recorded that killed millions of people across Europe, Africa, and the Americas. It has been a major driving force for the improvement of sanitation and safe water supply. The seventh pandemic was caused by the El Tor biotype, first isolated from pilgrims at the El Tor quarantine station in Sinai in 1906. It started in 1961 in South Asia, reached Africa in 1971, and is still ongoing. After more than hundred years, cholera spread to the Americas in 1991, and beginning in Peru, a large epidemic hit numerous Latin American countries with 1.4 million cases and more than 10,000 fatalities reported within 6 years.

Out of the 139 serogroups of *V. cholerae*, only O1 and O139 can cause epidemics. The serogroup O139, first identified in Bangladesh in 1992, possesses the same virulence factors as O1 and creates a similar clinical picture. Currently, the presence of O139 has been detected only in southeast and east Asia, but it is still unclear whether *V. cholerae* O139 will extend to other regions.

Since 2005, the re-emergence of cholera has been noted in parallel with the ever-increasing size of vulnerable populations living in unsanitary conditions. Cholera remains a global threat to public health and one of the key indicators of social development. While the disease is no longer an issue in countries where minimum hygiene standards are met, it remains a threat in almost every developing country. The number of cholera cases reported to the WHO during 2006 rose dramatically, reaching the level of the late 1990s. A total of 236,896 cases were notified from 52 countries, including 6,311 deaths, an overall increase of 79% compared with the number of cases reported in 2005. This increased number of cases is the result of several major outbreaks that occurred in countries where cases had not been reported for several years such as Sudan and Angola. It is estimated that only a small proportion of cases – less than 10% – are reported. The true burden of disease is therefore grossly underestimated.

The absence or the shortage of safe water and sufficient sanitation combined with a generally poor environmental status are the main causes of spread of the disease. Typical at-risk areas include periurban slums where basic infrastructure is not available, as well as camps for internally displaced people or refugees where minimum requirements of clean water and sanitation are not met. However, it is important to stress that the belief that cholera epidemics are caused by dead bodies after disasters, whether natural or manmade, is false. On the other hand, the consequences of a disaster—such as disruption of water and sanitation systems or massive displacement of population to inadequate and overcrowded camps—will increase the risk of transmission.

3.6 Vector-Borne Diseases

3.6.1 Chikungunya Fever

Chikungunya virus, an arbovirus belonging to the alphavirus group, is transmitted by various mosquitoes. The virus was first isolated in Tanzania in 1952 and since then has caused smaller epidemics in sub-Saharan Africa and parts of Asia with low public health impact. In 2005, the largest epidemic ever recorded started in east Africa, spread to Réunion and some other islands of the Indian Ocean, and then spread further to Asia, with more than 1.5 million cases in India alone so far. Characteristics of the disease are high fever and a debilitating polyarthritis, mainly of the small joints that can persist for months in some patients. Now, for the first time, severe and fatal cases have been observed that may be due to certain mutations of the epidemic strain (Parola et al. 2006).

The Asian tiger mosquito *Aedes albopictus* has proved to be an extremely effective vector in recent epidemics causing high transmission rates in big cities and leading to epidemics with high public health impact. This southeast Asian mosquito species has been shipped by transport of used tires and plants harboring water contaminated with larvae to other continents and, since 1990, *Ae. albopictus* has successfully spread in Italy and other parts of southern Europe. In August 2007, an outbreak of chikungunya fever occurred in northern Italy with more than 200 confirmed cases. The index case was a visitor from India who fell ill while visiting relatives in one of the villages and further transmission was facilitated by an abundant mosquito population during that time, as a consequence of seasonal synchronicity (Rezza et al. 2007).

3.6.2 Ross River Fever

Ross River virus (RRV) is another arbovirus of the alphavirus group that causes an acute disease with or without fever and/or rash. Most patients experience arthritis or arthralgia primarily affecting the wrist, knee, ankle, and small joints of the extremities (epidemic polyarthritis). About one-quarter of patients have rheumatic symptoms that persist for up to a year. The disease can cause incapacity and inability to work for months. It is the most common arboviral disease in Australia with an average of almost 5,000 notified cases per year. RRV is transmitted by various mosquito species and circulates in a primary mosquito–mammal cycle involving kangaroos, wallabies, bats, and rodents. A human–mosquito cycle may be present in explosive outbreaks which occur irregularly during the summer months in Australia and parts of Oceania. Heavy rainfalls as well as increasing travel and outdoor activities are considered as important factors contributing to the emergence of RRV epidemics.

3.6.3 *Japanese Encephalitis (JE)*

This flavivirus is transmitted by certain *Culex* mosquitoes and is a leading cause of viral encephalitis in Asia with 30,000–50,000 clinical cases reported annually. It occurs from the islands of the Western Pacific in the east to the Pakistani border in the west, and from Korea in the north to Papua New Guinea in the south. Only 1 in 50–200 infections will lead to encephalitis, which is, however, often severe with fatality rates of 5–30% and with a high incidence of neurological sequelae.

Despite the availability of effective vaccines, JE causes large epidemics and has spread to new areas during recent decades (e.g., India, Sri Lanka, Pakistan, Torres Strait islands, and isolated cases in northern Australia). JE is particularly common in areas where flooded rice fields attract water fowl and other birds as the natural reservoir and provide abundant breeding sites for mosquitoes such as *Culex tritaeniorhynchus*, which transmit the virus to humans. Pigs act as important amplifying hosts, and therefore JE distribution is very significantly linked to irrigated rice production combined with pig rearing. Because of the critical role of pigs, JE presence in Muslim countries is low.

3.6.4 *Crimean–Congo Hemorrhagic Fever (CCHF)*

Crimean–Congo virus is a bunyavirus causing an acute febrile disease often with extensive hepatitis resulting in jaundice in some cases. About one-quarter of patients present hemorrhages that can be severe. Fatality rates of 7.5–50% have been reported in hospitalized patients. CCHF is transmitted by *Hyalomma* ticks to a wide range of domestic and wild animals including birds. Human infection is acquired by tick bites or crushing infected ticks, and also by contact with blood or tissue from infected animals that usually do not become ill but do develop viremia. In addition, nosocomial transmission is possible and is usually related to extensive blood exposure or needle sticks. Human cases have been reported from more than 30 countries in Africa, Asia, southeastern Europe, and the Middle East. In recent years, an increase in the number of cases during tick seasons has been observed in several countries such as Russia, South Africa, Kosovo, and Greece. In Turkey, where before 2002 no human CCHF cases had been observed, a total of 2,508 confirmed cases, including 133 deaths, were reported between 2002 and June 2008. The emergence of CCHF has been associated with factors such as climatic features (temperature, humidity, etc.), changes of vector population, geographical conditions, flora, wildlife, and the animal husbandry sector.

3.6.5 *Rift Valley Fever (RVF)*

RVF is a mosquito-borne bunyavirus infection occurring in many parts of sub-Saharan Africa. It infects primarily sheep, cattle, and goats, and is maintained in nature by transovarial transmission in floodwater *Aedes* mosquitoes. It has been shown that infected eggs remain dormant in the dambos (i.e., depressions) of east

Africa and hatch after heavy rains and initiate mosquito–livestock–mosquito transmission giving rise to large epizootics. Remote sensing via satellite can predict the likelihood of RVF transmission by detecting both the ecological changes associated with heavy rainfall and the depressions from which the floodwater mosquitoes emerge.

Transmission to humans is also possible from direct and aerosol exposure to blood and amniotic fluids of livestock. Most human infections manifest themselves as uncomplicated febrile illness, but severe hemorrhagic disease, encephalitis, or retinal vasculitis is possible. In 1977, RVF has been transported, probably by infected camels to Egypt, where it caused major epidemics with several hundred thousand infections of humans. It has been suggested that introduction of RVF may be a risk to other potentially receptive areas such as parts of Asia and the Americas. Floods occurring during the El Niño phenomenon of 1997 in east Africa subsequently gave rise to large epidemics and further spread to the Arabian Peninsula. Most recent epidemics occurred in 2006 and 2007 following heavy rainfalls in Kenya, Somalia, and Sudan, causing several hundred deaths. Besides mosquito control, epidemics are best prevented by vaccination of livestock.

3.6.6 Leishmaniasis

Leishmaniasis, a protozoal transmitted by sandflies, has shown a sharp increase in the number of recorded cases and spread to new endemic regions over the last decade. Presently, 88 countries are affected with an estimated 12 million cases worldwide. There are about 1.5 million new cases of cutaneous and mucocutaneous leishmaniasis, a nonfatal but debilitating disease with 90% of cases occurring in Afghanistan, Brazil, Bolivia, Iran, Peru, Saudi Arabia, and Syria.

The incidence of visceral leishmaniasis (VL), a disease with a high fatality rate when untreated, is estimated at around 500,000 per year. The situation is further aggravated by emerging drug resistance (Table 3.4) and the deadly synergy of VL/HIV coinfection. Epidemics usually affect the poorest part of the population and have occurred recently in Bangladesh, Brazil, India, Nepal, and Sudan.

For many years, the public health impact of the leishmaniases has been grossly underestimated. They seriously hamper socioeconomic progress and epidemics have significantly delayed the implementation of numerous development programs.

The spread of leishmaniasis is associated with factors favoring the vector such as deforestation, building of dams, new irrigation schemes, and climate changes, but also with urbanization, migration of nonimmune people to endemic areas, poverty, malnutrition, and the breakdown of public health.

3.7 Emerging Resistance

Antimicrobial resistance of epidemiological relevance has emerged as a major problem in the treatment of many infectious diseases (Table 3.4). Resistance is no longer a problem that predominantly affects the chemotherapy of bacterial infections. It became increasingly important in parasitic and fungal diseases, and despite the short history of antiviral chemotherapy, it already plays a prominent role in the treatment of HIV infection and other viral diseases. Resistance is also a problem in some of the emerging infections and will further complicate their treatment and control.

Resistance of bacterial pathogens has become a common feature in *nosocomial infections*, especially in the ICU and in surgical wards. Currently, the number one problem in most hospitals is *S. aureus* resistant to methicillin (MRSA, see Chapter 22). However, common problems of resistance also extend to other major bacterial pathogens such as enterococci, various gram-negative enteric bacilli, and pseudomonas species. Resistance has developed not only to standard antibiotics (e.g., penicillins, cephalosporins, aminoglycosides, macrolides, or quinolones) but also to second-line antibiotics including carbapenems, glycopeptides, and newer quinolones. However, there is considerable geographic variation. In 2006, the European Antimicrobial Resistance Surveillance System (EARSS), a network of national surveillance systems, reported vancomycin-resistant rates among enterococci ranging from none in Iceland, Norway, Romania, Bulgaria, Denmark, and Hungary to 42% of *Enterococcus faecium* strains in Greece (EARSS 2006). A surveillance study conducted in the United States hospitals from 1995 to 2002 showed that 9% of nosocomial bloodstream infections were caused by enterococci and that 2% of *E. faecalis* isolates and 60% of *E. faecium* isolates were vancomycin resistant (Wisplinghof et al. 2004).

Rates and spectrum of antibacterial resistance of *E. coli* and other gram-negative enteric bacilli may differ considerably from one hospital to the other. In some important pathogens of hospital-related infections such as *Klebsiella*, *Enterobacter*, and *Pseudomonas* species, resistance to almost all available antimicrobials has been observed. This may complicate the choice of an effective initial chemotherapy considerably. Therefore, each hospital has to monitor the epidemiological situation of resistance regularly, at least for the most important bacteria causing nosocomial infections, such as staphylococci, enterococci, gram-negative enteric bacilli, and pseudomonas.

Even in *community-acquired infections*, there has been a considerable increase in resistance problems. At present, approximately 15% of pneumococcal isolates in the United States are resistant to penicillin, and 20% exhibit intermediate resistance. The rate of resistance is lower in countries that, by tradition, are conservative in their antibiotic use (e.g., Netherlands, Germany) and higher in countries where use is more liberal (e.g., France). In Hong Kong and Korea, resistance rates approach 80%. In addition, about one-quarter of all pneumococcal isolates in the United States are resistant to macrolides. This rate is even higher in strains highly resistant to penicillin, and increasingly there is multiresistance against other antibiotics such as cephalosporins.

The prevalence of meningococci with reduced susceptibility to penicillin has been increasing, and high-level resistance has been reported in some countries (e.g., Spain, United Kingdom). Although high-dose penicillin is effective in infections with strains of intermediate resistance, most national and international guidelines recommend broad-spectrum cephalosporins such as ceftriaxone as first-line drugs. However, in most developing countries, penicillin and chloramphenicol are the only affordable drugs.

In recent years, certain strains of community-acquired *S. aureus* with resistance to methicillin (cMRSA) have been observed which produce a toxin (Panton–Valentine leukocidin) that is cytolytic to PMNs, macrophages, and monocytes, and which are an emerging cause of community-acquired cases and outbreaks of necrotic lesions involving the skin or the mucosa, and in some patients also of necrotic hemorrhagic pneumonia with a high case fatality (Vandenesch et al. 2003).

Development of resistance is mainly determined by two factors:

- The genetic potential of a certain pathogen, i.e., mobile elements such as plasmids, transposons, or bacteriophages, genes coding for resistance, and mutation rate.
- The selection pressure caused by the therapeutic or the para-therapeutic application of antimicrobial drugs.

In the hospital these factors are supported by

- microbial strains that are highly adapted to this environment (e.g., rapid colonization of patients, resistance to disinfectants),
- an increasing percentage of patients who are highly susceptible to infections due to old age, multimorbidity, immunosuppression, extended surgery, and invasive procedures, and
- the frequent use of broad-spectrum antibiotics or combinations of antimicrobial drugs.

Another source of resistant bacteria has been identified in mass animal production and the use of antimicrobials as growth promoters (e.g., the glycopeptide avoparcin, the streptogramin virginiamycin) or as mass treatment in the therapy or the prevention of infections.

The inadequate use of antimicrobial drugs is also an important factor responsible for the development of resistance in community-acquired infections. This is especially true in developing countries where only a limited spectrum of antibiotics is available, where shortage of drugs often leads to treatment that is underdosed or too short, and where uncontrolled sale and use of antibiotics is commonplace. As a consequence, resistance of gonococci is extremely frequent in southeast Asia, and resistance of *Salmonella typhi*, *Shigella*, and *Campylobacter* to standard antibiotics is common. Some of the still effective second-line antibiotics have to be given parenterally or are not available because they are too costly.

A typical example of the consequences of insufficient chemotherapy due to lack of compliance and/or unavailability of drugs is the alarming increase in multiresistance and extreme resistance in TB (see Chapter 16). Resistance is also a problem in parasitic diseases such as malaria (see Chapter 21), leishmaniasis, or African trypanosomiasis. *Plasmodium falciparum* developed resistance against all major antimalarial drugs as soon as they were used on a broad scale. Resistance had contributed significantly to the increase in malaria-associated morbidity and mortality observed in many endemic areas (Wongsichranalai et al. 2002). A recent report on failures of the new artemisinin combination treatment for *P. falciparum* malaria at the Thai–Cambodian border supports fears of the development of resistance to this most promising class of drug at present (Dondrop et al. 2009).

Resistance against antiviral drugs has developed almost from the beginning of antiviral chemotherapy (Table 3.4). In the treatment of HIV infection, the risk of development of resistance has been drastically reduced by the combination of several drugs with different mechanisms of action (see Chapter 18). However, drug resistance remains the Achilles' heel of the highly active antiretroviral therapy (HAART) and may be at a considerable risk of expanding HAART to the developing world.

Table 3.4 Important resistance of infectious agents to antibiotics and chemotherapeutics

Agent/disease	*Frequent or significant resistances against*
Staphylococcus	Penicillin, methicillin, glycopeptides
Enterococcus	Glycopeptides, multiresistance
Enterobacteria (*E. coli*, *Klebsiella*, *Enterobacter* et al.)	Broad-spectrum penicillins, cephalosporins (ESBL)[a], quinolones, etc., multiresistance also against last-choice antibiotics
Pseudomonas spp.	Numerous antibiotics including last-choice antibiotics
S. typhi	Chloramphenicol, ampicillin, cotrimoxazole, quinolones, multiresistance in Thailand, Laos, Vietnam
Shigella	Ampicillin, tetracycline, cotrimoxazole, quinolones
Campylobacter	Quinolones
Pneumococci	Penicillin, cephalosporins, macrolides
Meningococci	Penicillins
Gonococci	Penicillins, tetracycline, quinolones
H. pylori	Nitroimidazoles
Cholera	Tetracycline, cotrimoxazole, quinolones (still rare)
Mycobacteria	INH, rifampicin, other antimycobacterials, multiresistance, and extreme resistance
Mycobacterium leprae	Dapsone
Plasmodia	Chloroquine, sulfa/pyrimethamine, mefloquine, quinine, atovaquone, multiresistance
Leishmania	Antimony drugs, especially in India and Sudan
Trypanosomes	Pentamidine, suramin, melarsoprol (especially east Africa)
Schistosomes	Praziquantel (Senegal, Egypt)
Fungi	Azol derivates, flucytosine, amphotericin B (still rare)
HIV	All antiretrovirals
HSV	Acyclovir
CMV	Ganciclovir and others
HBV	Lamivudine, adefovir, vaccine escape mutants

[a]Extended-spectrum beta-lactamases

Today, we have to realize that as we develop antimicrobial drugs, microbes will develop strategies of counterattack. Antimicrobial resistance occurs at an alarming rate among all classes of pathogens. Even in rich countries it causes real clinical problems in managing infections that were easily treatable just a few years ago. In life-threatening infections such as sepsis, nosocomial infections, or falciparum malaria, there is a substantial risk that the initial chemotherapy might not be effective. In addition, the delay caused by inadequate treatment might favor transmission to other people and support the spread of resistant pathogens (e.g., multiresistant TB). Last but not the least, surveillance and control and the necessity to use expensive second-line drugs or combinations of antimicrobials are enormous cost factors. For developing countries this is a major limitation in the treatment and control of infections caused by resistant agents. So, in many ways, emerging resistance contributes to the emergence of infectious diseases.

3.8 Outlook

Despite the availability of effective strategies for treatment and prevention, infectious diseases have remained a major cause of morbidity and mortality worldwide. However, the problems associated with infections are due to considerable changes.

In industrialized countries the mortality caused by infectious diseases has decreased tremendously during more than 100 years. However, during recent years, both mortality and morbidity associated with infections are increasing again. Ironically, this is closely associated with the advances in medicine which have contributed to profound changes in the spectrum of both patients and their infections. Advanced age, underlying conditions, and an altered immune response are common features in the seriously infected hospital patient today. Immunosuppressive therapy is frequently used to treat neoplastic and inflammatory diseases or to prevent the rejection of transplants. Some infections, most notably HIV/AIDS, cause immunosuppression by itself. In the compromised patient, infections are generally more severe or may be caused by opportunistic pathogens that will not harm the immunocompetent host. Antimicrobial treatment is often less effective in these patients and tends to be further complicated by antimicrobial resistance which may manifest itself or develop at a higher frequency in the immunocompromised patient. An increasing percentage of infections are hospital acquired or otherwise health care associated. It is estimated that nosocomial infections affect 1.7 million patients and contribute to approximately 100,000 deaths in US hospitals annually (Klevens et al. 2007). Considering the rising number of elderly and immunocompromised patients, a further increase in severe infections can be predicted.

In developing countries, the significance of infectious diseases has remained high for ages and despite the advances in medicine. Until now, infections are by far the leading cause of both disability-adjusted life years and life years lost. The reasons are obvious and mostly related to poverty and lack of development causing poor and unhealthy living conditions, inadequate health systems, and lack of resources for prevention and treatment. This is, of course, just an integral part of the general socioeconomic problems of developing countries. However, poor health conditions per se are an important obstacle to development, and infections such as HIV/AIDS in sub-Saharan Africa can be a major cause of lack of development, increasing poverty, and political instability.

Generally, the situation of many developing countries has not improved during the last two decades, and the gap between the first and the third world has increased. However, most of the mortality and morbidity associated with infectious diseases is avoidable. As laid down in the millennium goals, a major task of the world community will be to counteract the imbalance between the industrialized and the developing countries and to find strategies to ensure participation in the progress of modern medicine for all.

Developing countries also carry the main burden of diseases caused by newly emerging and re-emerging infections (Table 3.2 and 3.3). However, the consequences of economical and political crises on emerging infectious diseases are obvious in industrialized countries also—such as the return of diphtheria or the increase in TB and multiresistant TB after the breakdown of the former Soviet Union.

Today, all countries worldwide are affected by emerging infections as well as by emerging antimicrobial resistance. In the age of globalization, travel and transport of people, animals, and goods of all kinds have increased tremendously. As a consequence, infectious agents may travel over long distances and at high speed. This is clearly evident with influenza pandemics or outbreaks such as the SARS epidemic or with imported cases of viral hemorrhagic fever transmissible from person to person. The spread of antimicrobial resistance or the re-emergence of TB seems to be less spectacular, but the consequences may be at least as important in the long run.

Management and control of emerging and re-emerging infectious diseases can be very different from disease to disease and has to allow for all relevant factors of the populations at risk and of the specific disease including the ecology of the agent, its vectors, and reservoirs. However, some basic principles apply to all situations:

- Surveillance
- Information and communication
- Preemptive planning and preparedness
- Provision and implementation of
    - adequate treatment
    - adequate control and prevention
- international cooperation

Active and passive surveillance systems with rapid reporting and analysis of data are essential for the early detection of outbreaks, changes in epidemiology, and other events of public health concern (see Chapters 8 and 9). However, many resource-poor countries do not have functional surveillance systems.

In addition, reporting of infectious diseases may be neglected or delayed because of fears of stigma, international sanctions including trade and travel restrictions, or interference with tourism. Classical examples are plague and cholera, but also recent examples such as the BSE/vCJD crisis in the United Kingdom or SARS originating from China showed undue delays between first occurrence of cases and information to the public. Although, in outbreaks of new and unknown diseases it may be difficult, or even impossible, to predict or assess the magnitude of the problem and the potential consequences, timely and adequate information and communication is not only obligatory, according to international regulations, but also the best strategy to avoid rumors, misbeliefs, panic, or disregard.

In recent years, many countries have installed national plans of action for important epidemiological scenarios and outbreaks such as pandemic influenza, bioterrorism, import of viral hemorrhagic fevers transmissible from person to person, SARS, and comparable diseases or outbreaks. All member states of the World Health Assembly that have so far not been able to install functional surveillance and/or pre-emptive planning are obliged to do so within a maximum of 5 years after their ratification of the new International Health Regulations (WHO 2005).

Preparedness not only means surveillance and planning but also has to include the provision of facilities to adequately treat and, if necessary, to isolate patients with infectious diseases of public health importance and relevant epidemic potential and/or at risk of transmission to other persons including health-care workers. Task forces and high containment facilities for both laboratory diagnostic services and treatment of patients using barrier nursing have been set up in several countries. However, all health facilities of a certain level such as general hospitals should be prepared by their organization and structure to treat patients with infections of public health relevance such as multiresistant TB under appropriate isolation and barrier nursing conditions. This also applies to hospitals in resource-poor countries. Adequate training of health-care workers and strict management have been effective to control outbreaks of highly contagious infections within rural African hospitals lacking sophisticated technical equipments (CDC 1998).

Strategies for control and prevention may be quite different for various emerging infections. Effective vaccinations are available only for some infections and are usually lacking for newly emerging infections (Table 3.5). For the majority of emerging infections, control and prevention have to rely on information, education and exposure prophylaxis, interruption of transmission by vector control and control of reservoir hosts (e.g., rodents), and case finding with early diagnosis and treatment.

For diseases and outbreaks caused by infections of public health relevance that are transmissible from person to person, containment procedures including isolation and treatment of patients under condition of barrier nursing as well as tracking and surveillance of contacts are warranted by national and international health regulations. Here, international cooperation is essential to successfully contain outbreaks and epidemics such as the SARS epidemic in 2003.

Table 3.5 Availability and development of vaccines for emerging infectious diseases

Agent/disease	Available	Under clinical development	Remarks
B. burgdorferi	+		Withdrawn from the market
Chikungunya fever		+	
Cholera, *V. cholerae* 0139	+[1]		Oral rCTB[2] vaccine, protects against O1 and O139
Dengue fever		+	Quadrivalent vaccines
Filoviruses (Marburg/Ebola)		+	Phase I trials started recently
Hantavirus		+	Hantaan and Seoul virus vaccines
H. pylori		+	
Hepatitis C virus		+	
Hepatitis E virus		+	
HIV/AIDS		+	
Human papillomavirus	+		Two products (type 6/11/16/18; type 16/18)
New Influenza H1N1	+	+	
Influenza virus H5N1	+	+	
Japanese encephalitis	+	+	New cell culture vaccine
Lassa fever			
Leishmaniasis			
Malaria		+	
Plague[1]	+	+	Limited availability, new vaccines in clinical trials
Rift Valley fever	+		Veterinary vaccine in use, limited availability of human vaccine
Ross River fever		+	
Rabies	+		Plus rabies immunoglobulin for PEP
SARS coronavirus			
Sleeping sickness			
Tuberculosis	+[1]	+	New vaccines in clinical trial
West Nile virus		+	
Yellow fever	+		

[1]Partially effective
[2]Recombinant cholera toxin subunit B

3.9 Summary

Despite dramatic progress in their treatment and prevention, infectious diseases are still of enormous global significance with tremendous economic and political implications. Emerging and re-emerging infectious diseases as well as emerging antimicrobial resistance are major challenges to all countries worldwide. For the management of current and future problems, it will be most important to counteract the imbalance between the industrialized world, new economies, and developing countries, and to adequately and timely react to new threats on a global scale.

References

Boshart M, Gissmann L, Ikenberg H, Kleinheinz A, Scheurelen W, zur Hausen H (1984) A new type of papillomavirus DNA, its presence in genital cancer and in cell lines derived from genital cancer. EMBO J 3: 1151–1157

Centers for Disease Control (2008) West Nile virus. http://www.cdc.gov/ncidod/dvbid/westnile/htlm.

Centers for Disease Control (2007) Case information: hantavirus pulmonary syndrome case count and descriptive statistics. http://cdc.gov/ncidod/diseases/hanta/hps/

Centers for Disease Control (2006) Norovirus: technical fact sheet. http://www.cdc.gov/ncidod/dvrd/revb/gastro/norovirus-factsheet.htm

Centers for Disease Control and Prevention. (1998) World Health Organization: Infection Control for Viral Haemorrhagic Fevers in the African Health Care Setting. Centers for Disease Control and Prevention, Atlanta

Chua KB, Bellini WJ, Rota PA et al. (2000) Nipah virus: a recently emergent deadly paramyxovirus. Science 288: 1432–1435

Correa P, Fox J, Fontham E (1990) Helicobacter and gastric carcinoma. Serum antibody prevalence in populations with contrasting cancer risks. Cancer 66: 2569–2574

Danielova V et al. (2004) Effects of climate change on the incidence of tick-borne encephalitis in the Czech Republic in the past two decades. Epidemiol Mikrobiol Imunol 53 (4): 174–181

Dondrop AM, Nosten F, Yi P, et al. (2009). Artemisinin resistance in Plasmodium falciparum malaria. N Engl J Med 361: 455–467

Drosten C, Günther S, Preiser W, van der Werf S, et al. (2003) Identification of a novel coronavirus in patients with severe acute respiratory syndrome. N Engl J Med 348: 1967–1976

Dürst M, Gissmann L, Ikenberg H, zur Hausen H (1983) A papillomavirus DANN from a cervical carcinoma and its prevalence in cancer biopsy samples from different geographic regions. Proc Nat Acad Sci US 80: 3812–3815

European Antimicrobial Resistance Surveillance System (2006). Susceptibility results for *E. faecium* isolates. Available at: http://www.rivm.nl/earss/database/

Harit AK, Ichhupujani SG, Gill KS,Shiv Lal, Ganguly NK, Agarwal SP (2006) Indian J Med Res 123: 553–560

Hassler D, Zoller L, Haude M, Hufnagel HD, Sonntag HG (1992) Lyme-Borreliose in einem europäischen Endemiegebiet: Antikörperprävalenz und klinisches Spektrum. Dtsch Med Wochenschr 117: 767–774

Hofmann J, Meisel H, Klempa B, Vesenbeck SM, Beck R, Michel D, et al. (2008) Hantavirus outbreak, Germany 2007. Emerg Infect Dis 14: 850–852

Jones KE, Patel NG, Levy MA, Storeygard A, Balk D, Gittleman JL, Daszak P (2008) Global trends in emerging infectious diseases. Nature 451: 990–993

Kamar N, Selves J, Mansuy JM, et al. (2008) Hepatitis E virus and chronic hepatitis in organ-transplant recipients. N Engl J Med 358: 811–817

Klevens RM, Jonathan JR. Edwards JR, Richards CL et al. (2007) Estimating Health Care-Associated Infections and Deaths in U.S. Hospitals, 2002. Public Health Report 122: 160–166

Lam SK, Chua KB (2002) Nipah virus encephalitis outbreak in Malaysia. Clin Infect Dis 34 (Suppl 2): S48–51

Lindgren E, Jaenson TGT (2006) Lyme borreliosis in Europe: influences of climate and climate change, epidemiology, ecology and adaptation measures. WHO Regional Office for Europe, Copenhagen

Materna J, Daniel M, Danielova V (2005) Altitudinal distribution limit of the tick Ixodes ricinus shifted considerably towards higher altitudes in central Europe: results of three years monitoring in the Krkonose Mts. (Czech Republic). Cent Eur J Public Health 13 (1): 24–28

Mégraud F (1993) Epidemiology of Helicobacter pylori infection. Gastroenterol Clin North Am 22: 73–88

Mostashari F, Bunning ML, Kitsutani PT, Singer A (2001) Epidemic West Nile encephalitis, New York, 1999: results of a household-based seroepidemiological survey. Lancet 358: 261–264

Nash D, Mostashari F, Fine A, et al. (2001) Outbreak of West Nile virus infection, New York City area, 1999. N Engl J Med 14: 1858–1859

Organisation Mondiale de la Santé Animale (OIE) (2008). http://www.oie.int/eng/info/en_esbincidence.htm

Parola P, de Lamballerie X, Jourdan J, Rovery C, Vaillant V, Minodier P, Brouqui P, Flahault A, Raoult D, Charrel RN (2006) Novel chikungunya virus variant in travelers returning from Indian Ocean islands. Emerg Infect Dis 12: 1493–1499

Reyes GR, Purdy MA, Kim JP, Luk KC, Young LM, Fry KE, Bradley DW (1990) Isolation of a cDNA from the virus responsible for enterically transmitted non-A, non-B hepatitis. Science 247: 1335

Rezza G, Nicoletti L, Angelini R, Romi R, Finarelli AC, Panning M et al. (2007) Infection with Chikungunya virus in Italy: an outbreak in a temperate region. Lancet 370 (9602): 1840–1846

Robert Koch Institute (2001a). Waldarbeiter-Studie Berlin-Brandenburg 2000 zu zeckenübertragenen und andere Zoonosen. Epidem Bulletin 16: 109–110

Robert Koch Institute (2001b). Risikofaktoren für Lyme-Borreliose: Ergebnisse einer Studie in einem Brandenburger Landkreis. Epidem Bulletin 21: 147–149

Robert Koch Institute (2008a) Norovirus-Winterepidemie 2007/2008 übertrifft die Infektionszahlen der Vorjahre. Epidem Bulletin 6: 44–49

Robert Koch Institute (2008b) Zahl der Hantavirus-Erkrankungen erreichte 2007 in Deutschland einen neuen Höchststand. Epidem Bull 19: 147–152

Rothenbacher D, Bode G, Berg G et al. (1989) Prevalence and determinants of Helicobacter pylori infection in preschool children: a population-based study from Germany. Int J Epidemiol 27: 135–141

Schmaljohn C, Hjelle B (1997) Hantaviruses: a global disease problem. Emerg Inf Dis 3(2): 95–104

Shrestha MP, Scott RM, Joshi DM et al. (2007) Safety and efficacy of a recombinant hepatitis E vaccine. N Engl J Med 356: 895

Spach DH, Liles WC, Campbell GL, Quick RE, Anderson DE Jr, Fritsche TR. (1993) Tick-borne diseases in the United States. N Engl J Med 329:936–947

The National Creutzfeld-Jakob Disease Surveillance Unit (NCJDSU) (2008). http://www.cjd.ed.ac.uk//

Towner JS, Pourrut X, Albariño CG et al. (2007) Marburg virus infection detected in a common African bat. PLoS ONE 2: e764

Vandenesch F, Naimi T, Enright M, Lina G, Nimmo G, Heffernan H, Liassine N, Bes M, Greenland T, Reverdy M, Etienne J (2003). Community-acquired methicillin-resistant Staphylococcus aureus carrying Panton-Valentine leukocidin genes: worldwide emergence. Emerg Infect Dis 9: 978–984

Verhoef L, Boxman I, Duizer E, Rutjes SA, Vennema H, Friesema IHM et al. (2008) Multiple exposures during a norovirus outbreak on a river-cruise sailing through Europe, 2006. Eurosurveillance 13(4–6): 1–6

Warny M, Pepin J, Fang A, Killgore G, Thompson A, Brazier J, Frost E, McDonald LC (2005) Toxin production by an emerging strain of *Clostridium difficile* associated with outbreaks of severe disease in North America and Europe. Lancet 366: 1079–1084

Weiland T, Kuhnl P, Laufs R, Heesemann J (1992) Prevalence of Borrelia burgdorferi antibodies in Hamburg blood donors. Beitr Infusionsther 30: 92–95

Who (2008) Variant Creutzfeld-Jakob disease. http://www.who.int/mediacentre/factsheets/fs180/en/

WHO (2004a) Nipah virus outbreaks in Bangladesh. January-April 2004. Wkly Epidemiol Rec 23: 168–171

WHO (2004b) Severe Acute Respiratory Syndrome (SARS). Htttp://www.who.int/csr/sars/en

WHO (2005) Revision of the International Health regulations. www.who.int/csr/ihr

Wisplinghoff H, Bischoff T, Tallent SM, et al. (2004) Nosocomial bloodstream infections in US hospitals: analysis of 24 179 cases from a prospective nationwide surveillance study, Clin Infect Dis 39: pp. 309–317

Wit de M, Widdowson M, Vennema H, de Bruin E, Fernandes T, Koopmans M (2003) Large outbreak of norovirus: The baker who should have known better. J Infect 55(2): 188–193

Wongsichranalai C, Pickard AL, Wernsdorfer WH, Meshnick SR (2002) Epidemiology of drug-resistant malaria. Lancet Inf Dis 2: 209–218

Yob JM, Field H, Rashdi AM, Morrissy C, van der Heide B, Rota P, et al. (2001) Nipah virus infection in bats (order Chiroptera) in peninsular Malaysia. Emerg Infect Dis 7: 439–441

Chapter 4
Infectious Disease Control Policies and the Role of Governmental and Intergovernmental Organisations

Gérard Krause

Today, in an interdependent world, bacteria and viruses travel almost as fast as e-mail and financial flows. Gro Harlem Brundtland, Former Director General of the WHO (Brundtland 2003).

4.1 Introduction

Public health is generally regarded as the typical domain of national if not local governments, which takes into account local necessities arising from the epidemiologic situation, the health-care system and the government structures. Therefore in theory, public health policy is in the sovereignty of countries. However, the spread of infectious diseases has never been restricted to national borders; thus the principle of national sovereignty is largely theoretical. This is especially true in a world with unprecedented international mobility of goods and persons. Moreover, particularly public health actions in the field of infectious diseases within one country may well affect public health issues in other countries. One of the best recent examples is the Chinese management of the initial phase of the SARS epidemic, which was characterised by failing surveillance structures, insufficient control measures and restricted public information policy. Abba Ebban has described it as a paradox that in order for countries to effectively execute their public health sovereignty, they would consequently have to give up some of their sovereignty to intergovernmental organisations (Ebban 1995).

This chapter discusses the basic principles of public health sovereignty and what they mean in the context of the new International Health Regulations (IHR). This leads to a description of three very different organisations: The World Health Organisation, the US Centers for Disease Control and Prevention and the European

G. Krause (✉)
Department for Infectious Diseases Epidemiology, Robert Koch Institute, Nordufer 20, 13353 Berlin, Germany
e-mail: krauseg@rki.de

A. Krämer et al. (eds.), *Modern Infectious Disease Epidemiology*, Statistics for Biology and Health, DOI 10.1007/978-0-387-93835-6_4,

Centre for Disease Prevention and Control. The examples indicate that national governments have already ceded their sovereignty in public health policy to a considerable extent to intergovernmental organisations.

4.2 The International Health Regulations

The most prominent and recent process in which public health sovereignty has been ceded from countries to an international body is the adoption of the new International Health Regulations (IHR) by the 58th World Health Assembly (WHA) in May 2005, which entered into force in June 2007 (WHO 2005). The purpose of the IHR is to "prevent, protect against, control and provide a public health response to international spread of disease in ways . . . which avoid unnecessary interference with international traffic and trade" (WHO 2005). Compared to the previous IHR which were in place from 1969 to 2007, these new IHR have an expanded scope not only concerning the diseases and health hazards to be covered but also concerning the mandate of the World Health Organisation (WHO).

For various reasons, the old IHR did not motivate member states to inform the WHO about possible health threats of international concern: firstly, the scope of diseases covered by reporting regulation in the old IHR was limited to a few diseases such as cholera, plague and yellow fever. Secondly, there was virtually no standardization on how to define such threats and how to report them to the WHO, and there were hardly any internationally defined standards to assure that such threats come to the attention of national governments in the first place. Thirdly, a member state could expect little benefit for reporting a critical event. And fourthly, member states reporting such events ran the risk of suffering exaggerated control measures from other countries which might have additional adverse effects on the economy of the affected country or on the liberty and integrity of people travelling from or to such countries. The IHR 2005 aim to address these issues by radically expanding their scope not only to potentially any infectious disease but also to chemical and physical health hazards. In addition, IHR 2005 have a number of provisions to prevent other countries from taking exaggerated control precautions that could lead to the unjustified disadvantage of the reporting country or of free trade and travel in general.

In the literature, most attention is directed towards the fact that the IHR 2005 no longer limit themselves to infectious diseases and to the fact that a decision algorithm defines the notifiable entity of a public health emergency of international concern. The first may have strong organisational implications at the national level. The second is a tribute to the necessity of being able to detect unexpected threats such as SARS. Both issues however are more technical in nature and do not fundamentally touch the principle of member state sovereignty over national health policy issues (Fig. 4.1)

By ratifying the IHR 2005, member states have in fact ceded a considerable part of their respective sovereignty in national public health policy to the international

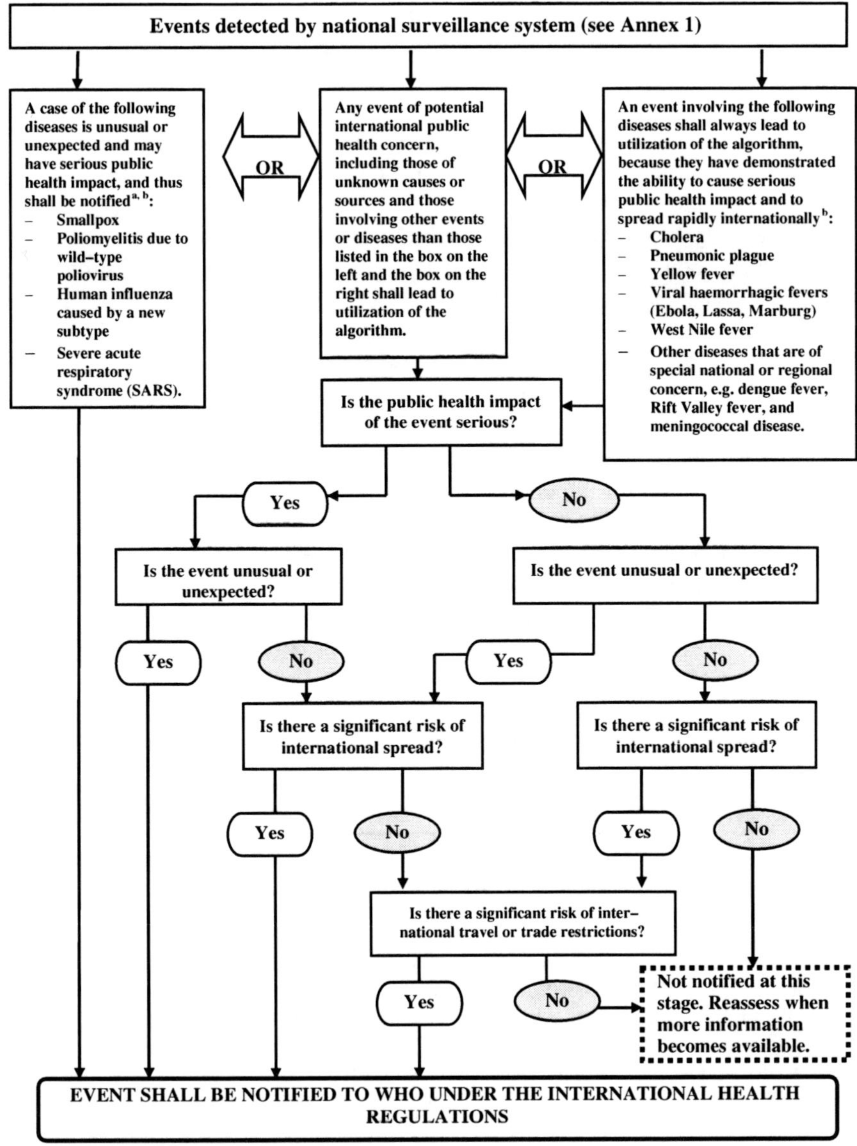

Fig. 4.1 Annex 2 of the International Health Regulations (http://www.who.int/csr/ihr/IHR_2005_en.pdf)

community. For this reason, Fidler has described this process as the step towards post-Westphalian public health (Fidler 2003), because the peace of Westphalia in 1648 after the Thirty Years' War had established an international political structure in which states gave up the full sovereignty of their territories to a systematic and binding supreme authority. Post-Westphalian public health, therefore, refers to the fact that international public health policy is no longer dominated by individual states' policies but rather that supranational structures and institutions do interfere in national health policy (Krause 2009). The following three examples will exemplify how aspects of the IHR 2005 may have considerable impact on national and international public health policy.

Core capacity requirements of the International Health Regulations: Annex 1 of the IHR 2005 defines a minimal set of core capacities which not only national but also intermediate and local public health services must provide in order to assure effective surveillance. It may be argued that member states of the World Health Assembly who have ratified the IHR would also naturally have the mandate to assure the implementation of these minimal standards. However, for federal governments whereby certain public health responsibilities and mandates are in the hands of local rather than national governments, this may not be the case. This so-called federalism dilemma is of significant importance as countries with federal governments make up about 40% of the world's population (Wilson et al. 2006). Wilson et al. have expressed concern that even if federal governments do have constitutional authorities to override jurisdiction of regional governments, in order to implement Annex 1, they may choose not to do so because of political reasons. The latter is of course true for any country (especially large ones) and not only for federations (Wilson et al. 2006) (Table 4.1).

Table 4.1 Annex 1 of the International Health Regulations (http://www.who.int/csr/ihr/IHR_2005_en.pdf)

Core capacity requirements for surveillance and response
1. States Parties shall utilise existing national structures and resources to meet their core capacity requirements under these Regulations, including with regard to
(a) their surveillance, reporting, notification, verification, response and collaboration activities and
(b) their activities concerning designated airports, ports and ground crossings.
2. Each State Party shall assess, within 2 years following the entry into force of these Regulations for that State Party, the ability of existing national structures and resources to meet the minimum requirements described in this Annex. As a result of such assessment, States Parties shall develop and implement plans of action to ensure that these core capacities are present and functioning throughout their territories as set out in paragraph 1 of Article 5 and paragraph 1 of Article 13.
3. States Parties and the WHO shall support assessments, planning and implementation processes under this Annex.
4. At the local community level and/or primary public health response level
The capacities
(a) to detect events involving disease or death above expected levels for the particular time and place in all areas within the territory of the State Party and

Table 4.1 (continued)

Core capacity requirements for surveillance and response
(b) to report all available essential information immediately to the appropriate level of health-care response. At the community level, reporting shall be to local community health-care institutions or the appropriate health personnel. At the primary public health response level, reporting shall be to the intermediate or national response level, depending on organisational structures. For the purposes of this Annex, essential information includes the following: clinical descriptions, laboratory results, sources and type of risk, number of human cases and deaths, conditions affecting the spread of the disease and the health measures employed and
(c) to implement preliminary control measures immediately.
5. At the intermediate public health response levels
The capacities
(a) to confirm the status of reported events and to support or implement additional control measures and
(b) to assess reported events immediately and, if found urgent, to report all essential information to the national level. For the purposes of this Annex, the criteria for urgent events include serious public health impact and/or unusual or unexpected nature with high potential for spread.
6. At the national level
Assessment and notification. The capacities
(a) to assess all reports of urgent events within 48 hours and
(b) to notify the WHO immediately through the National IHR Focal Point when the assessment indicates the event is notifiable pursuant to paragraph 1 of Article 6 and Annex 2 and to inform the WHO as required pursuant to Article 7 and paragraph 2 of Article 9.
Public health response. The capacities
(a) to rapidly determine the control measures required to prevent domestic and international spread;
(b) to provide support through specialised staff, laboratory analysis of samples (domestically or through collaborating centres) and logistical assistance (e.g. equipment, supplies and transport);
(c) to provide on-site assistance as required to supplement local investigations;
(d) to provide a direct operational link with senior health and other officials to rapidly approve and implement containment and control measures;
(e) to provide direct liaison with other relevant government ministries;
(f) to provide, by the most efficient means of communication available, links with hospitals, clinics, airports, ports, ground crossings, laboratories and other key operational areas for the dissemination of information and recommendations received from the WHO regarding events in the State Party's own territory and in the territories of other States Parties;
(g) to establish, operate and maintain a national public health emergency response plan, including the creation of multidisciplinary/multisectoral teams to respond to events that may constitute a public health emergency of international concern and
(h) to provide the foregoing on a 24-hour basis.

Many federal governments may already have local public health services in place strong enough to comply with the required core capacities. However, a great number of countries with notoriously poor public health infrastructure may simply not have the economic resources to implement and assure the provision of core capacities – regardless of how much political mandate the national government has over the local public health structure (Calain 2007). The IHR 2005 require the full compliance of the described public health infrastructure by June 2016 at the latest. While the rich countries with a strong infrastructure of private health services may in some ways compensate for deficiencies in public health infrastructure, those countries where this is not the case are most likely to be least capable of complying with the IHR requirements.

Particularly the Annex 1 of the IHR may thus be almost as utopian in nature as the WHO slogan "Health for all by the year 2000". In addition to the frustration of international milestones not being met by many countries, which would be most in need of reaching them, these IHR standards may additionally result in adverse effects. Setting up a system capable of complying with the core capacity requirements for surveillance and response in a country with non-existent or poor communication and transportation infrastructure may prove to be extremely costly. Furthermore, the realisation of these core capacities may divert already scarce funds away from essential public health services such as health education, vaccination and other primary health-care functions. On the other hand, it might be argued that these countries would continue to have insufficient public health services anyway regardless of whether Annex 1 of IHR existed or not. In this sense the IHR are also establishing a system capable of identifying the needs for assistance to member states in case of public health emergencies of international importance. By initiating and coordinating assistance, the WHO could prevent such events from spreading within the country and to others with equally limited resources to control them.

Impact of IHR on national public health surveillance and response infrastructure: In Article 9, the IHR now also give the WHO more flexibility in the use of medical intelligence in order to become fully aware of potential outbreaks before national governments choose to report these officially and voluntarily. In practice, the WHO had done so before the revision of the IHR. The Global Outbreak Alert and Response Network (GOARN) , which has been functioning since 1997, has collected information on outbreaks worldwide using unofficial sources such as media reports also (Tucker 2005). However, the difference now is that the IHR 2005 authorise the WHO to request verification from a State Party with reference to such information. Under certain circumstances this may exert considerable pressure upon the national surveillance and response infrastructure.

Impact of IHR on travel restrictions: Another important aspect of international public health policy concerns the measures taken by member states to control or prevent an outbreak. On the one hand, WHO recommendations might be perceived as too stringent and costly by member states and thus impossible to comply with. On the other hand, too "liberal" recommendations might be perceived by some states as insufficient, and these states might insist on additional measures. Since the IHR are also meant to accomplish best possible health protection while at the same time assuring least possible travel and trade restriction; very restrictive public health measures in one country may well have negative effects on people in other countries. For example, during the cholera outbreak in Zimbabwe in December (2008) the issue came up whether or not requirements for cholera vaccination at border crossing may expose more people to the risk of adverse vaccine effects which may outweigh the expected protective effect. The WHO recommended not to limit border crossing and also not to request cholera immunisations (WHO 2008). The IHR 2005 contain a clause that allows states to implement health measures other than those recommended by the WHO if they achieve the same or greater level of health protection and if they are neither more restrictive to international traffic nor more intrusive to persons (WHO 2005).

Core capacity requirements of the International Health Regulations, the authority of the WHO to request verifications on unofficial information and finally the influence of WHO recommendations are only examples to illustrate how the IHR have already taken away a substantial part of national sovereignty over public health policy. To what extent international public health policy is determined by national public health policy and vice versa also depends largely on the actors in this field. Three organisations, internationally active in infectious disease control, are portrayed briefly in order to illustrate their differences and also to display their interdependence.

4.3 The World Health Organisation

The WHO was founded in 1948 as a specialised agency of the United Nations. It has the mandate to direct and coordinate international health work (Aginam 2006). The World Health Assembly (WHA) is made up of representatives of over 190 member states and directs the policies of the WHO. The WHA can issue treaties and international regulations which may interfere directly with national, regional and even local public health policies. As discussed above, the WHA still functions very much in a Westphalian style of international governance, demonstrated by the fact that only representatives of member states can become members. However, the new IHR give the WHO the option of making use of informal, non-governmental information sources and thereby exerting considerable pressure upon member states to react to situations that may be of international public health importance.

Furthermore, the WHO Eleventh General Programme of Work entitled "Engaging for Health" also illustrates the role of the WHO in international public health policy. The Programme of Work covers the 10-year period from 2006 to 2015 and contains the following core functions:

- Providing leadership on matters critical to health and engaging in partnerships where joint action is needed;
- Shaping the research agenda and stimulating the generation, translation and dissemination of valuable knowledge;
- Setting norms as well as promoting and monitoring their implementation;
- Articulating ethical and evidence-based policy options;
- Providing technical support, catalysing change and building sustainable institutional capacity and
- Monitoring the health situation and assessing health trends.

Each of these functions has considerable impact on a country's public health policy. Particularly countries with a small or weak national public health infrastructure may on the one hand welcome such policy directions from the WHO, thus preventing them from having to reinvent the wheel. On the other hand, countries with an elaborate and detailed public health policy may feel pressured that public health policy coming from international organisations such as the WHO will stand in competition with their national concepts and might not be as well adapted to their national needs.

4.4 The Centers for Disease Control and Prevention, USA

The Centers for Disease Control and Prevention in Atlanta, USA, is primarily a national public health institute of the federal government. Many nations have similar national centres that use the acronym "CDC". This chapter therefore refers to the Atlanta-based CDC as the US-CDC. Like no other national public health institutions, the US-CDC is extremely productive in international public health activities. This is in full accordance with the organisation's mission which aims to promote health and quality of life by preventing and controlling disease, injury and disability by working with partners throughout the nation and the world ((CDC 2006). This mission leads to bilateral programmes that might only remotely affect public health issues within the United States. One of the numerous examples is the US-CDC Global Health Programme, which even includes projects with a very local focus such as a programme on intravenous drug users in Orel Oblast, Russia (Greenberg et al. 2005). It maintains various local offices mainly in Africa and Asia through which international public health programmes and research projects are coordinated. These bilateral projects are part of the global US-CDC strategy, which may contribute to public health in the United States by providing early and first hand information on emerging health threats and by establishing lines of communication and platforms for cooperations to facilitate US-CDC contribution to national control measures abroad. This is complemented by many other US-CDC activities that are not part of a global programme but may contribute perhaps even more strongly and permanently towards global public health policy. Often the US-CDC has a scientific leadership position in the field of infectious disease epidemiology and medical public health sciences in general. By hosting internationally renowned laboratory capacity, developing widespread surveillance standards such as the National Healthcare Safety Network (NHSN) and by playing an active role in the setting of research agendas, this federal government institution (which has hardly any regulatory or executive power to regulate the public health within the 50 states of its country) is in fact extremely influential not only within the United States but also in international public health policy.

The US-CDC's influence on international public health is a result of not only technical supremacy in multiple public health-related sciences but also an explicit national strategy documented in the Global Pathogen Surveillance Act. This bill of the US Congress links financial incentives of developing countries to participate in WHO surveillance networks with a privileged access and allows US-CDC participation in the investigation of outbreaks with access to surveillance data (Calain 2007). Of course this strategic interest is not unique to the US-CDC, but the effectiveness with which it pursues its goal is unequalled by any other national public health institute.

4.5 The European Centre for Disease Prevention and Control (ECDC)

Although public health is generally regarded as one area in which the sovereignty of European Union (EU) member states has not yet been ceded to bodies of the EU, the line has already been crossed in various ways. The European Commission is able to influence national public health policy of the member states and even more so of those countries that aim to become members of the EU. Since the 1960s, numerous EU regulations in the field of consumer protection, work safety and others have interfered directly or indirectly with public health policy at the national level (Schluter 1996). Regulations on tobacco prevention, for example, although primarily enacted in the framework of consumer protection in lieu of public health, do of course have public health implications. It is of note that this is an example of where health policy in one country does not actually concern other countries very much, compared to infectious diseases.

But even in the specific area of infectious disease control, EU member states have to comply with mandatory standards, which do affect national public health policies: Under decision 2119 of 1998 of the European Parliament (European Commission Communicable Disease Network Committee 1998), for example, member states may have to change their national system of infectious disease surveillance in order to comply with EU obligations of infectious disease reporting (Ammon and Faensen 2009). The European Centre for Disease Prevention and Control (ECDC) founded in May 2008 is likely to play an increasingly important role in international public health policy. However, for the time being the mandate of the ECDC is quite limited. As stated in its founding regulations of 2004, the mission of the ECDC is to identify, assess and communicate current and emerging threats to human health from communicable diseases (ECDC 2004). Similar to the US-CDC, the ECDC has neither executive nor regulatory power, but in strong contrast to the US-CDC, the ECDC is not designed to be the central provider of all competencies itself but instead aims to support, coordinate and build upon the existing competencies of Europe's national disease control agencies (ECDC 2004).

There is criticism that with this limited mission and subsequently limited budget and size, the ECDC will never be able to come near the role of an international reference body for disease control and thus to be influential in international public health policy (Grundmann and Goossens 2005). While it may be disputed whether the latter is a legitimate goal by itself, the question does remain to what extent the ECDC will be able to channel, harness and coordinate the existing expertise in the established national institutions of its EU member states. It is noteworthy that for laboratory expertise, the ECDC plans to rely on a network of high-level and reputed laboratories in the European member states, instead of building laboratory expertise in itself anytime soon. It remains to be seen whether this approach will detach laboratory science from epidemiology, as feared by some (Wigzell 2005). In contrast, several Asian countries plan to build a central Asian CDC with extensive laboratory capacities, following the model of the US-CDC (Tibayrenc 2005).

In certain fields, for example, in pandemic preparedness, it can be noted that the ECDC has been instrumental in facilitating a process of technical harmonisation in important areas of public health policy without formally interfering with national sovereignty (Haas and Straetemans 2009; Mounier-Jack and Coker 2006). Likewise, the ECDC has provided crucial support to member states in coordinating expertise from different countries in Europe, for example, in the risk assessment of the chikungunya outbreak in northern Italy in 2007, a viral disease mainly known as an arthropod-transmitted disease occurring in the tropics. By doing so the ECDC has not only helped Italy in controlling the outbreak but also facilitated risk assessment and preparedness decisions in other member states without interfering with their sovereignty (Depoortere and Coulombier 2006). However, the ECDC is also working in areas which might very well influence health policy in EU member states. Several networks and projects hosted at, or issued by, the ECDC deal with tremendous variety of immunisation schedules in the EU member states (Venice project 2007). The ECDC is generating guidance with respect to the use of new vaccines, such as, for example, vaccines against human papillomavirus infections (ECDC 2008). Although such guidance does not have the character of a recommendation, it is intended to support and thus likely to influence national policy decisions with respect to childhood immunisation schedules.

This description indicates that the mandate of the ECDC does not differ much from that of WHO–EURO, except for the fact that the first is focused on EU member states (currently 27), and for the time being it is focusing on infectious diseases, while the second covers the whole WHO–EURO region and all issues of public health. As early as 1995, Fiona Godlee, assistant editor of the *British Medical Journal*, warned that increasing activity of the European Union in the field of public health would be bound to create conflicts and duplications with the European Regional WHO Office (WHO–EURO) (Schluter 1996). In view of the Select Committee on Intergovernmental Organisations of the House of Lords, the founding of the ECDC in 2005 has made this risk more than obvious (Select Committee on Intergovernmental Organisations 2008). Zsusanna Jakab, director of the ECDC, however, sees more similarities between the constituencies and mandate of the ECDC and the US-CDC than between those of the ECDC and the WHO–EURO (Select Committee on Intergovernmental Organisations (2008). In practical terms, it seems that with the existence of the ECDC, WHO–EURO can concentrate more on those parts of its region that do not belong to the EU (Danzon 2004). In fact, WHO–EURO benefits from the ECDC as a competent partner that even includes data from non-EU countries in surveillance networks for TB and HIV.

In a way, it seems that both WHO–EURO and the ECDC can coexist quite well in mutual partnership and may in fact be able to address specific surveillance issues for the countries they primarily work with (Danzon 2004). It remains to be seen to what extent the mandate and capacity of the ECDC will gradually be expanded and how this might affect the ECDC's impact as a global player towards international public health policy.

4.6 Other International Players

The WHO, the US-CDC and the ECDC are of course only three of the many international players in the field of international public health policy. In fact, the World Trade Organisation, due to its regulatory power over the trade of goods, has tremendous impact on infectious disease control policies (Taylor 2002). There are a number of other United Nations Organisations with considerable legally binding power that have significant impact on national public health policy such as the Food and Agriculture Organisation, the World Organisation for Animal Health, the United Nations International Children's Emergency Fund or the United Nations Population Fund (Lazcano-Ponce et al. 2005). In addition to that, in the last few decades, the World Bank has increasingly taken health issues into its agenda, and due to its large funding capacity it is in a very prominent position to have a major impact on national health policies. Besides those international organisations of the United Nations, there are also other international bodies such as the European Commission which have a declared mandate to coordinate public health activities, if requested by the member states (Schreck et al. 2009). It is nearly impossible to oversee the interaction of all organisations involved in international health and Mbwe referred to this as the institutional labyrinth of international health (see Fig. 4.2) (Select Committee on Intergovernmental Organisations 2008).

Private foundations such as the Rockefeller Foundation, the Melinda and Bill Gates Foundation have budgets way beyond those of WHO's disease-specific programmes and have become driving forces, setting comprehensive international public health agendasWalt 1998 Moreover, non-governmental, non-profit organisations have focused agendas on health policy which may be highly influential even if they do not have large budgets: The International Society for Infectious Diseases, the International Union Against Tuberculosis, the International Union Against Venereal Diseases, Médecins Sans Frontiers, the Red Cross to name only a few of the numerous organisations with a significant role in international health policy (Taylor 2002). In addition to those mentioned above, one cannot overlook the pharmaceutical industry and other for-profit organisations as having a substantial influence on international health policy (Taylor 2002).

All these organisations may in fact have much greater impact – for better or for worse – on international and national public health policies than do governmental or intergovernmental organisations because of their very nature of being independent from government influence (Ronald 1997).

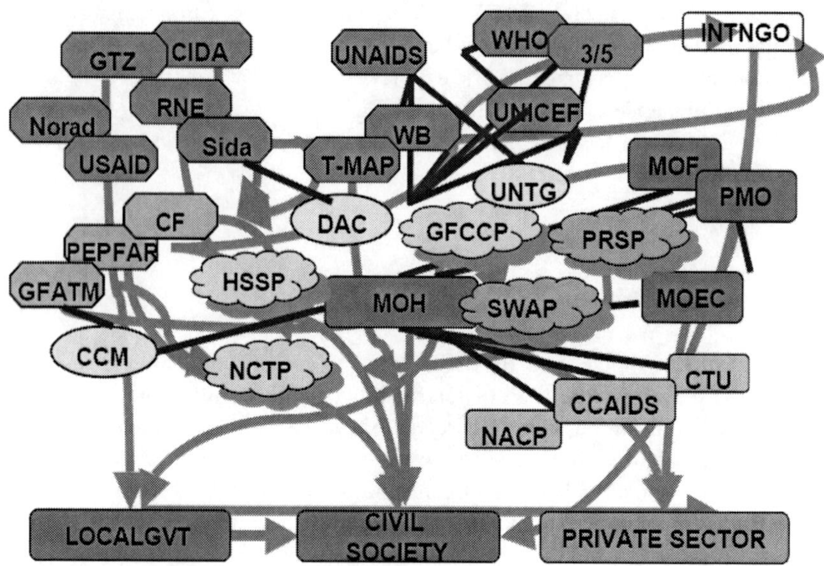

Fig. 4.2 Institutional labyrinth, Mbewe, WHO from Select Committee on Intergovernmental Organisations 2008

4.7 Conclusion

Multiple organisations play a role in shaping national public health policy. Such influence may certainly be beneficial when the vision of the institution that exerts its influence is concordant with the interests of the country accepting such influence. However, this need not necessarily be the case. Calain, for example, described in considerable detail how global surveillance initiatives have been heavily propagated in developing countries leading to undue distraction of attention and resources from highly prevalent diseases and to significant stress to already fragile health systems (Calain 2007).

International public health requires global health governance by a politically accountable institution. The WHO is not the sole organisation legitimised to fill this role. It is important, however, that the WHO regains and defends its leadership in setting the international public health agenda based on the interests of people of all member states, regardless of how influential individual governments and other organisations may be within and outside the WHA. For this purpose, the WHO should facilitate implementation of the IHR in member states. But perhaps more important than the formal mandate of the WHO received through IHR will be its capacity to expand its scientific authority and to stay clear of conflicts of interests. Similar expectations can be formulated for the ECDC, which in terms of mandate and capacity may become a hybrid between a sub-regional WHO office and a federal public health agency like the US-CDC. It will be interesting to follow how the increasing involvement of national and intergovernmental organisations in international public health policies might affect the scope and quality of infectious disease control in the future.

References

Aginam O (2006) Globalization of health insecurity: the World Health Organization and the new International Health Regulations. Med Law 25(4):663–672

Ammon A, Faensen D (2009) Surveillance von Infektionskrankheiten auf Europäischer Ebene. Bundesgesundheitsbl - Gesundheitsforsch - Gesundheitsschutz 52(2):176–82

Brundtland GH (2003) Global health and international security. Global Governance 9:417–23

Calain P (2007) Exploring the international arena of global public health surveillance. Health Policy Plan 22(1):2–12

Calain P (2007) From the field side of the binoculars: a different view on global public health surveillance. Health Policy Plan 22(1):13–20

CDC (2006) CDC Mission – To promote health and quality of life by preventing and controlling disease, injury, and disability. Available from: URL: http://www.cdc.gov/about/ organization/mission.html

Danzon M (2004) ECDC and WHO: a common mission for better health in Europe. Euro Surveill 9(12):2

Depoortere E, Coulombier D (2006). On behalf of the ECDE Chikungunya risk assessment group (Boutin J-P, Brooker S, De Valk H, Dieckmann S, et al.). Chikungunya risk assessment for Europe: recommendations for action. Eurosurveill Wkly; 11(19)

Ebban A (1995) The U.N. idea revisited. Foreign Aff 74(5):39–55

European centre for disease prevention and control (ECDC) (2008) Guidance for the introduction of HPV vaccines in EU countries

European centre for disease prevention and control (ECDC) (2004) Regulation (EC) No 851/2004 of the European Parliament and of the Council of 21 April 2004, 851/2004

European Commission Communicable Disease Network Committee (1998) Decision No 2119/98/EC of the European Parliament and of the Council

Fidler DP (2003) SARS: political pathology of the first post-Westphalian pathogen. J Law Med Ethics 31(4):485–505

Greenberg AE, Tappero J, Choopanya K, van GF, Martin M, Vanichseni S, et al. (2005) CDC international HIV prevention research activities among injection drug users in Thailand and Russia. J Urban Health 82(3 Suppl 4):iv24–iv33

Grundmann H, Goossens H (2005) Report of working group 1: public health challenges. Clin Microbiol Infect 11(Suppl 1):36–40

Haas W, Straetemans M (2009) Wie groß sind die Differenzen zwischen den europäischen Pandemieplänen, sind sie relevant und woher stammen sie? Bundesgesundheitsbl – Gesundheitsforsch – Gesundheitsschutz 52(2)(in print)

Krause G (2009) Infektionsschutz Europäisch - von staatlicher Sourveränität zu internationaler Vernetzung. Bundesgesundheitsbl - Gesundheitsforsch - Gesundheitsschutz 52(2):147–8

Lazcano-Ponce E, Allen B, Gonzalez CC (2005) The contribution of international agencies to the control of communicable diseases. Arch Med Res 36(6):731–738

Mounier-Jack S, Coker R (2006) Pandemic influenza: are Europe's institutions prepared? Eur J Public Health 16(2):119–120

Ronald A (1997) The role of international agencies in emerging infections. Ann Acad Med Singapore 26(5):616–619

Schluter P (1996) Legal requirements for health protection from the European viewpoint–uniform regulations or reciprocal recognition of public health norms? Zentralbl Hyg Umweltmed 199(2–4):105–18

Schreck S,, Strauss R., Lücking G, Krause G (2009) EU-Strukturen zur Überwachung und Bekämpfung von Infektionskrankheiten. Wer sie macht, wie sie entstehen und wie sie funktionieren?. Bundesgesundheitsbl - Gesundheitsforsch - Gesundheitsschutz 52(2):149–56

Select Committee on Intergovernmental Organisations (2008) Diseases Know No Frontiers: How effective are Intergovernmental Organisations in controlling their spread? Authority of the House of Lords

Taylor AL (2002) Global governance, international health law and WHO: looking towards the future. Bull World Health Organ 80(12):975–80

Tibayrenc M (2005) A hard lesson for Europeans: the ASEAN CDC. Trends Microbiol 13(6): 266–268

Tucker JB (2005) Updating the international health regulations. Biosecur Bioterror 3(4):338–347

Venice Project Work Package no. 3 (2007) Report on First survey of Immunisation Programs in Europe

Walt G (1998) Globalisation of international health. Lancet 351(9100):434–437

Wigzell H (2005) A European CDC? Science 307 (5716):1691

Wilson K , McDougall C, Upshur R (2006) The new International Health Regulations and the federalism dilemma. PLoS Med 3(1):e1

WHO (2008) Cholera in Zimbabwe. Disease outbreak News 2008 December. Available from: URL: http://www.who.int/csr/don/2008_12_02/en/index.html

WHO (2005) Revision of the International Health Regulations (WHA 58.3)

Part II
General Concepts and Methods

Chapter 5
Principles of Infectious Disease Epidemiology

Alexander Krämer, Manas Akmatov, and Mirjam Kretzschmar

In this chapter, principles and concepts of modern infectious disease epidemiology are presented. We delineate the role of epidemiology for public health and discuss the characteristics of infectious disease epidemiology. This chapter also includes definitions of important terms used in infectious disease epidemiology.

5.1 Definition and Aims of Epidemiology

Giving a universally valid definition of epidemiology is difficult. Epidemiology is not a science with a clearly defined field of application in contrast to anatomy or gastroenterology, which target specific parts or aspects of the human body. Rather it is a scientific method which can be applied to a broad range of health and medical problems, from infectious diseases to health care. Epidemiology is a constantly changing field of science, because new questions arise in population health and new statistical techniques are developed and adapted from other sciences. In times of modern information technologies and high-speed computers, new opportunities arise for data collection and storage on a large scale and for application of advanced bio-informatic and modelling techniques. In the era of globalization, many health problems are relevant on a global scale and intervention strategies have to be developed on an international level. In particular, for infectious disease epidemiology, global spread is increasingly important as demonstrated by the spread of the human immunodeficiency virus (HIV) and the pandemic spread of influenza A.

Definition: Epidemiology

The word "Epidemiology" is derived from Greek words meaning *study upon populations* (epi-upon, demos-people, logos-study).

A broader definition of epidemiology from *A Dictionary of Epidemiology* has been widely accepted. According to this definition, epidemiology is *the study*

A. Krämer (✉)
Department of Public Health Medicine, School of Public Health, University of Bielefeld, Bielefeld, Germany
e-mail: alexander.kraemer@uni-bielefeld.de

A. Krämer et al. (eds.), *Modern Infectious Disease Epidemiology*,
Statistics for Biology and Health, DOI 10.1007/978-0-387-93835-6_5,

of the distribution and determinants of health-related states or events in specified populations, and the application of this study to control of health problems (Last 2001).

The crucial point is that epidemiology concerns itself with populations or groups of population in contrast to clinical medicine, which deals with individuals (patients). Therefore, epidemiology describes health and disease in terms of frequencies and distributions of determinants and conditions in a population or in a specific group of a population. Epidemiology also includes the study of associations between specific diseases and factors to which populations are exposed. In this way, risk factors or protective factors which are associated with a health status of an individual or with some conditions can be identified. These associations can be identified because risk factors and diseases are not randomly distributed in populations but rather there are population groups where some diseases and associated factors occur more often than in other population groups. Commonly, risk factors are distributed by age and often also differ for men and women.

Based on the distribution of risk factors among different population groups, the concept of "vulnerable" population can be derived. This group is at higher risk for certain conditions because of the existence of a risk constellation favouring these conditions.

Epidemiological methods can be used to show statistical associations, but causal relationships have to be established by clinical and biological research. Epidemiological studies often aim at generating statistical evidence that identify factors, which play an important role in acquisition of infection and the development of a disease. Causality between these factors and the outcome might be more or less plausible or strong. Some criteria which demonstrate a possible causal relationship between identified factors and disease have been developed (causal criteria by Hill; Rothman and Greenland 2008). Based on epidemiological studies, specific hypotheses that tell us which potential factors may play a causal role in the development of certain diseases can be generated. Providing a final proof for the causality of these associations is a task of other sciences like clinical medicine or microbiology.

5.2 Epidemiology and Public Health

Epidemiology is the fundamental science of public health and provides the evidence on which public health professionals should base their decisions and strategies (Detels et al. 2002). In this way, epidemiology provides the tools for the control of diseases and health promotion. More specifically, some important tasks of epidemiology for public health are

- To elucidate the aetiology of a disease
- To describe the spectrum of a disease (what kind of symptoms occur and how frequently do they occur)

- To describe the natural history of a disease (what disease stages does a patient typically go through)
- To identify risk factors and protective factors (which factors enhance or prevent occurrence of a disease)
- To estimate disease burdens and health-care needs of a population
- To predict disease trends (to extrapolate from observations about time trends in risk factors and the future occurrence of the disease)
- To evaluate the effectiveness of interventions and public health programs

Spatial and temporal relations between the distribution of risk factors and the occurrence of disease can be established using surveillance methods and epidemiological studies. The information obtained in this way permits the identification of risk and protective factors and the analysis of time trends and spatial clustering of diseases. Knowledge of the spatial distribution and temporal trends of diseases is an important prerequisite for the effective application of preventive and interventive measures in order to reduce corresponding disease burdens. We want to illustrate the contributions of epidemiology to public health with the example of HIV/AIDS.

5.2.1 Example: Epidemiology and the HIV/AIDS Epidemic

A good example of the important role of epidemiology in collaboration with other relevant public health and medical disciplines is the research upon the AIDS epidemic. At the beginning of the 1980s, the syndrome of acquired immunodeficiency (AIDS) was for the first time described in the United States. It was observed in a group of homosexual men in California and New York who had opportunistic infections and specific tumours.

5.2.1.1 Elucidating the Aetiology

At that time, various theories explaining the aetiology of this syndrome were postulated. Through targeted epidemiological studies it was found that an infectious agent was responsible for this syndrome. Sexual contact was identified as an important transmission route, because homosexual men who had many sexual partners contracted the disease more frequently than those with only few partners. Later the human immunodeficiency virus (HIV) was characterised in the laboratory as the cause of the disease and an antibody test was developed. Epidemiological studies had to a certain extent a filter function for gaining insight into this new infectious disease by sorting a wide set of potential aetiological factors and elucidating the infectious nature of the disease. This hypothesis was then checked in the laboratory and proven through the identification of the infectious agent. Thereafter, epidemiology had not lost its important role in the investigation of the HIV epidemic. On the contrary, epidemiological studies continue to play a significant role for surveillance and prevention of this globally devastating infectious disease.

5.2.1.2 Describing the Spectrum of Disease for HIV/AIDS

The human immunodeficiency virus (HIV) can lead to the acquired immunodeficiency syndrome (AIDS), which is characterized by a potpourri of different symptoms and diseases, ranging from certain opportunistic infections and tumours to neurological illnesses. A common pathogenetic feature underlying these clinical conditions is the deficiency of the immune system caused by HIV, which primarily infects and destructs specific cells of the immune system ($CD4^+$ T lymphocytes). Aim of epidemiology is to study the distribution of these clinical manifestations depending on the population and its risk factors.

5.2.1.3 Describing the Natural History of HIV Infection

Epidemiological studies can be used to gain information on the natural history of a disease. The natural history of a disease refers to the course of the disease without treatment, which is usually not observed in clinical medicine. Using the antibody test, it became possible to study certain risk groups for HIV infection in the population by way of screening and to follow up persons with and without HIV infection over time in cohort studies in order to understand the risk factors and the natural history of the infection and to identify factors predicting AIDS development. The natural history of HIV infection in its initial stages is characterized by acute retroviral syndrome, which is accompanied by fever, substantial viral pathology and viremia, followed by a long-lasting latent period, where a relative equilibrium between HIV and the immune system of the infected individual exists despite active viral replication. Following an early clinical stage, full-blown AIDS may develop, which is marked by a collapse of the immune system. In the context of clinical epidemiology, the question arises at which phase and when treatment of HIV-infected patients should be applied.

5.2.1.4 Risk Factors and Protective Factors for HIV Infection

The aim of epidemiology is to identify risk and protective factors, which are associated with a disease, and to define frequencies and distributions of these factors in the population. The prevalence of relevant risk factors can then be reduced by the application of specific public health interventions. For the example of HIV, the identification of risk factors includes studies about sexual behaviour and behaviour related to intravenous injections, while the study of protective factors includes, for example, the effect of circumcision on HIV incidence.

5.2.1.5 Predicting Disease Trends

Backcalculation techniques and time series analysis can be used for the prediction of epidemiological trends. For the HIV epidemic, backcalculation approaches were much used up to the era of widespread use of antiretroviral therapy (Rosenberg et al.

1991; Seydel et al. 1994; Verdecchia and Mariotto 1995). Recently, incidence-based measures have gained in importance, since testing rates have increased and methods to detect early HIV infection have become available.

5.2.1.6 To Estimate Disease Burdens and Health-Care Needs of a Population

Due to their dynamic nature the burden of infectious diseases is hard to project. Nevertheless, it is estimated that in 2030, HIV/AIDS will be the third leading cause of death and the leading cause of disability-adjusted life years worldwide (Mathers and Loncar 2006). The authors estimate that 12.1% of all disability-adjusted life years will be due to HIV/AIDS in 2030. This has large implications for the need for health care, in particular the need for antiretroviral treatment (ART) worldwide and may jeopardize the aims of the WHO for providing ART for those living with HIV especially in low-income countries.

5.2.1.7 To Test the Effectiveness of Interventions

Extensive studies have been undertaken to evaluate the effectiveness of various prevention strategies to reduce HIV transmission. Prevention strategies that have been tested in large epidemiological studies were among others mass treatment for sexually transmitted infections (Korenromp et al. 2005) and the effect of circumcision on HIV transmission (Auvert et al. 2005; Gray et al. 2007). While mass treatment for sexually transmitted infections did not prove to be a strategy with lasting success, the results from the circumcision trials have been very promising (see also Chapter 18).

5.3 Characteristics of Infectious Disease Epidemiology

Infectious diseases are caused by pathogens that are transmitted either directly between persons or indirectly via a vector or the environment. They are therefore also called "communicable diseases", because their transmission relies on some form of contact between individuals of a population. The fact that transmission occurs makes the epidemiology of infectious diseases different from the epidemiology of non-communicable diseases for the important reason that the risk of contracting the disease depends on its prevalence in the population.

The spread of an infectious disease through populations is determined by characteristics of the infectious agent, the host, and the environment. Infectious agents are characterized by their biological properties, their host spectrum and natural occurrence; host characteristics are, for example, susceptibility to specific diseases, immune status, socio-demographic and contact behaviour. The interaction between host and pathogen is modulated among others by immune response, virulence of the pathogen, behavioural responses to disease symptoms and pathogen adaptation to treatment. Environmental factors determine the conditions under which the host–pathogen interaction takes place and influences pathogen survival and host behaviour. Environmental factors include physical factors (e.g. climate), biological factors (e.g. insects that transmit the infectious agent), as well as social factors such as sanitary conditions and quality of health-care services.

Definition: Infectious disease

An *infectious disease* is defined as a disease caused by an infectious agent or its toxic products. This agent can be transmitted by an infected person, an animal or a reservoir directly or indirectly through a vector (e.g. alternate host).

Just like other fields of epidemiology, infectious disease epidemiology is concerned with populations, instead of dealing with individual patients. At the centre of the focus of infectious disease epidemiology is the relationship between an infectious agent and its host, its routes of transmission and the environment in which transmission takes place. In contrast with non-communicable diseases, an infected individual (case) can be an initial source for further infections, thereby leading to chains of transmissions in a population. If these are clustered in time they will be recognized as an outbreak and will require localized intervention to break transmission chains. Inapparent and subclinical infections and carriers of infection may be sources for further infections without being identified as infectious cases. Some persons or population groups may be immune against an infection due to vaccinations or after prior exposure to the infection.

Important questions studied in infectious disease epidemiology concern the transmissibility and virulence of pathogens, the course of clinical or sub-clinical infections and the duration of protective immunity. Also, in contrast to the epidemiology of non-communicable diseases, in infectious disease epidemiology the study of human contact patterns play an important role. These can be contacts between humans, between humans and animals, between humans and vectors, or between humans and their environment. Epidemiological studies are conducted to determine why an infectious disease occurs endemically or epidemically and what causes differences in the occurrence of infections among populations and within populations.

In Page et al. (1995) the transmission of infectious disease is described by a chain of six elements that are needed in order for infection and disease to occur in an individual. This interaction is referred to as the "chain of infection" (Fig. 5.1). Each element must be present and lie in sequential order for an infection to occur. Intervention can target any of those six elements of the cycle.

The *portal of entry* is the way an infectious agent enters a susceptible host. The portal of entry is usually the same as the portal of exit from the host (Timmreck 1994). For example, measles virus exits the respiratory tract of the host and enters the respiratory tract of a new host. In the case of gastrointestinal infections an infectious agent is located in faeces and can be carried to the mouth of the new host by improperly washed hands. Other portals of entry are the skin (e.g. schistosomes), the mucous membrane (sexually transmitted diseases), the blood (HIV) and the transplacental mode of entry (toxoplasmosis).

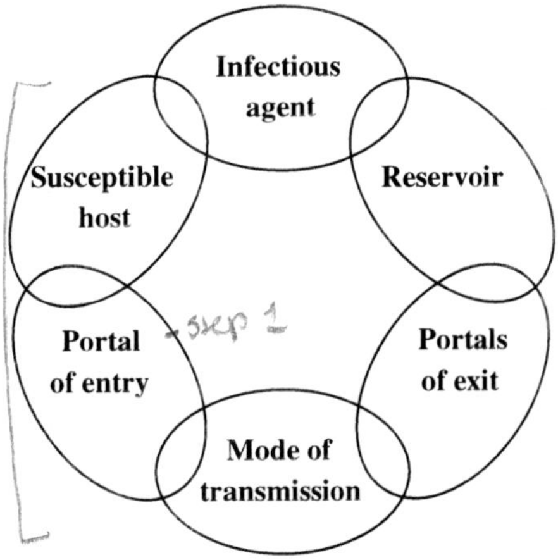

Fig. 5.1 The chain of infection

The *portal of exit* is the route by which the infectious agent leaves the host. The portal of exit is usually dependent on the localization of the infectious agent in the host. The most common portals of exit are respiratory tract (e.g. influenza, measles, mumps, and rubella), genitourinary tract (HIV, syphilis), gastrointestinal tract (hepatitis A, *Salmonella*), through skin (hepatitis B through needles), placenta (toxoplasmosis).

In the following we introduce some of the central concepts of infectious disease epidemiology.

5.3.1 Exposure

One of the central concepts of epidemiology is the *exposure* of an individual to a potential disease-causing agent or substance. In case of an infectious disease, their exposure to infectious agents – a pathogen – can lead to infection, but does not necessarily lead to disease. Infectious agents can be prions, viruses, bacteria, fungi or parasites. The disease can then be caused either by the pathogens themselves after replication in the infected host or by their toxic products. The exposure to an infectious agent depends on its transmission route. Different outcomes of an exposure to an infectious agent can be observed (Fig. 5.2). The outcome may or may not depend on the infectious dose or the inoculum size. For very infectious pathogens a small dose may result in infection of the host, while for less infectious pathogens higher doses of a pathogen are needed for infection. For example, exposure to hepatitis B virus via sexual contact has a much higher probability for resulting in infection than does exposure to HIV. For some infections the relationship between infectious dose and probability of infection can be quantified by dose–response relationships (Teunis et al. 1999).

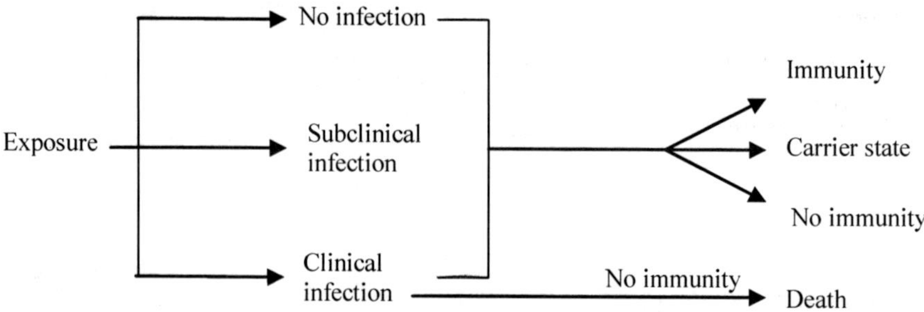

Fig. 5.2 The different outcomes of an exposure to an infectious agent (modified from Giesecke 1994)

5.3.2 *Infection*

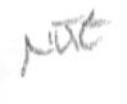

What is actually meant by *infection*? For most pathogens, infection describes the event that the pathogen can establish itself in the host individual and reproduce itself or some stages of its life cycle. For some pathogens one has to distinguish between colonization (a settlement of the pathogen on the skin or other body tissues), where an individual has no clinical signs or symptoms of disease, and invasive infection, when the pathogen permeates through certain barriers of the host like the skin or the mucous membrane and causes symptomatic infection. In pathology, an inflammation caused by an infectious pathogen (or other damaging agents) is characterized by following four phenomena: redness and hyperthermia of, e.g. affected skin areas followed by swelling, pain and loss or impairment of function.

Infections with different pathogens, but also with the same pathogen in different individuals, can differ widely in their natural history. Some infections are acute and exist only for a few hours, days or weeks (e.g. measles, mumps, influenza, diarrhoea), while others after a short acute phase can become chronic and might remain detectable for decades (e.g. hepatitis B and C, HIV). These differences reflect how the human immune system can deal with different pathogens, which in turn depends on a pathogen's genetic variability and on where it is localized in the host.

The *clinical* manifestations of an infection can also differ widely between individuals. An infection may lead to a carrier stage where an infected individual displays no symptoms. Nevertheless, the presence of pathogens can be detected in carriers by means of microbiological tests (serological tests or direct methods to detect the presence of pathogens). Carriers are of large importance for the spread of infections and for intervention, because they are not easily recognized or detected. A carrier of an infection is usually not aware of his/her infection and the risk they pose towards their direct contacts. Therefore, susceptible contact persons do not take precautions against being infected. It is difficult to target public health measures to prevent risky contacts and to identify sources of infection (e.g. hepatitis B infection, HIV). Under these conditions, only systematic screening of entire population groups may ensure that effective interventions are implemented.

Infections with symptomatic or clinical manifestations may display a large variability in symptoms. These symptoms can be very specific for some infectious diseases (e.g. typical rash and pox in smallpox) or they can be rather aspecific such as respiratory tract infections (fever and cough) or gastrointestinal infections (diarrhoea) such that a number of differential diagnoses are available. In the latter case a final diagnosis can be based only on laboratory testing of specimen.

Immunity after infection may or may not be protective against infection and may last for variable periods of time. Some infectious diseases confer lifelong immunity (e.g. measles), others confer some amount of immunity against severe symptomatic infection, but much less against sub-clinical infection (e.g. pertussis), and some confer no or negligible levels of immunity (e.g. Chlamydia infection). Finally, some pathogens invade the immune system itself and thereby not only limit the host's immune response against themselves but also enable other pathogens to invade the infected host (e.g. HIV and opportunistic infections). Immunity can be acquired either after natural infection or indirectly. Maternal antibodies protect the newborn child against many infections in the first few months of its life. After that, immunization for some infectious diseases is possible by vaccination. Also vaccine-induced immunity can be lifelong or temporary. In the latter case, repeated booster vaccinations are necessary to ensure protection against the infection.

5.3.3 Stages of Infection and Disease

During the course of an infection, different stages or time periods can be distinguished regarding the infectivity and manifestations of symptoms in the infected individual. The *latent period* is the time interval from infection to the start of the infectious period; the *incubation period* is the time interval from infection to the onset of clinical symptoms (Fig. 5.3). The *infectious period* is the time interval

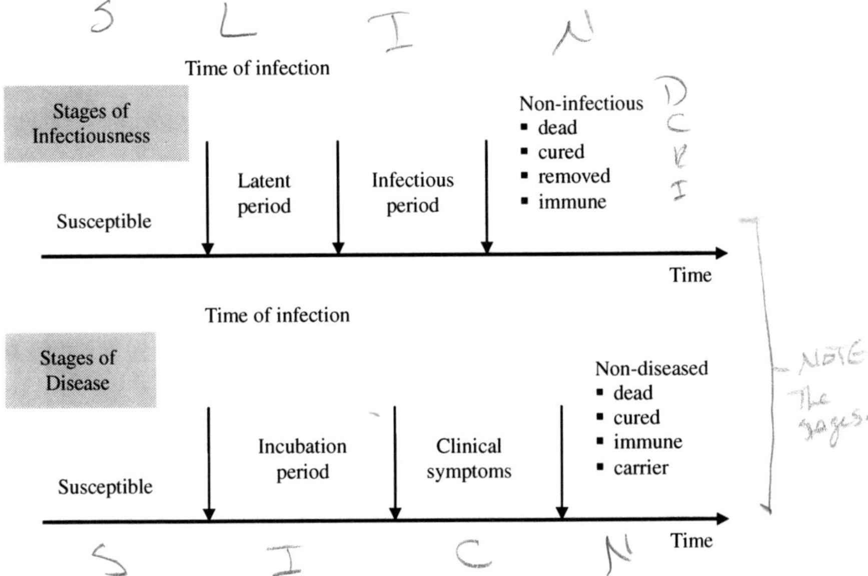

Fig. 5.3 Stages of infection and disease (modified according to Halloran 1998)

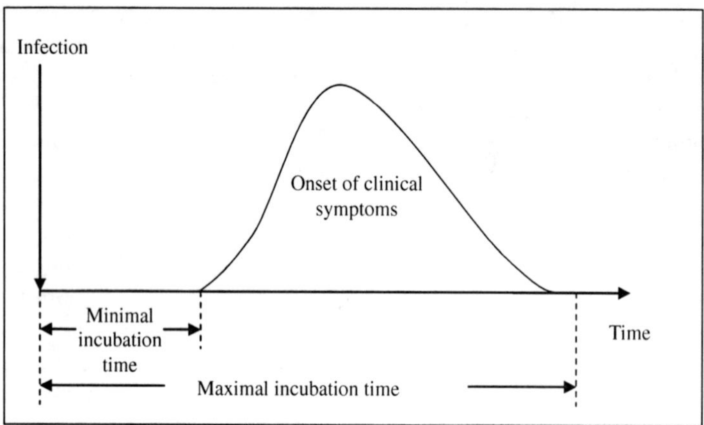

Fig. 5.4 Incubation time distribution

during which an infected person can transmit an infection to other susceptible persons.

For a specific infectious disease the incubation period may vary widely between individuals. Therefore, incubation periods are often better described as incubation time distributions with a minimal, a mean or median and a maximal incubation time (Fig. 5.4). In outbreaks one frequently observes several generations of an infection, i.e. clusters of cases with typical time intervals between their days of symptom onset (Fig. 5.5). The first case, or index case, in an outbreak is of great importance because he or she brings the infectious disease into the community. Secondary cases are those infected by the index case, tertiary cases those infected by a secondary case, etc. The typical time interval between the onset of symptoms in a case and the onset of symptoms in the cases infected by him/her is called the *generation interval* or *serial interval*. The distribution of this interval is determined by the durations of

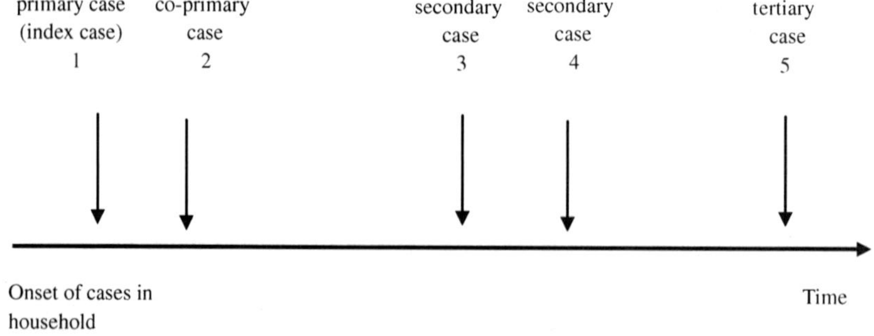

Fig. 5.5 Generations of an infection (modified according to Halloran 1998)

latent period and infectious period, and by the contact rates of infectious individuals (Fine 2003).

The reproduction number or *reproductive rate* of an infection is its potential to spread after invasion into a population. It depends on the proportion of immune persons in the population, the duration of the infectious period, the contact rates and the probability of transmission upon contact between an infected and a susceptible individual.

5.3.4 Virulence, Pathogenicity and Immunogenicity

There are different definitions of virulence in the literature, mostly based on the ability of a pathogen to cause host mortality. However, in many infectious diseases a virulence definition based on the death of a host is not useful, because we are more interested in the severity of symptoms rather than in death. In an absolute sense the capacity of a pathogen to cause symptoms is described as *pathogenicity*. By *virulence*, one usually refers to the pathogenicity of one (strain of a) pathogen in comparison with another. We therefore follow Casadevall and Pirofski (1999) in defining virulence as the relative capacity of a pathogen to cause damage in the host.

Pathogenicity and virulence are determined by the interaction between host and pathogen. Characteristics of infectious agents that affect virulence include their ability to proliferate, invade organisms and damage the host. These effects may be dependent on the infective dose, which is the number of organisms needed to cause an infection. A virulent pathogen can invade into the host organism with a small infectious dose. Characteristics of the host also play an important role in the ability of a pathogen to cause disease, that is, pathogenicity and virulence depend not only on the characteristics of the host such as resistance and immune system function but also on genetic factors, age, gender and other physiological conditions, e.g. pregnancy.

Immunogenicity is defined as the ability of a pathogen or a vaccine to evoke an immune response after an infection or a vaccination, which may lead to protection against re-infection with the same or similar pathogen. For some infections, immunity after natural infection is lifelong (measles or polio virus), while for others, immunity is temporary (pertussis) or strain specific (influenza). For some infections, immunity is acquired only after repeated re-infections and wanes if booster infections do not occur (malaria). For some infections, immunity is induced against symptomatic infection, but subclinical infection may still occur.

5.3.5 Routes of Transmission

An infectious agent may be transmitted to a susceptible host in many ways. These routes of transmission are classified as direct and indirect transmission (Giesecke 1994). Direct transmission includes direct skin-to-skin contact and close contact that permits transmission via droplets and aerosols. Droplet spread occurs by sneezing, coughing or talking at a short distance. Droplet spread is defined as direct transmission because it is transmitted by a direct spray over a few metres before droplets fall to the ground. Indirect transmission takes place through vectors or via the environment. A *vector* is an invertebrate animal that becomes infected from infected animals or persons and transmits the infection to other persons, e.g. the *Anopheles* mosquitoes that transmit malaria parasites from person to person. Vectors are typically insects or arthropods. Also, medical devices like injection syringes can act as vectors for disease transmission. Furthermore, environmental transmission occurs through water, food, soil, air, and solid surfaces depending on where a pathogen can best survive outside the host.

The *source of infection* is the initial point from which the infection passes to a person. In directly transmitted infections the source is an infected person. In indirectly transmitted infections, sources of infection can be different materials in the environment (e.g. objects, ground and water), contaminated or infected foods or infected animal vectors. A *reservoir* of infection is a living organism or a material in or on which an infectious agent lives and/or usually multiplies.

Examples of directly transmitted infections include sexually transmitted infections (transmission by mucous membrane contacts), toxoplasmosis (transmission through the placenta), HIV and hepatitis B (transmission by sexual contact and via blood), herpes virus type 1 infection (skin-to-skin contacts), and influenza [transmission by coughing and sneezing (droplet spread)]. Examples of indirectly transmitted infections are hepatitis A (faecal–oral transmission), *Salmonella* (food), malaria (mosquitoes) and schistosomiasis (water) (Table 5.1).

In addition to their main host (human or vertebrate animal), some pathogens have one or several intermediate hosts (e.g. arthropod), in which they multiply and develop. In case of malaria the human is an intermediate host and sexual proliferation of the pathogen takes place in the *Anopheles* mosquito.

A human can also become an accidental host by unusual contact with an infectious agent that has animals as the main host (e.g. hantavirus pulmonary syndrome). Any infection that is transmitted from an animal to a human is called *zoonosis*. It is believed that many newly emerging infections in humans evolve from zoonoses.

Table 5.1 Frequent media of transmission and transmission routes for some infectious agents

Transmission medium	Pathogen	Transmission route
Foods	*Salmonella*	Foodborne
	Campylobacter	Faecal–oral
	Hepatitis A	
Water	Cholera	Water-borne
Sputum droplets	Influenza	Close contact
Air/aerosols	Tuberculosis	Airborne
	Chickenpox, *Legionella* infection	
Organ transplants	Cytomegalovirus	Transplant-borne
Blood	HIV, hepatitis C	Blood-borne
Sperm, body fluids	Hepatitis B	Sexual contact

5.3.6 Endemic Infectious Diseases and Epidemic Outbreaks

An *outbreak* is defined as the occurrence of an infection in a population with an excess of cases in space and time above the expected level. An outbreak can be small – sometimes two linked cases constitute an outbreak – or it can affect large parts of the population. A larger outbreak that affects a considerable proportion of a population is also called *epidemic*. A global outbreak that affects many or all countries worldwide is called a *pandemic*.

If an infectious disease can establish itself permanently in a population, it is called *endemic*. For many endemic infections, the prevalence remains more or less constant over time as long as no changes occur in intervention or prevention strategies. By prevention or intervention one can aim at *elimination* of an endemic infection from a population. Elimination on a global scale is called *eradication*. Elimination occurs if there is no natural circulation of a pathogen any longer in a population; eradication is reached if a pathogen does not circulate at all any more in the human population. Smallpox is the only infectious disease for which eradication has been achieved at present.

Many endemic infectious diseases have seasonally fluctuating incidence rates (Fisman 2007). The seasonality is due to climate conditions, which influence pathogen survival in the environment, and human contact patterns, which fluctuate due to activity patterns (e.g. school holidays).

5.4 Challenges of Infectious Disease Epidemiology

Transnational migration, changes in human behaviour, rapid urbanization and newly emerging infectious diseases such as SARS and BSE (mad cow disease) are the challenges of modern infectious disease epidemiology (see Chapter 2). In times of globalization, transnational migration is of great importance for the spread of infectious diseases. The border cannot be seen as a barrier anymore as many infectious diseases have a long incubation period, which makes it difficult to control the spread of infectious diseases. On the other side, migrant populations are often marginalized in the society, which makes them vulnerable to certain diseases (Tselmin et al. 2007). Socio-economic inequalities also play an important role in the spread of infectious diseases. The poor population often lives in overcrowded households with inadequate sanitation conditions. These people usually have a worse nutritional status which makes them more vulnerable to infectious diseases. Individuals from low socio-economic classes also may have limited access to primary health care.

Population groups at risk for infectious diseases may benefit from educational interventions to improve knowledge, beliefs and attitudes concerning prevention. Such efforts are crucial to stop the spread of infections. Closer interaction between academic research and populations at risk can be achieved by using the *community-based participatory research* (CBPR) approach, which actively involves the community studied in the research (Israel et al. 1998). The benefits of this type of research are the following: (a) community members are considered to be the study partners and not just objects of research; (b) the knowledge of the community is used to better understand health problems in the community; (c) interventions can be directly conducted in the community. Close collaboration between communities and researchers is essential to develop adequate public health strategies that address community concerns (Kone et al. 2000). This approach is especially appropriate when research is conducted on sensitive issues such as HIV/AIDS or sexually transmitted diseases and has been successfully applied in infectious disease epidemiology.

Other challenges of infectious disease epidemiology lie in the rapid development of genetic typing methods, which allow a more detailed picture of how strains of pathogens are genetically related and along which routes they might have spread through a population. At present a wealth of genotyping data are already available, but epidemiological studies to understand the relationship between transmission risks and the distribution of genotypes are still scarce.

Another pressing area of research for infectious disease epidemiology comes from the ability of pathogens to escape intervention pressure by evolutionary adaptation. For example, the development of resistance of pathogens against treatments (antibiotic resistance, resistance against antiviral medication) is causing increasing problems not only in hospitals, where multiresistant strains of pathogens have become endemic, but also in the treatment of tuberculosis and chronic hepatitis B.

References

Auvert BD, Taljaard D, Lagarde E, Sobngwi-Tambekou J, Sitta R, and Puren A (2005) Randomized, controlled intervention trial of male circumcision for reduction of HIV infection risk: The ANRS 1265 Trial. PLoS Med. 2:e298

Casadevall A and Pirofski LA (1999) Host-pathogen interactions: redefining the basic concepts of virulence and pathogenicity. Infect Immun. 67:3703–3713

Detels R, Holland W, and McEwen J (2002) Oxford Textbook of Public Health. Oxford: Oxford University Press

Fine PE (2003) The interval between successive cases of an infectious disease. Am J Epidemiol. 158:1039–1047

Fisman DN (2007) Seasonality of infectious diseases. Annu Rev Public Health. 28:127–143

Giesecke J (1994) Modern Infectious Disease Epidemiology. London Sydney Auckland: Arnold

Gray RH, Kigozi G, Serwadda D, Makumbi F, Watya S, Nalugoda F, Kiwanuka N, Moulton LH, Chaudhary MA, Chen MZ, Sewankambo NK, Wabwire-Mangen F, Bacon MC, Williams CF, Opendi P, Reynolds SJ, Laeyendecker O, Quinn TC, and Wawer MJ (2007) Male circumcision for HIV prevention in men in Rakai, Uganda: a randomised trial. Lancet. 369:657–666

Halloran ME (1998) Concepts of infectious disease epidemiology. In KJRothman, S Greenland. Modern Epidemiology. Philadelphia: Lippincott-Raven,pp. 529–554

Israel BA, Schulz AJ, Parker EA, and Becker AB (1998) Review of community-based research: assessing partnership approaches to improve public health. Annu Rev Public Health. 19: 173–202

Kone A, Sullivan M, Senturia KD, Chrisman NJ, Ciske SJ, and Krieger JW (2000) Improving collaboration between researchers and communities. Public Health Rep. 115:243–248

Korenromp EL, White RG, Orroth KK, Bakker R, Kamali A, Serwadda D, Gray RH, Grosskurth H, Habbema JD, and Hayes RJ (2005) Determinants of the impact of sexually transmitted infection treatment on prevention of HIV infection: a synthesis of evidence from the Mwanza, Rakai, and Masaka intervention trials. J Infect Dis. 191 Suppl 1:S168–S178

Last JM (2001) A Dictionary of Epidemiology.Oxford: Oxford University Press

Mathers CD and Loncar D (2006) Projections of global mortality and burden of disease from 2002 to 2030. PLoS Med. 3:e442

Page RM, Cole GE, and Timmreck TC (1995) Basic Epidemiological Methods and Biostatistics. A Practical Guidebook. Boston London Singapore: Jones and Bartlett Publishers

Rosenberg PS, Biggar RJ, Goedert JJ, and Gail MH (1991) Backcalculation of the number with human immunodeficiency virus infection in the United States. Am J Epidemiol. 133:276–285

Rothman KJ, Greenland S and Lash TL, eds. (2008) Modern Epidemiology. 3rd. ed. Philadelphia: Lippincott Williams and Wilkins

Seydel J, Kramer A, Rosenberg PS, Wittkowski KM, and Gail MH. (1994) Backcalculation of the number infected with human immunodeficiency virus in Germany. J Acquir Immune Defic Syndr. 7:74–78

Teunis PF, Nagelkerke NJ, and Haas CN (1999) Dose response models for infectious gastroenteritis. Risk Anal. 19:1251–1260

Timmreck TC (1994) An Introduction to Epidemiology. Boston London Singapore: Jones and Bartlett Publishers

Tselmin S, Korenblum W, Reimann M, Bornstein SR, and Schwarz PE (2007) The Health Status of Russian-speaking Immigrants in Germany. Horm Metab Res. 39:858–861

Verdecchia A and Mariotto AB (1995) A back-calculation method to estimate the age and period HIV infection intensity, considering the susceptible population. Stat Med. 14:1513–1530

Chapter 6
Social Risk Factors

Klaus Krickeberg and David Klemperer

6.1 Introduction

Among risk factors for infectious diseases, *social* ones present a particular challenge due to the increasing importance of old and new infections on the one hand, and the complexity of social reality on the other. This is not a new phenomenon. Social risk factors for infectious diseases were a subject of much thought throughout, roughly, the early nineteenth century up to the First World War although rigorous epidemiologic methods were of course still rudimentary. Modern public health originated during that period even before the discovery of specific micro-organisms as infective agents (Rosen 1993). In addition to organizing public health services, the main preoccupation of health authorities was *hygiene*, and hygiene then amounted, in modern epidemiologic terms, to the fight against the principal biological risk factor, which is the exposition to the known or suspected infective agent (see Chapter 5). However, social factors like poverty, malnutrition, deficient water supply, crowded housing, and dangerous occupations played an equally important role.

As it is well known, the interest in infectious diseases in general, and in their social risk factors in particular, waned in the sequel, especially after the Second World War, partly as a consequence of over-reliance on antibiotics in spite of early evidence of resistance phenomena (see Chapter 3). Hygienic standards even declined in many places. Then, in the last one or two decades, several phenomena contributed to a resurgence of activities around infectious diseases. More and more people, both in the medical professions and outside, became aware of the dangers of resistance of infective agents or their hosts to drugs or insecticides. Nosocomial infections became more frequent (see Chapter 22). Finally, several *new* infectious diseases emerged (see Chapter 3). Still, this renewed interest in infectious diseases has not yet led to a large coherent body of studies on their social risk factors.

There are several ways of looking at the influence of social risk factors on the distribution and spread of an infectious disease in a given population. What is indeed

K. Krickeberg (✉)
Formerly, Universitè de Paris V, France; Bielefeld, Germany
e-mail: krik@ideenwelt.de

A. Krämer et al. (eds.), *Modern Infectious Disease Epidemiology*,
Statistics for Biology and Health, DOI 10.1007/978-0-387-93835-6_6,

the meaning of a statement like "Poor people tend to suffer more than rich ones from tuberculosis"? The classical epidemiologic interpretation (see Chapter 11) makes use of input (exposition) and outcome variables that are defined for *persons.* Thus, for every individual person in the population at hand the input, or risk, variable would describe the degree of poverty of that person, and the outcome variable would represent some feature of his or her state of health connected with tuberculosis. An epidemiologic study of relations between these two variables would be *person based.*

However, already in the early times of social epidemiology it appeared sometimes to be necessary or more natural to deal with *communities* in the sense of *groups*, or *sets,* of people, and not with individual persons as the underlying *units* of concepts and studies. One would, for example, describe the degree of poverty of a family or a block of dwellings or an entire geographical area by a certain indicator, and similarly speak of the situation of tuberculosis in such an entity. Sometimes, a community-based study will be conducted if only information concerning the underlying communities as a whole can be obtained, but not data about their individual members. As a rule such a study will provide a rougher picture of the action of the factor "poverty" than a person-based investigation. In other settings, the unit "community" will be in the centre of interest from the start. Moreover, as we will see later, there are social risk factors that can only be defined for groups of people and have no meaning for individual persons. Finally, in a "multilevel" approach, both person-based and community-based concepts on various levels are being investigated.

The challenge with which we are now confronted is to study the effect of social factors more systematically, using modern epidemiologic concepts, and at the same time to keep in mind the relevance and usefulness of the results for public health policy. In the following, after having reviewed the main concepts (Sections 6.2, 6.3, and 6.4), we will try to convey an idea about the kind of past and present work in this area by presenting typical examples, arranged by sources of information and methods of study (Sections 6.5, 6.6, 6.7, 6.8, and 6.9). We then summarize the methodological issues and point out some desirable future directions of research (Section 6.10). Finally, in Section 6.11, we will mention some implications for health policy, knowing fully well that many or most of them will appear unrealistic at this point in time, or controversial, or both.

6.2 Pathways

The exposition to an infective agent is, by definition, a necessary condition for the corresponding infectious disease to manifest itself in an individual. With a few exceptions, it is not a sufficient one, although in the beginning of modern medical bacteriology the third Henle–Koch postulate (Susser 2001) seemed to claim that. Infectious diseases are indeed, like non-infectious ones, mostly multi-factorial. Given the type of agent and the intensity of the exposition of a specific person, both the first manifestation and the course of the disease still depend on additional factors such as genetic disposition, acquired immunity, and the general state of physical and mental health of the subject including stress, fatigue, and concomitant infections.

Factors of this kind act more or less *directly* on the disease, but they are not easy to define rigorously or to measure. For simplicity of reference, we will call them the *biological* variables, subsuming mental factors in this category. They are influenced, in turn, by factors that *can* be quantified and measured and that normally act indirectly through the biological ones. We can classify these factors with indirect action by the following scheme, which applies to infectious as well as non-infectious diseases and in essence goes back to antiquity:

- environmental factors
- social factors
- lifestyle-related factors
- iatrogenic factors

where of course the dividing lines still need to be made precise. It is *these* factors that enter into public health policy. Hence, from the viewpoint of public health, it is *their* epidemiologic action in which we are interested even when we cannot completely elucidate the underlying mechanisms.

Regarding social factors, they do not only act directly on biological variables, but they interact with each other, too. They may also have an influence on environmental, lifestyle, or iatrogenic factors, which in turn affect biological variables. Finally, they influence the *transmission* of the infection within a population as it is sometimes being modelled mathematically (see Chapter 12). Thus the overall picture of the action of social risk factors is, finally, fairly complicated and modern studies try to tackle the problem by following this action along the various *paths* it may take.

One also attempts to uncover *causal* effects in some sense. Causation research may use, among others, the full machinery of the mathematical–statistical analysis of dependencies as presented, e.g. in Cox and Wermuth (1996). It is widespread in the study of social risk factors for non-infectious diseases (Chandola and Marmot 2005), but less so for infectious diseases because of the preponderance of the factor "infection" which has been diverting the attention from others. The papers by Krieger (1994, 2001) discuss basic aspects of the epidemiologic reasoning involved and in particular of the search for causes; they contain extensive bibliographies (see also Section 6.6).

6.3 Outcome Variables

Let us first try to gain an overview of the variables we are going to deal with. The particular outcome variables to be studied are determined by the fact that we are treating *infectious* disease epidemiology. In any person-based study concerning a given infectious disease we will naturally be interested in one or several variables of any of the following types:

- The presence of antibodies.
- A clinically diagnosed infection.

- An infection defined and diagnosed by biological, chemical or physical procedures, e.g. blood, sputum, or urine examination in the laboratory or X-rays.
- Various aspects of the evolution of the disease like hospitalization, time to recovery, fatal issue, etc.
- Direct health consequences of infections such as dental caries, periodontal problems or virus-induced cancers.

A community-based investigation will use corresponding outcome variables that describe the state of health in a population, e.g. an incidence, prevalence or mortality in a city or country. Such a variable is usually obtained by averaging the values of an underlying person-defined variable over such and such population, but dealing directly with this original individual-level variable may be either not feasible or not the focus of attention.

6.4 Social Risk Factors

There will probably be less agreement about the exposure variables or determinants, to be studied, i.e. about the concept of a *social risk factor*. Let us start again with person-based concepts. In the older literature one encounters the expression "demographic variables", which stands for age, sex, marital status, place of residence, religion, race (ethnicity), education, occupation, etc. Many of these variables appear in the descriptive epidemiology of classical health statistics. In modern social epidemiology we find a more differentiated view of risk factors (Bourdieu 1979). Variables like age, sex, marital status, number of children or nationality are sometimes called *horizontal* social factors because a priori they do not imply the idea of a hierarchy, i.e. of "upper" and "lower" classes. In contrast, there are *vertical* variables tied to the idea of social status such as education, profession, income, housing, and to some extent also previous migration. Variables like gender or ethnicity or place of residence may belong to one or the other category depending on the context. Vertical variables are the social risk factors in the narrower sense, and it is them that we are investigating when we are looking at social inequality and injustice and their influence on infectious diseases.

Similar remarks apply to social risk factors defined for communities. They focus on exposure patterns within groups of people and not on individual-level factors and may be of manifold nature. Certain social risk factors such as *segregation* or the existence of particular *social networks* and of *social capital* cannot even be reasonably defined for single persons; they are relations *between* members of a group of people.

6.5 Routine Health Statistics

Descriptive epidemiology is often identified with classical medical statistics. This amounts to the regular, e.g. monthly or yearly, cross-sectional study of some of the "demographic" social risk factors listed above such as age, sex, place of residence and others. By studying the geographical factor on the scale of entire nations or regions, we gain a global view of the distribution of the incidence or prevalence of infectious diseases over the world, of their relative weight and of their "burden". This is the subject of Chapter 1. A somewhat more detailed description is provided by WHO publications (Murray et al. 2004), which, however, largely reflect the reports received from Ministries of Health and other national administrations. These reports, in turn, are based on national health information systems (Krickeberg 2007) that are often unreliable. They derive their information mainly from hospital and health centre records (see Chapter 8). Systematic statistical control and correction mechanisms for these systems are rare both at the national and the WHO level.

For particular infectious diseases like malaria, tuberculosis or leprosy, specialized information systems exist in some countries; see, e.g. the recent description of the Tuberculosis–Leprosy Management System in Malaysia where the social factor "migration" is taken into account (Dony et al. 2004). Another part of descriptive routine information on infectious diseases comes from epidemiologic surveillance; see Chapter 9 for more details and examples. Particular features of the evaluation of information containing a geographical component are presented in Chapter 11.

An analysis of existing health statistics can only yield very crude and limited insights into the action of social factors on infectious diseases. The units of study are necessarily fairly large communities like provinces of a given country. Very few social risk factors are being taken into account. Let us look at a typical "*Health Statistics Yearbook*", e.g. the one edited by the Vietnamese Ministry of Health for the year 2003. There, incidences or prevalences of infectious diseases are mostly given for the eight regions of the country. For tuberculosis, malaria, leprosy and AIDS they are also provided by province, and the resulting inter-provincial comparisons are presented in the form of maps. There is only one socio-economic factor in addition to the geographic one; it concerns malnutrition of children. Hence a study of a factor like income would necessitate the concomitant use of tables of per capita income in every province in 2003.

A good example of such a simultaneous use of several "official" sources of indicators (WHO, UNDP and others) is the study of Hobdell et al. (2003) about the relation of oral diseases and socio-economic status. Its aim is not *intra-* but *inter-*country comparisons; thus the underlying units are countries. The outcomes are measured, in addition to (non-infectious) oral cancer prevalence, by the prevalence of dental caries and periodontal diseases. Socio-economic risk factors appear in the form of country indicators such as the Human Development Index, Mean Years of Schooling, Gross National Product per capita, or the Gini Index, which describes unequal distribution of income in a country. It turns out that many of these risk factors are strongly associated with dental caries and even more with destructive periodontal disease (but very little with oral cancer). A community study of this kind leaves of course open the question of pathways of action: to which extent do the socio-economic factors studied act on factors known to favour, e.g. periodontal disease, such as access to water, toothbrushes and toothpaste, tobacco, and psychosocial stress? Do they also act in some other way? To answer such questions, finer studies are required.

6.6 Classical Studies

The influence of social conditions, in particular of vertical risk factors, on infectious diseases has been suspected, observed and mentioned for a long time. For example, in the Middle Ages leprosy was known to be endemic particularly among the poor (Rosen 1993, p. 39). Typhoid fever was called "jail fever" in England in the sixteenth and seventeenth centuries, because it seemed to be an inevitable consequence of going to prison (Rosen 1993, p. 65). In the nineteenth century, merely stating hypotheses and describing observations gradually made way for more and more rigorous studies based on the quintessence of all epidemiologic research, namely the comparison of groups defined by different levels of exposure. Virchow's classical report (Virchow 1848) on a typhoid fever epidemic in Upper Silesia (which was in fact louse-borne typhus as we know by now) marks a transition. He carefully describes factors such as topography, history, ethnicity and culture, dwellings, hygiene and nutrition as well as outcomes, but the paucity of health statistics and the short duration of his mission do not yet allow a comparative study.

The subsequent development and the state of knowledge and consciousness on the eve of the First World War are very well presented in the three chapters of the classical book by Mosse and Tugendreich (1913) devoted to, respectively, sexually transmissible diseases, general infectious diseases and tuberculosis. We are going to review the chapter on tuberculosis written by M. Mosse. It is the most substantial and interesting of the three, which is not surprising since tuberculosis had then been the most studied infectious disease in relation to social factors – as it probably still is.

In 1913, the necessity of comparing populations seems to have been widely recognized. Most of the papers summarized in this chapter describe investigations that might be looked upon, from a modern point of view, as record-based retrospective cohort studies, that is, they draw on official health statistics or hospital records and present, for various levels of the risk factors, corresponding data on morbidity or mortality. Questions around what we would now call "hospital bias" are being discussed in this context. Statistical material from health insurances in the United States and Germany is also already being exploited. A few other studies give data on risk factors for various levels of an outcome variable, which amounts to a rudimentary case–control study, but they are methodologically deficient and do not provide any insight. There are both person- and community-based studies.

Modern concepts of epidemiology appear. For example, the word "factor" is used from the beginning in the sense of "social risk factor", and the chapter is organized accordingly, with horizontal risk factors first and vertical ones afterwards. Pathways are already being considered and so is the relation of specific social factors with others.

The fundamental idea of a *confounder* plays both implicitly and explicitly an important role although the term itself is not yet used. Mosse talks about "veiling" *(Verschleierung)* and later points out the role of the factor "age" as a possible confounder, or criticizes the lack of stratifications by age in certain studies. In a pioneering paper published in 1906, Newsholme deals with the decrease of general mortality in England and tries to identify those social factors that contribute *specifically* to diminishing TB mortality. He concludes that these specific factors are "housing" and "isolation of patients in sanatoria". His method consists of comparing the temporal evolution of mortalities in several countries. A study by Dörner starting with data from 1852 shows that for a fixed income level, the factor "housing" has an important influence on TB incidence. An interesting discussion in the same realm of confounding factors tries to explain why alcoholics seem to be less prone to TB morbidity and mortality than the general population. Schmid in 1899 eliminates the possible confounder "working in agriculture or not" in a study of the action of the geographical factor "altitude" by stratification.

Let us look at some particularly valuable studies described by Mosse, starting with risk factors related to "income" or "wealth". Sørensen divided the Danish population in the 1880s into three social groups, stratified by age and sex, and found striking differences of TB mortality. For the same outcome variable, a community study by Neef covering the same period investigates the factor "average income in a district of the city of Breslau"; Bertillon around 1909 picks six districts *(arrondissements)* of Paris from "very rich" to "very poor"; and Marié-Davy defines an exposure variable for all 20 "arrondissements" of Paris by "number of windows per person", resulting in a very clear inverse relation with TB mortality in the period 1858–1902.

The influence of the factor "profession" on TB morbidity and mortality is the subject of several studies, some of them based on insurance records. A remarkable analysis by Tobler gives TB mortality in Switzerland for the period 1889–1900 in many professions, stratified by age, with farmers displaying the lowest and stonemasons the highest death rates. Very "modern" is also a paper published in 1912 by the Statistical Office of the city of Halle (Germany), which attempts to disentangle the action of the factors "profession" and "social standing", the first one having a markedly higher influence.

The modernity of the book by Mosse and Tugendreich contrasts with some papers published recently but written in the spirit of the middle of the nineteenth century. We quote Zahraoui-Mehadji et al. (2004) as a deterrent. Its purpose was to measure the risk of infection by HIV, hepatitis B and C and syphilis incurred by traditional barbers in the Casablanca region of Morocco. The four corresponding outcome variables were well defined in serological terms. A sample of 150 male barbers was selected. While HIV serology turned out to be negative for all of them, the other three outcome variables were positive for many. Regarding the risk factor studied here, it was clearly the factor "occupation". However, since a sample was taken only from the particular occupation "traditional barber", comparison with other occupations was impossible and the public health recommendations made on the basis of this work are standing on shaky grounds.

We are now going to jump to the present and try to shed some light on the state of the field by reviewing a few selected investigations, starting with the methodologically simplest ones.

6.7 Studies Centring Round a Single Dichotomous Risk Factor

They form the next higher level of epidemiologic sophistication. In a series of papers from Israel, the influence of the social factor "Jewish or Bedouin" on some infectious disease-related outcome variables was investigated by various methods, largely based on hospital records. The article by Levy et al. (1998) is a characteristic example. The target population of this study consists of all children under 15 years of age in the Negev region, and the risk factor determines the two complementary subpopulations to be compared, viz. Jewish and Bedouin children, respectively. The authors remark that these two population groups have equal access to tertiary health care in the only regional hospital, free from financial barriers, and they thus discard a conceivable confounder. The groups differ by lifestyle and religion. The Jewish lifestyle is largely urban and industrialized whereas the Moslem Bedouins are in transition from their traditional nomadic life to settlement. The main outcome variable is "hospitalization for infectious diseases". The study consists in estimating, in each of the two populations, the frequency of such hospitalizations during the period 1989–1991, expressed as numbers of hospitalizations due to infectious diseases per 10,000 child years. There were 15,947 hospitalizations for any cause during that period, documented by computerized hospital records. The number of children in each population group and in any year of the period in question was obtained from population statistics. Per 10,000 child years there were 250 hospitalizations for infectious diseases of Bedouins and 121 of Jews. For hospitalizations because of diarrhoea, the corresponding figures were 114 and 32, respectively, and for pneumonia, 55 and 19. These differences were even more pronounced in infants, especially for diarrhoea. For infectious diseases again, paediatric intensive care hospitalizations were over 2.5 times more frequent for Bedouin children than for Jewish ones, and in-hospital mortality was near to 6 times higher.

Technically speaking, this is again a *record-based cohort* study. A recent example of several *case–control* studies conducted in parallel treats the outcome variable "new case of avian influenza" in Vietnam (Pham Ngoc Dinh et al. 2006). Each of the social risk factors "the patient *prepared* dead or sick poultry less than 8 days before onset", "there *was* such poultry in the household in this period", and "there is no indoor water source in his house", turned out to have a significant influence, while certain others did not. In addition, a multiple logistic regression was done.

The AIDS epidemic has naturally given rise to a large number of studies, to which we will come back in Section 6.9. In Africa, the factor "migration" has been the focus of much interest, continuing a line of research that started in 1949 for syphilis and gonorrhoea (Kark 1949). Not surprisingly, migration always turned out to be an influential risk factor. The particular "circular" nature of the migration at hand where workers return regularly to their fixed home was more and more taken into account. Earlier investigations centred around HIV infections contracted by the male migrant worker while away, and infections of his female partner were considered as having originated from him after his return. A recent more refined cross-sectional study in a rural district of South Africa (Lurie et al. 2003) succeeded in separating this "inside" pathway from infections outside a regular partnership by sampling 168 couples and recording for each of them, in addition to the variable "migrant", *which* of the two partners was positive or negative. Strictly speaking, this was a community study, the "communities" being couples. There were only 9% "positively concordant" couples but 21% "discordant" ones, and in 29% of discordant couples it was the female partner who was infected. Migrant couples were more likely than non-migrant ones to have at least one partner infected and to be discordant.

6.8 Community Studies

It is natural that questions about pathways and causal relations should be treated, and perhaps even answered, via community studies. Here, the key problem that poses itself right in the beginning is how to *define*, in a given setting, the appropriate exposure variables in a rigorous and quantitative manner. We are going to present three recent community studies on risk factors for tuberculosis mortality or incidence that illustrate basic and methodological aspects, and also provide a good introduction to the literature. They differ in the definitions of outcomes and risk factors as well as in the statistical methods used for evaluating the data.

Recall first that the units of community studies are groups of people. The first study (Ferreira Antunes and Alves Waldman 2001) and the second one (Kistemann et al. 2002) define outcomes and exposures in such a group essentially as averages of the corresponding variables for the members of the group whereas the third one (Acevedo-Garcia 2001) deals with a more sophisticated concept derived from the *distribution* of risk factors *within* the group. The first two studies employ classical statistical procedures, whereas the third one takes a Boolean approach.

The units of the study Ferreira Antunes and Alves Waldman (2001) are the 96 districts of the Brazilian Metropolis, São Paulo. The outcome variables are defined as suitably standardized annual mortality rates by tuberculosis for the years 1994–1998. One of the main purposes was to estimate the percentage of tuberculosis deaths attributable to a HIV co-infection; the result was 22%. In addition, the analysis revealed the following associations of tuberculosis mortality with social risk factors: a certain social development index (not to be made precise here): negative association; mean number of dwellers per bedroom: positive; mean number of dwellers per dwelling: no association; population density: no association; mean number of rooms per household: negative; recent immigration from abroad or other Brazilian states: positive. The associations are defined by a simultaneous autoregressive analysis that takes the spatial distribution of the districts into account. The authors also suggest some interpretations of these results in terms of possible pathways. For instance, the positive association of tuberculosis deaths with bedroom overcrowding in contrast to the absence of association with district-level overcrowding may indicate that prolonged contact is needed for disease transmission, and the negative correlation with the household size is consistent with respiratory transmission. Immigrants may contribute to higher tuberculosis mortality both because they bring along relatively more new sources of transmission than there are in the population already in place, and because their economic and social status is lower.

The article by Kistemann et al. (2002) on tuberculosis incidence in the large German city of Cologne pursues similar purposes and uses similar methods. Its list of social risk factors is more detailed, though, and hence there is a more refined discussion of possible pathways and causal relations. Regarding immigration, it is interesting to note that deprivation of immigrants already settled rather than high prevalence at the moment of arrival seems to be the decisive factor. In general settings, material deprivation acts both through poor housing conditions and the associated increased exposure to the infective agent, and by lowering immunocompetence, but in Cologne where crowded housing is not a severe problem the first factor contributes relatively little.

In the study by Acevedo-Garcia (2001) a unit is determined by a common ZIP (postal) code in the state of New Jersey, USA, and an ethnic group (non-Hispanic whites, African-Americans, Hispanics, Asians), which amounts to $591 \times 4 = 2{,}364$ units. All of them are included in the study; thus formally, as in the two papers discussed before, we have a census-like cross-sectional survey. Only one outcome variable is investigated, its value for a given ZIP code and a given ethnic group being defined as the average annual tuberculosis incidence over the years 1985–1992 in this “unit”.

The essential idea of the concept of risk factors on the level of these units is to take into account the distribution of risks within the ZIP code area in question. To this end, the partition of the ZIP area into (street-) blocks is used. For example, in order to define the exposure to *poverty* in the ZIP area 08544 among Asians, consider, in each block in that ZIP area, the proportion of poor people, suitably determined. By exposure to poverty in that unit the author means, then, the *average,* or *expected,* value of this proportion if we select a block at random from the ZIP area 08544, the probability of selecting a given block being the proportion of Asians living in this block to all Asians in the whole ZIP area 08544. Exposure to dilapidated (i.e. rented) and to overcrowded housing is defined analogously. In the paper (Acevedo-Garcia 2000) it is argued that these factors may have an *indirect* effect on the transmission of tuberculosis. Aspects of *segregation* that may act *directly* are described by factors that are defined along the same lines: isolation (contact with members of the same ethnic group), contact with immigrants and concentration (partial and total density, e.g. per square kilometre).

As the author remarks, an epidemiologic study can be analysed in two ways. The first, usual, route is regression, which means starting from the exposure variables and finding their relative contribution to the outcomes. The second method, which she employs here, focuses on the outcomes first and tries to identify *configurations* of risk factors that favour a given outcome. Outcomes are categorized as *no, low, high* and *very high* tuberculosis incidence. Risk factors are dichotomized in order to define configurations as in Boolean algebra. For each outcome category and each ethnic group, the frequency of ZIP areas that display a certain configuration among all ZIP areas in the same outcome category and ethnic group is given for several important configurations. This allows comparisons between outcome categories and reveals in some cases significant differences, too lengthy to be described here.

In a similar vein, the cross-sectional study by (Tellez et al. 2006) involves a blend of individual-level and community-level risk factors. The outcome is caries severity. From the start, only African-American families in Detroit, MI, USA who live in neighbourhood clusters of essentially the same low-income status are considered. The study thus focuses on social factors other than poverty. After accounting for individual characteristics of persons, there is still significant variation between clusters. In particular, caries severity increases with a higher number of grocery stores and decreases with a higher number of churches.

We close this section with an example of a community study of a very different kind, namely by mathematical modelling (see Chapter 12). For a change, this work showed that a particular behaviour of an outcome variable was *not* the result of the influence of a certain social factor contrary to what had been suspected. Mosse and Tugendreich (1913) quote a study from Denmark that described a periodicity of the incidence of syphilis with a period of around 16 years and suggest that this might be due to a corresponding periodicity of socio-economic factors. Similar periodicities were observed later in other countries too. This lead to a long controversy until Grassly et al. (2005) showed that the underlying cause was in fact the dynamics of building up immunities within the population.

6.9 Surveys on the Literature

In the year 2004, two expository articles appeared that might guide the reader further through the meanders in our field. The first one (Myer et al. 2004) although restricted to South Africa, is particularly interesting and useful by presenting the history, by referring to concrete settings and by critically analysing the basic issues. It concerns non-infectious as well as infectious diseases; however, given the context of South Africa, the latter play indeed the main role.

The survey by Poundstone et al. (2004) covers only HIV infections but mentions most facets of modern social epidemiology of infectious diseases in general. In particular, it reviews attempts to establish categories of social determinants. Thus, one might distinguish *individual*, *social* and *structural* level factors. Social-level factors fall into one of the categories: *cultural context*, *social networks*, *neighbourhood effects* and *social capital*. However, it is not always clear for which units of study they are defined.

In contrast to these two surveys, the purpose of the article by Justin et al. (2007) is not to provide an overview, nor to evaluate or analyse. It counts and compares the number of papers or citations devoted to such and such subject during such and such period between 1966 and 2005 as found by various search strategies. There is even a p-value for a hypothesis of the type “the number of citations has increased”!

6.10 Discussion

The idea that social factors and in particular social injustices influence the state of health is, for infectious diseases, very old and particularly prominent. However, it is precisely for infectious diseases that it cannot easily be formulated in exact terms and supported by correct studies. The reason may be found in the complex dual aetiology of infectious diseases. On the one hand, there is the main, and necessary, factor, which is the infection by the pathogen. Within and between given populations, it may follow complicated ways of transmission. On the other hand, there are many more factors including social ones, both on a person and a population level, and they interact with each other in addition to influencing the process of infecting individual persons and the circulation of pathogens in populations. Social factors are tied to environmental, lifestyle and iatrogenic ones. Moreover, behaviour is to some extent conditioned by genetic structures as we are discerning now in a more and more precise manner. Some of these many determinants may also act directly on certain infectious diseases. Thus it is not easy to isolate the action of a given social factor and to eliminate numerous possible confounders.

We have seen that on the eve of the First World War the study of social risk factors for infectious diseases using simple person-based concepts and models had already made much progress. It placed the individual into the centre of interest; typical risk factors were income, profession and housing. Population-based notions appeared only in very elementary forms, and mostly derived from person-based ones.

A fresh impetus came only much later, partly under the influence of work on non-infectious diseases (Cassel 1976; Marmot et al. 1991; Marmot and Wilkinson 1999; Chandola and Marmot 2005). In some countries, research in this area had also been hampered by political pressure when a field like social epidemiology was suspicious and notions like social class and social injustice amounted to heresy; see Leibfried and Tennstedt (1980) for Germany during the Nazi regime and Krieger (1994) for the United States during the McCarthy era.

The fundamental idea underlying all of modern epidemiology of investigating the influence of factors by comparing the outcomes for different levels, or values, of these factors is still valid. However, the emphasis has now shifted to social factors of a much more complex structure, belonging, for example, to the categories *social networks, social environments* and *social capital;* see Badura (2006) for a survey. They are mostly defined for populations and hard to quantify. It is not easy to translate ideas on the pathways along which they act alongside the transmission mechanism into hypotheses that can be tested. Mathematical modelling of the flow of infections in relation to social factors is also difficult. In this area, most of the work is still to be done; the studies that we have presented are just first attempts.

6.11 Implications for Public Health Policy

The general conclusions to be drawn from observations on social determinants of diseases, and in particular infectious ones, are old, and may nowadays appear almost obvious. They amount to changing the social environment, eliminating absolute and reducing relative poverty and promoting education for the less well-to-do. In Great Britain, the Chadwick report of 1834 lead to the "Poor Law Amendment

Act" (Rosen 1993, p. 176). An even more outspoken report of the Poor Law Commission appeared in 1842 (Rosen 1993, p. 187). In Germany, Virchow's conclusions (Virchow 1848) were quite explicit and insisted in particular on the disastrous effects of the lack of instruction, which he attributed in part to the Catholic Church. In the United States, the City Inspector of the New York Board of Health, John C. Griscom, published a study in 1845 on the sanitary conditions of the "labouring population" as factors that should be changed in order to improve the health situation (Rosen 1993, p. 213).

However, alleviating poverty and raising the level of education depend on political willingness and is everywhere a slow process with many ups and downs even where it is explicitly declared a goal to be attained. Thus, in the first place, progress in fighting infectious diseases has come from public hygiene, in particular sewage disposal, clean water supplies, and food control, and from vaccination programmes. The social factor "instruction" played an indirect role in the form of health education, which led to better personal hygiene. To some extent, the studies mentioned above also contributed to exerting pressure for eliminating the worst excesses in crowded and unhealthy living quarters. Later on, the general improvement of living standards such as housing, nutrition and working conditions certainly played a role in reducing morbidity and mortality by infectious diseases although it is hardly possible to quantify this effect.

Implications of insights into the action of more *specific* social factors are a matter of the recent past and sparse. They concern, for example, *screening* and *prevention*, and here some studies have led to actions that had not been obvious from the beginning. This is particularly true for AIDS. Thus, the study by Lurie et al. (2003) described in Section 6.7 gave rise to the recommendation to extend preventive measures to the wives of migrant workers. The report on trends of AIDS incidence and prevalence in Uganda (Green et al. 2006) discusses and compares general preventive strategies that had been influenced by the knowledge of the action of social factors. The studies on social risk factors for tuberculosis described in Section 6.8 also lend themselves to applications both to surveillance and prevention. Thus Ferreira Antunes and Alves Waldman (2001) deduce from their results a reduced effectiveness of certain existing control programmes.

References

Acevedo-Garcia, D. (2000) Residential segregation and the epidemiology of infectious diseases . Soc. Sci. Med. 51, 1143–1161

Acevedo-Garcia, D. (2001) Zip code-level risk factors for tuberculosis: Neighborhood environment and residential segregation in New Jersey, 1985–1992. Am. J. Public Health 91, 734–741

Badura, B. (2006) Social capital, social inequality, and the healthy organization. In: Noack, H. and Kahr-Gottlieb, D. (eds.), Promoting the public's health. The EUPHA 2005 conference book, Verlag für Gesundheitsförderung, Gamburg, 53–60

Bourdieu, P. (1979) La distinction. Editions de Minuit, Paris

Cassel, J.(1976) The contribution of the social environment to host resistance. Am. J. Epidemiol. 104, 107–123

Chandola, T. and Marmot, M. (2005) Social epidemiology. In: Ahrens, W. and Pigeot, I. (eds.), Handbook of Epidemiology. Springer, Berlin Heidelberg, 893–916

Cox, D. and Wermuth, N. (1996) Multivariate Dependencies: Models, Analysis and Interpretation. Chapman & Hall, London

Dony, J.F., Ahmad, J. and Khen Tiong, Y. (2004) Epidemiology of tuberculosis and leprosy, Sabah, Malaysia. Tuberc. (Edinb.) 84 (1–2), 8–18

Ferreira Antunes, J.L. and Alves Waldman, E. (2001) The impact of AIDS, immigration and housing overcrowding on tuberculosis deaths in Sao Paulo, Brazil, 1994–1998. Soc. Sci. Med. 52, 1071–1080

Grassly, N.C., Fraser, F. and Garnett, G.P. (2005) Host immunity and synchronized epidemics of syphilis across the United States. Nature 433, 417–421

Green, E.C., Halperin, D.T., Nantulya V. and Hogle, J.A. (2006) Uganda's HIV prevention success: The role of sexual behavior change and the national response. AIDS Behav. 10 (4), 335–346

Hobdell, M.H., Oliveira, E.R., Bautista, R., Myburgh, N.G., Lalloo, R., Narendran, S. and Johnson, N.W. (2003) Oral diseases and socio-economic status (SES). Br. Dent. J. 194 (2), 91–96

Justin, M. C., Wilson, M.L. and Allison, E.A. (2007) Analysis of social epidemiology research on infectious diseases: historical patterns and future opportunities. J. Epidemiol Community Health 61, 1021–1027

Kark, S.A. (1949) The social pathology of syphilis in Africans. S. Afr. Med. J. 23, 77–84

Kistemann, T.h., Munzinger, A. and Dangendorf, F. (2002) Spatial patterns of tuberculosis incidence in Cologne (Germany). Soc. Sci. Med. 55, 7–19

Krickeberg, K. (2007) Principles of health information systems in developing countries. Health Inf. Manag. J. 36 (3), 8–20

Krieger, N. (1994) Epidemiology and the web of causation: Has anyone seen the spider? Soc. Sci. Med. 39, 887–903

Krieger, N. (2001) Theories for social epidemiology in the 21st century: an ecosocial perspective. Internat. J. Epidemiol. 30, 668–677

Leibfried, S, and Tennstedt, F. (1980). Berufsverbote und Sozialpolitik 1933. Die Auswirkungen der nationalsozialistischen Machtergreifung auf die Krankenkassenverwaltung und die Kassenärzte. 2nd. Ed. Series: Arbeitspapiere des Forschungsschwerpunktes Reproduktionsrisiken, soziale Bewegungen und Sozialpolitik, University of Bremen, Bremen

Levy, A., Fraser, D., Vardi, H. and Dagan, R. (1998) Hospitalizations for infectious diseases in Jewish and Bedouin children in southern Israel. Eur J Epidemiol 14 (2), 179–186

Lurie, M., Williams, B.G., Zuma, K.D.K., Mkaya-Mwamburi, D. et al. (2003) Who infects whom? HIV-1 concordance and discordance among migrant and non-migrant couples in South Africa. AIDS 17 (15), 2245–2252

Marmot, M.G., Smith, G.D., Stansfeld, S., Patel, C., North, F., Head, J., et al. (1991) Health inequalities among British civil servants: the Whitehall II study. Lancet 337(8754), 1387–1393

Marmot, M.G. and Wilkinson, R.G. (1999) Social Determinants of Health. Oxford University Press, Oxford

Mosse, M. and Tugendreich, G. (eds.), (1913) Krankheit und soziale Lage (Disease and social condition). Lehmanns, München. Reprinted 1981 WiSo Med, Göttingen, 3rd Ed.

Murray, C.J.L., Lopez, A.D., and Mathers, C.D. (2004) The global epidemiology of infectious diseases. WHO global burden of disease and injury series 1, WHO, Geneva

Myer, L., Ehrlich, R.I. and Susser, E.S. (2004) Social epidemiology in South Africa. Epidemiol. Rev. 26, 112–123

DinhP.N., LongH.T., TienN.T.K., HienN.T., Mai Le T.Q., Phong LeH., Tuan LeV., Van TanH., NguyenN.B., Van TuP. and PhuongN.T.M. (2006) Risk factors for human infection with avian influenza A H5N1, Vietnam, 2004. Emerg. Infect. Dis. 12 (12), 1841–1847

Poundstone, K.E., Strathdee, S.A. and Celentano, D.D. (2004) The social epidemiology of human immunodeficiency virus/Acquired immune deficiency syndrome. Epidemiol. Rev. 26, 22–35

Rosen, G. (1993) A history of public health. Expanded Edition. The John Hopkins Press, London

Susser, M. (2001) Glossary: causality in public health science. J. Epidemiol. Community Health 55, 376–378

Tellez, M., Sohn, W., Burt, B.A. and Ismail, A.I. (2006) Assessment of the relationship between neighborhood characteristics and dental caries severity among low-income African-Americans: a multilevel approach. J. Public Health Dent. 66 (1), 30–36

Virchow, R. (1848) Mittheilungen über die in Oberschlesien herrschende Typhusepidemie (Informations on the present typhoid fever epidemic in Upper Silesia). Archiv für pathologische Anatomie und Physiologie und für klinische Medizin II (1–2)

Zahraoui-Mehadji, M., Baakrim, M.Z., Laraqui, S., Laraqui, O., El Kabouss, Y., Verger, C., Caubet, A. and Laraqui, C.H. (2004) Infectious risks associated with blood exposure for traditional barbers and their customers in Morocco [in French]. Santé 14 (4), 211–216

Chapter 7
Molecular Typing and Clustering Analysis as a Tool for Epidemiology of Infectious Diseases

Sylvia M. Bruisten and Leo Schouls

7.1 Introduction

This chapter describes the mechanism of typing procedures of human pathogens and gives some examples to substantiate the added value of typing and clustering analysis in epidemiology. Three steps need to be discerned in the process toward molecular clustering analysis. First, the pathogen must be recognized and identified (the diagnostic step). Second, the typing of the pathogen genome is performed and third, the clustering of the specific type with other known or newly identified types is needed for added epidemiological information.

For many infections, public health services monitor the transmission pattern of a disease and the possibility of outbreaks by performing active case finding (see Chapter 8). The ensuing data of both the index patients and their (possible) contacts are entered in local or central databases or in national registries. Traditionally, epidemiological data are obtained by subjecting patients to structured questionnaires – filled out by either themselves or by trained nurses or other public health workers. Studies of pathogen dissemination that rely solely on these self-reported behavioral data can yield incomplete or incorrect information. For example, for sexually transmitted infections (STI), the sensitive nature of the questions inhibits truthful answers. Nevertheless, identification of high-risk populations to whom prevention and intervention should be tailored is essential in infectious disease control. In the last decades, additional possibilities have emerged for contact tracing and for establishing patterns of transmissions of certain pathogens by using molecular typing techniques. Classical epidemiological data and the typing data should be analyzed together to interpret the data (Tenover et al. 1995). These typing tools work only for those cases in which the pathogen itself can be recovered from the infected person, which introduces a bias with respect to behavioral data. Molecular typing also requires genetic polymorphism within a species. Polymorphism will arise because pathogens adapt to different environments. For example, bacteria have

S.M. Bruisten (✉)
Cluster Infectious Diseases, Public Health Service of Amsterdam, Amsterdam, The Netherlands
e-mail: sbruisten@ggd.amsterdam.nl

A. Krämer et al. (eds.), *Modern Infectious Disease Epidemiology*,
Statistics for Biology and Health, DOI 10.1007/978-0-387-93835-6_7,

to cross barriers for initial colonization, and subsequent survival requires specific virulence traits that are subject to variation. Characterization of the polymorphic traits and subsequent cluster analysis should reveal if distinct types or clusters of strains are associated with particular disease manifestations, for example, in the case of the "hamburger bacterium," *Escherichia coli* type O157:H7 (Noller et al. 2006). Another example is the different serovars of *Chlamydia trachomatis* with diverse disease manifestations such as the ocular serovars A and B, the urogenital serovars C–F, and the lymphogranuloma-causing serovar L (Klint et al. 2007; Spaargaren et al. 2005; Hamill et al. 2007). Strains and clusters can, however, also be associated with distinct host risk groups, as was shown to occur for hepatitis A virus (Tjon et al. 2007). Typing may also aid to identify the source of an infection (person to person or environmental) and in case of a hospital (nosocomial) infection, typing can be used to assess preventative measures and treatment. In addition, typing may help to assess the effects of human intervention, such as antimicrobial treatment or vaccination, on the composition of the pathogen population.

Molecular methods are increasingly applied to aid the control of infectious diseases, both for detection and for typing of the pathogen. For detection purposes, the polymerase chain reaction (PCR) has a crucial role, but other nucleic acid amplification techniques are also increasingly used. Molecular typing and subsequent storage of this molecular data, as well as clinical and epidemiological data in libraries, can be helpful in identifying transmission routes within and among populations.

Typing is helpful in individual cases for

a. aiding in source tracing to elucidate whether there is transmission from patient to patient or from an environmental source to patient
b. revealing phenotypical properties of the pathogen: drug resistance, infectivity, virulence
c. assessing treatment effectivity: relapse or possible reinfection
d. identifying sampling and laboratory errors

Typing is helpful for public health issues:

e. Libraries help to decide which isolates belong to a nosocomial or a community-acquired outbreak
f. Vaccination issues: does the (live) vaccine strain cause disease or is it the wild-type pathogen?
g. Intervention efficacy: do strains mutate and escape treatment or vaccination?

Epidemic and endemic clones need to be recognized and their geographical spread should be informative about the nature of the outbreak. Nowadays, several techniques for typing of pathogens are available. In this chapter, we introduce these typing methods and discuss their value for providing additional epidemiological information.

7.2 Attributes for Successful Typing

Typing methods not only should be practical but also need to be highly standardized to facilitate (inter)national comparison and data exchange. Ideally, typing methods should be easy to perform, rapid, reliable, highly discriminatory, and suitable for large-scale and widespread use (van der Zee et al. 1999). Reproducibility is also of great importance, because variation in typing results of samples repeatedly taken from the same person should ideally reflect biological variation due to different sampling sites or different time points of sampling, and not technical variation. Another important characteristic of typing is the discriminatory power that depends on both the variation of the typing marker used within the pathogen population and the typing procedure itself. Different formulas based on Simpson's index of diversity are in use to calculate this discriminatory power (Blanc 2004; van Belkum 2007).

Phenotypic typing methods such as biotyping (e.g., the ability to ferment certain sugars), serotyping (reactivity with type-specific antibodies), phage typing (sensitivity for bacteriophages), antibiogram typing (determining the resistance of a panel of antibiotics), and multilocus enzyme electrophoresis (MLEE) generally show less discriminatory power than do genotypic methods. In addition, the phenotypic characterization may vary due to variations in growth conditions. Genotypic methods encompass both fragment-based (i.e., PFGE, PCR–RFLP, AFLP, VNTR) and sequence-based methods (i.e., MLST, Spa typing, microarray).

In bacteria, and also in other microbes such as viruses, fungi or parasites, genetic variations can be divided into three categories (Arnold 2007):

a. Small local changes in the nucleotide sequences (single nucleotide polymorphisms or SNPs)
b. Intragenomic rearrangements (including insertions, deletions, and duplications)
c. Acquisition of DNA sequences from other microorganisms or even from other living beings such as the host (horizontal gene transfer and recombination)

A small glossary is added at the end of this chapter. It contains definitions of terms used here.

7.3 Genotyping Methods

7.3.1 Plasmid Typing

One of the oldest methods to genotypically characterize bacteria is plasmid profiling (Snipes et al. 1989). Such methods have proven to be particularly useful if there is suspicion of dissemination of a particular resistance gene or set of genes (Singh et al. 2006). However, as plasmids are mobile genetic elements, they cannot be easily used in epidemiological linking studies.

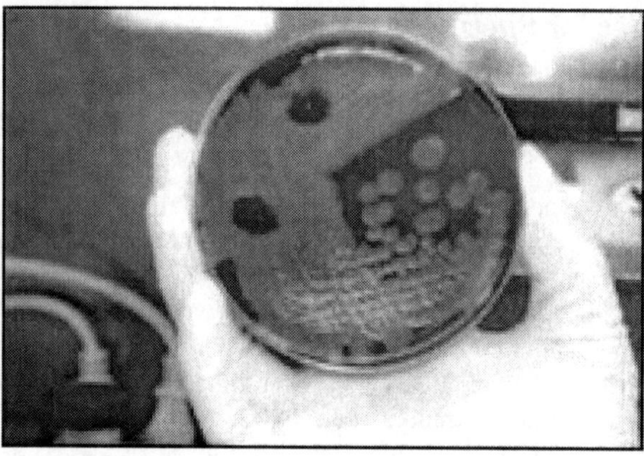

Fig. 7.1 Bacterial culture to obtain an isolate (from Wikipedia website, http://en.wikipedia.org/wiki/Microbiological_culture). A culture of *Bacillus anthracis*

The fragment-based typing (FBT) techniques mostly apply to bacteria and can be subdivided into those that make use of sequence variation in the total genome and those that target particular genes or repeat elements. For both approaches it is usually required that the bacteria are first cultured on agar or in broth to start with pure cultures (Fig. 7.1). This will ensure that ample DNA is available. If the typing needs to be performed directly on patient samples, specific PCR amplification usually precedes or is part of the typing procedure. For the principle of PCR, see the website http://users.ugent.be/~avierstr/principles/pcr.html

Fragment-based methods are relatively simple to perform and rather inexpensive. However, the discriminatory power and the reproducibility, especially between laboratories, can vary extensively.

7.3.2 RFLP, PFGE, and Ribotyping

In the last few decades a typing technique called restriction fragment length polymorphism (RFLP) has been used extensively to characterize bacterial isolates. In RFLP, total bacterial DNA is isolated from pure cultures and cleaved with restriction enzymes that recognize short double-stranded sequences. The generated fragments are separated on gels and in the early applications of this technique the patterns were visualized by staining. However, due to the complexity of the bacterial genomes, this technique yields hundreds of bands, too many to use for reliable typing. Therefore, these banding patterns are often simplified by hybridizing the separated fragments with specific DNA probes. A "probe" is an oligonucleotide with a sequence that is known to be complementary to the generated fragment. To accomplish this, the DNA bands are transferred from the agarose gel onto a membrane and used for hybridization. This technique is called Southern blot hybridization or DNA fingerprinting (Snipes et al. 1989). For many bacterial pathogens the ubiquitous but specific *16S rRNA* genes are used as probes (ribotyping), for example, for MRSA, enterococci, and *Mycobacteria.* The *16S rRNA* gene is usually present in several copies in the bacterial genome. For example, in *E. coli* there are seven copies, and as a result the complex banding pattern of hundreds of bands is reduced to only seven bands, making comparison easier and much more reliable. It is important to realize that in ribotyping and other RFLP-based variations in banding, the profiles are caused by insertions, deletions, and inversions of relatively large segments of DNA and by simple mutations in the restriction enzyme recognition sequence. Often a high degree of polymorphism is associated with repetitive DNA elements. Members of the mycobacterium complex (for example), can be typed very well using insertion sequences (IS) such as the IS6110 element (Arnold 2007; (Reisig et al. 2005; van Embden et al. 1993). The variable number (0–25) of IS6110 copies are dispersed over the mycobacterium genomes and they can be detected by hybridization with specific DNA probes. The IS6110 typing has been proven to be reliable and reproducible within a laboratory if highly standardized protocols for DNA isolation, restriction analysis by gel separation, and hybridization are used (van Embden et al. 1993; Behr and Mostowy 2007). However, exchange of DNA profiles for inter-laboratory comparison is difficult. For example, for tuberculosis outbreaks in Houston, Texas, a US metropolitan area with very high case rates, studies were performed using combined molecular typing with IS6110-based fingerprints, classical epidemiology, and network analysis to reconstruct an outbreak network (Klovdahl et al. 2001). A network is defined as a set of nodes connected together by links of one kind or another. The data were also used to quantify the relative importance of different actors (persons and places), which played a role in the tuberculosis outbreak, showing that the majority of the cases were men who had sex with other anonymous men. These homosexual men were thus proven to be part of a large outbreak and without the IS6110 typing data, their links would have remained uncovered (Klovdahl et al. 2001).

Another widely used approach to reduce the number of bands for RFLP analyses is a typing method called pulsed-field gel electrophoresis (PFGE). In PFGE the extracted whole genome bacterial DNA is digested by restriction enzymes that recognize rare cutting sites (Snell and Wilkins 1986). For example, the restriction enzyme *HindIII* cuts the *Staphylococcus aureus* genome into more than 1,000 fragments (as was used for ribotyping of MRSA). In contrast, the restriction enzyme *SmaI* which is used for PFGE, yields only approximately 25 fragments (Fig. 7.2). These DNA fragments obtained with a rare cutting enzyme are very large (50–100 kb), too large for conventional gel separation. Using special electrophoresis equipment (CHEF, Clamp) with alternating electrical fields, these large fragments can be separated very reproducibly with typical running times of 30–50 hours. PFGE is still considered the gold standard technique for the typing of bacterial strains as it can assist in establishing clonal relationships. However, PFGE is technically demanding and the interchangeability of typing patterns among laboratories is limited because small technical variations in electrophoresis conditions result in different banding patterns.

Fig. 7.2 Example of a PFGE gel

Dendrogram of PFGE pattens of 31 isolates of *S. aureus* from Dutch patients. MRSA, methicillin resistant *S. aureus*; MSSA, methicillin sensitive *S. aureus*

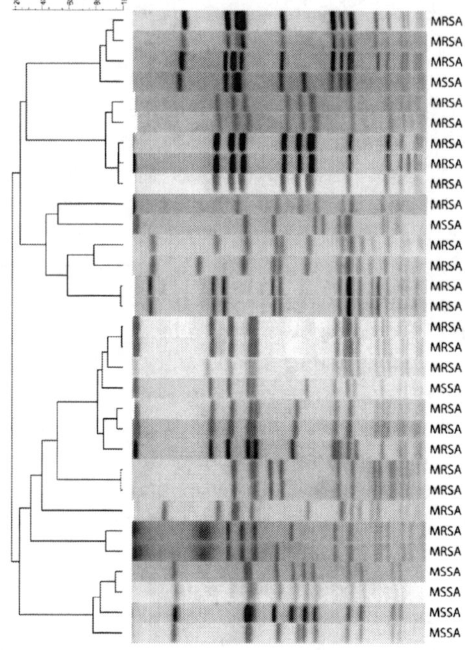

7.3.3 PCR–RFLP

Using PCR-based typing has the advantage that typing can be performed even if very little DNA is available. In some cases where culture of the pathogen is impossible, PCR–RFLP may provide the only method to characterize the agent. However, in most cases it is still necessary to first culture the pathogen to have sufficient pure starting material. In PCR–RFLP, a specific genomic part (a gene or an intergenic region) is amplified and the PCR product is subsequently cleaved with certain restriction enzymes (as in RFLP). The cleaved PCR products are either visualized on gels or separated with an automated sequencer in the fragment analysis mode. The idea is then to screen for the presence of different restriction recognition sites by comparing banding patterns. Only a part of the genome is now used for typing and care should be taken to choose an informative part in order to have a high discriminatory power.

7.3.4 RAPD and AP-PCR

For outbreaks, and particularly for nosocomial outbreaks, it is essential to have typing results at short notice, and for this purpose a "quick and dirty" typing technique

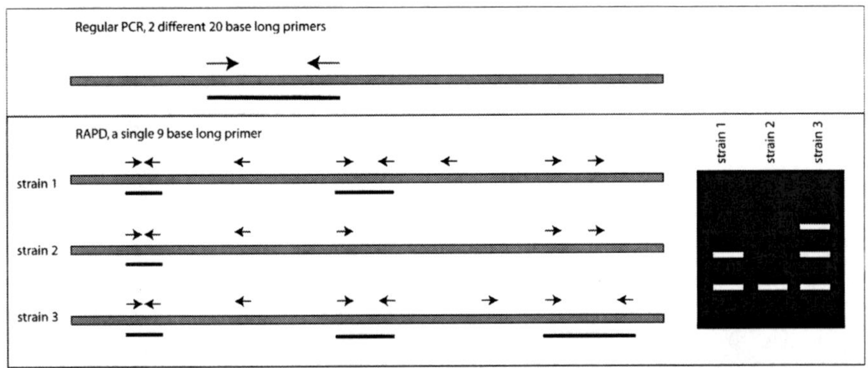

Fig. 7.3 Principle of RAPD. Lines in *below arrows* show PCR products for different strains 1, 2, and 3. The accompanying (*white*) bands on the (*black*) gel are shown for each strain

is available, termed the random amplified polymorphic DNA (RAPD) or the arbitrarily primed PCR (AP-PCR) (Williams et al. 1990). RAPD requires the availability of pure DNA from cultures, however, and the isolation and purification of DNA is a step that limits the speed of typing. Short nonspecific oligonucleotides (8–12 nucleotides) are used to serve both as forward and as reverse primer to generate random PCR products. Informative AP-PCR typically yields a number of PCR products ranging from 300 to 2500 base pairs that can be visualized on agarose gels (Fig. 7.3). In a multicenter study by van Belkum et al. (1995), the AP-PCR typing performance was assessed with respect to reproducibility and discriminatory power using 60 well-defined *Staphylococcus* strains (van Belkum et al. 1995). These *S. aureus* strains were collected at five documented outbreaks and also included sporadic cases. The DNA samples were centrally isolated and distributed to seven laboratories. Each laboratory used the same set of three random primers for AP typing but still, even in these controlled circumstances, the inter-laboratory variation was extensive. Although the outbreaks could be recognized in the resulting clusters as also established by PFGE, the general conclusion is that AP-PCR should not be used for *S. aureus* outbreak analysis if performed in different laboratories (Deplano et al. 2000; van Belkum et al. 1995). In general, the AP-PCR method is suited only for comparison of small numbers of isolates that are processed simultaneously. It is not suitable for longitudinal comparison, not even within the same laboratory (van Belkum et al. 2007).

7.3.5 AFLP

The benefits of RFLP and the sensitivity of PCR can be combined as was devised in amplified fragment length polymorphism (AFLP) (Vos et al. 1995). This high-resolution genomic fingerprinting method starts with purified pathogen DNA that is cleaved with two specific restriction enzymes. One of the two restriction enzymes, e.g., *MseI,* yields many small fragments and the other, e.g., *EcoRI*, yields relatively few, larger fragments (Koeleman et al. 1998). After the cleavage with the restriction enzymes, two types of synthetic oligonucleotides (linkers), one that fits at the *MseI* cut end and the other that fits only at the *EcoRI* end, are ligated ("collated") onto the PCR fragments. Subsequently, PCR amplification with two different primers that hybridize either of the two linkers is performed and the primer that anneals with the *EcoRI* linker carries a 5′-fluorescent label. Using AFLP, only those small fragments that are cut by *MseI* at one end and by *EcoRI* at the other end are amplified and visualized. The resulting PCR products ranging from 50 to 500 base pairs are separated on an automated DNA sequencer. It is also possible to use "selective" primers; these primers contain one extra nucleotide at their 3′-end which limits the number of PCR fragments formed, thereby further reducing the complexity of the profile. AFLP was also used for typing members of the *Mycobacterium tuberculosis* complex and many polymorphic markers for the different subspecies were identified (van den Braak et al. 2004). Although AFLP yields a high-resolution typing technique, interpretation of profiles is notoriously difficult due to the variation in the intensity of bands. This problem is caused by the variation in ligation and PCR. As a result, inter-laboratory exchange of AFLP data is virtually impossible.

Comparison of typing performance of AP-PCR (= RAPD), PFGE, and AFLP was described in a study of nosocomial outbreaks of Legionnaires disease in Germany (Jonas et al. 2000). *Legionella pneumophila* strains were obtained from both patient bronchoalveolar lavages and environmental sources. All three typing procedures found one predominant genotype that was associated with the hospital outbreaks. The discriminatory power differed however, with AP-PCR being the least and AFLP the most discriminating method. Because of this, and its simplicity and reproducibility, Jonas et al. concluded that AFLP was the most effective typing technique (Jonas et al. 2000). Of course this is open to debate and always depends on the epidemiological questions that need to be answered.

7.3.6 MLVA

The last fragment-based typing technique described here is called MLVA and is based on the variation in the number of tandem repeats. Tandem repeat loci are made up of two or more identical or nearly identical short DNA sequences that are not interspersed with any intervening DNA sequence. Tandem repeats are the result of errors of the DNA polymerase, which incorrectly copies these segments by a mechanism called slipped strand mispairing. The DNA polymerase stumbles in certain regions in the genome and as a result some DNA regions are duplicated or deleted. This malfunction of the DNA polymerase may happen several times and will cause some regions to be multiplied several times and the size of these tandem repeat units may range from 3 to 100 bp. These stutter regions result in variation in the number of repeats; hence their name "variable number of tandem repeats" (VNTR) loci (van Belkum et al. 1998). See also Fig. 7.4.

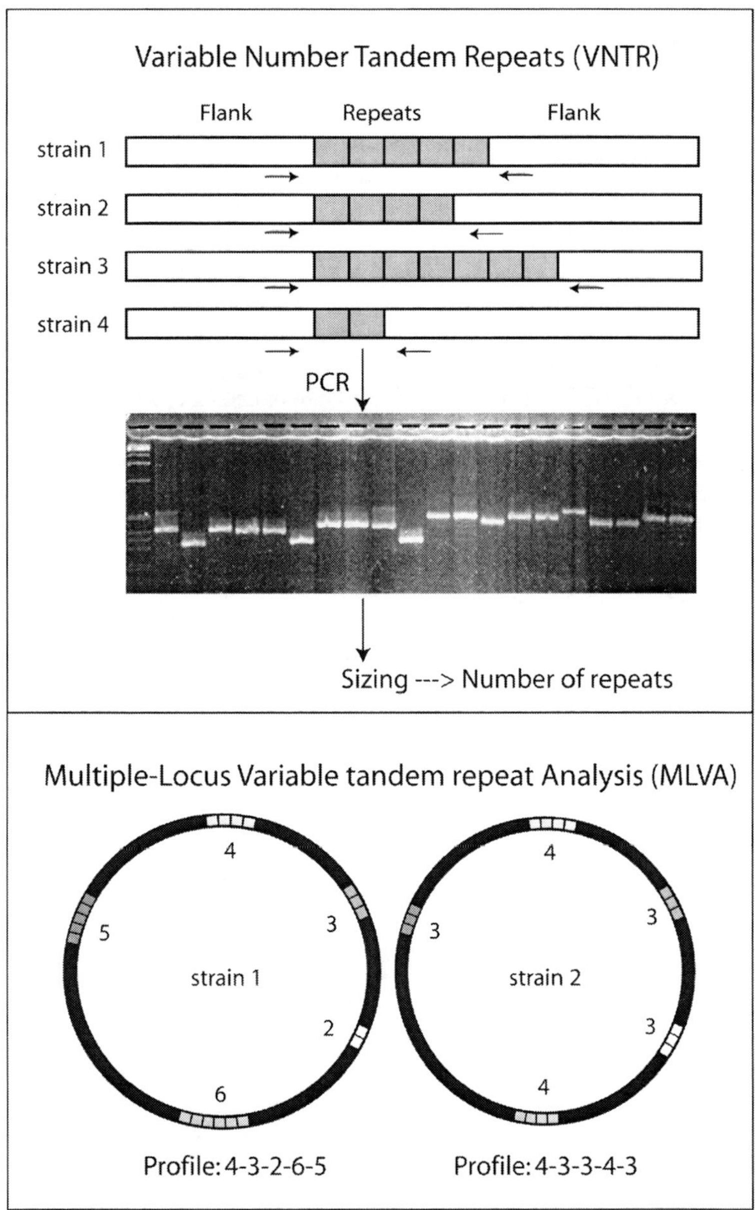

Fig. 7.4 Variable number of tandem repeats (VNTRs). VNTRs are polymorphic DNA sequences composed of different numbers of a repeated "core" sequence arranged sequentially. The size of the core sequence can vary from 8 to 100 bp in different VNTRs, and the number of repeats present at a VNTR locus also varies widely. Although many different VNTRs have been identified in genomes of both human and pathogen origin, their function is not currently known

The polymorphism in repeat loci is utilized in a typing method called multiple-locus VNTR analysis (MLVA) (Fig. 7.4). MLVA is a method that utilizes variation in 4–15 regions of tandemly repeated DNA in the genome (van Belkum et al. 2007). By performing PCRs spanning these repeats, the size of the product can be assessed by gel electrophoresis or by sequencing analysis. From the PCR product size, the number of repeats can be deduced. By combining the number of repeats of several repeat loci, a multidigit, specific strain code is obtained and these profiles can be used for clustering analysis. The use of automated DNA sequencers to perform the sizing of the PCR product makes MLVA a very reliable method and the numerical nature of the data makes it suitable for inter-laboratory exchange. The first published study on the use of MLVA was in 1993 and in this study, van Belkum et al. used the variation in various VNTR loci of *Haemophilus influenzae* (van Belkum et al. 1994). For *Mycobacteria*, MLVA (MIRU, mycobacterium interspersed repeat units-VNTR) was successfully used to type members of the tuberculosis complex (van Deutekom et al. 2005; Behr and Mostowy 2007). Given its technical simplicity, MLVA may have a successful future as it performed well compared to other genotyping methods for a variety of bacterial species so far (Schouls et al. 2006; Schouls et al. 2004; Lindstedt 2005; Francois et al. 2005; Noller et al. 2006).

Many fragment-based typing techniques are available today and for some purposes it may be needed to combine typing techniques to provide answers. For example, IS 6110 typing for TB characterization may not be discriminatory if less than five IS6110 copies are present. In TB typing studies, combinations of IS6110, spoligotyping (see below), MIRU-VNTR, and/or AFLP were used (Bauer et al. 1999; van Deutekom et al. 2005; Behr and Mostowy 2007).

7.4 Hybridization Arrays

7.4.1 Spoligotyping

Spoligotyping is an acronym for *sp*acer *oligo typing* and is a variation of the reverse line blot hybridization technique (Kamerbeek et al. 1997). In reverse line blotting, oligonucleotide probes are bound covalently to a membrane in parallel lines and hybridized with biotin-labeled PCR products in parallel lines, perpendicular to the oligonucleotide lines (Fig. 7.5). The intersections of the lines, where PCR products hybridize, are visualized by enhanced chemiluminescence. This generates easy to read fingerprints that are comparable to barcode patterns. For example, spoligotyping is used as a technique that analyzes a genomic region present in *M. tuberculosis* where virtually identical 36-bp direct repeats are interspersed with unique 35–40-bp spacer regions. Primers that recognize the direct repeats are used to amplify the direct repeat region including the spacer sequences between these variable repeats (Fig. 7.5). The resulting mixture of PCR products is used in a reverse line blot hybridization using immobilized spacer-specific oligonucleotide probes (Kamerbeek et al. 1997). Because some MTC members such as *M. leprae* are not cultivable, spoligotyping is of general use for all MTC members. The

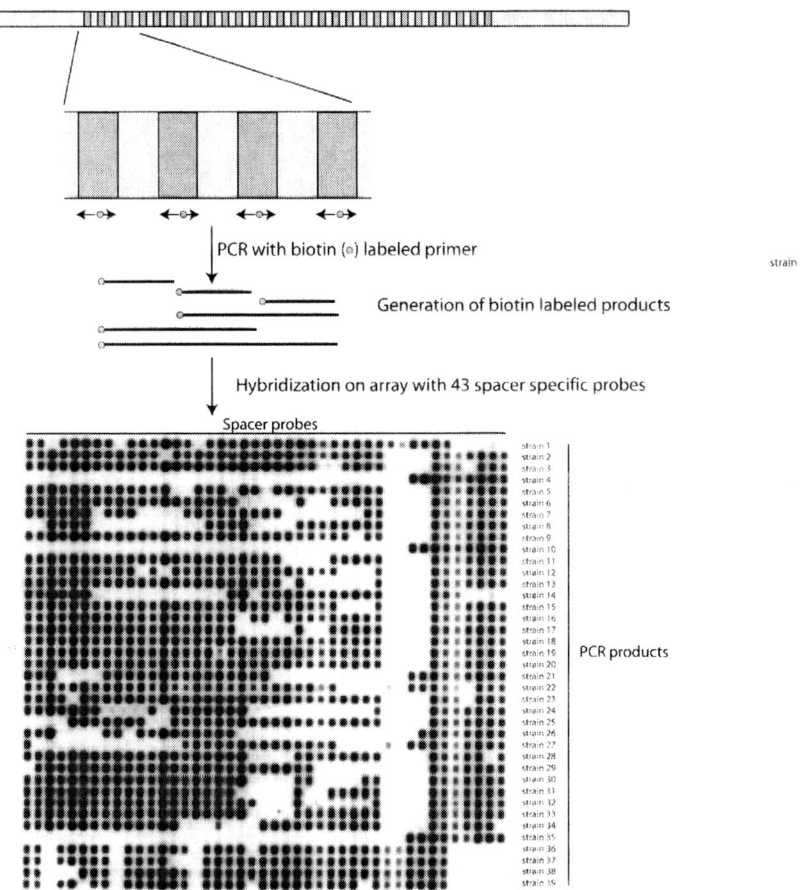

Fig. 7.5 Spoligotyping. Spacer oligonucleotide typing (spoligotyping) is a molecular method used to differentiate, for example, *M. tuberculosis complex* isolates. This method is based on the analysis of polymorphisms in the *M. tuberculosis complex* direct repeat (DR) chromosomal region consisting of identical 36-bp DRs alternating with 35-to 41-bp unique spacer sequences. The method is PCR based and is hence more rapid and easier to perform than the standard typing technique based on IS6110 profiling. Spoligotyping can also be performed directly from *M. tuberculosis* organisms, even those that are nonviable or that are found in tissues in paraffin-embedded blocks or in archeological samples

discriminative power of spoligotyping for typing MTC is lower than that of IS6110 fingerprinting (Kremer et al. 2005; van der Zanden et al. 2002). However, Bauer et al. found spoligotyping to be very useful to discriminate low copy number IS6110 MTC strains in Denmark, where tuberculosis caused by this type of strain increased in the last decade, supposedly due to influx of immigrants with tuberculosis (Bauer et al. 1999).

7.4.2 Microarrays

Microarray analysis can be used to perform full-length typing of genomes, even of large bacterial or parasitic genomes. Whole genome arrays detect the presence or the absence of similar DNA regions in sufficiently related microorganisms, allowing genome-wide comparison of their genetic contents (Garaizar et al. 2006). In this technique, called comparative genomic hybridization (CGH), fluorescently labeled genomic DNA of a microorganism is hybridized with a very large collection of DNA probes fixed on a solid support. The probes can be PCR products or synthetic oligonucleotide probes that are usually about 70 base pairs in length and are mostly specific for all the open reading frames (ORFs or genes) present in the bacterial genome of interest. The probes, which are designed based on the strain from which a genome sequence is available, can be deposited on support materials such as nitrocellulose membranes, but mostly glass slides are used. The latter support material permits the deposition of up to 10^4–10^5 probes. Differences between strains are expressed as the presence or the absence of genes that are present in the indicator strain, i.e., the strain from which the probe sequences were derived. If short oligonucleotide probes are used, it is also possible to detect single nucleotide polymorphisms (SNPs), for which probes covering over 10^5 polymorphisms can be used in a single hybridization, permitting excellent discrimination between different strains of a species (Garaizar et al. 2006). The major drawback of CGH is that only already known genes are tested. New genes, not present in the strain used to design the microarray, will never be detected. The costs for the microarray technology are relatively high, for the time being too expensive for routine typing.

7.5 Sequence-Based Typing (SBT) Analysis

In recent years, DNA sequence-based typing has started to replace the fragment-based typing methods because SBT has fewer problems with reproducibility and portability. DNA sequence data have the major advantage that they are unambiguous and independent of the method used to obtain the DNA sequence. This has resulted in portable methods that yield robust data that are highly suitable for inter-laboratory exchange.

Viral genomes are rather small compared to bacterial genomes. For example, the hepatitis B virus (HBV) genome is only around 3,200 base pairs in size and the hepatitis A virus (HAV) is 7,500 base pairs in size. Typing viral pathogens is often performed by sequencing parts of the genome (either coding/genes or non-coding). The sequenced regions need to be polymorphic to discriminate within a species. Choosing regions that are conserved will not give enough discriminatory power and regions that are highly variable will lose the link in the dissemination chain, making them unsuitable for epidemiological purposes. The discriminatory power has to be assessed by first validating the chosen region. Suitable genetic regions are, for example, genes or parts thereof that encode surface structures, such as the S-gene in HBV and the VP genes in HAV. Variability in genes encoding surface structures is mostly caused by the selective immune pressure of the host. Too much variability would not be suitable for clustering analysis, with every infected host having its own strain of virus. On the other hand, choosing genomic regions that are too conserved in sequence will yield very large clusters, linking persons who never were in contact. To find out which level of variation suits the epidemiological questions best, it is absolutely required to validate the typing method by linking it to sound classical epidemiological information.

7.5.1 SLST

This "single-locus sequence typing" (SLST) was found useful in molecular epidemiological studies of hepatitis A, B, and C viruses in our laboratory and some examples are given below in the paragraph dealing with cluster analysis. For hepatitis B virus, an international database HepSEQ is accessible at http://www.hpa-bioinfodatabases.org.uk/hepatitis/main.php

In recent years, single-locus sequence typing has also been used to type bacterial pathogens. One of the currently best known pathogens for which SLST has been utilized is *S. aureus* and in particular methicillin-resistant *S. aureus* (MRSA). In *S. aureus* the gene encoding the immunoglobulin G–binding protein A contains a tandem repeat region that is variable both in number of repeats and in the DNA sequence of these repeats. In the so-called Spa-(*Staphylococcal protein A*) sequence typing, a PCR product encompassing the repeat region is sequenced and the sequence is used to create profiles representing the composition of the repeat region (Harmsen et al. 2003). This results in the assignment of Spa types, each of which has its own Spa profile. As an example, Spa type t073 has an Spa profile of r08r16r02r16r13r17r34r16r34. The profile shows that this Spa type contains nine tandem repeats and in addition the composition of the specific repeats. In the given profile, for instance, r08 represents the sequence **G**A**G**GAAGAC**AA**CAACAA**G**CCTGGT and r16 is similar to this but differs at the positions in bold **A**A**A**GAAGAC**GG**CAACAA**A**CCTGGT. Currently more than 200 different repeat sequences and nearly 3,500 Spa types have been identified in the *S. aureus* genomes.

7.5.2 MLST

For bacteria the best known sequence-based typing is *m*ulti*l*ocus *s*equence *t*yping (MLST) in which the DNA sequence of a set (mostly seven) of housekeeping genes is determined by sequencing polymorphic 400–500 base pair segments of each of these genes. Housekeeping genes are encoding components that are essential for the bacterium (Maiden et al. 1998). As a result these genes are always present and change only slowly over time. In MLST each of the resulting housekeeping gene sequences is assigned an allele number. Allele numbers are consecutive numbers that have been assigned to the sequence variants of each housekeeping gene and thus do not reflect the degree of similarity between alleles. Each strain can be characterized as a sequence type (ST), representing an allelic profile, which is an ordered string of allele numbers separated by dashes, e.g., ST-100 in *Neisseria meningitidis* represents allelic profile 6-6-9-1-26-36-32. MLST is a portable, unambiguous, and highly discriminating genotyping system that can be used for many bacterial species and even for some other microorganisms such as *Candida albicans*. However, some bacterial species, e.g., *M. tuberculosis*, are too clonal, rendering MLST useless as a typing technique. Although the availability of pure cultures is required to perform MLST, isolation and purification of DNA are not. The major disadvantages of the MLST are its labor-intensive nature and the high costs associated with sequencing. In order to characterize a single isolate, one needs to perform seven PCRs and subsequently 14 sequence analyses (two directions per PCR product). The MLST approach has been successful for the unambiguous characterization of isolates of many bacterial species and other microorganisms and a number of libraries can be accessed over the Internet (www.mlst.net, website visited November 2007).

7.5.3 Whole Genome Sequencing

MLST allows clustering of isolates using an unambiguous DNA sequence and has been a major step forward in genotyping methodology. However, seven gene sequences obtained with MLST for *L. pneumophila* represent only 0.1% of the total genome. Increasingly the full-length DNA sequences of organisms, particularly of bacterial species, are being determined. Many of these sequences are available in the public domain, e.g., in GenBank:

http://www.ncbi.nlm.nih.gov/sites/entrez

At the time of the writing of this chapter, 634 microbial genomes have been completely sequenced and are available online

http://www.ncbi.nlm.nih.gov/sites/entrez and

http://www.integratedgenomics.com

Sequencing of another 965 microbial genomes is in progress and the number will rapidly expand due to the fact that new high-throughput sequencing methods have become available. It is now possible to sequence a complete bacterial genome within a week's time. Comparison of complete genome sequences is the ultimate genotyping method. However, costs of sequencing a complete bacterial genome are still too high to use this ultimate form of genotyping.

7.5.4 SNP Genotyping

Single nucleotide polymorphisms (SNPs) can be used successfully for genome-wide typing. It involves the determination of the nucleotide base that is known to be variable at a defined position in the genome in a given isolate. It is a more efficient typing method than full genome sequencing not only because of lower costs to perform but also because the results can be easily shared by different users if standard sets of SNPs per pathogen are analyzed (van Belkum et al. 2007). Variable positions useful for typing must have been discovered prior to the application of SNP genotyping. Once a set of SNPs has been selected, different SNP genotyping methods such as Sanger sequencing or pyrosequencing can be applied. Newer methods are being developed at a fast pace, for example, mini-sequencing and Luminex technology (van Belkum et al. 2007; Syvanen 2005; Dunbar 2006). Mini-sequencing uses primers and a mixture of all four dideoxynucleotides, each with their specific fluorescent label. Each primer borders an SNP region and is extended by only a single base, and the incorporated base can be discriminated by fluorescence after capillary electrophoresis. In pathogens with highly homologous genomes, such as *E. coli* O157:H7, *M. tuberculosis*, *Salmonella enterica* serotype Typhi, and *Bacillus anthracis*, SNP genotyping methods can be very helpful to quickly discriminate them (van Belkum et al. 2007).

7.6 Cluster Analysis

Epidemic histories can be assessed by constructing phylogenetic trees and subsequent cluster analysis. In a phylogenetic tree, or dendrogram, groups can be assigned by distinguishing clusters defined by a distance measure, such as the percentage nucleotide difference (which is a crude distance measure). These clusters are then, by consensus, defined as specific genotypes. For a conserved sequence region (i.e., for HAV), a genetic distance of >15% may indicate different genotypes, but genetic differences between 15 and 5% indicate different "sub-genotypes" (in case of HAV: 1A and 1B). So, clusters may represent either (sub)-genotypes or even groups of strains with less genetic distance between them.

In general, to use typing information for answering epidemiological questions, information collected in libraries needs to be structured by performing cluster analysis. To determine which of the ensuing strains are found in a particular outbreak, or a specific high-risk group, it is necessary to combine clinical and conventional epidemiological information with the typing data. To this end, different clustering of the genetic typing data must be performed based on the variation of genetic distance measures. Then the resulting clustering structure has to be compared to epidemiological data and analyzed for corresponding structural properties. For example, if a very fine genetic distance measure is used to define clustering, only small clusters will be found. These small genetic differences would have arisen by chance, as mutations occur at all times in all genomes of living beings, but they may also reflect pressures of the host immune response, generating polymorphism between source and contact strains. However, a small genetic distance that reflects only one or two mutations may point to the presence of the same epidemic strain. A clustering based on a coarser distance measure might be able to bring larger epidemiological structures to the foreground, such as transmission clusters that connect cases within a specific risk group.

Algorithms are needed to construct clusters starting from an available typing library. The BURST algorithm (http://eburst.mlst.net/) first identifies mutually exclusive groups of related genotypes in the population (typically an MLST

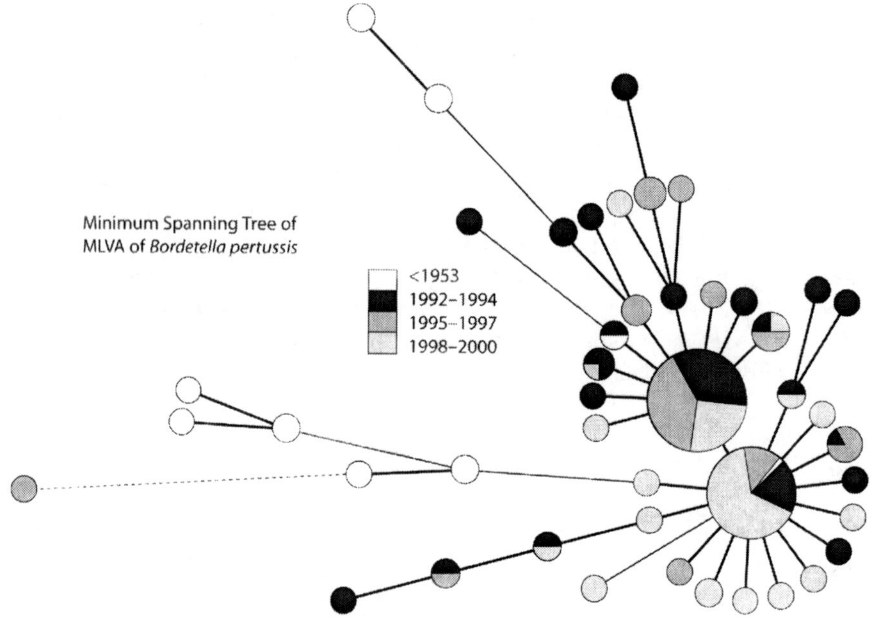

Fig. 7.6 Minimum spanning tree. Example for *B. pertussis*, the causative agent of whooping cough

database) and attempts to identify the founding genotype (sequence type or ST) of each group. The algorithm then predicts the descent from the founding genotype to the other genotypes in the group, displaying the output as a radial diagram, centered on the predicted founding genotype. The presentation of such a grouping is called a minimum spanning tree (MST) and software packages are available to construct these MSTs. In Fig. 7.6 the size of the circles corresponds to the amount of strains; colors may indicate certain properties of strains or their hosts.

The MSTs may depict either single-locus variations (the profile varies at one locus) or dual-locus variations (the profile varies at two loci), by connecting the circles. The MST procedure is based on an old algorithm that has been adapted for clustering character-based data such as MLST and MLVA.

7.6.1 Cluster Analysis for Nosocomial and Community-Acquired Outbreaks

Community-acquired outbreaks can be studied using previously built databases that contain typing data connected to epidemiological data. A database such as PulseNet for foodborne infections proved very successful in aiding source tracing and pointing out reservoirs of infection. PulseNet participants perform standardized molecular subtyping by pulsed-field gel electrophoresis to distinguish foodborne disease-causing bacteria such as *E. coli* O157:H7, *Salmonella*, *Shigella*, *Listeria*, or *Campylobacter* (website: http://www.cdc.gov/pulsenet/). The PulseNet network initially started in 1996 in the United States, but nowadays these PFGE-based databases have been developed and made accessible also in Canada, Latin America, Japan, and Europe (http://www.pulsenet-europe.org/) and in other parts of the world.

Viral foodborne infections by noroviruses, which cannot be cultured, are widespread. An example of the additional use of typing is given in Koek et al. (Koek et al. 2006). In this study, we describe the molecular epidemiology of a group of nine outbreaks associated with a catering firm and two outbreaks, 5 months apart, in a hospital in Amsterdam, the Netherlands. All outbreaks were typed to confirm their linkage, and the hospital-related cases were studied to see if the two outbreaks were caused by one persisting norovirus strain or by a reintroduction after 5 months. For the outbreaks associated with the catering firm, one norovirus genogroup I strain was found which was identical in sequence among customers and employees of the caterer. This was not the strain that predominantly circulated in 2002/2003 in and around Amsterdam, which was the norovirus genogroup II4 "new variant" (GgII4nv) strain. In the Amsterdam hospital, the two outbreaks were caused by this predominant GgII4nv type, and we argue that NV was most likely reintroduced in the second outbreak from the Amsterdam community.

7.6.2 Cluster Analysis and Linkage to Risk Groups

From DNA sequences it is possible to create phylogenetic trees and to determine the reliability of the tree branchings by bootstrapping. Bootstrap values >90% indicate that a (sub)cluster can be discerned with a high probability. This way of typing and clustering is mostly used for viruses with rather small genomes.

7.6.2.1 Human Immunodeficiency Virus

The structure of sexual contact networks can be reconstructed from interview data and in some cases this provided valuable insights into the spread of the infection. For HIV-1 however, the long period of infectivity and the anonymous sexual contacts made the interpretation very difficult, producing discrepancies in the networks. Using viral genotype data from large sets of HIV-1 *pol* and *gag* sequences, which were initially collected to monitor therapy resistance to antivirals, enabled Lewis and colleagues recently to derive the network structure of HIV-1 transmission among homosexual men in London (Lewis et al. 2008; Pilcher et al. 2008). Nine large clusters were discerned on the basis of genetic distance. Dated phylogenies with a molecular clock-like calculation indicated that 65% of the HIV-1 transmissions took place between 1995 and 2000 and that 25% occurred within 6 months after infection. The quantitative description, also called "phylodynamics" (Grenfell et al. 2004), is important for parametrization of epidemiological models and in designing intervention strategies (Lewis et al. 2008).

Many HIV phylogeny studies have been published and others are still in progress. A recent Chinese study is informative for the use of phylogenies in typing sequences from HIV-1-infected drug users in the Yunnan Province, which borders Myanmar and Tibet, countries known to be involved in illegal drug transports (Zhang et al. 2006). Recombinant circulating HIV-1 strains of types BC and AE were found to circulate codominantly among the 321 HIV-1-infected and analyzed persons. The type BC strain was strongly associated with intravenous drug behavior, whereas the type AE strain was mainly sexually transmitted. This last type AE appears to be on the rise and forms a threat to the general population. Aids education and prevention efforts in the general population are therefore urgently needed (Zhang et al. 2006).

7.6.2.2 Hepatitis A Virus

Clustering analysis in hepatitis A epidemiology is given in Tjon et al. 2007. In Amsterdam, the Netherlands, the patterns of introduction and transmission of hepatitis A virus (HAV) were investigated from 2001 to 2004 and HAV strains were divided according to two risk groups: (1) travelers and their contacts, who were most often infected with HAV subgenotype 1B strains, and (2) homosexual men and their contacts, who were shown to have subgenotype 1A strains. Among travelers many sporadic cases were found, and the clusters were small and limited in time but introduced frequently into the population, mostly in the second half of each calendar year, indicating a seasonal pattern of introduction and transmission after the summer holidays. These introductions were especially by Dutch children from parents originating from hepatitis A-endemic countries, like Morocco. Among men who have sex with men (MSM), the clusters were bigger and remained present for a longer time; sporadic cases were few, and introduction of new strains occurred only occasionally but throughout the year. Our findings indicate that travelers frequently import new HAV strains into Amsterdam, but they are limited in the extent and season of their spread. In contrast, HAV is endemic among the male homosexual and bisexual population, and the same strain spreads to many individuals without a seasonal pattern.

Large outbreaks of hepatitis A have also occurred elsewhere in Europe affecting MSM in countries such as Denmark, Germany, Norway, Spain, Sweden, and the United Kingdom during the period 1997–2005. An international collaboration was formed between these countries to determine if the strains involved in these outbreaks were genetically related. Part of the genetic regions coding for HAV capsid genes were sequenced and compared. The majority of the HAV strains found among homosexual men from different European countries formed a closely related cluster, named MSM1, belonging to genotype IA. Different HAV strains circulated among other risk groups in these countries during the same period, indicating that specific strains were circulating among MSM exclusively. Similar strains found among homosexual men from 1997 to 2005 indicate that these HAV strains have been circulating within this group for a long time. The homosexual communities across Europe are probably large enough to sustain continued circulation of HAV strains for years, resulting in an endemic situation among MSM (Stene-Johansen et al. 2007).

7.6.2.3 Neisseria gonorrhoeae

Bacterial typing also needs validation of cluster formation. In London and Sheffield, UK, sexual links were described and compared among people with gonorrhea, caused by the sexually transmitted *N. gonorrhoeae*. Most cases concerned homosexual men and fewer female sex workers. In Sheffield, large, linked heterosexual networks identified were associated with local contacts but the networks in London were more difficult to trace back, due to anonymous contacts (Day et al. 1998). Subsequently, the use of gonococcal *opa* typing, based on the polymorphisms of the *opa* genes, suggested a highly connected population in Sheffield where almost 80% of cases had shared profiles. In London the *opa* typing could also link infections that would otherwise have remained unlinked, and typing may thus aid interventions to control endemic gonorrhea (Ward et al. 2000). In Amsterdam, the Netherlands, *N. gonorrhoeae* strains were also collected for several years and patients were subjected to a questionnaire pertaining to sexual risk behavior and sexual partners in the 6 months prior to the diagnosis (Kolader et al. 2006). The *N. gonorrhoeae* isolates were all genotyped using PCR–RFLP of the *porin* and *opa* genes. There were 11 clusters of ≥ 20 patients; in seven clusters, almost all patients were MSM, three clusters contained mainly heterosexual men and women, and one cluster was formed by equal proportions of MSM and heterosexual male and female patients. However, the various clusters also differed in characteristics such as types of coinfections, numbers of sexual partners, Internet use to seek sexual partners, and locations of sexual encounters. Molecular epidemiology by typing of gonococcal isolates thus revealed core groups and clusters of MSM and heterosexual patients that probably indicate distinct transmission networks (Kolader et al. 2006).

7.6.2.4 Methicillin-Resistant *S. aureus*

An example of the additional use of clusters containing different sequence types (STs) as defined by MLST is given here for methicillin-resistant *S. aureus* (MRSA). MRSA originated through the transfer of the mobile resistant determinant staphylococcal cassette chromosome *mec* (SSC*mec*) into sensitive *S. aureus* isolates. Community-associated (CA) MRSA have been reported all over the world. The prevalence of MRSA is less than 1% in the Netherlands because of the "search and destroy" policy in hospitals affected with MRSA. In the case where two indiscriminate isolates are found, costly measures are taken such as very strict hygiene, cohorting of patients and staff in hospitals, closing of wards, and postponing or rescheduling surgery. All those in contact with the index patients are screened for MRSA carriage. Quick typing results are required to save time and money to keep the Dutch prevalence low. The MRSA prevalence in hospitals is much higher, however, in surrounding countries such as the United Kingdom, France, and south European countries, with prevalences up to 30%. Since 2003 a new clone of CA MRSA has been found in farm animals (pigs and veal calves) and in humans in direct contact with these animals (Voss et al. 2005). The first recognized case with pig MRSA was a six-month-old girl who was found MRSA positive in a Dutch hospital. She was the daughter of a pig farmer (Huijsdens et al. 2006). In a still ongoing outbreak in the Netherlands and Belgium, this MRSA strain was found to be "untypeable" by PFGE, which was considered to be the gold standard typing procedure. PFGE failed to give adequate answers because the *SmaI* enzyme could not cleave the DNA derived from outbreak-associated SA strains. Spa (Staphylococcus protein A) typing (see above) and MLST showed that strains of this MRSA clone belong to a number of closely related Spa types, all of which correspond to MLST ST-398 (Voss et al. 2005).

7.7 Limitations of Typing

The first limitation of molecular typing is that the specific nucleic acid content (usually the genome) of the pathogen is not always available for analysis. For example, in the case of whooping cough, the patient shows prolonged respiratory symptoms due to the toxins that were excreted by the etiological agent, the bacterium *Bordetella pertussis*. However, these symptoms often become apparent only after the pathogen itself was cleared by the time samples are taken, resulting in negative culture. People may carry the pathogen, but due to clearance or (partial) immunity the pathogen is present in such a low load that isolation does not succeed even though transmission may still occur.

There are several assumptions concerning the use of molecular typing techniques for the interpretation of outbreak data (Singh et al. 2006):

1. Isolates associated with an outbreak are of recent progeny of a single precursor or clone
2. All outbreak-associated descendants have the same genotype
3. Epidemiologically unrelated isolates have different genotypes

For frequently used techniques such as AP-PCR, PFGE and also AFLP, the reproducibility suffers inevitably because the electromobility of the DNA fragments varies between lanes in gels and between runs on separate days. But the variation between laboratories is even more extensive due to differences in DNA isolation procedures and the use of different gel instrumentation.

The major disadvantages of PFGE are the need for specific equipment, the complexity of performing the assay, and above all, the lengthy time to complete the results (van Deutekom et al. 2005). Nevertheless, the discriminatory power of PFGE is high, so replacing this technique will require at least the same index of discrimination. Also MLST clearly has its limitations. If housekeeping genes that do not show enough polymorphism are chosen, for example, in homomorphic, recently introduced pathogens, it may not be possible to separate outbreaks from other, sporadic, cases. Similarly, VNTR loci used for MLVA may be invariable or display hypervariability. The rate of change in the number of repeats may differ between the VNTR loci, influencing the stability of an MLVA pattern. For example, for *E. coli* O157:H7 (the hamburger bacterium), the TR2 locus showed a much higher degree of variation than the other six loci tested (Noller et al. 2006).

The microarrays are presently only sporadically used for typing because of the comparatively low availability of complete genome arrays and the high cost per reaction (Garaizar et al. 2006). Another limitation is that the genetic reservoir may be unstable. Mutations could arise even in clonal strains being induced during culture due to longer duration or temperature variation. Conventional assays such as PFGE or IS typing will not detect this because their discriminatory power is much less compared to full genome microarray analysis.

Typing guidelines have been described to decide when strains or isolates are indistinguishable (Tenover 1995; van Belkum 2007). It is clear however that these rules pertain to the typing method that was chosen because the underlying biological phenomena are not the same. In case of fragment-based typing, the absolute number of band differences or percentage similarity is often taken into account to define relatedness. The absolute number may differ with the possibility that more mutational events lead to less banding differences. The percentage similarity is independent of banding patterns but it is clearly influenced by the level of tolerance in band position. Therefore reference samples should be included in each analysis for normalization (for example, for PFGE). Sequence-based typing methods do not need such reference samples but the quality of the sequences has to be thoroughly checked (van Belkum et al. 2007).

It is important to realize that the genetic markers used for typing usually do not reflect the virulence of isolates. Some markers may be mere coincidental indicators for hypervirulent genotypes or genogroups. The results obtained by genotyping are often used as a starting point for further investigation into the pathogenic properties of subgroups of microorganisms.

7.8 Concluding Remarks

New molecular typing methods have substantially helped to better understand epidemiological observations. It must be emphasized however that typing results never stand alone and need to be interpreted in the context of all available demographical, clinical, and other epidemiological data (van Belkum et al. 2007). In general, the sequence or character-based typing techniques such as MLST and MLVA are superior in that their data can be documented unambiguously, allowing direct comparison of results between laboratories, and it is expected that these methods will prevail in the near future. The PCR-based nature of MLVA gives it a speed that is presently not matched by other typing techniques with equal reproducibility. The few handling steps make it amenable for complete automation and adaptable to future fragment separation techniques (Lindstedt 2005). The typing data are stored in publicly accessible databases or libraries on the Internet, which increasingly also contain epidemiologically relevant information. Building such databases relies on the standardization or at least the harmonization of typing methods (Harmony website: http://harmony-microbe.net/index.htm). A clean working hypothesis must be formulated to guide the choice of the typing method, since different questions may require answers with different levels of discriminatory power. Translating typing results into clinical practice is a very important endpoint of a typing exercise. Real-time typing may now be feasible, but next to speedy typing results, the feedback to all parties involved (in an outbreak) is of major importance. It is also essential that it is clear-cut what appropriate action is needed once indistinguishable isolates are encountered, as happens in the case of an outbreak. Thus, multidisciplinary work provides the basis for outbreak investigation, disease control, and pathogen surveillance.

Acknowledgment The authors wish to thank Prof. Dr. R.A. Coutinho for his valuable comments to improve the readability for non-laboratory trained persons.

Definitions

Adapted from (Tenover et al. 1995; van Belkum et al. 2007)

Isolate: An isolate is a pure culture of bacteria or virus from a primary patient sample. In the molecular era it may however also be a DNA sample isolated from the infected site containing the full genomic content of the pathogen.

Strain: A strain is an isolate or a group of isolates that can be distinguished from other isolates of the same genus and species by phenotypic or genotypic characteristics. A strain is a descriptive subdivision of a species.

Epidemiologically related strains: These isolates are cultured from specimens collected from patients or their excretions (feces, fomites), or from the environment during a discrete time frame, or from a well-defined (geographical) area as part of an epidemiologic investigation that suggests that the isolates may be derived from a common source.

Genetically related strains (clones): These isolates are (almost) indistinguishable from each other by one or a variety of genetic tests, supporting the suggestion that they are derived from a common ancestor.

Cluster or clonal complexClonal complexdefinition: The term cluster is used to indicate isolates with identical or highly similar DNA typing results (fingerprints) but also the group of persons (patients) from whom these isolates were derived.

Outbreak strain: Outbreak strains are isolates of the same species that are epidemiologically related *and* genetically related. Such isolates are presumed to be clonally related since they have common genotypes and phenotypes.

Epidemic strain: Isolates that are frequently recovered from infected patients in a particular health-care setting or community and that are genetically closely related, but for which no direct or epidemiologic relation can be established. Their common origin may be more temporally distant from those of outbreak strains.

References

Arnold C. (2007) Molecular evolution of Mycobacterium tuberculosis. Clin Microbiol Infect 13: 120–128

Bauer J, Andersen AB, Kremer K, and Miorner H (1999) Usefulness of spoligotyping To discriminate IS6110 low-copy-number Mycobacterium tuberculosis complex strains cultured in Denmark. J Clin Microbiol 37: 2602–2606

Behr MA, and Mostowy S (2007) Molecular tools for typing and branding the tubercle bacillus. Curr Mol Med 7: 309–317

Blanc DS. (2004) The use of molecular typing for epidemiological surveillance and investigation of endemic nosocomial infections. Infect Genet Evol 4: 193–197

Day S, Ward H, Ghani A, Bell G, Goan U, Parker M et al. (1998) Sexual histories, partnerships and networks associated with the transmission of gonorrhoea. Int J STD AIDS 9: 666–671

Deplano A, Schuermans A, Van Eldere J, Witte W, Meugnier H, Etienne J et al. (2000) Multicenter evaluation of epidemiological typing of methicillin-resistant Staphylococcus aureus strains by repetitive-element PCR analysis. The European Study Group on Epidemiological Markers of the ESCMID. J Clin Microbiol 38: 3527–3533

Dunbar SA (2006) Applications of Luminex xMAP technology for rapid, high-throughput multiplexed nucleic acid detection. Clin Chim Acta 363: 71–82

Francois P, Huyghe A, Charbonnier Y, Bento M, Herzig S, Topolski I et al. (2005) Use of an automated multiple-locus, variable-number tandem repeat-based method for rapid and high-throughput genotyping of Staphylococcus aureus isolates. J Clin Microbiol 43: 3346–3355

Garaizar J, Rementeria A, and Porwollik S (2006) DNA microarray technology: a new tool for the epidemiological typing of bacterial pathogens? FEMS Immunol Med Microbiol 47: 178–189

Grenfell BT, Pybus OG, Gog JR, Wood JL, Daly JM, Mumford JA, and Holmes EC (2004) Unifying the epidemiological and evolutionary dynamics of pathogens. Science 303: 327–332

Hamill M, Benn P, Carder C, Copas A, Ward H, Ison C, and French P (2007) The clinical manifestations of anorectal infection with lymphogranuloma venereum (LGV) versus non-LGV strains of Chlamydia trachomatis: a case-control study in homosexual men. Int J STD AIDS 18: 472–475

Harmsen D, Claus H, Witte W, Rothganger J, Claus H, Turnwald D, and Vogel U (2003) Typing of methicillin-resistant Staphylococcus aureus in a university hospital setting by using novel software for spa repeat determination and database management. J Clin Microbiol 41: 5442–5448

Huijsdens XW, van Dijke BJ, Spalburg E, van Santen-Verheuvel MG, Heck ME, Pluister GN et al. (2006) Community-acquired MRSA and pig-farming. Ann Clin Microbiol Antimicrob 5: 26

Jonas D, Meyer HG, Matthes P, Hartung D, Jahn B, Daschner FD, and Jansen B (2000) Comparative evaluation of three different genotyping methods for investigation of nosocomial outbreaks of Legionnaires′ disease in hospitals. J Clin Microbiol 38: 2284–2291

Kamerbeek J, Schouls L, Kolk A, van Agterveld M, van Soolingen D, Kuijper S et al. (1997) Simultaneous detection and strain differentiation of Mycobacterium tuberculosis for diagnosis and epidemiology. J Clin Microbiol 35: 907–914

Klint M, Fuxelius HH, Goldkuhl RR, Skarin H, Rutemark C, Andersson SG et al. (2007) High-resolution genotyping of Chlamydia trachomatis strains by multilocus sequence analysis. J Clin Microbiol 45: 1410–1414

Klovdahl AS, Graviss EA, Yaganehdoost A, Ross MW, Wanger A, Adams GJ, and Musser JM (2001) Networks and tuberculosis: an undetected community outbreak involving public places. Soc Sci Med 52: 681–694

Koek AG, Bovee LP, van den Hoek JA, Bos AJ, and Bruisten SM (2006) Additional value of typing Noroviruses in gastroenteritis outbreaks in Amsterdam, The Netherlands. J Clin Virol 35: 167–172

Koeleman JG, Stoof J, Biesmans DJ, Savelkoul PH, and Vandenbroucke-Grauls CM (1998) Comparison of amplified ribosomal DNA restriction analysis, random amplified polymorphic DNA analysis, and amplified fragment length polymorphism fingerprinting for identification of Acinetobacter genomic species and typing of *Acinetobacter baumannii*. J Clin Microbiol 36: 2522–2529

Kolader ME, Dukers NH, van der Bij AK, Dierdorp M, Fennema JS, Coutinho RA, and Bruisten SM (2006) Molecular epidemiology of Neisseria gonorrhoeae in Amsterdam, The Netherlands, shows distinct heterosexual and homosexual networks. J Clin Microbiol 44: 2689–2697

Kremer K, Arnold C, Cataldi A, Gutierrez MC, Haas WH, Panaiotov S et al. (2005) Discriminatory power and reproducibility of novel DNA typing methods for Mycobacterium tuberculosis complex strains. J Clin Microbiol 43: 5628–5638

Lewis F, Hughes GJ, Rambaut A, Pozniak A, and Leigh Brown AJ (2008) Episodic sexual transmission of HIV revealed by molecular phylodynamics. PLoS Med 5: e50

Lindstedt BA (2005) Multiple-locus variable number tandem repeats analysis for genetic fingerprinting of pathogenic bacteria. Electrophoresis 26: 2567–2582

Maiden MC, Bygraves JA, Feil E, Morelli G, Russell JE, Urwin R et al. (1998) Multilocus sequence typing: a portable approach to the identification of clones within populations of pathogenic microorganisms. Proc Natl Acad Sci USA 95: 3140–3145

Noller AC, McEllistrem MC, Shutt KA, and Harrison LH. (2006) Locus-specific mutational events in a multilocus variable-number tandem repeat analysis of Escherichia coli O157:H7. J Clin Microbiol 44: 374–377

Pilcher CD, Wong JK, and Pillai SK (2008) Inferring HIV transmission dynamics from phylogenetic sequence relationships. PLoS Med 5: e69

Reisig F, Kremer K, Amthor B, van Soolingen D, and Haas WH. (2005) Fast ligation-mediated PCR, a fast and reliable method for IS6110-based typing of Mycobacterium tuberculosis complex. J Clin Microbiol 43: 5622–5627

Schouls LM, van der Heide HG, Vauterin L, Vauterin P, and Mooi FR (2004) Multiple-locus variable-number tandem repeat analysis of Dutch Bordetella pertussis strains reveals rapid genetic changes with clonal expansion during the late 1990 s. J Bacteriol 186: 5496–5505

Schouls LM, van der Ende A, Damen M., and van de Pol I (2006) Multiple-locus variable-number tandem repeat analysis of Neisseria meningitidis yields groupings similar to those obtained by multilocus sequence typing. J Clin Microbiol 44: 1509–1518

Singh A, Goering RV, Simjee S, Foley SL, and Zervos MJ (2006) Application of molecular techniques to the study of hospital infection. Clin Microbiol Rev 19: 512–530

Snell RG, and Wilkins RJ (1986) Separation of chromosomal DNA molecules from *C. albicans* by pulsed field gel electrophoresis. Nucleic Acids Res 14: 4401–4406

Snipes KP, Hirsh DC, Kasten RW, Hansen LM, Hird DW, Carpenter TE, and McCapes RH (1989) Use of an rRNA probe and restriction endonuclease analysis to fingerprint *Pasteurella multocida* isolated from turkeys and wildlife. J Clin Microbiol 27: 1847–1853

Spaargaren J, Schachter J, Moncada J, de Vries HJ, Fennema HS, Pena AS et al. (2005) Slow epidemic of lymphogranuloma venereum L2b strain. Emerg Infect Dis 11: 1787–1788

Stene-Johansen K, Tjon G, Schreier E, Bremer V, Bruisten S, Ngui SL et al. (2007) Molecular epidemiological studies show that hepatitis A virus is endemic among active homosexual men in Europe. J Med Virol 79: 356–365

Syvanen AC (2005) Toward genome-wide SNP genotyping. Nat Genet 37 Suppl: S5–S10

Tenover FC, Arbeit RD, Goering RV, Mickelsen PA, Murray BE, Persing DH., and Swaminathan B (1995) Interpreting chromosomal DNA restriction patterns produced by pulsed-field gel electrophoresis: criteria for bacterial strain typing. J Clin Microbiol 33: 2233–2239

Tjon G, Xiridou M, Coutinho R, and Bruisten S (2007) Different transmission patterns of hepatitis A virus for two main risk groups as evidenced by molecular cluster analysis. J Med Virol 79: 488–494

van Belkum A, Duim B, Regelink A, Moller L, Quint W, and van Alphen L. (1994) Genomic DNA fingerprinting of clinical Haemophilus influenzae isolates by polymerase chain reaction amplification: comparison with major outer-membrane protein and restriction fragment length polymorphism analysis. J Med Microbiol 41: 63–68

van Belkum A, Kluytmans J, van Leeuwen W, Bax R, Quint W, Peters E et al. (1995) Multicenter evaluation of arbitrarily primed PCR for typing of Staphylococcus aureus strains. J Clin Microbiol 33: 1537–1547

van Belkum A, Scherer S, van Alphen L, and Verbrugh H (1998) Short-sequence DNA repeats in prokaryotic genomes. Microbiol Mol Biol Rev 62: 275–293

van Belkum A, Tassios PT, Dijkshoorn L, Haeggman S, Cookson B, Fry NK et al. (2007) Guidelines for the validation and application of typing methods for use in bacterial epidemiology. Clin Microbiol Infect 13 Suppl 3: 1–46

van den Braak N, Simons G, Gorkink R, Reijans M, Eadie K, Kremers K et al. (2004) A new high-throughput AFLP approach for identification of new genetic polymorphism in the genome of the clonal microorganism Mycobacterium tuberculosis. J Microbiol Methods 56: 49–62

van der Zanden AG, Kremer K, Schouls LM, Caimi K, Cataldi A, Hulleman A et al. (2002) Improvement of differentiation and interpretability of spoligotyping for Mycobacterium tuberculosis complex isolates by introduction of new spacer oligonucleotides. J Clin Microbiol 40: 4628–4639

van der Zee A, Verbakel H, van Zon JC, Frenay I, van Belkum A, Peeters M et al. (1999) Molecular genotyping of Staphylococcus aureus strains: comparison of repetitive element sequence-based PCR with various typing methods and isolation of a novel epidemicity marker. J Clin Microbiol 37: 342–349

van Deutekom H, Supply P, de Haas PE, Willery E, Hoijng SP, Locht C et al. (2005) Molecular typing of Mycobacterium tuberculosis by mycobacterial interspersed repetitive unit-variable-number tandem repeat analysis, a more accurate method for identifying epidemiological links between patients with tuberculosis. J Clin Microbiol 43: 4473–4479

van Embden JD, Cave MD, Crawford JT, Dale JW, Eisenach KD, Gicquel B et al. (1993) Strain identification of Mycobacterium tuberculosis by DNA fingerprinting: recommendations for a standardized methodology. J Clin Microbiol 31: 406–409

Vos P, Hogers R, Bleeker M, Reijans M, van de Lee T, Hornes M et al (1995) AFLP: a new technique for DNA fingerprinting. Nucleic Acids Res 23: 4407–4414

Voss A, Loeffen F, Bakker J, Klaassen C, and Wulf M (2005) Methicillin-resistant Staphylococcus aurcus in pig farming. Emerg Infect Dis 11: 1965–1966

Ward H, Ison CA, Day SE, Martin I, Ghani AC, Garnett GP et al. (2000) A prospective social and molecular investigation of gonococcal transmission. Lancet 356: 1812–1817

Williams JG, Kubelik AR, Livak KJ, Rafalski JA, and Tingey SV (1990) DNA polymorphisms amplified by arbitrary primers are useful as genetic markers. Nucleic Acids Res 18: 6531–6535

Zhang Y, Lu L, Ba L, Liu L, Yang L, Jia M et al. (2006) Dominance of HIV-1 subtype CRF01_AE in sexually acquired cases leads to a new epidemic in Yunnan province of China. PLoS Med 3: e443

Chapter 8
Epidemiologic Surveillance

Ralf Reintjes and Klaus Krickeberg

8.1 Introduction

Not every topic admits a precise definition but ours does:

Epidemiologic surveillance is the collection, transfer, analysis, and interpretation of information related to cases of diseases, which is done systematically and routinely.

Thus surveillance is to be distinguished from studies set up ad hoc in order to investigate a particular epidemiologic problem. In the present chapter, we restrict ourselves to surveillance of infectious diseases. The information may be in the form of *data* or of statistical *indicators* such as incidences or prevalences. Its *content* can be fairly wide. In addition to general data on infected persons and their diseases, there may be data on symptoms, serological and other laboratory data, data concerning pathogens recovered from patients and patients' behaviour, and information on the presence of vectors as well as on general risk factors.

Epidemiologic surveillance works in many ways but always within a well-defined *system.* Such a system consists of the sources of the information, the mechanisms for collecting and transmitting it, and procedures of analysis. Data originate in the first place in physicians' practices, hospitals, and other health facilities including laboratories, but additional information may flow from various other sources like statistical offices, health insurance, and vector surveillance. Mechanisms for collection, transmission, and analysis vary considerably – both by their organization and by the technical means employed. A surveillance system can operate on a local level, for example, in a city, or on a regional, national, or international scale.

Surveillance is used for monitoring the time trends in the occurrence and distribution of diseases in populations and of factors that may have an influence on them. Information derived from disease surveillance is used for policy decisions regarding immediate interventions, general health strategies, health management, and the structure of the health system. The discovery and management of disease outbreaks,

---

R. Reintjes (✉)
Department of Public Health, Hamburg University of Applied Sciences, Hamburg, Germany
e-mail: ralf.reintjes@haw-hamburg.de

A. Krämer et al. (eds.), *Modern Infectious Disease Epidemiology*,
Statistics for Biology and Health, DOI 10.1007/978-0-387-93835-6_8,

formerly also called "epidemic surveillance" and described in Chapter 9, is normally based on an existing system of routine surveillance supplemented by special investigations and interventions.

In the following sections, we look at the various facets of surveillance systems in a more detailed and concrete manner. After a short historical sketch (Section 8.2), technical issues (Sections 8.3, 8.4, and 8.5) and then, on this basis, the most important question, namely the objectives and applications of surveillance (Section 8.6), are discussed. Finally, some examples of specific surveillance systems are presented (Section 8.7) and some useful sources for further study indicated (Section 8.8).

8.2 History

Epidemiologic surveillance of infectious diseases is relatively young. It could indeed not exist before health authorities existed to whom reports would be made, which was hardly the case before the late 18th century (Rosen 1993, Chapter 5). An exception were the reports on mortality based on death certificates, which gave rise to the first health statistics in the 17th century, due to John Graunt (Rosen 1993, Chapter 4). In order to be comparable on a wide scale they necessitated an international classification of causes of death and later of general morbidity. This was initiated at the International Statistical Congress in 1853, then continued by the International Statistical Institute, and finally taken over by the World Health Organization (WHO) in the form of the present International Classification of Diseases (ICD).

Surveillance really got started with the obligation imposed on physicians and hospitals to report cases of "notifiable" communicable diseases to health authorities. The oldest notification system is the one in England and Wales, which began with the "Infectious Disease Act" of 1889.

Surveillance in the sense of the general definition stated at the beginning evolved only after World War II. The definition given by Langmuir (1963) and affirmed in 1968 at the 21st World Health Assembly still restricts its scope to "...the number of incident cases ...." The general concept appears in a paper by the Centers for Disease Control and Prevention (1986).

While the classical system of notifications was more or less the same all over the world as far as the basic ideas are concerned, the subsequent development took different forms in different countries. The form of their health systems determined that of their surveillance systems to a large extent. In centralized state-run health systems, one attempted to build all-embracing *health information systems* that consisted of regular, for example, monthly, reports from the basic health facilities upwards through the hierarchy of district health offices and provincial health departments to the Ministry of Health. In some countries, especially in the former or presently socialist ones, these systems were, or still are, quite elaborate; in others, in particular in the developing world, they often remain fairly rudimentary. In any case, in principle, they cover almost all aspects of activities, from consultations and treatments to preventive work, health education, and administrative and economic matters. Information on infectious diseases is just one part. Sometimes special subsystems were set up to deal with particular diseases such as tuberculosis, malaria, or AIDS; see, for example, the system in Vietnam (Section 8.7, below).

In comparison, surveillance in countries that have decentralized and mainly private health systems is usually organized in a much less systematic and comprehensive way. It consists of different parts constructed ad hoc for specific purposes.

8.3 Sources of Information

The main primary sources of data and of indicators are the following:

1. Persons and households.
2. Schools, workplaces, and similar institutions.
3. Population registers.
4. Death certificates.
5. Health facility records.
6. Health insurance records.
7. Laboratory records.
8. "Sentinel" records.
9. Monitoring reservoirs and evolution of vectors.

Let us elaborate a bit; examples are given in Section 8.7.

The first type of source, persons and households, is mostly exploited in special surveys and studies. Surveillance systems based directly on them are indeed rare because people cannot be expected to regularly file reports about their health situation to any authority. The only possible surveillance is the so-called active one (Section 8.5). In such a surveillance system, health officials pay routine visits to the sources in question in order to collect the information.

Schools, homes for the elderly, restaurants, factories, and other institutions are subject to epidemiologic surveillance in many countries. Again, in most cases, only active surveillance can work.

Population registers belong to routine demographic information systems that exist in some form in most countries. For example, in Europe, these systems often arose from registers of births, marriages, and deaths that were first kept by parishes. Nowadays birth and death registrations are almost universally integrated into the general civil administration.

Death certificates are ideally written by a physician and then forwarded either to a health administration or to the general civil administration or both. They normally contain information about the main, and sometimes about secondary, causes of death classified according to ICD-10 codes.

Health facility records are the main source of information. On the level of primary health care, there are, depending on the structure of the health system, patient records of the general practitioner or registers of consultations in a health station, in a polyclinic, or in the outpatient ward of a hospital. On the secondary and tertiary level, we have a multitude of documentations in hospitals. There are, for example, the classical books of entry and exit (discharge) of patients. Each ward has case registers, and often the hospital keeps a central, or master, index of patients. In industrialized countries, most hospitals routinely use centralized electronic hospital information systems, which integrate data from all of these sources.

Patient-based surveillance may also be restricted to a particular group of persons, for example, pregnant women or drug addicts.

Laboratories are, next to case notification and case reporting from health facilities, the most important source of information for infectious disease surveillance. They may be part of a polyclinic or a hospital, or independent. The normal independent laboratory serves the general practitioners and small clinics in its neighbourhood. In addition there are reference laboratories for special tasks on a national, regional, or global scale such as the various WHO reference laboratories. By their very nature, laboratories are obliged to keep precise records that are mostly case- or patient(person-) based.

A *sentinel* is an institution set up for the purpose of observing, recording, and reporting health-related information. It may be a small station, also called a surveillance site, built especially to this end. It can also be an already existing station that will be especially equipped or a single general practitioner designated for this task. Sentinels are practically always organized in the form of sentinel *networks*. Their function is to obtain needed information if getting it from the "normal" general surveillance system based on health facilities is impossible, or too expensive, or too slow. Sometimes, especially in developing countries, they function as a source for *integrated* surveillance that handles information of very varied nature and serves several purposes. Other sentinel surveillance systems may cover only a specific disease.

Instead of *fixed* sentinels, there is sometimes a scheme of taking *varying* samples from the target population. Some systems of sero-surveillance work like this (see Sections 8.5 and 8.7).

Sources of information on animal reservoirs, hosts, and vectors that may be relevant for observing and controlling infectious diseases vary very much depending on local conditions. There are many that work on a routine basis and thus enter into the realm of our definition of surveillance.

Every surveillance system is meant to monitor health-related information that concerns a certain *target population* or *target area* in which we are interested and that needs to be specified in advance, for example, all inhabitants of a given province of a certain country or a certain animal population. The question then arises whether the sources of information that we are actually using are *representative* of the entirety of existing sources in the habitual sense of statistics, i.e. up to an error that is considered acceptable. In the usual notification systems as well as in comprehensive health information systems, this is the case since *all* available sources are being taken into account, at least in theory. A sentinel system, however, is normally exploiting only a sample of sources. Hence it must include a statistical estimation of sampling errors, including those due to various biases. On the other hand, it may in fact yield more precise information, for example, in the form of indicators, because it is less prone to measuring errors when collecting data and usually also has more material and personnel at its disposal.

8.4 Form and Content of Information

Information transmitted within a surveillance system is either in the form of *individual data* or in that of *indicators* computed from a set of data.

Individual data concern, for example, single cases of a communicable disease to be reported in a notification scheme. Case definition is an integral and fundamental part of the scheme. In general, it follows the ICD-10, but in notifications from the primary level, the available laboratory facilities do not always suffice to distinguish, for example, between amoebic and bacterial dysentery. In addition to the tentative or confirmed diagnosis we might have data like place and time of the case, personal data of the patient and his contacts, and certain risk factors. Depending on the "target" disease, other data may need to be reported, for example, in the case of rabies a bite by a suspect animal.

Data from laboratories concern, among others, the results of diagnostic tests and more details about the infective agent obtained, e.g. by molecular typing (see Chapter 7).

We distinguish between *nominative* notifications, which allow the receiver of the information to identify the patient, and *non-nominative* ones.

Side effects of curative or preventive treatments are also usually reported in the form of data concerning individual cases. Other examples of data appear in the surveillance of animal populations, a current one being that of birds having been diagnosed with avian influenza H5N1 virus infection.

In *syndromic* surveillance, taken up in the following section, the information handled concerns observed symptoms and even more distant clues to the occurrence of cases such as sales of over-the-counter medication and ambulance rides.

However, most information treated within a surveillance system has the form of indicators concerning groups of people such as incidences, prevalences, mortalities, and case fatality rates. They are mostly derived from individual case records by *aggregation* (also called account consolidation in bookkeeping). This is particularly true for comprehensive health information systems, which, however, cover only fairly basic information. When deriving incidences or prevalences from reported results of laboratory tests, the question of the sensitivity, specificity, or predictive values of the tests used comes up.

In more specialized surveillance systems we find the statistics of other features of case management, for example, *compliance* with a certain drug treatment such as the "standard" or the "short" treatment of tuberculosis (Chapter 16), with a multi-drug treatment of an HIV infection (Chapter 18), or with oral rehydration of children dehydrated by diarrhoea (Chapter 17). Drug *resistances* of pathogens like those against antibiotics or against the current malaria treatments, and resistance of vectors against insecticides, are being reported in the form of individual or of aggregate data depending on circumstances. In *sero-surveillance*,, one deals with aggregate data on the immunity of human populations against vaccine-preventable diseases. There may also be indicators about the distribution of risk factors as in the *behavioural* (second generation) HIV surveillance (see Section 8.7).

8.5 Mechanisms of Surveillance

A surveillance system consists, in the first place, of methods for collecting information and then of procedures to transmit it to those who might analyse and use it. The analysis is sometimes already integrated into the system, at least in part. Let us look at the mechanisms for doing all of this.

Most of the relevant information is buried in some records kept at the sources listed above. The question is how to extract and transmit it. We distinguish two basic categories of methods: *passive* and *active* surveillance. In passive surveillance, information is taken from the records, sometimes processed locally by aggregation and then reported to those for whom it is meant, following established rules. The receivers, usually higher health authorities, do not intervene. This is the normal procedure in, for example, the notification of particular communicable diseases or the comprehensive health information systems mentioned in Section 8.2.

On the other hand, in active surveillance, those who are carrying it out have to collect the information by themselves. This may be done by routine telephone calls to "sentinel" practitioners as in the early European systems (Section 8.7) or by contacting clinics, hospitals, and laboratories regularly. Direct visits by health officials to health facilities also imply the many advantages of personal contacts. Another example is the active search for cases of chronic infectious diseases like tuberculosis, malaria, or leprosy, which is sometimes done systematically, especially in developing countries. Here, health workers visit households regularly, thus exploiting the source no. 1 listed in Section 8.3.

Naturally, passive surveillance requires as a rule fewer human and financial resources than does an active one, but the information transmitted is often full of gaps and marred by errors, and usually arrives slower except in very well-organized and automated systems. For ways to build efficient health information systems, see Krickeberg (2007).

One also distinguishes between *mandatory* surveillance on the one hand, also called *statutory* or *compulsory* surveillance, and *voluntary* surveillance on the other hand. In a mandatory system, the collection and transmission of information is regulated by laws and decrees. Most comprehensive health information systems as well as infectious disease notification systems are of this type.

The accessibility of data at the various sources is sometimes described by the *iceberg* metaphor. The emerging part represents the accessible information, which depends on the mechanism of surveillance. The classical iceberg phenomenon derives from the fact that cases appear in the registers of health facilities only if the patient had a contact with the health system. Furthermore, even when the patient sought medical care, his case may not have been diagnosed or diagnosed but not reported. In order to find the "hidden" cases, active surveillance may be used, and to estimate the "under water" prevalence, a sample survey in the population is needed. The immune status of populations is not monitored within the standard health facility-based surveillance and requires additional sero-surveillance.

When describing and distinguishing surveillance systems, the time dimension must also be taken into account. In *concurrent* surveillance, data is collected, recorded, and transmitted at the moment it originates or very shortly afterwards. The notification of certain communicable diseases falls into this category and more generally any surveillance that requires urgent action. Most surveillance is *retrospective*, although not over long time spans, by exploiting, for example, registers of consultations only weekly or monthly.

The means of *transmitting* information is part of the mechanisms of a surveillance system. Here, anything imaginable has been used. A voluntary health worker in a developing country may make regular oral reports to his communal health station. Mail is of course widely employed, but reports may be handed over as well at the occasion of routine meetings of health officials. Active surveillance is largely based on personal visits to the sources by those collecting data. The telephone is still an important tool whereas e-mail and Internet have replaced telegraph and telex.

As a second step in the surveillance mechanism, after the collection of indicators from the sources and some initial handling and transmission, so-called *health reporting systems* were organized recently in many places and on many levels, either locally, nationally, regionally (e.g. European), or globally (WHO). They take the information from existing basic systems, arrange it further, process it in a coherent fashion, analyse it, store it in the form of databases, and publish it in view of the various objectives to be enumerated in the following section. An example in the United States described by Pascual et al. (2003) is the reporting system on tetanus, which uses the Centers for Disease Control and Prevention (CDC) notification system as its basis. More common are reporting systems that concern several diseases, in fact both infectious and non-infectious ones, founded on various bases. The description of the system of the WHO (WHO Data and Statistics 2008) lists many national systems in addition. For Europe, see Europa – Public Health-Health Information (2008).

By "spatial surveillance", one refers to a system where data and indicators include geographical information, for example, about a case, an incidence, or a finding of a pathogen, and where spatial analysis is essential in the evaluation; see Chapter 10 and the book by Lawson and Kleinman (2005). Similarly, if both the location and the time of every registered case are recorded and if this data is entered into the analysis, one speaks of "spatio-temporal surveillance".

Fairly recently, the term "syndromic surveillance" has entered the arena to designate one more scheme for reporting and analysing data from health facilities. It is, in fact, both very old and very new. It is old because often, especially in developing countries, diagnoses are recorded and reported that base themselves exclusively on some clinical symptoms, i.e. on a clinical syndrome. Incidences are computed and published on this base. Such a syndromic surveillance ought to include correction methods in order to derive estimates of the "true" incidences as opposed to the reported ones (Krickeberg 1994). New syndromic surveillance is more related to outbreak investigation and is to some extent motivated by the fear of terrorist attacks by pathogenic micro-organisms. The objective here is to identify the nature of cases rapidly on the basis of reported syndromes and other observations (Lawson and Kleinman 2005).

8.6 Objectives of Surveillance

The objectives of epidemiologic surveillance of infectious diseases were sketched in a general way at the end of Section 8.1. Let us scrutinize them now in a more concrete fashion.

The purpose of notifications of specific communicable diseases is to elicit rapid intervention. Such interventions may be the isolation of infected persons and perhaps of their contacts, or quarantine of entire groups of people, or preventive vaccinations. Smallpox has been a notifiable disease from the beginning and it was by rapidly vaccinating everybody around a diseased person (ring vaccination) that it was finally eradicated (Fenner 1988).

The classical active surveillance, or screening, of school children, for example, by a tuberculin test or for caries (which is in principle an infectious disease!) aimed in the first place at early treatment, but also at obtaining epidemiologic knowledge and at containing, for example, the spread of tuberculosis.

As mentioned before, outbreak investigation of epidemics may make use of routine surveillance too; its objectives will be treated in the following chapter.

In the last 50 years or so, many more objectives were added to these classical ones. In the first place, beyond the old statistics of causes of death, the indicators on general morbidity obtained via comprehensive or partial health information systems allow health officials to monitor the distribution and extent of infectious diseases across geographical areas and population groups, and their evolution in time. This, in turn, is an important component of the basis for managing the health system, for example, for drawing up yearly budgets. It also gives rise to publications like annual Health Yearbooks that provide a general picture of the health situation of a region or a country. It is indispensable for planning particular health strategies on the one hand and the structure of the health system on the other. Finally, it may help to evaluate measures for preventing and controlling infectious diseases.

Regarding demographic surveillance, its main traditional objective has been to calculate *rates*. Indicators like total number of new cases during a given period, or of existing cases at a given moment, are converted into incidence or prevalence rates by dividing them by the respective number of inhabitants.

In the recent past, other types of surveillance systems appeared in response to the need for information of a different nature. In sero-surveillance, the degree of immunity of the target population is monitored in order to complement the normal disease surveillance, to plan and to evaluate vaccination strategies, and to serve as a basis for mathematical modelling. Analogous objectives have led to surveillance systems of the type sketched at the end of Section 8.4, such as surveillance of compliance and behaviour of patients, of general changes in the health behaviour of the population, of changes in other risk factors, of new drug resistances and secondary effects, of resistance of pathogens and vectors, and of appearance of new forms of pathogens. The objective is always to continuously adapt the health strategies being used to newly observed situations. In addition, the results of surveillance give rise to epidemiologic and biomedical studies and insights concerning, for example, the aetiology of specific diseases and other causal relations, their pathways and seasonal or long-term trends, various risk factors including social ones, and other characteristics (for further details, see Chapter 4, 7, and 14).

For every surveillance system the question naturally arises as to what extent it attains its objectives, in other words, the issue of its *evaluation*. Given the multitude of objectives, it is not possible to enter into details here; see Centers for Disease Control (2001) and Chapter 3 of the book by Lawson and Kleinman (2005). The general ideas and statistical methods are similar to those of the evaluation of a clinical test as expressed by the concepts of *sensitivity, specificity*, and *predictive values:* Which fraction of the existing cases is being reported by the system and what is the extent of underreporting? How many affirmative reports about cases are unfounded? What can we infer from reported incidences, prevalences, or mortalities about the true ones?

8.7 Some Examples of Specific Surveillance Systems

Notification Systems. We are going to have a look at the mandatory notification system in England and Wales, mentioned in Section 8.2 (McCormick 1993), because it is the oldest one. In the present system, cases from a list of 30 diseases are to be reported immediately by the attending physician to a local health authority. The reports are nominative. The local health authorities forward this information weekly in a non-nominative way to the Health Protection Agency in Colindale, North London. The list comprises the following diseases including case definitions: acute encephalitis; anthrax; cholera; diphtheria; dysentery; enteric fever; food poisoning; leprosy; leptospirosis; malaria; measles; mumps; rubella; meningitis (meningo- and pneumococcal); viral meningococcal septicaemia (without meningitis); haemophilus influenzae; ophthalmia neonatorum; paratyphoid fever; plague; poliomyelitis; relapsing fever; scarlet fever; smallpox; tetanus; typhus; tuberculosis; viral haemorrhagic fever; viral hepatitis (types A, B and C); pertussis; yellow fever. They are categorized according to different levels of "urgency."

The systems in most other countries are basically similar. Another example would be in the United States CDC's National Notifiable Disease Surveillance

System (2008). However, in this system, only the notification to state health authorities is mandatory, whereas the notification by the states to CDC is voluntary and governed by state legislation.

General "comprehensive" health information systems. They are defined in Section 8.2. Lippeveld et al. (2000) presented their typical structure and the problems from which they suffer. Krickeberg (1999) described the example of the entirety of the health information systems in Vietnam.

Surveillance of particular infectious diseases. For certain diseases, special surveillance systems outside the general notification scheme have been developed. Some are sentinel systems as in the examples mentioned below. Others are run by a specialized central institution, for example, by a malaria or tuberculosis institute in a developing country (Krickeberg 1999). They rely on passive reporting along hierarchical paths from commune over district and province level to the central institute in question; hence their structure is usually similar to that of a general health information system. Depending on the country, they may actually or in theory be integrated into it, or be independent. A more recent example is the Tuberculosis–Leprosy Management System in Malaysia sketched in Section 6.5.

Looking at developed countries, Norway has had a central Tuberculosis Registry organized similarly to a Cancer Registry since 1962; see Norwegian Institute of Public Health (2008). It also keeps a central Registry of Vaccinations.

As illustrated in Section 8.5 by the reporting system for tetanus in the United States (Pascual et al. 2003), for many notifiable diseases there exist a specific *reporting system* for transmitting, analysing, and exploiting the information on the notified cases.

Health information systems for "vertical" programmes. These are programmes in developing countries organized "top-down" such as CDD (Control of Diarrhoeal Diseases), ARI (Acute Respiratory Infections), HIV/AIDS, MCH (Mother and Child Health), and EPI (Expanded Programme on Immunization). Every one of them uses an information system, which is implemented and operated by the organization that runs the programme, for example, a central health institute, the UNICEF, or a non-governmental organization. In general it is independent of the general health information system of the country from which it borrows, however, the hierarchical structure. Its objectives are planning and evaluating the programme and, above all, its management. Naturally, there is a strong *surveillance* component. For examples, see Krickeberg (1999). The large number of these information systems, together with those described before, frequently leads to "over-surveillance", which becomes a heavy burden on the health system and its personnel (Krickeberg 1999, Lippeveld et al. 2000).

Surveillance in schools, work places. Surveillance systems that take their sources in schools (as sketched in Section 8.6) are old and widespread but are usually limited to a few diseases. In some European countries, more comprehensive syndromic surveillance systems have been set up recently.

Surveillance in places of work is part of occupational hygiene and very varied, depending on the type of work and the social structure of the country in question. Surveillance in restaurants, cafeterias, etc. is performed within the administrative structures of food control and also takes very many forms. Hence we will not present particular examples. Its role in outbreak investigations is described in Chapter 9.

Sentinel stations. The "International Network of field sites with continuous Demographic Evaluation of Populations and Their Health in developing countries" (INDEPTH ; 2002) counts fixed stations in many countries. They have a fairly wide area of responsibilities as indicated by their name, where surveillance of trends of the situation of infectious diseases and their risk factors plays a prominent role.

In many European countries a fixed sample of general practitioners is selected for surveillance of specific infectious diseases. Reporting was originally done by telephone and is now done by Internet or e-mail; see, for example, Weinberg et al. (1997). The British system described by Hawker et al. (2005) comprises about 70 physicians. Other examples are the European Influenza Surveillance Scheme (2008) and the European Network on Imported Infectious Disease Surveillance (2009) (see Section 21.2.1).

Surveillance of nosocomial infections. An example is given in Chapter 22.

Sero-surveillance. This is, in the first place, the surveillance of the immune status of the population for infectious diseases, mostly vaccine-preventable ones, which lead to sero-conversion of infected individuals. It started in several countries with single sample surveys that are evolving over time into a surveillance system by being repeated in a more or less systematic fashion. There exist two basically different sampling methods. In the system in England and Wales (Osborne et al. 2000) and the one in Australia modelled after it, sera samples that had been submitted for diagnostic testing and would otherwise have been discarded are used. In the United States (Gergen et al. 1995) and the Netherlands (de Melker 1998), population-based random sampling is employed. The former method is of course much cheaper, which enabled those systems to advance more towards regular surveillance, for example, in Australia by a yearly survey in specific age groups and one across the entire age range every 5 years. On the other hand, population-based random sampling makes it possible to include certain additional risk factors and is less prone to bias (see also Chapter 14).

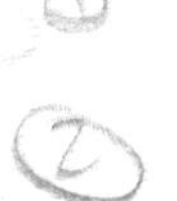

Another type of sero-surveillance singles out particular risk groups as its target populations. For example, potential blood donors are being examined for HIV or HCV.

The European Sero-Epidemiology Network (ESEN) (Osborne et al. 1997) was established in 1996 mainly in order to standardize sero-surveillance in its member states. ESEN also serves as the framework of ad hoc surveys, for example, about pertussis toxin antibodies between the years 1994 and 1998 and their relation to historical surveillance and vaccine programme data (Pebody et al. 2005).

Vector surveillance. Hosts of rabies such as foxes, stray dogs, bats, and wildlife have been subject to surveillance for a long time. For the present, see WHO Expert Consultation on Rabies 2004 (2005). National health administrations often do some surveillance of rats as hosts of fleas that might be vectors of *Yersinia pestis* by requiring reports from beer and food factories, large restaurants, and the like.

Surveillance of mosquitoes that carry malaria, yellow fever, or dengue is usually integrated into the reporting network of the institution entrusted with general control of the disease in question; see "Surveillance of particular infectious diseases". There are various schemes for catching mosquitoes (sampling plans) and for examining their status of infection.

Surveillance of pathogens. For an example from hospitals, see Chapter 22 on nosocomial infections (microbiologic tools are described in Chapter 7).

The example of the surveillance of *Chlamydia trachomatis* in Sweden (Söderblom et al. 2006) illustrates several general aspects. Infections by this pathogen belong to the 60 notifiable diseases in Sweden. In the late 2005 and early 2006, an unexpected fall by about 25% of the reported incidence of sexually transmitted cases was noticed in the county of Halland. It then turned out that there indeed existed cases that could not be detected by the standard laboratory test (AR) used for diagnosis. An investigation in all of Sweden followed. A *Chlamydia* genetic variant was identified where the genomic target region of the test AR had suffered a deletion and which therefore did not respond to that test. This variant can, however, still be discovered by another test (BD), which uses a different target region. Thus, constant monitoring of the tests is necessary. Moreover, the basic issue of an "evolution driven by diagnostic methods" comes up since a genetic variant that is not detected and treated may spread more easily than others. See also Chapter 20 for the epidemiology of *Chlamydia* infections.

Pathogen surveillance for some vaccine-preventable infections such as those caused by meningococci C, pneumococci, or human papillomaviruses serves to detect strain replacement, shifts in strain composition, and virulence factors. It is also important for monitoring antibiotic and antiviral resistance. For details, see the relevant WHO documentation.

Surveillance of efficacy and side effects of curative and preventive treatments. This belongs to the domain of therapeutic trials including those of immunizations and other preventive treatments. Surveillance has the form of post-marketing surveillance (phase IV trials) of drugs and surveillance of vaccination efficacy and side effects after the implementation of an immunization programme. It is a huge area apart; hence no example will be given here (see, however, Chapter 14).

Second-generation surveillance. This concept stems from the surveillance of AIDS and its pathogen HIV. There, systems using different sources and mechanisms, dealing with various types of information, and pursuing several objectives were advocated and tried out. Second-generation surveillance now means building efficient systems that combine the two basic forms of AIDS/HIV surveillance. One of them is usually called *biological* surveillance and deals with the distribution of cases over risk groups and geographical areas, and with the occurrence of opportunistic infections, CD4 counts, viral loads, and the like. Data on other sexually transmittable diseases may be included. *Behavioural* surveillance concerns general risk factors (see Chapter 18), behaviour in the strict sense being the most prominent one. The mechanisms may be based either on sentinels, mostly clinics and hospitals, or on multiple rounds of population-based sample surveys. For details, see Rehle et al. (2004) and Reintjes and Wiessing (2007).

Spatial surveillance. This had been defined at the end of Section 8.5. Chapter 10 presents some examples. The book by Lawson and Kleinman (2005) describes several more, in particular in its Chapter 7.

Syndromic surveillance. The System of the New York City Department of Health and Mental Hygiene (Heffernan et al. 2004) which started in 2001 uses daily electronic reports on certain syndromes from consultations in emergency departments of hospitals in order to spot outbreaks as early as possible. Not surprisingly, most respiratory and fever type syndromes occur during peak influenza activity, and diarrhoeal and vomiting syndromes are mainly observed during periods of suspected norovirus and rotavirus transmission. For other examples see Lawson and Kleinman (2005).

8.8 A Guide to Further Study

Many books on epidemiology or public health contain a chapter on surveillance, most of it concerning infectious diseases, for example American Public Health Association (2000), Hawker et al. (2005), Nelson and Masters Williams (2007), Thomas and Weber (2001), Webber (2005), and Rothman and Greenland (1998).

The volumes edited by Teutsch and Churchill (2000) and Reintjes and Klein (2007) provide a general, practical overview on surveillance. Statistical methods are treated in Brookmeyer and Stroup (2004) on an intermediate level; there is also a long list of selected sources of information. The book by Lawson and Kleinman (2005), although in principle restricted to spatial and syndromic surveillance, touches in fact upon most issues of modern surveillance in developed countries and emphasizes the mathematical and statistical techniques. On a less technical level, Nsubuga et al. (2006) deal with surveillance in developing countries.

References

American Public Health Association (2000) Control of communicable diseases manual. American Public Health Association, Washington, DC

Brookmeyer, R and Stroup, D, eds. (2004) Monitoring the health of populations: Statistical principles and methods for public health. Oxford University Press, Oxford

CDC's National Notifiable Disease Surveillance System (2008) www.cdc.gov/ncphi/diss/nndss (accessed 29 February 2008)

Centers for Disease Control (1986) Comprehensive plan for epidemiologic surveillance. Centers for Disease Control, Atlanta, Georgia

Centers for Disease Control (2001) Updated guidelines for evaluating public health surveillance systems: Recommendations from the Guidelines Working Group. MMWR 50 (13), 1–35

de Melker HE, Conyn-Van Spaendonck MA (1998) Immunosurveillance and the evaluation of national immunization programmes: A population-based approach. Epidemiol Infect 121, 637–643

Europa – Public Health-Health Information (2008) http://ec.europa.eu/health/ph_information/information_en.htm (accessed 24 February 2008)

European Influenza Surveillance Scheme (2008) www.eiss.org (accessed 10 January 2008)

European Network on Imported Infectious Disease Surveillance (2009) www.tropnet.eu (accessed 7 April 2009)

Fenner F (1988) Smallpox and its eradication (History of International Public Health, No. 6). World Health Organization, Geneva

Gergen PJ, McQuillan GM, Kiely M, Ezzati-Rice TM, Sutter RW and Virella G (1995) A population based serologic survey of immunity to tetanus in the United States. New Engl J Med 332, 761–766

Hawker J, Begg N, Blair I, Reintjes R and Weinberg J (2005) Communicable disease control handbook, 2nd ed., Blackwell Science, Oxford

Heffernan R, Mostashari F, Das D, Karpati A, Kulldorf M and Weiss D (2004) Syndromic surveillance in public health practice, New York City. Emerging Infect Dis 10, 858–864

INDEPTH (2002) INDEPTH, health and demography in developing countries, vol. 1: Population, health and survival at INDEPTH sites. IDRC, Ottawa

Krickeberg K (1994) Health information in developing countries. Frontiers in Mathematical Biology. Lecture Notes in Biomathematics 100, 550–568

Krickeberg K (1999) The health information system in Vietnam in 1999. Assignment report for the joint programme of Vietnam and the European Committee on Health Systems Development. Available from the author on request

Krickeberg K (2007) Principles of health information systems in developing countries. Health Inf Manag J 36 (3), 8–20

Langmuir AD (1963) The surveillance of communicable diseases of national importance. N Engl J Med 268, 182–192

Lawson AB and KleinmannK, eds. (2005) Spatial and syndromic surveillance for public health. Wiley, Chichester

Lippeveld Th, Sauerborn R and Bodart C, eds. (2000) Design and implementation of health information systems. World Health Organization, Geneva

McCormick A (1993) The notification of infectious diseases in England and Wales. Commun Dis Rep CDR Rev 3, 19–25

Nelson KE and Masters Williams CF (2007) Infectious disease epidemiology: Theory and practice. Jones and Bartlett, Sudbury

Norwegian Institute of Public Health (2008) www.fhi.no (accessed 28 January 2008)

Nsubuga P et al. (2006) Public health surveillance: A tool for targeting and monitoring interventions. Chapter 53, in: Jamison, DT et al. Disease control priorities in developing countries. Oxford University Press, New York

Osborne K, Weinberg J and Miller E (1997) The European sero-epidemiology network. Euro Surveill 2, 29–31

Osborne K, Gay N, Hesketh L, Morgan-Capner P and Miller E (2000) Ten years of serological surveillance in England and Wales: Methods, results, implications and action. Int J Epidemiol 29, 362–368

Pascual FB, McGinley EL, Zanardi L., Cortese MM, Murphy TV (2003) Tetanus surveillance – United States, 1998–2000. MMWR CDC Surveill Summ 52 (3), 1–8

Pebody RG et al. (2005) The seroepidemiology of *Bordetella pertussis* infection in Western Europe. Epidemiol Infect 133, 159–171

Rehle Th, Lazzari S, Dallabetta G and Asamoah-Odei E (2004) Second-generation HIV-surveillance: better data for decision making. Bulletin WHO 82, 121–127

Reintjes R and Klein S, eds. (2007) Gesundheitsberichterstattung und Surveillance: Messen, Entscheiden, Handeln. Verlag Hans Huber, Bern

Reintjes R and Wiessing LG (2007) 2nd-generation HIV surveillance and injecting drug use: uncovering the epidemiological surveillance ice-berg. Internat J Public Health 52, 166–172

Rosen G (1993) A history of public health. Expanded Edition. John Hopkins Press, Baltimore
Rothman KJ, Greenland S and Lash TL, eds. (2008) Modern Epidemiology. 3rd ed. Philadelphia: Lippincott Williams and Wilkins
Söderblom T, Blaxhult A, Fredlund H and Herrmann B (2006) Impact of a genetic variant of Chlamydia trachomatis on national detection rates in Sweden. Euro Surveill 11 (12) E0612071
Teutsch SM and Churchill RE, eds. (2000) Principles and practice of public health surveillance. 2nd ed. Oxford University Press, New York
Thomas JC and Weber DJ, eds. (2001) Epidemiologic methods for the study of infectious diseases. Oxford University Press, Oxford
Webber R (2005) Communicable disease epidemiology and control: A global perspective. 2nd ed. CABI Publishing, Oxfordshire
Weinberg J, Nohynek H and Giesecke J (1997) Development of a European electronic network on communicable diseases: the IDA-HSSCD programme. Euro Surveill 2 (7), 51–53
WHO Data and Statistics (2008) www.who.int/research/en (accessed 3 March 2008)
WHO Expert Consultation on Rabies 2004 (2005) WHO Technical Report Series 931. WHO, Geneva

Chapter 9
Outbreak Investigations

Ralf Reintjes and Aryna Zanuzdana

9.1 Introduction

The aim of outbreak epidemiology is to study an epidemic in order to gain control over it and to prevent further spread of the disease. Generally outbreak means a "sudden occurrence," while in the epidemiological sense an outbreak is defined as a sudden increase in the disease frequency, related to time, place, and observed population. Thousands of outbreaks among humans and animals have been reported and investigated during the last two centuries, among them the most numerous being outbreaks of cholera, plague, malaria, smallpox, influenza, SARS, measles, salmonella, chikungunya, and various foodborne outbreaks.

Traditionally, outbreak investigations are an essential part of infectious disease epidemiology. During the 18th and 19th century, epidemics of different diseases were widespread in Europe. Epidemiologists like Edward Jenner (1749–1823), who, as a country doctor, had observed the devastating epidemic of smallpox in England in the late 18th century, based on his observation had introduced a preventive vaccination against it, and John Snow (1813–1858), who had found contaminated water to be the cause of the cholera outbreak in London in the 1850s, undoubtedly created the fundamentals of modern outbreak investigations (Gordis 2009).

Today there are new challenges for studies of infectious diseases. On the one hand, due to global and regional changes in the environment, industry, food processing, transportation of goods and food, and behavioral changes, new infectious diseases emerge. On the other hand, people are confronted with already forgotten diseases, which are no longer considered to be a danger to public health (Dwyer and Groves 2001). Chapter 3 provides a comprehensive overview of emerging and reemerging infectious diseases. Furthermore, the increasing density of populations, growing megacities in the developing world, an increasing number of subpopulations at risk, and other socio-demographical factors influence the way communicable diseases spread (see Chapter 2). Considering the changing

R. Reintjes (✉)
Department of Public Health, Hamburg University of Applied Sciences, Hamburg, Germany
e-mail: ralf.reintjes@haw-hamburg.de

A. Krämer et al. (eds.), *Modern Infectious Disease Epidemiology*,
Statistics for Biology and Health, DOI 10.1007/978-0-387-93835-6_9,

nature of modern infectious diseases, outbreak investigations play a crucial role in understanding their nature and subsequent control.

This chapter provides information on the objectives and the use and planning of outbreak investigations as well as on methods of conducting and reporting an outbreak. In addition, we provide simple examples of how to apply different study designs to investigate an outbreak.

9.2 Defining an Outbreak

The term "outbreak" is most commonly associated with a number of cases significantly higher than the background expected number of cases in a particular area over a given period of time. Beyond a simple increase in the number of cases, there can be an indication of an outbreak when the same exposure (risk factor) causes a *cluster* of cases (two and more cases simultaneously) with the same disease; the number of disease cases in a cluster must not necessarily be higher than expected (Ungchusak 2004). For instance, a cluster of five cases with hemolytic uremic syndrome (HUS) was identified in one community in southwest France in 2005. The outbreak investigation showed that all patients had consumed one brand of frozen beef burgers in the week before the onset of symptom. *Escherichia coli* O157:H7 (E. coli 0157:H7) was identified as the cause of the disease (King et al. 2008). An outbreak investigation should also take place even if only one case of an *unknown or an unusual* disease occurs and if this disease is life threatening [e.g., avian flu and severe acute respiratory syndrome (SARS)] (Timmreck 1994).

Typical for any outbreak is that it occurs suddenly and requires direct measures to be taken. A well-conducted outbreak investigation may serve several aims. First of all, an outbreak investigation serves the detection and elimination of a potential epidemic's cause and provides postexposure prophylaxis to affected individuals. Next, outbreak investigations often result in discovering new infections and diseases. The last quarter of the 20th as well as the first years of the 21st century was rich regarding the discovery of new etiologic agents and diseases, among which were *Legionella* spp. and *legionellosis*, toxic shock syndrome associated with tampon use, *E. coli* 0157:H7 – potentially causing fatal hemolytic uremic syndrome, Ebola virus (which was sensationalized in the news media) – causing viral hemorrhagic fever, and severe acute respiratory syndrome (SARS), just to name a few (see Chapter 3 and Weber et al. 2001; Dwyer and Groves 2001; Hawker et al. 2005; Towner et al. 2008; Oxford et al. 2003). The recent outbreak of influenza A (H1N1), which started in Mexico in April 2009, led to the raise of the highest level of influenza pandemic alert (phase 6) by the World Health Organization.

Outbreak analysis may deliver information about the spread of a well-known pathogen to new geographical areas. Infectious agents may be introduced into new areas with immigrants, tourists, imported animals, and contaminated food and goods (Weber et al. 2001). Successful outbreak investigations contribute to the development of knowledge about infectious diseases by identifying new modes of transmission. For example, *E. coli* O157:H7 infection had previously been associated with eating undercooked hamburger meat; however, numerous outbreak investigations registered *E. coli* O157:H7 transmission via unpasteurized cheese and apple drinks, swimming pools, lakes, municipal water, and person-to-person transmission (Center for Disease Control and Prevention 1993; Cody et al. 1999; Honish et al. 2005; Bruneau et al. 2004; Belongia et al. 1993; Weber et al. 2001).

Finally, outbreak investigations serve as a basis for the development of public health regulations and prevention guidelines. Scientific knowledge makes it possible to draw general conclusions, detect new trends, and show ways to new prevention measures. The study of outbreaks is therefore an important component of public health practice.

The investigation of an outbreak makes simultaneous use of epidemiological, microbiological, toxicological, and clinical methods in order to develop and test hypotheses about the causes of the outbreak. In the following sections, the most important methodological aspects of planning and conducting an outbreak investigation are described and explained using examples.

9.3 Suspicions of an Outbreak and Risk Communication

Outbreak investigations differ from other types of epidemiological studies, particularly in the way that they often start without clear hypotheses and require the use of descriptive analysis in order to analyze the situation in terms of time, place, person, and scope of the problem (Brownson 2006).

An outbreak can be suspected if data from several cases display common characteristics (e.g., occurrence of many cases of a disease in the same period of time, in the same area, and with similar manifestations). In order to assess *the existence of an outbreak*, diagnosis of the suspected cases should be confirmed and then the number of detected cases should be compared with the baseline rate for the disease and setting. Possible biases which can influence the evaluation of an outbreak must be taken into account; first of all, changes in reporting practices, changes in population size, improved diagnostic procedures or screening campaigns (detection bias), or increased interest of the public and media in certain diseases (Gerstman 2003). Often it might also be helpful to interview several representative cases. That can help to understand the clinical picture of the disease and obtain additional information about the affected individuals. The collection of epidemiological data is important for the development of prevention and control measures. Based on the initial information, an epidemiological investigation can be planned and control measures can be implemented immediately to stop further transmission of a disease (Dwyer and Groves 2001).

In case of a confirmed outbreak, the relevant public health authorities should be notified immediately and all important findings should be shared with involved individuals and parties. It is important to carefully record data and maintain both internal and external communication. Internal communication concerns the team of outbreak investigators, whereas external communication concerns selection and presentation of the information to the news media as well as the contact of stakeholders. Investigators should avoid unnecessary speculation and identify key points to communicate and provide relevant background information of the epidemic as well as methods of its evaluation and control (Weber et al. 2001).

General control and prevention measures can already be implemented at the initial stage of the outbreak investigation. For instance, suspicious foods can be taken out of the trade, sick individuals who commercially have to deal with manufacturing or processing of groceries are restricted from their respective activities, or the population can be informed about risk-bearing products.

9.4 Descriptive Analysis

The main components of an outbreak investigation are summarized in the flowchart in Fig. 9.1. These steps need not necessarily be performed in the described sequence. Moreover, several steps, as many authors emphasize, often occur simultaneously (Gerstman 2003; Weber et al. 2001). The sequence and completeness of these steps would most likely depend on the urgency of the situation, the availability of human and other resources, and the process of obtaining data (Dwyer and Groves 2001).

In outbreak investigations, descriptive epidemiology is given one of the key roles. It illustrates an outbreak using the three standard variables, time, place, and person, and makes it possible to set up specific hypotheses about causes and sources of

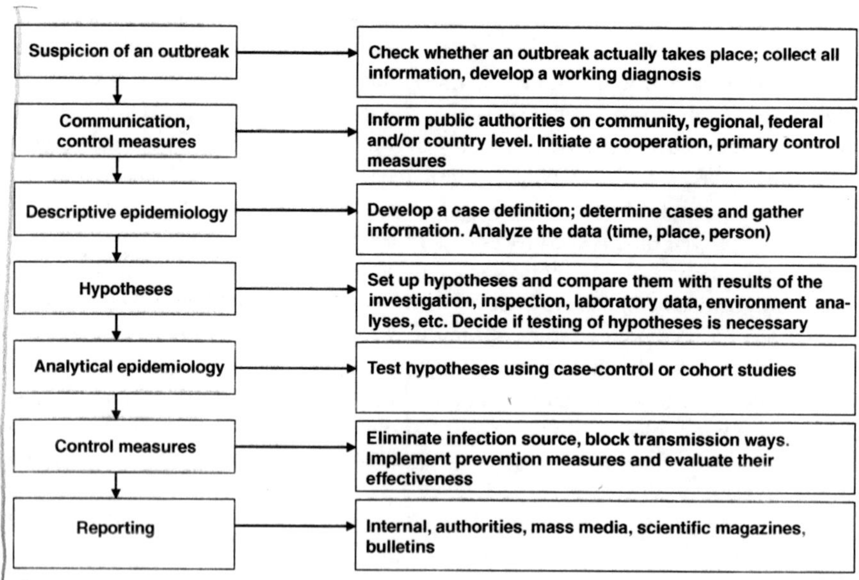

Fig. 9.1 Flowchart for outbreak management

infection and modes of transmission. The components of the descriptive process are discussed in the following sections.

9.4.1 Case Definition

It is essential to establish a simple and workable case definition for both the description of an outbreak and a possible analytical investigation. In the present context, the epidemiological case definition also includes orienting variables related to time, place, and person. This is in addition to clinical and, where appropriate, laboratory medical criteria. The case definition must be applied equally to all cases under investigation from the beginning. Obviously, early or preliminary case definitions can be based only on information about signs and symptoms of a disease or an infectious agent. For example, a primary definition of a foodborne outbreak can be formulated as follows:

> A case of illness is defined as any vomiting, diarrhea, abdominal pains, headache, and fever that developed after attending an event X.

This definition does not imply any common risk factors for affected individuals, and thus emphasizes the *sensitivity* to detect disease cases. However, as the investigation goes on, the case definition should be reviewed and refined to increase *specificity*. The previous case definition of a foodborne outbreak may then be reformulated as:

> A case of illness is defined as vomiting or diarrhea with onset within 4 days (96 hours) of consuming food served at the event X.

Here the definition has higher specificity and aims to exclude cases of gastroenteritis or other illnesses (Dwyer and Groves 2001).

Investigators can sometimes divide cases into "definite" (e.g., confirmed in a laboratory), "probable" (e.g., cases who have objective signs and symptoms contained in the case definition), and "possible" ("suspect") (e.g., cases who have subjective signs and symptoms contained in the case definition) (Weber et al. 2001).

The following definition was formulated for "possible" cases in the outbreak of the influenza A (H1N1): "Defined as an individual with an acute febrile respiratory illness (fever >38°C) with onset of symptoms:

- Within 7 days of travel to affected areas; or
- Within 7 days of close contact with a confirmed or a probable case of influenza A (H1N1)."

One of the definitions for "probable" cases of the influenza A (H1N1) ran as following: "An individual with a clinically compatible illness or who died of an unexplained acute respiratory illness that is considered to be epidemiologically linked to a probable or a confirmed case.

"Definite" case of the influenza A (H1N1) would be "an individual with laboratory confirmed Influenza A (H1N1) virus infection by one or more of the following tests:

- Real-time polymerase chain reaction (RT-PCR);
- Viral culture;
- Four-fold rise in Influenza A (H1N1) virus specific neutralizing antibodies" (European Centre for Disease Prevention and Control 2009; World Health Organization 2009a, 2009b).

9.4.2 Finding Cases and Collecting Information

Usually investigators know only about a part of the cases which occur during an outbreak. The main reasons for that are the following:

- Not all sick individuals visit a physician. Many of them feel no need to do so.
- Physicians do not always send a sample to a laboratory for microbiological analysis.
- Laboratory investigations do not always succeed in identifying a causal pathogen.
- Not all positive findings are reported to the public health department.
- Some patients avoid being reported.

Thus, in addition to the cases already known, there are cases which might have been missed or overlooked, and investigators should search for them. Only then the extent of an outbreak can be objectively estimated and the outbreak population defined. Hence, active search for cases might be carried out using certain case-finding techniques, for example:

- Searching in surveillance data and laboratory data (e.g., summaries of illnesses, morbidity reports from local health departments)
- Surveying physicians, personnel of clinical microbiological laboratories, and hospitals to check logs about diseases or diagnoses typical for the current outbreak
- Questioning known outbreak cases to find secondary cases (e.g., based on guest or participant lists of an event), public announcements in the local press, radio, and other mass media (More about surveillance systems in Chapter 8).

After all the cases are identified, comprehensive information about them is collected. The individuals can either be interviewed personally (or per telephone) or given a standardized questionnaire to fill in. Regardless of the type of disease, the following basic information is necessary to describe the general pattern of it to the population at risk (Gerstman 2003; Dwyer and Groves 2001):

- Case identification (name, address, etc.),
- Demographical background,
- Clinical information (disease onset, time of exposure to the infectious agent, signs, manifestation, laboratory test results), and
- Potential risk factors (exposure or factors that might influence the probability of disease).

Following the collection of this information on cases, it is possible to structure the data in terms of *time, place, and person*. The goal of the descriptive epidemiology here is to find answers to the following questions: What do the patients have in common? Is there any increasing frequency in relation to sex, age groups, occupation as well as to demographical or geographical variables and variables related to time? In order to simplify answering these questions, it is often helpful to present the collected data in diagrams, tables, and maps and to calculate the attack rate.

9.4.3 Time: Epidemic Curves of Outbreaks

For the purpose of graphical description of cases by time of onset of illness, an epidemic curve can be drawn in which the occurrence of cases is shown over an appropriate time interval. Graphically, such a curve is constructed by putting the number of cases on the y-axis and the date of onset of illness on the x-axis. An epidemic curve helps to keep track of the time course of the events and gives clues about ways of transmission, exposure, and incubation period of the investigated disease. Disease cases, whose time course strongly deviates from that of the other cases ("outliers"), can give important clues to the source of infection (Gordis 2009). An epidemic curve can also help in distinguishing between common and propagated source epidemics.

Four examples of typical epidemic curves are given in Fig. 9.2a–d, modified from Checko (1996). Examples A and B represent an epidemic curve for *a propagated (continuing or progressive) source outbreak*. Propagated outbreaks depend on transmission from person to person or continuing exposure from a single source (Gerstman 2003). Curve A illustrates an outbreak (e.g., measles, influenza, or chickenpox) with a single exposure and index cases (index cases are those that first come to the attention of public health authorities) (Friis and Sellers 2004). Curve B shows the incidence of secondary and tertiary cases, typical, for example, for hepatitis A (secondary cases are those who acquire disease from contact with primary cases and tertiary cases are those who acquire disease from contact with secondary cases). In such a propagated outbreak, as it is shown in part B, there first occurs an increase in cases after exposure, then a fall in the incidence of cases; later there occurs a second increase in cases eventually infected by person-to-person transmission from primary cases. Curves C and D of Fig. 9.2 are examples of *common source outbreaks*. In such outbreaks most cases are exposed to one risk factor. Part C is a possible example for

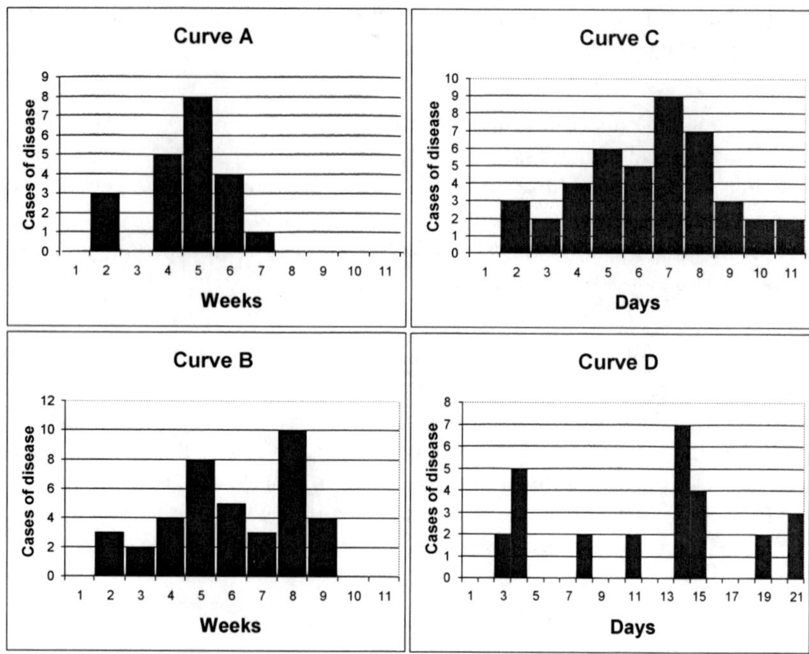

Fig. 9.2 (**a–c**) Examples of epidemic curves; (**a** and **b**) propagated or continuing source outbreak; (**c** and **d**) common source outbreak. Source: Modified from Checko 1996

an outbreak when the number of cases rises suddenly and then slowly falls again. This is characteristic of a common source outbreak with a point exposure when the population at risk is exposed simultaneously within a short period of time. In this instance the epidemic ends, unless secondary cases occur, which is typical for food-borne outbreaks. Another example of the point source outbreak is Legionnaires' disease, which broke out among people who attended a convention of the American Legion in Philadelphia in 1976 (Arias 2000).

In part D there is a continued (intermittent) exposure of individuals; cases of disease occur suddenly after the minimum incubation period, but do not disappear completely, because more individuals continue to be exposed to the source of infection.

9.4.4 Place: Spatial distribution

The spatial description of an outbreak can provide useful evidence about the geographical distribution of the cases, the size of an outbreak, and under special circumstances about the underlying source. For example, this might give information about specific locations within closed environments (e.g., a hospital), sites of routine activities (e.g., fast-food restaurant, public pools), or the place where affected individuals live (Weber et al. 2001). It is practical to present geographical information in the form of maps, for example, dot density maps and choropleth maps. Dot density maps may serve to graphically present the geographical extent of the problem and provide information on clustering. Probably the most famous dot density map was drawn by John Snow, showing the cholera deaths near the Golden Square in London (where the outbreak occurred) in 1854 (McLeod 2001). From his map, one could recognize the connection between clustering of cholera cases around the Broad Street pump, thus, the water-borne nature of the infectious agent (Gerstman 2003). However, the disadvantage of dot density maps is that they do not provide any information concerning the number of people at risk in a mapped area, which can be confusing when populations of these areas are unequal in size. Another option is to build a map, which shows area-specific disease rates, for example, disease attack rates per 100 inhabitants showing epicenters of an epidemic.

In any case, visual representations are beneficial to understand more about the spread of an outbreak of disease. In addition to the above mentioned, there are more complex methods [e.g., Geographic Information Systems (GIS)], which combine both geographical and other information. For advanced treatment of these methods, please see Chapter 10.

9.4.5 Person: Portraying the Outbreak Population

Person-based variables can be used for portraying the outbreak population. An increasing frequency of cases in a certain population group can point to groups at high risk (for example, increased occurrence of cases among workers in a certain part of a factory or among visitors of a local restaurant). Person-based factors include demographical characteristics (age, sex, ethnicity), marital status, personal activities (occupation, habits, leisure activities, knowledge, attitudes, and behavior), genetic factors, physiological conditions (nutritional status, distresses, pregnancy, etc.), current diseases, and immune condition (Gerstman 2003). Furthermore, investigations of specific diseases, like STDs or HIV/AIDS, require the use of variables related to sexual behavior, sexual practices, number of sexual partners, and in specific cases also intravenous drug use.

CB

Exhibit 9.1 Use of mathematical methods in outbreak investigation

The elementary analysis of data as sketched above is meant to detect a *possible* outbreak but does not lead to a definitive statement about its existence. We *suspect* an outbreak if the epidemic curve looks unusual, in particular, if we find incidences that are significantly higher than expected if there is no outbreak. Such a purely qualitative judgment may suffice in a relatively simple and clear-cut setting as in the following examples of food poisoning, especially if supported by an a posteriori epidemiological analysis of the kind made there. In many situations, however, given the consequences of actions to be taken depending on the result of the investigation, a more precise decision rule will be necessary. We have to state what we mean by "significantly higher than expected."

If we base our conclusion exclusively on the epidemic curve, which amounts to disregarding the spatial component of the data on cases, the problem may be formulated as follows: how can we determine a "threshold value" t such that, in the *absence* of an outbreak, an incidence exceeding t for a given period has a "very small" probability. We will then declare that there is an outbreak if the epidemic curve passes to values above t. What we mean by a "very small" probability needs to be defined in advance, depending on the risk we are willing to face for overlooking an outbreak.

Mathematically, this approach bears some similarity with the so-called theory of dams. There we are interested in the probability that a dam built to contain water in a reservoir, e.g., for an electrical power station, will overflow during a given period of the future, given data from the past. Some research along these lines was indeed done within the framework of outbreak investigations but has not gained much importance because it became increasingly clear that the larger part of relevant information is usually contained in the spatial component of the data on cases. This led to the so-called cluster analysis, both for noninfectious and infectious diseases. The basic idea is similar to the one formulated before, namely to describe in a rigorous quantitative way what kind of clustering is, in the absence of an outbreak, still to be considered as "normal" and arising purely by random effects. We cannot enter into details here; some of the methods are presented in Chapter 11. There is an introductory text by Waller and Gotway (2004). For an advanced treatment, see the book by Lawson and Kleinman (2005), especially its chapter by Kulldorff on "Scan Statistics for Geographical Disease Surveillance: An Overview."

9.5 Analytical Epidemiology

To remind the reader, the goal of an outbreak investigation is fundamentally not only to identify and describe the causative agent but also, more specifically, to find a pathogen source of the disease and modes of transmission in order to develop control and prevention measures. In outbreak investigations, analytical studies are applied mainly in order to assess the centre, source, and cause of infection independently from laboratory methods.

The first important and probably the most difficult step in the analytical epidemiology is formulating and testing hypotheses. A formal testing of hypotheses can under certain circumstances be omitted, provided all the collected information clearly supports the generated hypotheses. In case some important issues remain unclear, further investigations are needed.

It is characteristic of analytical epidemiological studies to use a comparison group that allows quantifying a possible association between specific exposures and the disease under investigation. The two most frequently used study designs are case–control studies and cohort studies. Methodological aspects of these and other types of epidemiological studies are presented in Chapter 11.

9.5.1 Formulating a Hypothesis

Based on the findings of the descriptive analysis of the cases, the laboratory analysis, inspections carried out on site, and clinical investigations, the researchers are able to set up qualified hypotheses about the cause of infection, possible source of the pathogen, modes of transmission, and specific exposures. After developing the first hypotheses, a list of potential risk factors related to the infection can be developed. For instance, collected information may strongly suggest that members of a certain community supplied by a specific water system are at high risk to get ill or visitors of some event may report a disease with common manifestations (Gregg 2002).

9.5.2 Assessing Risks: Historical Cohort Studies

The choice of an appropriate study design may depend on various factors, like timing of the investigation, available resources, experiences of investigators, the size of the affected population, the exposure prevalence, and disease incidence (Gerstman 2003). If an outbreak occurs in a limited, closed population group (for example, participants of a celebration, a party, or patients of a hospital), the historical cohort study can be preferred to other study designs. In such a study the total population is divided into persons who were exposed to the potential risk factor and persons who were not exposed to the risk factor. After that the risk-specific attack rates are calculated and compared in both groups. The risk-specific attack rate is normally presented as a percentage:

$$\text{Attack rate} = \frac{\text{No. of cases in the population at risk}}{\text{Total } N \text{ of people at risk}} \times 100$$

The attack rate does not explicitly take a time variable into account, but as soon as the period from the exposure to the onset of most cases is known, the time is implicitly included in the calculation of the attack rate (Gordis 2009).

An example of a hypothesized foodborne outbreak is given below. A foodborne disease outbreak (FBDO) is defined as an incident in which two or more persons experience a similar illness resulting from the ingestion of a common food (Center for Disease Control and Prevention 2008). The example provides the calculation of attack rates and the identification of food or drink items which could possibly have caused the outbreak. In case of such an outbreak, first, investigators list all food and drinks served at the dinner. Next, they divide guests into those who consumed a certain food or drink and those who did not. After that the attack rate in each of the groups is calculated using the formula for attack rate given above. The next step is to find a difference in attack rates between the two groups. The food or drink items which show the biggest differences in attack rates can be responsible for an outbreak of disease (Friis and Sellers 2004). Exhibit 9.2 summarizes the steps in the reporting of a foodborne outbreak, as recommended by the US Centers for Disease Control and Prevention (Center for Disease Control and Prevention 2008).

Exhibit 9.2. Guidelines for reporting in investigations of a foodborne outbreak

Investigation of a foodborne outbreak:
reported information and guidelines

1. *Report type* (final or preliminary report during an outbreak)
2. *Number of cases* (laboratory/confirmed and presumptive cases; if necessary estimated number of cases)
3. *Dates* (dates where the first and the last known case patients got ill; dates of the first and the last known exposure; attached epidemic curve)
4. *Location of exposure* (use of country-specific cities' name abbreviations)
5. *Approximate percentage of cases in each age group* (identification of patterns of age distribution, age groups most affected)
6. *Sex of cases*
7. *Investigation methods*
8. *Implicated food(s)*
   - The contaminated ingredient(s)
   - Reasons for suspecting the food (e.g. laboratory analysis)
   - Methods of preparation
9. *Etiology* (identification of bacterium, virus, parasite, or toxin, according to the standard taxonomy)
11. *Contributing factors* [evidence of contamination, proliferation (increase in numbers), and survival factors responsible for the outbreak]
12. *Symptoms, signs, and outcomes* (number of patients with outcomes)
13. *Incubation period* (the shortest, the median, and the longest incubation period measured in hours or days)
14. *Duration of illness* (the shortest, the longest, and the median duration of illness measured in hours or days)
15. *Possible cohort investigation* (report of attack rate with formula)
16. *Location of food preparation*
17. *Location of exposure* (where food was eaten)
18. *Traceback* (if any traceback investigation)
19. *Recall* (recall of any food product related to the outbreak)
20. *Available reports* (if any additional reports)
21. *Agency reporting the outbreak* (contact information)

For advanced reading and downloading the reporting form for foodborne outbreaks, please refer to the Center for Disease Control and Prevention electronic materials, available at http://www.cdc.gov/foodborneoutbreaks/toolkit.htm

9.5.2.1 Example of a Cohort Study in a Hypothetical Foodborne Outbreak

After participating in a wedding dinner, many of the guests became ill with symptoms like nausea, vomiting, and diarrhea. All 150 persons who participated in the wedding meal were asked about the food and drink they had consumed and whether they got sick after that. The investigators suggested that some food or drink could have been contaminated with staphylococcal bacteria. Using the case definition the

Table 9.1 Analysis of a cohort study

Risk factor present	Disease, N=50	No disease, N=100	Food-specific attack rate (%)
Ate food X	45	40	45/85=53
Did not eat food X	5	60	5/65=7.7

attack rates for specific food (for example, food X) was calculated and compared (Table 9.1).

Out of a total of 85 individuals who ate food X, 45 got sick (attack rate 45/85=53%). The attack rate of those who did not eat food X was 5/65 or 7.7%. Food X was assumed to be a possible risk factor for the disease, because of the following reasons:

- Food-specific attack rate among those who ate food X was high (53%).
- Food-specific attack rate among those who did not eat food X was low (7.7%), and therefore the difference ("risk difference") between the attack rates was high (45.3%).
- The majority of the cases ate food X (45/50 or 90%).

In addition, the relative risk (RR), i.e., the ratio of attack rates, can be calculated:

$$\text{RR} = \frac{\text{Attack rate ate food X}}{\text{Attack rate did not eat food X}} = \frac{53}{7.7} = 6.9$$

A relative risk of 6.9 indicates that individuals who ate food X had a 6.9 times higher probability to get ill than those who had not eaten that food. Statistical significance tests can be used to assess that this association was not found due to chance exclusively (see also Chapter 12).

9.5.3 Secondary Attack Rate

When a disease spreads from the initial case to other persons, for example, to family members, the secondary attack rate can be calculated. It generally refers to the spread of disease in a family, household, dwelling unit, or another community or group. Here we would like to emphasize the use of definitions of initial cases. If a few cases of a disease occur at about the same time after an exposure, then the first case which gets the attention of the public health authorities is referred to as *an index case*, while the other ones are called *coprimary cases* (Friis and Sellers 2004). A coprimary case is by definition very close in time to an index case; therefore it is considered to belong to the same generation of cases. Therefore a secondary attack rate is defined as follows (Friis and Sellers 2004):

$$\begin{matrix}\text{Secondary}\\ \text{attack rate}\end{matrix} = \frac{\text{Number of new cases in group} - \text{initial cases}}{\text{Number of susceptible persons in the group} - \text{initial cases}} \times 100$$

For instance, three cases of measles occurred in a group of 17 children in a summer camp, and it was assumed that exposure took place outside of the camp. Out of these three cases the first one registered by the camp health authorities was considered to be the index case and two other the coprimary cases. Ten days after the first measles symptoms were noticed in the initial cases, further 11 children in the group got ill.

Thus the secondary attack rate was

$$(11 - 3)/(17 - 3) \times 100 = 57.1\%$$

9.5.4 *Case–Control Study*

A case–control study should be the preferred study design in an outbreak investigation under at least the following three circumstances (Dwyer et al. 1994). First, if the initial population is very large and only a part of the population at risk can be sampled. Second, if the initial population at risk is not defined well enough to determine a cohort to be followed. Finally, a nested case–control study can be applied within a studied cohort when additional hypotheses should be tested. In a case–control study the distribution of exposures in the group of cases is compared with that in a group of healthy individuals (controls). The aim of case–control studies is to find differences in the risk factors to which two examined groups (cases and control persons) were exposed in the past. The questionnaire used to interview persons is identical in both groups.

9.5.4.1 Example of a Case–Control Study in a Hypothetical Foodborne Outbreak

We now look at the above example (Table 9.1) from the angle of a case–control study. This means, in particular, that the two groups of "cases" and "controls" involved had been sampled from larger populations of unknown size.

Ninety percent of all cases ate food X, compared to only 40% of the control persons (Table 9.2). This suggests that consumption of food X is associated with the disease.

Table 9.2 Analysis of a case–control study

Exposure	Cases	Controls
Ate food X	45	40
Did not eat food X	5	60
Percentage exposed	*90%*	*40%*

We compare the odds of the food consumption in the group of the cases (45/5) to the odds of the food consumption in the group of the control persons (40/60). The odds ratio is therefore equal to

$$\text{Odds ratio} = \frac{\frac{P1(E)}{1-P1(E)}}{\frac{P2(E)}{1-P2(E)}} = \frac{45/5}{40/60} = \frac{45 \times 60}{5 \times 40} = 13.5$$

An odds ratio of 13.5 hints at a strong association between falling ill and having consumed the food X. Similar to cohort studies it is possible to calculate the potential influence of chance with the help of statistical tests.

9.5.5 Proving Evidence for Causal Associations

A statistical association asserted on the basis of an analytical epidemiological study does not mean a causal association.

The likelihood of a cause and effect relationship increases if the following statements are true:

- The exposure preceded the illness. The suspected causation is biologically plausible; in other words, it is consistent with modern biological knowledge.
- The results correspond to those from other investigations, established and known facts about the disease.
- The value of risk or chance (measured by relative risk or odds ratio) is high, which increases the probability of causal association.
- There is evidence which reveals a dose–response association (the risk increases with the consumed quantity of the suspected infectious cause) (For more about postulates for causation, see Gordis 2009 and Hill 1965).

9.6 Control Measures and Reporting

As has already been mentioned in Section 9.1, the main goal of an outbreak investigation is to stop a current outbreak and to avoid future outbreaks or epidemics. In order to stop an outbreak, the infectious source must be removed or transmission ways should be blocked. To avoid further spread of the infection it is necessary that the conditions that caused the outbreak are eliminated with the help of suitable long-term measures and structural changes. The investigation cannot be considered as completed until the preventive measures have been taken and they have been proven to be effective.

Specific measures that can be implemented to control the infectious source are, e.g., callback of contaminated products, closing of a manufacturing plant, cleaning or disinfection, removing persons from the infective source, treating the infected persons. In order to block the transmission, measures such as vaccination or improvement of hygiene, interruption of animate or inanimate environmental transmission, information and educational campaigns can be taken.

Obviously, any outbreak investigation should be completed by the writing of a report and dissemination of results to the involved parties. Detailed guidelines for writing reports of outbreak investigations can be found elsewhere; however, the following remarks should be taken into account (Ungchusak 2004; Arias 2000; Gregg 2002).

First, the results of the investigations should be carefully documented and sent in the form of a detailed interim and final report to all authorities involved as well as to the administrative staff of the affected facility and the infection control center or committee (Weber et al. 2001; Arias 2000). Study findings should also be reported in the form of oral briefings or reports to all informants, interested local, state, and federal public health departments. In addition, the community of people where the outbreak occurred and study participants should be given feedback about the outcome of the investigation; the public can be informed through the news media. The scientific content of the investigation should be made accessible to specialists through publications in scientific journals and bulletins so that everyone can profit from the experience and insights gained.

During the pandemic of influenza A (H1N1), the World Health Organization provided the guidelines document for preparedness and response encouraging not only governments but also communities, families, and individuals to take active part in mitigating the global and local effects of the pandemic. During an outbreak, civil society groups should play a mediator role between government and communities, taking part in health communication and raising awareness. Taking preventive measures at the level of families and individuals such as regular hand washing, covering sneeze and cough, and isolating ill individuals is crucially important as well. It is furthermore necessary that each household takes care of its own safety in terms of access to precise and update information, medicines, water, and food. Recovered individuals should make use of their illness experience and reach out to other affected people to provide them with information and support (WHO 2009).

9.7 Conclusions

In the light of increasing frequencies of epidemics and outbreaks, a systematic and targeted action is needed in order to collect evidence and support decision-making processes. An outbreak investigation requires an application of methods of descriptive and, where appropriate, analytical epidemiology. The outbreak investigation and management includes several steps, among them most important are the establishment of the case definition and case-finding techniques, collection of data, and description of cases in terms of time, place, and affected person. Usually an analysis is required. Although associations found in an outbreak investigation cannot automatically be considered as causal, the simultaneous use of a well-planned epidemiological investigation and clinical and laboratory evidence will almost always provide valid information about causes and modes of transmission of diseases which will be helpful for decision making.

References

Arias KM (2000) Quick reference to outbreak investigation and control in health care facilities. Jones and Bartlett Publishers, Sudbury, MA

Belongia EA, Osterholm MT, Soler JT, Ammend DA, Braun JE, MacDonald KL (1993) Transmission of Escherichia coli O157:H7 infection in Minnesota child day-care facilities. JAMA 17; 269(7):883–888

Brownson RC (2006) Outbreak and cluster investigations. In: Brownson RC and Petitti DB eds. Applied epidemiology theory to practice, 2nd ed. Oxford University Press, Oxford

Bruneau A, Rodrigue H, Ismäel J, Dion R, Allard R (2004) Outbreak of E. coli O157:H7 associated with bathing at a public beach in the Montreal-Centre region. Can Commun Dis Rep 30(15):133–136

Center for Disease Control and Prevention (2008) OutbreakNet team: Foodborne disease surveillance and outbreak investigation toolkit. Available online at: http://www.cdc.gov/foodborneoutbreaks/toolkit.htm. (Accessed on: 01.12.2008)

Centers for Disease Control and Prevention (1993) Preliminary report: foodborne outbreak of Escherichia coli O157:H7 infections from hamburgers – Western United States, 1993. Morb Mortal Wkly Rep 42(4):85–86

Checko PJ (1996) Outbreak investigations. In: Bowlus B, ed. Infection control and applied epidemiology. Mosby-Year Book, St. Lois, Missouri

Cody SH, Glynn MK, Farrar JA, Cairns KL, Griffin PM, Kobayashi J, Fyfe M, Hoffman R, King AS, Lewis JH, Swaminathan B, Bryant RG, Vugia DJ (1999) An outbreak of Escherichia coli O157:H7 infection from unpasteurized commercial apple juice. Ann Intern Med 130(3): 202–209

Dwyer DM, Groves C (2001) Outbreak epidemiology. In: Nelson KE, Williams CF. Infectious disease epidemiology: theory and practice, 2nd ed. Jones and Bartlett Publishers, Sudbury

Dwyer DM, Strickler H, Goodman RA, and Armenian HK (1994) Use of case-control studies in outbreak investigations. Epidemiol Rev 16(1): 109–123

European Centre for Disease Prevention and Control (2009) Influenza A(H1N1)v pandemic 2009–2010. http://ecdc.europa.eu/en/Health_topics/novel_influenza_virus/2009_Outbreak/ (latest access June, 2009)

Friis RH , Sellers TA (2004) Epidemiology for public health practice, 3rd ed. Jones and Bartlett Publishers, Sudbury

Gerstman BB (2003) Epidemiology kept simple: an introduction to traditional and modern epidemiology, 2nd ed. Wiley-Liss, New York

Gordis L (2009) Epidemiology, 4th ed. Elsevier, USA

Gregg MB (2002) The principles of an epidemic field investigation. In: Detels R, McEwen J, Beaglehole R, Tanaka H. Oxford textbook of public health, 2, The methods of public health, 4th ed. Oxford University Press, New York

Hawker J, Begg NT, Blair I, Reintjes R, Weinberg J (2005) Communicable Disease Control Handbook. 2nd edition. Blackwell Publishing, Oxford

Hill AB (1965) The environment and disease: Association or causation? Proc R Soc Med 58:295–300

Honish L, Predy G, Hislop N, Chui L, Kowalewska-Grochowska K, Trottier L, Kreplin C, Zazulak I. (2005) An outbreak of E. coli O157:H7 hemorrhagic colitis associated with unpasteurized gouda cheese. Can J Public Health 96(3):182–184

King LA, Mailles A, Mariani-Kurkdjian P, Vernozy-Rozand C, Montet MP, Grimont F, Pihier N, Devalk H, Perret F, Bingen E, Bingen E , Espié E, and Vaillant V (2009) Community-wideoutbreak of Escherichia coli O157:H7 associated with consumption of frozen beef burgers. Epidemiology and infection, 137(6): 889–896

Lawson AB and Kleinman K eds. (2005) Spatial and syndromic surveillance for public health. Wiley, Chichester

McLeod KS (2001) Our sense of Snow: the myth of John Snow in medical geography. Soc Sci Med 52(11):1751–1754

Oxford JS, Bossuyt S, Lambkin R (2003) A new infectious disease challenge: Urbani severe acute respiratory syndrome (SARS) associated coronavirus. Immunology 109 (3): 326–328

Timmreck TC (1994) An introduction to epidemiology. Jones and Bartlett Publishers International, London

Towner JS, Sealy TK, Khristova ML, Albariño CG, Conlan S, Reeder SA, Quan PL, Lipkin WI, Downing R, Tappero JW, Okware S, Lutwama J, Bakamutumaho B, Kayiwa J, Comer JA, Rollin PE, Ksiazek TG, Nichol ST (2008) Newly discovered Ebola virus associated with hemorrhagic fever outbreak in Uganda. PLoS Pathog 4 (11): e1000212

Ungchusak K (2004) Principles of outbreak investigation. In: Detels R, McEwen J, Beaglehole R and Tanaka H. Oxford textbook of public health, 4th ed. Oxford University Press, Oxford

Waller LA and Gotway CA (2004) Applied spatial statistics for public health data. Wiley Interscience, New York

Weber DJ, Menajovsky LB, Wenzel R (2001) Investigation of outbreaks. In: Thomas JC, Weber DJ eds. Epidemiologic methods for the study of infectious diseases. Oxford University Press, New York

World Health Organization (2009) Pandemic influenza preparedness and response. A WHO guidance document. WHO, Geneva. http://www.who.int/csr/disease/influenza/pipguidance 2009/en/index.html (accessed June, 2009)

World Health Organization (2009) Influenza A (H1N1). http://www.who.int/csr/disease/swineflu/en/ (accessed June, 2009)

Chapter 10
Geographic Information Systems

Patrick Hostert and Oliver Gruebner

10.1 Introduction

There is a wealth of publications expanding on geoinformation analysis in health sciences. Facing globalisation and the "urban millennium", interdisciplinary research focusing on the interface between infectious disease epidemiology (IDE) and geoinformation analysis is gaining importance in this context (Kraas 2007; Martinez et al. 2008; UN-Habitat 2006). While it is not feasible to adequately cover the full range of conceptual frameworks and practical approaches in this chapter, we shall focus on the most common techniques and give examples illustrating the potential of geographic information systems (GIS) in IDE. Disease transmission is comprehensively covered in Part III. We hence focus on the relevant methodological issues, being well aware of the fact that an in-depth knowledge on disease transmission is mandatory for effective spatial modelling.

A few application-specific definitions shall serve as a starting point:

- Geographic information system (GIS) for IDE: A GIS for IDE-related research comprises a collection of compatible hardware, software (or algorithms) and methods for analysing spatial patterns of diseases, their mechanisms (risk factors, transmission) and for producing maps and reports of spatialised disease information. The science related to implementing and applying spatial methods with GIS is referred to as "GI Science".
- Geoinformation analysis in IDE means spatial analysis based on GIS techniques
  - for finding patterns of infectious diseases;
  - focusing on understanding broad-scale (e.g. global) and fine-scale (e.g. local) drivers of infectious diseases transmission and
  - allowing spatially explicit modelling to explore future scenarios on the spread of infectious diseases.

P. Hostert (✉)
Geography Department Geomatics Lab, Humboldt-Universität zu Berlin, Berlin, Germany
e-mail: patrick.hostert@geo.hu-berlin.de

A. Krämer et al. (eds.), *Modern Infectious Disease Epidemiology*,
Statistics for Biology and Health, DOI 10.1007/978-0-387-93835-6_10,

- Remote sensing in IDE: The use of airborne or satellite imagery for analysing spatial patterns of factors with relevance for IDE and infectious disease transmission. Remote sensing-based image analysis can in this context be regarded as a component of geoinformation analysis.

This chapter is divided in three major sections:

1. We explain the conceptual framework for solution building based on geoinformation analysis in the IDE context.
2. We introduce the most important principles of geoinformation processing for IDE, covering both GIS and remote sensing data analysis.
3. The future development of GI-based IDE research is sketched.

10.2 A Conceptual Framework for GI Science in the IDE Context

Spatial patterns of infectious diseases obviously depend on the spatial patterns of underlying processes. Hence, analyses based on spatially explicit methods are necessarily based on an in-depth knowledge of pathogenetic processes and the related biological background. Research on pathogenesis is always research on the exposure of individuals to potential pathways of infectious diseases; the spatial patterns of processes or factors related to a population at risk are mapped and analysed. A related conceptual framework supports theory building through spatial analysis, theory confirmation or rejection or theory application in a spatially explicit context, i.e. with map-based analyses.

The first step in spatial analysis will hence always be disease mapping, i.e. the spatially explicit representation of disease prevalence or incidence. While a spatial representation is generally helpful for visual interpretation and raising awareness, the detection of disease clusters with methods of cluster analysis is the starting point for further research. Spatial autocorrelation theory is the background for analysing the interdependencies between different regions of a given study area: Tobler's first law says that "everything is related to everything else, but near things are more related to each other" (Tobler 1970). Based on this assumption, the deviation of spatial distributions of incidences from theoretically expected clusters on local to global scales is examined.

Once clusters are identified, the focus is on estimating the exposure of a cohort to a risk factor within space[1] and time[2]. If the pathogenesis is well known, we may

---

[1] "Space" may also cover non-metric variables, such as social distances of family members, then referred to as "social space". We solely expand on metric space here, i.e. real-world distances based on map coordinates.

[2] Aspects of time-related analysis are beyond the scope of this chapter. Time is often represented by two or more data sets from different time periods. The simplest case is a spatially explicit

directly try to identify spatial linkages between incidence patterns and their underlying causes. In the case that the pathogenic background is unidentified, different hypotheses on transmission pathways have to be tested on significance in a spatial context before an in-depth analysis can be performed.

After pathogens and the etiological background of an infectious disease are known, we can approach spatial pattern analyses on different levels: We might initially want to further explore the spatial context of transmission pathways. Scrutinising transmission pathways includes as different foci as the analysis of vector or host habitats in the case of vector-borne diseases, social or socioeconomic indicators related to living or working conditions in the case of social diseases (compare Chapter 6) or the distribution of potential environmental threats in the case of environmental diseases (e.g. water holes with high pollution levels). Such questions can be tackled empirically (based on map operations) or by modelling (based on analytical models).

The most advanced approaches in spatial analysis of infectious diseases relate to simulation models. Spatially explicit predictions on the future development of a disease (forecasting) or scenario building that incorporates potential interventions in the form of "what–if" relationships can be realised in different ways. Fully integrated approaches, i.e. models completely implemented in a GIS environment, are consistent in terms of data management and there is no need to build interfaces between different software packages. However, many solutions rely on coupled models, as underlying epidemiological processes are often difficult to represent in a GIS environment, while at the same time spatial models (e.g. cellular automata or agent-based approaches) are best employed in a GIS.

10.3 Principles of Geoinformation Processing

Section 10.2 illustrated the importance of relating spatial analysis to the knowledge of pathogenesis. We now focus on a more technical question: How can spatially related analyses be practically performed and relevant results extracted from spatial data, i.e. based on GIS?

A GIS is by definition a system for entry, management, analysis and display of spatially related data. In most cases, it is a combination of a spatial database, a (geo-) visualisation and a (geo-) processing tool.

Related tools will be explained here, whereas the more technical aspect of data input is spared.

10.3.1 Data and Databases

Different types of health-related spatial data sets can support spatial data analysis in the IDE context. First, spatialised epidemiological data need to be explored:

"from-to-analysis" over time, while more sophisticated time-series analysis tools might be utilised, if a time series is dense enough.

- data on mortality
- data on morbidity
- data on disease prevalence, distribution, etc.

Second, spatial data sets of potential explanatory variables need to be derived or collected, e.g. through GPS surveys, such as spatialised data on

- health infrastructure and healthcare facilities;
- social infrastructure (e.g. availability and accessibility to education, health insurance and social networks);
- technical infrastructure (e.g. water, sanitation/sewage, (storm water) drainage, electricity, solid waste management, road and railway network and public transport);
- census, socioeconomic and lifestyle variables (e.g. age, sex, income, family size, population density, livelihood activities and nutrition);
- housing (e.g. tenancy, housing quality, housing density, water supply, electricity and sanitary facilities);
- environment (e.g. topography, groundwater information or climatological data);
- ecology (e.g. monitoring information on pollution or vegetation);
- land use and land cover (e.g. satellite data analysis, serving – for example – as important variable in vector habitat analysis).

In a GIS database, the real world is abstracted and geographically represented by a universal GIS data model[3]. A GIS data model comprises spatial features (in vector- or raster-based formats) and thematic information associated with those features (attributes). Vector-based features are, for example, points for wells or sampling locations, lines for streets and areas (polygons) for housing plots. It can also include raster data such as satellite imagery, results from raster image analyses or digital elevation models. For describing the geographic objects, attributes are usually added and stored as tabular data linked to the geographic objects. Like in non-spatial databases, content-related relationships can be considered. In doing so, the data model may be designed with respect to certain purposes, e.g. a health data model which considers interdependencies of a cohort and its living conditions. Information about the social infrastructure and housing as well as on socioeconomic variables might be stored with respect to direct and indirect health impacts. For example, indoor or outdoor pollution might have a direct impact on the health status of the people if they are confronted with this at work, at home or on the everyday trip to reach a special location like the working place. People living in poor housing conditions (slums or squatter settlements) sharing one room with the whole family as well as one tube well and a latrine with other families are exposed, e.g. to infectious and other diseases and this must be considered in the health data model. The health data model can then be integrated into the GIS data model relating attribute

[3]A data model is an abstract model describing how data are structured. Data models are used to integrate different kinds of information putting them into a thematic, semantic or – in the case of spatial data – in a geometric-topological structure.

information to the spatial information, e.g. where to find those observations in the geographical context (geographic coordinates) and what is surrounding those observations (technical infrastructure, data on environment, ecology, land use and land cover). Returning to the example above, poor housing conditions in combination with highly densified built-up areas might constitute a high potential for spreading of infectious diseases.

Many data sets with relevance in IDE are collected as point data and do not provide continuous information. Point data are, for example, related to the location of clinics, to the housing of a person at threat or to water holes as potential source of infection. Today, coordinate information is often collected based on global positioning system (GPS) surveys or on information extracted from Google Earth. In any case, we need to understand which positional inaccuracies go along with the data collection method and how these influence analyses based on the respective data set. From a geographical point of view, these factors are closely connected to the question of the targeted scale of analysis (from local to global) that should be taken into account when designing a data collection campaign. Furthermore, we should be aware of spatial autocorrelation that inhibits spatial data sets when sampling designs ignore certain minimum distances between sampling locations.

We should be prepared for the fact that many – at a first glimpse – continuous data sets covering complete test areas, do not necessarily tell the analyst all details of data quality and aggregation. As the analyst is often different from the data collecting person, it is not always stated how the underlying information relates to the respective areal units, e.g. districts or catchments. Such aggregation units are not necessarily designed to serve IDE studies. GIS provide powerful tools to document data sets with so-called metadata that help analysts understand how data were collected, aggregated or processed and who has processed a data set. Metadata on spatial data enables finding, evaluating and effectively sharing data with others. For example, health survey information may be aggregated on the postcode level for privacy reasons although it is originally sampled at household level. If well documented, such data sets can be disaggregated to gain deeper insight into the distribution and accuracy of the underlying spatial data, assumed not to offend privacy rights (Matisziw et al. 2008). The preferable solution is to design field surveys in a way that we can derive different aggregation levels depending on the respective question at hand. GIS offers to guide this process based on a particular data set. It is possible to stratify a given test area based on survey distribution, locations of health-care centres and clinics or in nested scales that can represent different aggregation levels.

10.3.2 Geovisualisation

GIS can also be regarded as a set of intelligent maps, representing geographic information in a defined spatial coordinate system. Maps act as the main user interface for most GIS applications. On the map data sets are visualised with so-called layers representing vector or raster data sets (Fig. 10.1). With layers the data can be visually organised and numerous tasks such as advanced data compilation, analyses and

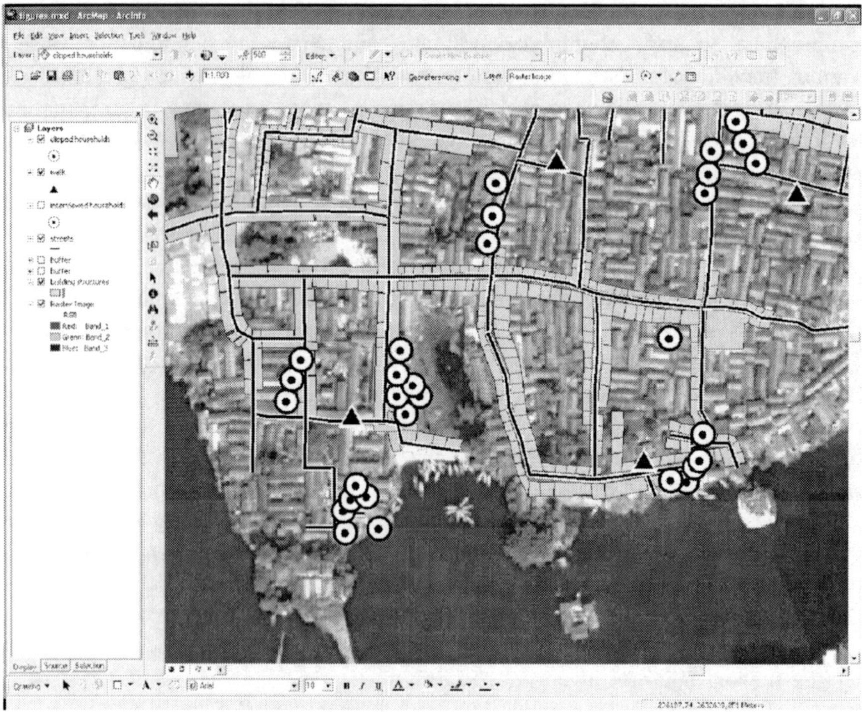

Fig. 10.1 Layer in ArcGIS. The content table on the *left side* shows the layers which are visually represented through signatures and overlayed on the raster layer

spatial database queries can be performed (see Section 10.3.3). GIS also assist in cartographic designing of maps of initial results or the final outcome of a study. Health or disease mapping is usually the first step of spatial analysis in IDE. Visualising disease incidence and prevalence in a spatial context is crucial for further investigation like testing for clusters or spatial disease modelling. Underlying point data, for example, can be visualised with dot or dot density maps[4] and choropleth maps[5] in the case of underlying areal data (Rezaeian et al. 2007).

Yet, the final product is often also a map-based visualisation along with extracted spatial statistics. Traditional static maps as well as dynamic maps may be provided with interactivity offering more information than visually representable at one time.

[4] A dot density map is a thematic map which uses symbols such as dots to represent the quantity and distribution of certain occurrences in space. Depending on the purpose and scale of the map, symbols may represent a single entity, e.g. one dot for one person or a group, e.g. one dot for 100 people.

[5] A choropleth map is used for data which are aggregated on area level. The polygons on the map representing a certain area may be shaded according to their attribute values linked to that area, like disease prevalence in different wards or population density.

The interested reader is referred to Kraak and Brown (2001) for a more complete overview. Time series are either represented by several maps of the same geographic area at a different point in time or by a dynamic map. The latter may display the starting point of a diffusion process and guide the user through time by interactively selecting the desired point in time (state of diffusion). A diffusion process might also be displayed by a cartographic animation, i.e. an animated map sequence visualising dynamic processes over time (Dransch 2000; Kraak 1999). The outcome does not necessarily have to be a printed or online published map. It can also serve as input variables for other applications, such as web-based information systems for infectious disease surveillance, forecasting and warning or any other model.

10.3.3 Map Operations and Analytical Models in GIS

GIS can also be understood as a set of data analysis tools for geoprocessing to extract information from existing data sets by applying analytic operations. Important geoprocessing tools in the IDE context include

- interpolation methods;
- topological analysis;
- proximity analysis;
- overlay analysis;
- spatial autocorrelation analysis;
- analytical models.

Interpolation methods deriving spatially continuous information from spatially discontinuous point data are needed to relate point sampling data on diseases with explanatory information sampled at different locations. The same applies when connecting point data with information that has been produced in a continuous way (compare Section 10.3.4). "Kriging", for example, is an established method to produce such continuous map surfaces from point data sets (Cromley and McLafferty 2002). Kriging takes into account the existing underlying spatial structure of georeferenced information (distances among samples or observations). Statistically optimal estimates and their standard errors for locations with missing data (no-sample locations) can be derived, combining the actual and estimated data as a smoothed surface or raster data structure (Boulos 2004; Moore and Carpenter 1999).

Topological analysis works with vector layers (that visualise vector data sets) and refers to the fact that each vector feature (point, line or polygon) "knows" its geographic coordinate and its neighbouring features (adjacency) according to the spatial data model. It is possible to track all connected features with topology, e.g. shared borders between adjacent polygons or connected point locations. For example, when a point is connected with a line and this line is connected with another point, topology can infer that both points are also connected (connectivity). Topology can also be used to detect features lying in a polygon (containment). Additionally, attribute data from the attribute table can be used in a spatial database query, like: "Which housings are adjacent to an industrial area with recorded blood cancer or respiratory disease cases?"

Proximity analysis works with so-called buffers that are drawn around a point, line or polygon. Consider study sites where the local information about wells and housing is mapped and combined in GIS with surveyed health and census information. In this case proximity analysis with buffers helps the analyst, for example, to answer questions like "How many residents live within a 50 m radius around this well?" or "Which surveyed households are falling into the catchments area of a certain well?" (Fig. 10.2, Fig. 10.3). In proximity analysis thematic information can be used to stratify data. Considering the previous example, residents may be divided into age groups or quartiles of age distributions might be used to derive buffer zones with equal proportions of certain age groups.

Overlay analysis works with different data types including vector or raster layers. Relationships between these data sets can be discovered and new layers with a higher level of information content are created. Vector (topological) overlay functions are, for example, "intersect", "union" and "clip". "Intersect" is used to combine two data sets and to preserve those features and attributes falling in the

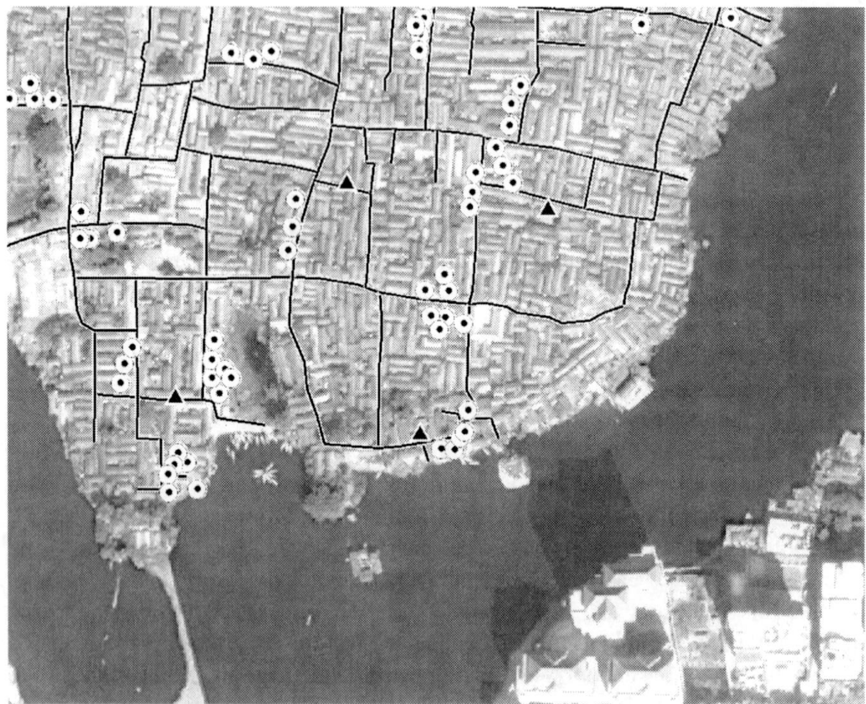

Fig. 10.2 Vector layer of wells (*triangles*) and GPS-based health survey locations (points: interviewed households) overlaid on satellite raster image of a slum in Dhaka, Bangladesh

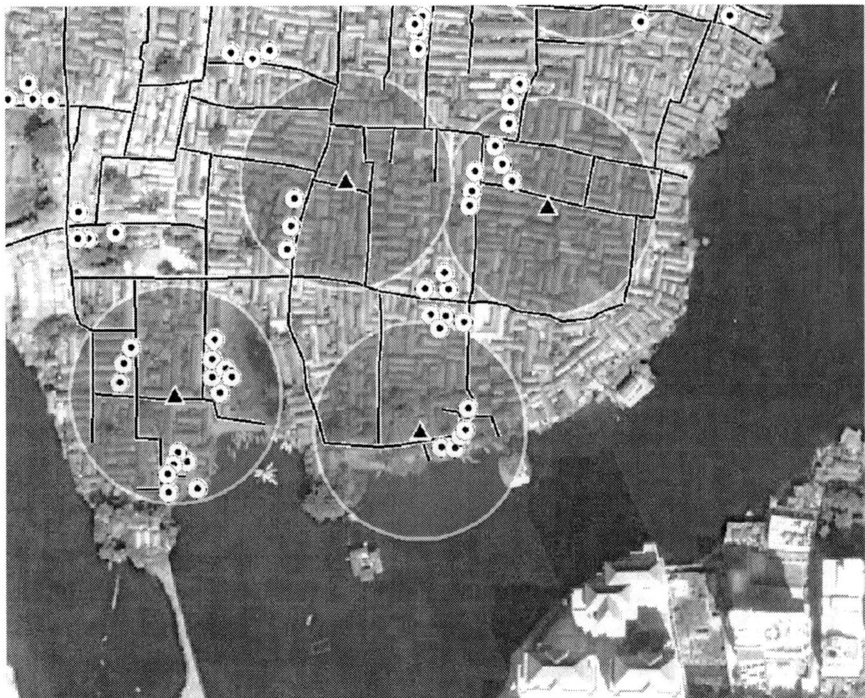

Fig. 10.3 Buffer of 50 m around each well, showing surveyed households which are falling into the wells' catchments area

spatial extent of both layers, while "union" generally keeps all features of both data sets. With "clip", one portion of a layer is cut by using another layer as a kind of "cookie-cutter" (Fig. 10.4). For detailed information on how these functions work and how they are used refer to Longley et al. (2006). Raster overlay deals with cell values from different raster grid scenes that can be combined via mathematical operations (map algebra) to generate new values of cells at corresponding positions in a new grid layer (Boulos 2004; Boulos et al. 2001).

Spatial autocorrelation analysis is used to discover in how far given observations can be regarded as spatially independent or clustered (Tobler 1970). Test statistics are therefore used in IDE to detect significant deviations from theoretically or empirically predicted dispersion patterns of diseases in space and time (for a complete overview refer to Albert et al. (2000), Cromley and McLafferty (2002), Waller and Gotway (2004) and Lawson and Kleinman (2005)). Test statistics with different capabilities in detecting different kinds of clusters can be implemented in GIS. Moran's I (Moran 1950), for example, is well established for continuous data-like information extracted from satellite imagery. For discontinuous data, like health information gathered by household surveys, the spatial scan statistics (SatScan) (Kulldorff 1997) is good at detecting localised clusters and

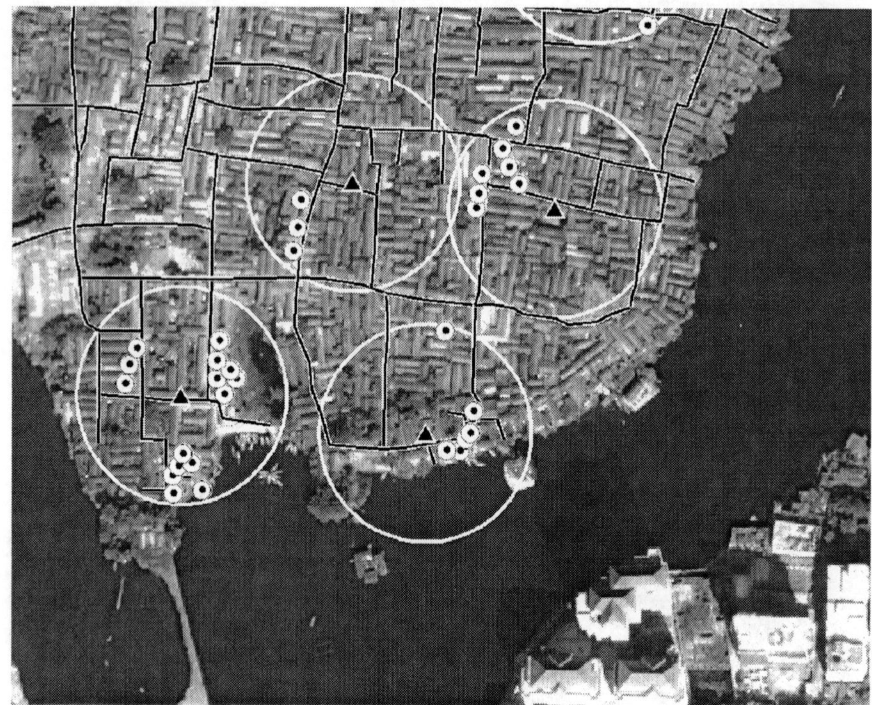

Fig. 10.4 Only households falling into the catchments area are shown after clipping

Tango's Maximized Excess Events Test (MEET) (Tango 2000) supports detecting global clustering (Kulldorff 1997; Song and Kulldorff 2003; Tango and Takahashi 2005). There are many more test statistics for global clustering detection, like Besag–Newell's R (Besag and Newell 1991), Cuzick–Edwards' k-nearest neighbours (k-NN) (Cuzick and Edwards 1990), Swart's entropy test (Swartz 1998) or Whittemore's test (Whittemore et al. 1987), but for all it is true that their power is highly dependent on the parameters chosen, i.e. the user should be aware of the respective boundary conditions of each test (Boulos 2004; Kulldorff et al. 2006; Tango and Takahashi 2005; Wang 2006) (for applications in infectious disease surveillance, see also Chapter 8).

Once clusters of disease incidences are identified, these need to be related to potential explanatory variables in a spatially explicit way. For example, an infectious disease associated with climatic variables is likely to be spatially correlated with relevant climatic drivers (Kleinschmidt et al. 2000). This can easily be tested empirically, i.e. supported by the previously described methods of overlaying, buffering, etc.

More sophisticated analyses to examine the causes of an infectious disease can be performed based on analytical models. Environmental modelling is a powerful application in GIS to analyse habitat, lifecycle and transmission pathways of vectors to predict the dispersion of a virus like dengue or malaria. Land cover information from remotely sensed data (e.g. vegetation, water and housing density), field survey data concerning land use, water and air quality, wind speed and direction as well as expert knowledge about the pathogen itself and its lifecycle can be included in a GIS-based model. Data about the health status of the residents in certain areas are then utilised to validate and iteratively enhance such a model (Gong et al. 2006; Heinrich et al. 2005; Kleinschmidt et al. 2000).

With a validated model for different points in time, simulations can be derived to calculate spatially explicit scenarios. In doing so, many "what–if" questions can be answered: For example, how will habitats of *Aedes aegypti* change if the average temperature rises about 0.5°C in this area and how will that influence yellow and dengue fever in South America? (Barcellos et al. 2005) Another example discussed these days is the potential dispersion of malaria vivax in Germany due to global climate change (Schmidt and Schröder 2007). GIS may also support surveillance and monitoring systems in identifying potential and actual habitats for ticks transmitting lyme disease (Daniel et al. 2004; Zeman and Lynen,2006). What will happen if a human population in densified quarters like slums or squatter settlements amidst a megacity agglomeration faces an infectious disease outbreak? Which transmission paths would the vectors probably take? Will the disease disperse to surrounding residential areas? (Ali et al. 2003; De Castro et al. 2004; Tatem and Hay 2004).

An operational analytical model in a GIS comprises specific processing steps that are defined in a process flow chart. Such a model is designed to be transferable, i.e. to work under similar boundary conditions, but with different data sets and in different locations (Boulos 2004; Boulos et al. 2001). Models are often implemented in a GIS environment by coding a software tool and accordingly extending and customising the GIS software package. Depending on the software, different application programming interfaces (APIs) exist, enabling developers to code their own GIS applications, e.g. geoprocessing models (Stevens et al. 2007; Zhang et al. 2007).

10.3.4 The Role of Remote Sensing

Remote sensing-derived data become increasingly available in different regions of the world and at multiple scales. GI science increasingly integrates remote sensing-derived information in the analysis process. Moreover, methods from GIS are more and more integrated with digital image processing methods. Lillesand et al. (2003) provide an introduction in remote sensing and image interpretation. For details on digital image processing in remote sensing Richards and Jia (2005) is suggested as an introductory reading.

Remote sensing from airborne and satellite platforms provides spatially continuous data at different scales. The above described problems of point data and their spatial representativity can hence be avoided. While the mere image data can serve as a cartographic base map or image backdrop for visualisation, we are usually interested in problem-specific information derived from remote sensing imagery.

Raw image data are turned into information layers via image interpretation or digital image processing. This can in turn be integrated in complex IDE analysis approaches or modelling scenarios.

We hence need to define how IDE-related research can be supported with remote sensing-derived information products. Such a strategy always starts with identifying epidemiologically relevant indicators that can be tackled from a remote sensing point of view. These are very diverse and equally diverse can be the appropriate processing strategies. With respect to IDE, it is useful to differentiate generic remote sensing analyses (resulting in so-called baseline products) and problem-specific maps that are explicitly designed to support the analysis of a certain IDE-related case.

Typical remote sensing-derived information for IDE studies comprises land use and land cover, vegetation type or habitat maps, water maps or diverse structural surface properties, e.g. information on infrastructure or corridors (vegetation, airflow, etc.). Also, more sophisticated products may be derived, as, for example, indicators on housing structures in slum areas or indirect estimates of population density in cases where adequate statistical data are missing or erroneous. In other words, remote sensing can provide information urgently needed on the explanatory side of the equation concerning IDE processes.

Any image processing is based on the analysis of pixel-wise recorded spectral reflectance or emission from the Earth's surface (Lillesand et al. 2003). It is hence important to note that only those surface properties or phenomena can be distinguished, which correspond with the spatial (i.e. pixel size) and spectral resolution (observed wavelength region) of the respective sensor. If remotely sensed features on the Earth's surface comply with these necessities, we are able to cover large areas synoptically, to acquire repetitive data and to produce continuous information layers for analyses in IDE.

In the context of this chapter, only a few basic nonetheless important image analysis concepts are presented:

- generating maps of land cover;
- Vegetation analysis and
- monitoring through multitemporal data analysis Multitemporal data analysis.

Automatic image classification leading to land cover classes (or any thematic classes of interest that can be distinguished from remote sensing data) builds the backbone of most remote sensing data analyses. Image data are either clustered into spectrally similar classes in an unsupervised way, i.e. we only have to specify a few basic parameters like a clustering algorithm and the number of desired classes. The classifier will then automatically group the most similar pixels into a common class. Or image data are classified in a supervised way, i.e. the analyst has to define spectral training samples before a classification algorithm is chosen that compares the spectral properties of these sample classes with every image pixel. Each pixel is then assigned to the most similar spectral class. Classified imagery often builds the basic input for more sophisticated thematic analyses or modelling approaches, e.g. for vector habitat maps relating habitat needs to certain land cover or for characterising water pollution levels from remotely sensed data.

The second huge field of remote sensing applications is vegetation analysis. Vegetation behaves spectrally different from any other surface on Earth due to its pigment and water content, as well as its cell structure. These characteristics lead to very specific reflectance properties in the visible and near infrared wavelength regions, which are routinely scanned by most of today's Earth observation remote sensing systems. Indices relating visible and near infrared reflectance properties are therefore well suited to detect and characterise photosynthetically active vegetation. In the simplest case, ratios calculated from the visible and near infrared spectral domain (so-called vegetation indices) allow characterising vegetation vitality. It is, for example, possible to separate different vegetation structures being important for analysing disease transmission pathways by combining vegetation index values with classified image data.

Multitemporal data analysis is an important aspect when including remote sensing imagery in IDE-related studies. Specifically, satellite data are obtained on a regular basis (e.g. with daily re-visiting cycles in the case of spatial coarse resolution sensors or bi-weekly re-visiting time for high-resolution sensors). Spatial very high-resolution sensors (i.e. metre resolution) are designed as pointing devices scanning specified target regions of the world on demand. Multitemporal remote sensing data analysis supports IDE studies by enabling change detection, on daily, monthly or yearly basis – depending on the phenology of the observed phenomenon and the information needs for solving a specific research question. The spatial extent of short-term events such as floodings may be analysed, as well as the long-term phenological cycle of vegetation serving as habitat for specific vectors. In many cases, multitemporal remote sensing-based maps are the only available input for IDE modelling. This holds especially true for global scale studies or in remote areas with poor statistical data and lacking base maps.

10.4 Conclusion and Future Perspectives

In the future, public bodies, health organisations and epidemiological research centres will strengthen their efforts to build up extended databases for IDE applications. This applies specifically to developing countries. Such databases include thematic data, i.e. information on disease incidence and prevalence, but also spatialised information. Spatially explicit data are needed at different levels: Coordinates related to reported infected diseases should be recorded (household location, working place, activity profiles); basic cadastral data sets need to be build up in a timely and accurate manner providing the mandatory spatial background information; remote sensing-derived information should be further exploited to enhance analysis capabilities, specifically where other information is scarce.

With such data at hand, spatial decision support systems in IDE can help urban planners and decision makers to find the right location for hospitals and health-care facilities. Risk areas may be declared and programmes started to prevent population at risk from being exposed. Mosquito prevention programmes in southern latitudes, for example, could be better coordinated by exactly knowing (locating) potential breeding sites.

The previous sections underpin the need of a close collaboration between epidemiologists and geographers. Analysing spatial patterns in IDE is far from trivial and encompasses great responsibilities, specifically when research output is an important contribution to decision support systems and integrated disease modelling. Wrong or inadequate conclusions from spatial data analysis may not only yield enormous costs, but also constitute an immediate threat for public health, i.e. through inadequate warnings on pandemic hazards. Strengthening the application of GIS and GI science in IDE-related research will certainly reduce the probability of inadequate conclusions.

References

Albert DP, Wilbert MG and Levergood B, eds. (2000) Spatial analysis, GIS, and remote sensing: applications in the health sciences, Chelsea

Ali M, Wagatsuma Y, Emch M and Breiman RF (2003) Use of a Geographic Information System for defining spatial risk for dengue transmission in Bangladesh: Role for Aedes Albopictus in an urban outbreak. Am J Trop Med Hyg, 69: 634–640

Barcellos C, Pustai AK, Weber MA and Brito MRV (2005) Identification of places with potential transmission of dengue fever in Porto Alegre using Geographical Information Systems. Revista Da Sociedade Brasileira De Medicina Tropical, 38: 246–250

Besag J and Newell J (1991) The detection of clusters in rare diseases. J R Stat Soc Ser A (Stat Soc), 154: 143–155

Boulos MNK (2004) Towards evidence-based, GIS-driven national spatial health information infrastructure and surveillance services in the United Kingdom. Int J Health Geogr, 3: 1

Boulos MNK, Roudsari AV and Carson ER (2001) Health geomatics: An enabling suite of technologies in health and healthcare. J Biomed Inform, 34: 195–219

Cromley EK and McLafferty SL (2002) Gis and public health, New York

Cuzick J and Edwards R (1990) Spatial clustering for inhomogeneous populations. J R Stat Soc Ser B (Methodol), 52: 73–104

Daniel M, Kolar J and Zeman K (2004) GIS tools for tick and tick-borne disease occurrence. Parasitology, 129: S329–S352

De Castro MC, Yamagata Y, Mtasiwa D, Tanner M, Utzinger J, Keiser J and Singer BH (2004) Integrated urban malaria control: A case study in Dar Es Salaam, Tanzania. Am J Trop Med Hyg, 71: 103–117

Dransch D (2000) Begriffe und Grundprinzipien der Animation. In: Buziek, G, Dransch, D. and Rase, W.-D. (eds.), Dynamische visualisierung, Berlin, NY, 5–14

Gong P, Xu B and Liang S (2006) Remote sensing and geographic information systems in the spatial temporal dynamics modeling of infectious diseases. Sci China C-Life Sci, 49: 573–582

Heinrich J, Gehring U, Cyrys J, Brauer M, Hoek G, Fischer P, Bellander T and Brunekreef B (2005) Exposure to traffic related air pollutants: self reported traffic intensity versus GIS modelled exposure. Occup Environ Med, 62: 517–523

Kleinschmidt I, Bagayoko M, Clarke GPY, Craig M and Le Sueur D (2000) A spatial statistical approach to malaria mapping. Int. J. Epidemiol, 29: 355–361

Kraak M-J (1999) Cartography and the Use of Animation. In: Cartwright, W, Peterson, M.P. and Gartner, G. (eds.), Multimedia cartography, Berlin, NY

Kraak M-J and Brown A (2001) Web cartography, Padstow, Cornwall

Kraas F (2007) Megacities and global change: key priorities. Geogr J, 173: 79–82

Kulldorff M (1997) A spatial scan statistic. Commun Stat Theory Methods, 26: 1481–1496

Kulldorff M, Song C, Gregorio D, Samociuk H and DeChello L (2006) Cancer map patterns: Are they random or not? Am J Prev Med, 30: S37–S49

Lawson AB and Kleinman K, eds (2005) Spatial and Syndromic Surveillance for Public Health, Chichester

Lillesand TM, Kiefer RW and Chipman JW (2003) Remote Sensing and Image Interpretation. Wiley, New York 784 .

Longley PA, Goodchild MF, Maguire DJ and Rhind DW, eds (2006) Geographic information systems and science. Wiley & Sons, New York 472 .

Martinez J, Mboup G, Sliuzas R and Stein A (2008) Trends in urban and slum indicators across developing world cities, 1990–2003. Habitat Int, 32: 86–108

Matisziw TC, Grubesic TH and Wei H (2008) Downscaling spatial structure for the analysis of epidemiological data. Comput Environ Urban Syst, 32: 81–93

Moore DA and Carpenter TE (1999) Spatial analytical methods and geographic information systems: Use in health research and epidemiology. Epidemiol Rev, 21: 143–161

Moran PAP (1950) Notes on continuous stochastic phenomena. Biometrika, 37: 17–23

Rezaeian M, Dunn G, St Leger S and Appleby L (2007) Geographical epidemiology, spatial analysis and geographical information systems: a multidisciplinary glossary. J Epidemiol Community Health, 61: 98–102

Richards JA and Jia X (2005) Remote sensing digital image analysis. Springer, Berlin, Germany 439

Schmidt G and Schröder W (2007) Flächenhafte Szenarien zur potenziellen Ausbreitung von Malaria vivax in Niedersachsen in Abhängigkeit steigender Lufttemperaturen. In: Strobl, J, Blaschke, T. and Griesebner, G. (eds.), Angewandte geoinformatik 2007. Beiträge zum 19. Agit-Symposium, Heidelberg, 670–680

Song C and Kulldorff M (2003) Power evaluation of disease clustering tests. Int J Health Geogr, 2: 9

Stevens D, Dragicevic S and Rothley K (2007) iCity: A GIS-CA modelling tool for urban planning and decision making. Environ Model Software, 22: 761–773

Swartz JB (1998) An entropy-based algorithm for detecting clusters of cases and controls and its comparison with a method using nearest neighbours. Health Place, 4: 67–77

Tango T (2000) A test for spatial disease clustering adjusted for multiple testing. Stat Med, 19: 191–204

Tango T and Takahashi K (2005) A flexibly shaped spatial scan statistic for detecting clusters. Int J Health Geogr, 4: 11

Tatem AJ and Hay SI (2004) Measuring urbanization pattern and extent for malaria research: A review of remote sensing approaches. J Urban Health-Bull NY Acad Med, 81: 363–376

Tobler WR (1970) A computer model simulation of urban growth in the Detroit region. Eco Geogr, 46: 234–240

UN-Habitat (2006) State of the world's cities 2006/2007. UN-Habitat, Nairobi

Waller LA and Gotway CA (2004) Applied spatial statistics for public health data, Hoboken, New Jersey

Wang F (2006) Quantitative methods and applications in Gis, Boca Raton, New York

Whittemore AS, Friend N, Brown BW and Holly EA (1987) A test to detect clusters of disease. Biometrika, 74: 631–635

Zeman P and Lynen G (2006) Evaluation of four modelling techniques to predict the potential distribution of ticks using indigenous cattle infestations as calibration data. Exp Appl Acarol, 39: 163–176

Zhang JT, Pennington DD and Liu XH (2007) GBD-Explorer: Extending open source java GIS for exploring ecoregion-based biodiversity data. Ecolog Inform, 2: 94–102

Chapter 11
Methods and Concepts of Epidemiology

Rafael Mikolajczyk

11.1 Introduction

The purpose of this chapter is to review the basic concepts of epidemiology, including definitions of measures of disease occurrence and measures of association, brief descriptions of study designs and ethical principles of epidemiological research. Additionally, the theory and criteria of causation, systematic and random errors in epidemiological studies and methodological issues related to diagnostic tests are discussed. The concepts are outlined and some examples are given.

11.2 Definitions of Epidemiological Terms

11.2.1 Measures of Disease Occurrence

Terms used to quantify the occurrence of a disease in a population are listed in Table 11.1.

Table 11.1 Measures of disease occurrence

Measure	Description
Prevalence	Number or proportion of persons with a specific disease at a specific time point in the population
Incidence	Number or proportion of persons developing a specific disease during a time period
Morbidity	Ambiguously used: prevalence or incidence
Mortality	Number or proportion of persons dying during a time period
Fatality rate	Proportion of persons dying from a specific disease among all persons with the disease
Attack rate	Proportion of cases developing the disease among all persons who were exposed to the disease

R. Mikolajczyk (✉)
Department of Public Health Medicine, School of Public Health, University of Bielefeld, Germany
e-mail: rafael.mikolajczyk@uni-bielefeld.de

A. Krämer et al. (eds.), *Modern Infectious Disease Epidemiology*,
Statistics for Biology and Health, DOI 10.1007/978-0-387-93835-6_11,

For frequent diseases, *prevalence* can be provided in percentages; for rare diseases, prevalence can be presented as the number of cases per 1,000, 100,000, or even 1 million within the population. For example, 5.6 persons with chronic hepatitis C per 1,000 persons of the population on January 1, 2006. The prevalence can be age or gender specific; in such cases, additional information such as "per 1,000 women aged 20–30" should be included. Prevalence can be defined at a given time point (*point prevalence*), for example, when all participants in a telephone survey are asked about having a specific disease. *Period prevalence* is defined as the cumulative number of cases observed during a given time period.

In contrast, *incidence* is the number of new cases with a specific illness occurring during a given time period (for example, 10 new HIV infections per 10,000 inhabitants during the year 2005). The time period can be flexibly specified as a daily, weekly, monthly, or yearly incidence, depending on how much variability is present in the number of cases observed over time. For example, providing only yearly incidence for a disease with a strong seasonality like influenza will not capture the information about the temporally overcrowded doctor offices during influenza season. While prevalence is important for assessing the need of treatment in the population, incidence provides information about the dynamics of the spread of infection and is the most important measure during outbreaks or epidemics. *Mortality* is the incidence of deaths.

The term *morbidity* is used inconsistently: most often to indicate prevalence but sometimes also to indicate incidence.

Case fatality describes how many of infected persons die because of the disease. It does not provide any information about the duration of the disease before death, so in chronic infections the deaths can spread over long period of time, while in the case of acute infections like influenza or SARS they are concentrated in short period of time – despite possibly the same case fatality.

Attack rate is the fraction of persons acquiring an infection among all persons who were exposed to the infection. The attack rate depends on the composition of the population, especially with regard to immunity.

11.2.2 Measures of Association

Measures of association commonly used in epidemiology to assess the relationship between exposure and outcome are presented in Table 11.2 and Fig. 11.1.

Table 11.2 Measures of association

Measure	Description
Absolute risk	Probability of a specific outcome
Relative risk (risk ratio)	Ratio of absolute risks in two distinct, mutually exclusive subgroups with different exposure status
Absolute odds	Chance of a specific outcome (if 1 person gets the disease and 9 do not, then the odds is 1:9)
Odds ratio (relative odds)	Ratio of two absolute odds in two distinct, mutually exclusive subgroups with different exposure status

Exposure / Outcome	1	2	Sum
Yes	a	b	All sick cases
No	c	d	All healthy cases
Sum	All cases with exposure 1	All cases with exposure 2	All tests / all cases

Outcome can be a disease or death, exposure can be any risk behaviour or any characteristic of the person (like gender or age group). The letters "a" to "d" indicate numbers of cases in each cell – for example "a" - the number of persons with the disease and exposure status 1. The information to fill the table for a concrete research question can be obtained from routine statistics or from epidemiological studies.

Absolute risk for persons with exposure 1: a/(a+c)

Relative risk for exposure 1 compared to exposure 2: $\dfrac{a/(a+c)}{b/(b+d)}$

Odds ratio for exposure 1 compared to exposure 2: $\dfrac{a/c}{b/d} = \dfrac{a \times d}{b \times c}$

Fig. 11.1 Figure for illustration of relative risk and odds ratio

The *absolute risk* of a disease can be different among persons with a specific exposure (risk factor) than among persons without this exposure, for example, the risk of acquiring HIV can be different for males and females. *Relative risk* provides information regarding how many times higher or lower the risk is among individuals with one exposure status compared to individuals with another exposure status. For example, in a given population the risk of having HIV infection can be 3.2 times higher for males than females. In the simplest scenario, the *relative risk* can be calculated from a two-by-two table displayed in Fig. 11.1.

While the two-by-two table can be constructed whenever there is a dichotomous outcome and exposure, the measures of absolute and relative risks are not always meaningful. For example, when the study population consists of persons who were selected because they have a given disease and compared to another group who does not have the disease (see case–control study below), absolute risk of having the disease cannot be obtained from these data. In such a study, the relative risk as a ratio of two absolute risks cannot be calculated either. However, even if the absolute risk is not known, the two-by-two table contains useful information. The information can be used to calculate *absolute odds* and *odds ratio*. Both measures are calculated from the inner cells of the table (see Fig. 11.1). *Odds* is the chance of disease, i.e. the ratio of sick to healthy persons – for example, if in a population there are 100 HIV-infected individuals and 900 noninfected individuals, the odds of being infected is 1/9. Risk of being infected is 100/(100+900)=1/10, which is close to the odds, but not identical. (The lower is the prevalence of the disease in the population, the closer are odds and risks to each other.)

Both these measures – relative risk and odds ratio – apply to a disease status at one given time point. Two further measures of association are absolute hazard and corresponding hazard ratio, which measure the occurrence of disease over time. If a

given exposure not only causes a disease but also accelerates its development, then these findings would be better conveyed by hazard ratio than risk ratio or odds ratio.

A different concept – not directly used for analysis but for interpretation of the relative risk – is the *population attributable risk.*

> *Population attributable risk* (PAR) is the fraction of cases with a disease which can be avoided if the risk factor is totally removed from the population.

PAR can be calculated according to the formula PAR = PE(RR–1)/(1+PE (RR–1)), where PE is the prevalence of the risk factor and RR is the relative risk associated with the risk factor (Greenland and Robins 1988). The measure is very appealing for presenting the public health impact of a specific risk behaviour or intervention, for example, PAR of 30% for intravenous drug use for hepatitis B means that when this behaviour can be removed as a risk factor, 30% of cases of hepatitis B infection can be prevented. Similarly, increasing vaccination coverage would lead to a decrease in the incidence of the specific disease and this can be reported as PAR (see Chapters 12 and 14). While the calculation of PAR for non-communicable diseases follows the above formula, additional considerations are required for communicable infectious diseases. For communicable diseases, the removal of a given risk factor often results not only in directly avoided infected cases (primary cases) but also in a reduction in the risk of infection for other persons in the population (secondary cases) who would be otherwise infected by primary cases. These effects may not be proportional, and removing a specific risk factor can result in smaller or larger effect on the incidence than in the above formula.

11.3 Populations, Study Samples and Random Error

All the above definitions are based on the assumption that there is a "true" value of the incidence, the prevalence and the association between risk and outcome in a given population. Population might be defined widely as all inhabitants of a country or more specifically as a group of individuals with special characteristics, for example, intravenous drug users. In some simple cases we might know the incidence of cases in the whole population based on registries, like, for example, the death certificate registry; however, in the case of most diseases and risk factors, it is not feasible to assess them in the whole population. In such cases, for the purpose of specific study, smaller groups might be sampled from the population and assessed more in depth. Since subjects of the study are only a subgroup of the population, by chance the study might have recruited more individuals with a given disease than the prevalence in the population. This is based on the same principle as obtaining four times heads in a row while flipping the coin although the "true" proportion is 50%. This is called *sampling error*, a subtype of *random error* encountered in epidemiological studies. Another potential source of random error is non-sampling error, which can be introduced by the uncertainty in measurement. Non-sampling error would lead to different results when the study is repeated in the same sample; sampling error would provide different results if a new study sample is recruited from the population. Historically, the first solution to deal with sampling error was testing of significance, with results from the test reported as p values. More recently, there has been a trend towards reporting the confidence intervals for the results (Armstrong 1998). While both results are often reported together, confidence intervals provide more information about the studied relationship. Confidence intervals not including a "zero effect" (which is 1 for odds ratio or relative risk) can have the same interpretation as a significance test; they allow the rejection of the tested hypothesis. But additionally, a narrow confidence interval demonstrates that the study is big enough to provide precise information and therefore the size of the observed effect is relatively certain. Modern statistical analysis provided solutions to many specific problems and while sampling error is not avoidable, it can be usually quantified. Other types of error will be discussed later.

11.4 Common Types of Epidemiological Studies

The purpose of epidemiological studies is to provide estimates for measures of disease occurrence in the population and information about the relationship between risk factors and disease using specifically selected samples of the population. There are three main study designs: survey, case–control study and cohort study (including randomized clinical trial) (Table 11.3) (von Elm et al. 2007).

Table 11.3 Selected types of epidemiological studies

Type	Description
Survey	Collection of data at a single time point in a sample of the population
Case–control study	Selection of the sample revolves around the disease status, i.e. participants are included if they have a disease (cases), while a comparison group without this disease is selected (controls)
Cohort study	Collection of data performed over time in the same defined group of participants with different exposure status; information about different time points is either obtained from existing records or reported by participants at different occasions
Randomized clinical trial	Persons meeting specified inclusion criteria are enrolled in the study and randomized into subgroups receiving different treatments
Meta-analysis	Joint analysis of previous studies based typically on published results only, but sometimes also on original data (individual data meta-analysis)

A *survey*: a study in which information concerning each participant is collected only once and the participants are selected to reflect the studied population. It can be used to estimate the prevalence of disease and of risk factors. The estimate of incidence can be obtained only based on retrospective information about when the disease started. Similarly, information about changes in the risk behaviour can be obtained only retrospectively. Therefore, for the current risk behaviour and disease status, it is not clear whether disease preceded the risk behaviour or not (Hernan and Robins 2006; Martin 2008). Some persons might adapt a healthy lifestyle after developing the disease. Although retrospective information about behaviour before the onset of a disease can be obtained in a survey, its accuracy depends on the memory of the participant and the quality of reporting which can be subject to reporting bias (Hartman et al. 2002). Surveys can be conducted through personal interviews, mailed questionnaires or on the phone. In particular, the two latter forms are relatively cheap and easy to implement, making the survey design a very attractive research method when information needs to be quickly obtained and should be representative for the population. In some cases, the researcher might not be interested in the whole population, but in a specific subgroup like intravenous drug users or prostitutes, he or she would still attempt to obtain a good representation of this subgroup in the study sample. On the other hand, survey design can also include the collection of biological samples. In the epidemiology of infectious diseases, biological samples are collected in serological surveys assessing for HIV status (Montana et al. 2008) or vaccination against childhood diseases in the population (Nardone et al. 2003). Surveys can be used to link seroprevalence of antibodies and information about risk behaviours, but again the possibility has to be considered that the current behaviours might not be related to the disease at all or that the behaviours might have been influenced by knowledge of the disease status.

Case–control studies can provide neither prevalence or incidence estimates nor information about absolute or relative risk. However, case–control studies allow the comparison of exposure status in persons with a disease (cases) and healthy participants (controls) using odds ratios. The case–control design is especially advantageous when risk factors for a very rare disease have to be investigated. Instead of recruiting a very large population for a longitudinal study with the expectation that some cases of the rare disease will occur over time in the study population, for the case–control study, persons who developed the disease are selected. For example, rare complications of vaccinations can be studied in case–control studies. While the identification of cases may sometimes pose diagnostic difficulties, the main challenge in a case–control study is the selection of controls. The aim in selecting controls is choosing individuals representative of the population from which the cases originated (Wacholder et al. 1992a; Wacholder et al. 1992b). Many approaches have been proposed to the selection of controls: hospital controls, controls having a different disease with similar symptoms, best friend controls (Lopes et al. 1996). All these approaches can be seen as convenience samples. A better approach, but more demanding and expensive, is to use population-based controls. In order to make the cases and controls more similar to each other, for example, in terms of gender or age, the researcher might perform *matching* – either as frequency matching (the number of controls in the same age group matched to the number of controls) or as individual-based matching (one or more controls are matched to each individual case for all requested characteristics) (Wacholder et al. 1992c).

Cohort study: a distinction should be made between an open cohort which is defined by a specific framework (for example, all inhabitants of a specific town) and allows new entries (younger inhabitants who reach the age for inclusion in the study or people who move into the studied area) and a more traditional closed cohort for which a defined group of participants is selected and only loss to follow-up but no new entries are allowed (Philippe 2001). Cohort studies can provide information about the incidence occurring over time as well as the prevalence of the disease at a given time point. To address the problem of changing cohort size over time (due to deaths or loss to follow-up), incidence can be measured as *incidence density*, where the sum of the times each participant contributed to the study during the specific period is in the denominator. Apart from the above distinction, the cohort study itself can be either retrospective or prospective. A prospective cohort study is by far the most demanding and the most expensive study design. Retrospective cohort studies have the advantage of using existing records for a defined population. These studies are often used to identify occupational hazards due to biochemical exposures. However, while more convenient, retrospective studies are restricted to routinely collected information, which may not include many questions of interest. Through the longitudinal character, cohort studies can provide clear information about the sequence of exposure and disease. A drawback is that only very common diseases can be studied with moderate cohort size and the less frequently a disease occurs, the larger the cohort has to be. Another practical problem can be the very long duration of a cohort study when development of the disease occurs over a long process. In infectious disease epidemiology, cohort studies are commonly used to assess the transmission or the progression of the disease. Prospective cohort studies were used to study stages of AIDS (Badri et al. 2006) or seroconversions among HIV serodiscordant couples (Bunnell et al. 2006).

Randomized clinical trials (RCTs) recruit participants who meet predefined inclusion and exclusion criteria and then randomly allocate them into groups which receive different interventions (Moher et al. 2001). At minimum, there are two groups of participants, one in which the intervention is conducted and one placebo group, but RCTs can also test several interventions against each other or against standard therapy or placebo treatment. The control group is necessary because of the subjectivity of human perception which might result in a mistaken impression that the treatment is more effective than in the reality. Two other mechanisms to ensure objectivity of RCTs are randomization and blinding. Randomization should ensure that the studied groups are comparable and the selection of patients is not influenced by the expectations of the researcher (Kang et al. 2008). Different techniques can be used for randomization and it was shown that less rigorous randomization, possibly including incomplete concealment of the randomization sequence, can affect results of the study (Schulz et al. 1994; Schulz et al. 1995; Schulz and Grimes 2002a). To further improve the objectivity, RCTs apply blinding, which means, at minimum, that patients do not know whether they receive active medication or placebo, or that neither patients nor their doctors (double blinding) know the group of the patient (Schulz and Grimes 2002b). Sometimes, triple blinding is also used, which means that during the analysis of the data, anonymous codes are used and only after the results are obtained the meaning of the codes is revealed. While there is a strong agreement about the necessity of blinding in RCTs, the blinding is not always correctly performed and reported in publications (Haahr and Hrobjartsson 2006).

In the control group, placebo therapy is used, but some problems arise if the application of placebo has its own effects (Hrobjartsson and Gotzsche 2001). Another difficulty is when the intervention involves manipulations which are obvious to the patient. In such case, application of placebo infusions, needle insertion outside of areas used in standard acupuncture or even surgical scars are sometimes used to blind the patient (called *sham* procedures (Sutherland 2007)). While testing against placebo is usually the most desirable way to obtain information about the true effectiveness of the treatment, this option is unethical when effective treatment for the studied question already exists because a treatment which is considered to be effective cannot be withheld from the patient. In some cases, when the new medication is not expected to be more effective, but, for example, have fewer side effects or simpler administration, a new medication can be tested in *non-inferiority trials* in comparison with the standard medication (Piaggio et al. 2006). Non-inferiority trials require substantially larger sample sizes than trials oriented towards demonstrating a difference in treatments, but are increasingly common in modern pharmaco-epidemiology.

A subtype of randomized clinical trials is the *cross-over trial*, which is especially oriented towards the assessment of physiological processes. In these trials, participants are randomized for a given sequence of intervention or placebo (Putt and Ravina 2002). In the simplest case, a participant, after being in the placebo group, switches to the intervention group and vice versa. In more complex studies, several different medications can be applied sequentially. The advantage of cross-over trials is that patient's values under treatment can be compared with his/her own values under placebo; however, their use is limited if the patient can be cured or his condition permanently changes.

While originally designed for simple one-step interventions, clinical trials can also be used for the assessment of *complex interventions* (Campbell et al. 2000). Complex interventions are defined as a specified sequence of treatments which might be applied in different combinations to individual patients. Studies assessing the effectiveness of complex interventions usually require a large sample size.

All the above types of trials are person based in which the unit of evaluation is a single person. A specifically epidemiological type of an intervention trial is a *community-based intervention* (Doyle et al. 2008). In this type of studies, groups of participants rather than individual patients are randomized; these groups can be based on geographic or other criteria (for example, minorities can be studied in specific settings which do not follow a geographic distribution). When the intervention is applied, the results are evaluated as rates on the level of randomization units.

Another type of epidemiological studies is systematic review, which is a joint evaluation of several, possibly all existing studies addressing a specific question. It is called *meta-analysis* when statistical methods are also used to obtain a combined estimate from all included studies. Meta-analysis can be based either on published estimates or on originally collected data from several studies (more on systematic reviews and meta-analyses in Blettner et al. 1999).

Some additional study designs are also used in specific fields. For example, *nested case–control studies* can be used to address more specific questions based on cases and controls recruited from an existing cohort study (Ernster 1994; Cologne et al. 2004). To study the effects of transient exposures (stress events, jogging in the morning or vaccination) as triggers of certain diseases, *case cross-over design* was proposed (Maclure 1991; Maclure and Mittleman 2000; Park et al. 2004; Reintjes et al. 2005). In this study the exposure of the participant at some earlier time point is compared with the exposure during the time window in which the exposure could potentially trigger the disease. A methodological innovation in recruiting survey participants from the so-called hidden populations [for example, populations with illegal (like intravenous drug users) or socially stigmatized behaviours (prostitutes, homosexual men)] is *respondent-driven sampling* (Heckathorn 1997; Heckathorn 2002). This method is based on the idea of "snowball" sampling: the participant is asked to recruit further persons from the same population, but advanced methodologies are used to convert the derived estimates into representative estimates for the whole studied populations (Heckathorn 2007). Developmental psychologists invented the *accelerated longitudinal design* also called cohort sequential or mixed longitudinal design (Prinzie and Onghena 2005). This design uses multiple cohorts which are overlapping with respect to age at the end of the study. The information from the separate cohorts is combined to evaluate the trajectory over the whole age spectrum of the participants, which can be several times larger than the duration of the observation period (Miyazaki and Raudenbush 2000).

11.5 Ethic in Epidemiological Research

The most crucial ethical requirement for clinical or epidemiological studies is the *informed consent*, which assures that study participants are informed about possible consequences of the study, understand them and agree to participate in the study (World Medical Association 1964). Historically, the debate about ethical aspects of research and informed consent was triggered by a study of syphilis infection in the African-American population in Alabama from 1932 to 1972 (Jones 1993). In order to assess the natural course of the syphilis infection in untreated patients, no treatment was provided to the participants, even after an effective treatment was developed and introduced in the general population. Over the course of the study, 28 participants died directly of syphilis, 100 died of complications, 40 infected their wives and 19 of their children had been born with congenital syphilis. While this drastic example is surely an issue of the past, epidemiological studies bear the potential of abuse, especially when conducted in disadvantaged populations. Recent reviews of informed consent practices and whether patients are able to understand them indicate a further need of improvement (Flory and Emanuel 2004; Sugarman et al. 2005; Hill et al. 2008).

To assist the researchers in the planning of studies, *ethical approval* by *institutional review boards* is provided. This practice is standard in many developed countries, but in some developing countries these control mechanisms might be deficient (Bhutta 2002; Creed-Kanashiro et al. 2005; Marshall 2005; Sumathipala et al. 2008).

11.6 Causality in Epidemiological Research

Seminal work on the criteria of causality for associations observed in epidemiological studies was conducted by a British medical statistician Austin Bradford Hill (1897–1991). He proposed a list of nine criteria, of which only one was logically necessary but none was sufficient. More recently, a theoretical work on the scientific foundations of epidemiology, including the understanding of causation, was requested (Susser and Susser 1996a; Krieger, Zierler 1997). In a recent review, Parascandola and Weed (Parascandola and Weed 2001) identified five definitions of causation used by epidemiologists:

- *Production*: a given variable is understood as a cause when it creates or produces a specific outcome; this definition was repeatedly criticized because it applies an equally unclear concept of production to define the causation.
- *Necessary cause*: only the logically necessary conditions are understood as causes. This definition is strongly influenced by the notion of scientific determinism. If in some cases the expected outcome does not occur in the exposed participant, this has to be attributed to other, not yet known deterministic causes.
- *Sufficient-component cause*, in which several variables play a role as component causes and jointly form a sufficient cause. This definition was proposed by Rothman and Saunders (Rothman and Greenland 2002) and follows older philosophical traditions. Parascandola and Weed (Parascandola and Weed 2001) argue that this definition is also based on the concept of scientific determinism, since for a specific patient it implies that he/she either has the sufficient cause or not.
- *Probabilistic causation* is opposed to the deterministic understanding of science. According to this definition, cause is a variable or a characteristic which increases the risk of disease. This definition can be used to accommodate the concepts of sufficient cause (which raises the probability of outcome to 1) and necessary cause (which raises the probability of outcome above 0) (Parascandola and Weed 2001).
- *Counterfactuals*: the definition is based on the idea of comparing the outcomes under two contrasting scenarios, one including a specific effect and one excluding it. The definition is not directly opposed to the concept of necessary and sufficient cause and can also be combined with both the scientific determinism and the probabilistic causation. It is also not opposed by the other definitions but rather adds a specific aspect of understanding the causal relationship.

While Parascandola and Weed (Parascandola and Weed 2001) argue in favour of the probabilistic causation, they also stress that distinction should be made between defining causation and recognizing a cause. For the latter the counterfactual definition can be very helpful.

Another issue which received recent attention is the understanding of proximate and distal or direct and indirect causes (Susser and Susser 1996a). Susser and Susser (Susser and Susser 1996b) proposed that after the era of risk behaviours assessed in the individual patient, social structures on the one side and genetic epidemiology on the other side will receive more attention in the 21st century. The effects of social structures were studied in social epidemiology but now they will be combined with molecular knowledge in multilevel models. The different levels of these models are also associated with a different understanding of causation (Parascandola and Weed 2001; Susser 2001).

11.7 Systematic Error in Epidemiological Studies

While the issue of causation is related to the more general understanding of epidemiological research, at the technical level the issue of a correct measurement of associations in epidemiological studied receives a lot of attention.

> *Systematic error (Bias)* is a phenomenon which causes a distortion of the result – the measured effects are either too small or too large.

Bias can occur in the study at different stages: during planning, conducting the study, analysing the data or publishing the results. Extensive lists of possible bias were published in the literature *(Good* 1962; *Sackett* 1979; *Hartman et al.* 2002*)*. Some forms of bias are rather obvious and easily understood, but others require technical knowledge and reflection. Probably the most commonly discussed bias refers to the selection of participants for the study: in any study related to health, persons with a special interest in this area are more likely to participate. This might not affect the ill cases in a case–control study, but it may affect the selection of controls. If controls are the most healthy individuals from the population, they might have fewer risk factors – and in such a case the association between specific risk factors and the disease might appear too strong. While the selection bias may not be avoidable, the researcher should be aware of the direction in which such bias would affect the results. If the bias would affect the results towards a zero effect (odds ratio or relative risk of 1), and the effect still can be observed, then the researcher can propose that the effect is "at least" that large. When the direction in which the bias is most likely to affect the results is towards a smaller effect and no effect is observed in the study, the study is inconclusive, but such "negative" study will also receive less attention. The truly difficult case is when the bias is towards a larger effect and a positive effect is found in the study. Given this relationship, epidemiologists try to keep unavoidable errors in the direction which does not support the study hypothesis, and in such a case at least a conservative estimate of the effect can be obtained. Finally, it has to be kept in mind that each study has its own potential in providing systematically distorted results.

11.8 Methodological Issues of Diagnostic Tests

Assessment of any disease is based on diagnostic tests, which is a specific area of measurement error. There are four basic terms which refer to diagnostic tests: sensitivity, specificity, positive and negative predictive value (Fig. 11.2).

Test / Disease	Positive	Negative	Sum
Yes	True positive	False negative	All sick cases
No	False positive	True negative	All healthy cases
Sum	All positive tests	All negative tests	All tests / all cases

Sensitivity = True positive/all sick cases
Specificity = True negative/all healthy cases
Positive predictive value (PPV) = True positive/all positive tests
Negative predictive value (NPV) = True negative/all negative tests

Fig. 11.2 Figure for illustration of sensitivity, specificity, positive and negative predictive value

Sensitivity is the ability of the test to detect sick cases. Some of the detected cases have the disease in reality, but others might be incorrectly classified as sick. *Specificity* is the ability of the test to distinguish between false-positive and truly negative cases.

A method which diagnoses all sick cases as sick and does not include any healthy cases in this group would be a perfect test and has a 100% sensitivity and a 100% specificity. However, in many cases either due to technical limitations of the test or due to overlapping values in both healthy and ill subjects, the sensitivity and the specificity are interconnected. Increasing sensitivity (i.e. detecting more of the diseased cases) results in a decreased specificity of the test (along with the higher detection of true cases, the number of false-positive tests also increases). Balancing sensitivity and specificity by selecting an appropriate cut-off for positive test is therefore based on the rationale of the test. For example, a screening test should have a high enough sensitivity to detect a high fraction of the sick cases. But since many of the cases might be incorrectly classified as positive, a second test can be used to confirm the result. This second test should have high specificity in order to discard the truly negative cases, after which only the truly positive cases should remain. Since the second test is used only in the subgroup which had positive results in the first test, the requirements on its sensitivity are not as high. This relationship points towards the fact that the performance of the test depends on the prevalence of the disease in the sample: when the disease is very rare, along with the truly positive cases, there will be many false-positive cases.

Two other measures were proposed to provide information which incorporates the prevalence of the disease in the population:

> *Positive predictive value* is the probability of being ill when the test is positive.
> *Negative predictive value* is the probability of being healthy when the test is negative.

Tests with the same sensitivity and specificity will have a lower positive predictive value in a population where the disease is less frequent as compared to a population with a higher prevalence. This relationship is the opposite for the negative predictive value.

Test characteristics also affect the estimates of prevalence or incidence of a disease: when a real-world test is used, neither specificity nor sensitivity can be 100%. Therefore some cases will be falsely classified as sick while not having the disease and some others will be classified as healthy although they have the disease. When the sensitivity and the specificity are known, they can be used to correct the prevalence estimate. (For further reading on sensitivity and specificity, see Loong 2003.)

11.9 Outlook on the Use of Mathematical Modelling in Infectious Disease Epidemiology

For many research questions, infectious disease epidemiology uses the same methods as general epidemiology. For example, the estimates of prevalence can be obtained from surveys and that of incidence from cohort studies. However, the situation is more complicated for analytical studies, i.e. studies assessing risk factors of being infected. For communicable diseases, the probability of getting an infection depends not only on behavioural or genetic factors but also on the prevalence of the disease. This dependency requires the use of special statistical methods or mathematical models to obtain accurate results. Especially models designed to predict future spread of the disease should consider the relationship between risk of getting an infection and prevalence of this infection. When a fast investigation is necessary (as in outbreak investigation, see Chapter 9), conducting the analysis without taking into account the potential dependency between infected persons could be an option providing initial results. However, when not an immediate intervention, but estimation of the impact of specific risk factors is necessary, it should be performed taking into account the potential dependency between infected persons. To address this issue, statistical models incorporating dependency and dynamic transmission models were developed. Solutions to the dependency issue based on dynamic transmission models are presented in Chapter 12.

References

Armstrong BG (1998) Effect of measurement error on epidemiological studies of environmental and occupational exposures. Occup Environ Med 55(10): 651–6

Badri M, Lawn SD and Wood R (2006) Short-term risk of aids or death in people infected with HIV-1 before antiretroviral therapy in South Africa: A longitudinal study. Lancet 368(9543): 1254–9

Bhutta ZA (2002) Ethics in international health research: A perspective from the developing world. Bull World Health Organ 80(2): 114–20

Blettner M, Sauerbrei W, Schlehofer B, Scheuchenpflug T and Friedenreich C (1999) Traditional reviews, meta-analyses and pooled analyses in epidemiology. Int J Epidemiol 28(1): 1–9

Bunnell R, Ekwaru JP, Solberg P, Wamai N, Bikaako-Kajura W, Were W, Coutinho A, Liechty C, Madraa E, Rutherford G and Mermin J (2006) Changes in sexual behavior and risk of HIV transmission after antiretroviral therapy and prevention interventions in rural Uganda. Aids 20(1): 85–92

Campbell M, Fitzpatrick R, Haines A, Kinmonth AL, Sandercock P, Spiegelhalter D and Tyrer P (2000) Framework for design and evaluation of complex interventions to improve health. Bmj 321(7262): 694–6

Cologne JB, Sharp GB, Neriishi K, Verkasalo PK, Land CE and Nakachi K (2004) Improving the efficiency of nested case-control studies of interaction by selecting controls using counter matching on exposure. Int J Epidemiol 33(3): 485–92

Creed-Kanashiro H, Ore B, Scurrah M, Gil A and Penny M (2005) Conducting research in developing countries: Experiences of the informed consent process from community studies in Peru. J Nutr 135(4): 925–8

Doyle J, Armstrong R and Waters E (2008) Issues raised in systematic reviews of complex multisectoral and community based interventions. J Public Health (Oxf) 30(2): 213–5

Ernster VL (1994) Nested case-control studies. Prev Med 23(5): 587–90.

Flory J and Emanuel E (2004) Interventions to improve research participants' understanding in informed consent for research: A systematic review. Jama 292(13): 1593–601

Good IJ (1962) A classification of fallacious arguments and interpretations. Technometrics 4(1): 125–32

Greenland S and Robins JM (1988) Conceptual problems in the definition and interpretation of attributable fractions. Am J Epidemiol 128(6): 1185–97.

Haahr MT and Hrobjartsson A (2006) Who is blinded in randomized clinical trials? A study of 200 trials and a survey of authors. Clin Trials 3(4): 360–5

Hartman JM, Forsen JW, Jr., Wallace MS and Neely JG (2002) Tutorials in clinical research: Part iv: Recognizing and controlling bias. Laryngoscope 112(1): 23–31

Heckathorn DD (1997) Respondent-driven sampling: A new approach to the study of hidden populations. Social Problems 44(2)

Heckathorn DD (2002) Respondent-driven sampling ii: deriving valid population estimates from chain.Referral samples of hidden populations. Soc Probl 49(1): 11–34

Heckathorn DD (2007) Extensions of respondent-driven sampling: Analyzing continuous variables and controlling for differential recruitment. Sociol Methodol 37(1): 151–207

Hernan MA and Robins JM (2006) Estimating causal effects from epidemiological data. J Epidemiol Community Health 60(7): 578–86

Hill Z, Tawiah-Agyemang C, Odei-Danso S and Kirkwood B (2008)Informed consent in Ghana: What do participants really understand? J Med Ethics 34(1): 48–53

Hrobjartsson A and Gotzsche PC (2001) Is the placebo powerless? An analysis of clinical trials comparing placebo with no treatment. N Engl J Med 344(21): 1594–602

Jones JH (1993) Bad blood: The Tuskegee syphilis experiment. New York, Free Press

Kang M, Ragan BG and Park JH (2008) Issues in outcomes research: An overview of randomization techniques for clinical trials. J Athl Train 43(2): 215–21

Krieger N and Zierler S (1997) The Need for epidemiologic theory. Epidemiology 8(2): 212–4

Loong TW (2003) Understanding sensitivity and specificity with the right side of the brain. Bmj 327(7417): 716–9

Lopes CS, Rodrigues LC and Sichieri R (1996) The lack of selection bias in a snowball sampled case-control study on drug abuse. Int J Epidemiol 25(6): 1267–70

Maclure M (1991) The case-crossover design: a method for studying transient effects on the risk of acute events. Am J Epidemiol 133(2): 144–53

Maclure M and Mittleman MA (2000) Should we use a case-crossover design? Annu Rev Public Health 21: 193–221

Marshall PA (2005) Human rights, cultural pluralism, and international health research. Theor Med Bioeth 26(6): 529–57

Martin W (2008) Linking causal concepts, study design, analysis and inference in support of one epidemiology for population health. Prev Vet Med 86(3-4): 270–88

Miyazaki Y and Raudenbush SW (2000) Tests for linkage of multiple cohorts in an accelerated longitudinal design. Psychol Methods 5(1): 44–63

Moher D, Schulz KF and Altman DG (2001) The consort statement: revised recommendations for improving the quality of reports of parallel-group randomised trials. Lancet 357(9263): 1191–4

Montana LS, Mishra V and Hong R (2008) Comparison of HIV prevalence estimates from antenatal care surveillance and population-based surveys in sub-Saharan Africa. Sex Transm Infect 84 Suppl 1 : i78–i84

Nardone A, Pebody RG, van den Hof S, Levy-Bruhl D, Plesner AM, Rota MC, Tischer A, Andrews N, Berbers G, Crovari P, Edmunds WJ, Gabutti G, Saliou P and Miller E (2003) Sero-epidemiology of mumps in western Europe. Epidemiol Infect 131(1): 691–701

Parascandola M and Weed DL (2001) Causation in epidemiology. J Epidemiol Community Health 55(12): 905–12

Park T, Ki M and Yi SG (2004) Statistical analysis of Mmr vaccine adverse events on aseptic meningitis using the case cross-over design. Stat Med 23(12): 1871–83

Philippe P (2001) Density incidence and cumulative incidence: A fundamental difference. Internet J Intern Med 2(2)

Piaggio G, Elbourne DR, Altman DG, Pocock SJ and Evans SJ (2006) Reporting of noninferiority and equivalence randomized trials: An extension of the consort statement. Jama 295(10): 1152–60

Prinzie P and Onghena P (2005). Cohort Sequential Design. B. Everitt and D. Howell, (eds.),. Encyclopedia of statistics in behavioral science. John Wiley & Sons

Putt ME and Ravina B (2002) Randomized, placebo-controlled, parallel group versus crossover study designs for the study of dementia in Parkinson's disease. Control Clin Trials 23(2): 111–26

Reintjes R, Kajueter H, Ehrhard I, van Treeck U and Ammons A (2005) Applying a case-crossover study design to examine transient exposures in the transmission of *N. Meningitides*. Eur J Epidemiol 20(7): 629–33

Rothman K and Greenland S (2002) Modern epidemiology. Lippincott-Raven, Philadelphia, PA.

Sackett DL (1979) Bias in analytic research. J Chronic Dis 32(1–2): 51–63.

Schulz KF, Chalmers I, Altman DG, Grimes DA and Dore CJ (1995) The methodologic quality of randomization as assessed from reports of trials in specialist and general medical journals. Online J Curr Clin Trials Doc No 197: [81 paragraphs]

Schulz KF, Chalmers I, Grimes DA and Altman DG (1994) Assessing the quality of randomization from reports of controlled trials published in obstetrics and gynecology journals. Jama 272(2): 125–8

Schulz KF and Grimes DA (2002a) Allocation concealment in randomised trials: Defending against deciphering. Lancet 359(9306): 614–8.

Schulz KF and Grimes DA (2002b) Blinding in randomised trials: Hiding who got what. Lancet 359(9307): 696–700

Sugarman J, Lavori PW, Boeger M, Cain C, Edsond R, Morrison V and Yeh SS (2005) Evaluating the quality of informed consent. Clin Trials 2(1): 34–41

Sumathipala A, Siribaddana S, Hewege S, Lekamwattage M, Athukorale M, Siriwardhana C, Murray J and Prince M (2008) Ethics review committee approval and informed consent: An analysis of biomedical publications originating from Sri Lanka. BMC Med Ethics 9: 3

Susser M (2001) Glossary: Causality in public health science. J Epidemiol Community Health 55: 376–8

Susser M and Susser E (1996a) Choosing a future for epidemiology: i. eras and paradigms. Am J Public Health 86(5): 668–73

Susser M and Susser E (1996b) Choosing a future for epidemiology: Ii. From black box to Chinese boxes and eco-epidemiology. Am J Public Health 86(5): 674–7

Sutherland ER (2007) Sham procedure versus usual care as the control in clinical trials of devices: Which is better? Proc Am Thorac Soc 4(7): 574–6.

von Elm E, Altman DG, Egger M, Pocock SJ, Gotzsche PC and Vandenbroucke JP (2007) The strengthening the reporting of observational studies in epidemiology (strobe) statement: Guidelines for reporting observational studies. PLoS Med 4(10): e296

Wacholder S, McLaughlin JK, Silverman DT and Mandel JS (1992a) Selection of controls in case-control studies. I. Principles. Am J Epidemiol 135(9): 1019–28

Wacholder S, Silverman DT, McLaughlin JK and Mandel JS (1992b) Selection of controls in case-control studies. II. Types of controls. Am J Epidemiol 135(9): 1029–41

Wacholder S, Silverman DT, McLaughlin JK and Mandel JS (1992c) Selection of controls in case-control studies. III. Design options. Am J Epidemiol 135(9): 1042–50

World medical association declaration of Helsinki. ethical principles for medical research involving human subjects [Http://Www.Wma.Net/E/Policy/Pdf/17c.Pdf] Website

Chapter 12
Mathematical Models in Infectious Disease Epidemiology

Mirjam Kretzschmar and Jacco Wallinga

12.1 Introduction

The idea that transmission and spread of infectious diseases follows laws that can be formulated in mathematical language is old. In 1766 Daniel Bernoulli published an article where he described the effects of smallpox variolation (a precursor of vaccination) on life expectancy using mathematical life table analysis (Dietz and Heesterbeek 2000). However, it was only in the twentieth century that the nonlinear dynamics of infectious disease transmission was really understood. In the beginning of that century there was much discussion about why an epidemic ended before all susceptibles were infected with hypotheses about changing virulence of the pathogen during the epidemic. Hamer (1906) was one of the first to recognize that it was the diminishing density of susceptible persons alone that could bring the epidemic to a halt. Sir Ronald Ross, who received the Nobel prize in 1902 for elucidating the life cycle of the malaria parasite, used mathematical modeling to investigate the effectiveness of various intervention strategies for malaria.

In 1927, Kermack and McKendrick published a series of papers in which they described the dynamics of disease transmission in terms of a system of differential equations (Kermack and McKendrick 1991a; Kermack and McKendrick 1991b; Kermack and McKendrick 1991c). They pioneered the concept of a threshold quantity that separates different dynamic regimes. Only if the so-called basic reproduction number is above a threshold value can an infectious disease spread in a susceptible population. In the context of vaccination this leads to the concept of herd immunity, stating that it is not necessary to vaccinate the entire population to eliminate an infectious disease. This theory proved its value during the eradication of smallpox in the 1970s. Vaccination coverage of around 80% worldwide in combination with ring vaccination was sufficient for eradication of this virus.

M. Kretzschmar (✉)
Julius Centre for Health Sciences and Primary Care, University Medical Centre Utrecht, Utrecht, The Netherlands; Center for Infectious Disease Control, RIVM, Bilthoven, The Netherlands
e-mail: mirjam.kretzschmar@rivm.nl

A. Krämer et al. (eds.), *Modern Infectious Disease Epidemiology*, Statistics for Biology and Health, DOI 10.1007/978-0-387-93835-6_12,

Only towards the end of the twentieth century did mathematical modeling come into more widespread use for public health policy making. Modeling approaches were increasingly used during the first two decades of the AIDS pandemic for predicting the further course of the epidemic and for trying to identify the most effective prevention strategies. But the real impact of mathematical modeling on public health came with the need for evaluating intervention strategies for newly emerging and re-emerging pathogens. In the first instance it was the fear of a bioterrorist attack with smallpox virus that sparked off the use of mathematical modeling to combine historical data from smallpox outbreaks with questions about vaccination in modern societies (Ferguson et al. 2003). Later the outbreak of the SARS virus as a newly emerging pathogen initiated the use of mathematical modeling for analyzing infectious disease outbreak data in real time to assess the effectiveness of intervention measures (Wallinga and Teunis 2004).

Analysis of historical data about pandemic outbreaks of influenza A have led to the important insight that the basic reproduction number of influenza has been low in historical outbreaks, but the serial interval is short (Mills et al. 2004). This implies that in principle an outbreak of influenza can be stopped with moderate levels of intervention, but measures have to be taken very rapidly in order to be effective. In contrast, for an infection such as measles with a high basic reproduction number, very high levels of vaccination coverage are needed for elimination. Such insights gained from mathematical analysis are extremely helpful for designing appropriate intervention policy and for the evaluation of existing interventions.

12.2 Basic Concepts in Mathematical Modeling

The central idea about transmission models, as opposed to statistical models, is a mechanistic description of the transmission of infection between two individuals. This mechanistic description makes it possible to describe the time evolution of an epidemic in mathematical terms and in this way connect the individual level process of transmission with a population level description of incidence and prevalence of an infectious disease. The rigorous mathematical way of formulating these dependencies leads to the necessity of analyzing all dynamic processes that contribute to disease transmission in much detail. Therefore, developing a mathematical model helps to focus thoughts on the essential processes involved in shaping the epidemiology of an infectious disease and to reveal the parameters that are most influential and amenable for control. Mathematical modeling is then also integrative in combining knowledge from very different disciplines like microbiology, social sciences, and clinical sciences.

For many infections – such as influenza and smallpox – individuals can be categorized as either "susceptible," "infected" or "recovered and immune." The susceptibles that are affected by an epidemic move through these stages of infection (Fig. 12.1).

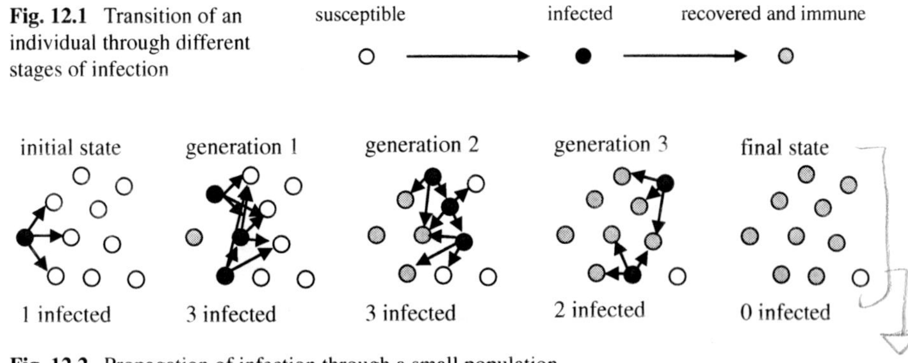

Fig. 12.1 Transition of an individual through different stages of infection

Fig. 12.2 Propagation of infection through a small population

A key quantity in infectious disease epidemiology is the reproduction number, denoted by the symbol R, which is defined as the number of secondary cases that are infected by one infectious individual. As an example we can sketch the typical course of an epidemic if the reproduction number $R = 3$ (here the generation time equals the duration of infectivity; Fig. 12.2).

In the illustration of Fig. 12.2, the number of new infections increases in the first generation by a factor equal to the reproduction number R. The number of available susceptible individuals is depleted in the course of the epidemic. When the last infected person fails to contact any susceptible person, the epidemic dies out.

The infection attack rate is the total proportion of the population that is eventually infected during the epidemic, and it is denoted by A. This infection attack rate is completely determined by the reproduction number R and the contact process that describes who contacts whom (Fig. 12.3). To illustrate the basic shape of the relation between the reproduction number R and the infection attack rate A, we suppose that infectious contacts are made at random.

This provides us with a simple and robust relation that indicates what would happen if a new infection were to hit a completely susceptible population: if the

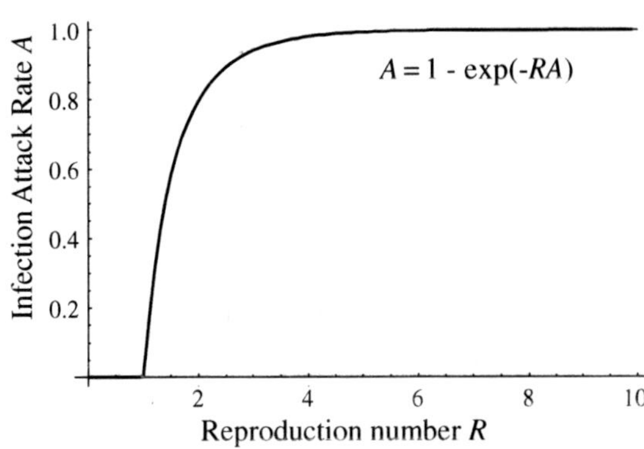

Fig. 12.3 The attack rate A as a function of the reproduction number R

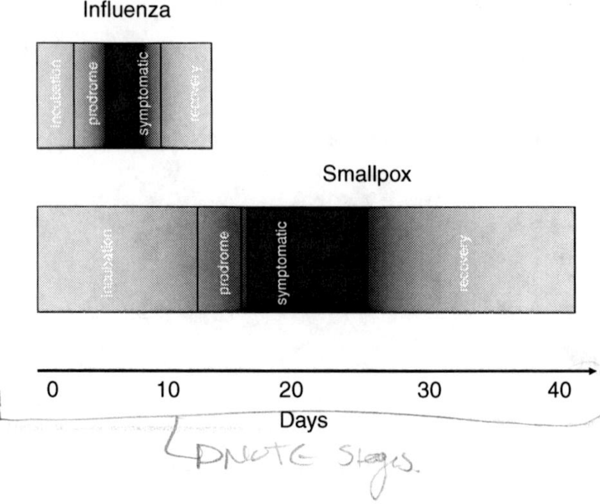

Fig. 12.4 Differences in duration of the infectious period and varying infectiousness during the course of an infection for influenza and smallpox. *Dark gray* and *black* areas symbolize periods with medium to high infectiousness, *light gray* no or low infectiousness

new infection is like influenza, with a reproduction number of about $R = 1.5$, we expect that more than half of the population will be infected; and if the new infection is like smallpox, with a reproduction number of about $R = 5$, we expect that almost the entire population will be infected during an epidemic without interventions.

To capture the epidemic dynamics over time, we need to incorporate the natural course of infection of an individual host. As time proceeds, an infected host moves from the incubation period through the prodromal phase and the infectious period to recovery and immunity (Fig. 12.4). For influenza and smallpox, such timelines are depicted in Fig. 12.4. The duration of the incubation period and the relative infectiousness in the stages before symptom onset (the prodromal phase) and the symptomatic stage are crucial in determining the success of control strategies such as contact tracing and isolation of symptomatic cases.

The timelines determine another epidemiological key quantity, the generation time T. This generation time is defined as the typical duration between the time of infection of a source and the time of infection of its secondary case(s). For influenza, the generation time is in the order of $T = 3$ days. For smallpox, the generation time is in the order of $T = 20$ days.

The chain reaction nature of the epidemic process leads to exponential growth in real (calendar) time during the initial phase of the epidemic, once the number of infected individuals has become large enough to avoid chance events that lead to an early extinction of the epidemic. The exponential growth rate r is determined by the precise timelines of infection. There is a lower limit to the growth rate r that is set by both the reproduction number R and the generation time T (specifically, $r > \ln(R)/T$).

To illustrate the strength of this basic approach to epidemic modeling, we use it to assess the impact of border closure on epidemic spread. The number of infected persons that will try to cross the border from an infected country into a country that is not yet infected will increase exponentially with a growth rate r. Closing the borders will stop most infected persons, but a proportion p might slip through. Therefore, closing the borders will result in a reduction by a factor p of the exponential growth of number of imported cases. This reduction corresponds to a delay in the exponential growth of the number of imported cases (specifically, the delay is at most $(-\ln p / \ln R)\ T$). Therefore, border closure will only postpone the import of cases for a few generations of infection. For example, if closure was to reduce all of those infected travelers who would ordinarily have crossed the border to 1%, the introduction of an influenza epidemic may be delayed by about a month, and the introduction of a smallpox epidemic may be delayed by about 2 months.

The key epidemiological variables that characterize spread of infection are the generation time T and the reproduction number R. If a novel infection starts spreading, such as SARS in 2003, these key variables are unknown. But even if an outbreak of a more familiar infection occurs, such as norovirus, we might be groping in the dark about the precise values of these key variables. Yet, if modeling is to be helpful in infectious disease control, it is crucial to have the best possible estimates for the generation time and the reproduction number, along with other quantities such as the incubation time and hospitalization rate. Estimation would be easy if we had perfect information about the outbreak. If we would know exactly who had infected whom, and if we know precisely who was infected when, we could simply measure the duration of each time interval from infection of a case back to time of infection of its source, and the distribution of the length of these time intervals would inform us about the generation interval. Similarly, we could simply count for each infected individual how many others were infected by this individual, and the distribution of such counts would inform us about the reproduction number. Of course, in a real world such information is not available and we have to deal with incomplete observations, proxy measures, and reporting delays. But real-time estimating procedures have been proposed that attempt to reconstruct the likely patterns of who infected whom, and who was infected when, from the incomplete data and proxy measures, using standard statistical techniques for dealing with missing data and censoring (Wallinga and Teunis 2004; Cauchemez et al. 2006). The main message is that during an outbreak it is important to collect data on cases (time of symptom onset) and about the relation between cases (existence of an epidemiological link). The more accurate this data is, the more useful it is to estimate the key model ingredients, the generation time T and the reproduction number R, and the more helpful this data can be in predicting the likely future course of the epidemic without intervention and the required control effort to curb the epidemic.

Many of the above ideas can be formalized mathematically in the so-called SIR model that describes the dynamics of different states of individuals in the population in terms of a system of ordinary differential equations. The variables of the system are given by the compartments described above: the group of susceptible persons (denoted by S), the group of infected persons (denoted by I), and the group of removed persons (removed from the process of transmission by immunity) (denoted by R). The mathematical model provides a precise description of the movements in and out of the three compartments. Those movements are birth (flow into the compartment of susceptible individuals), death (flow out of all compartments), transmission of infection (flow from S into I), and recovery (flow from I into R) (Fig. 12.5).

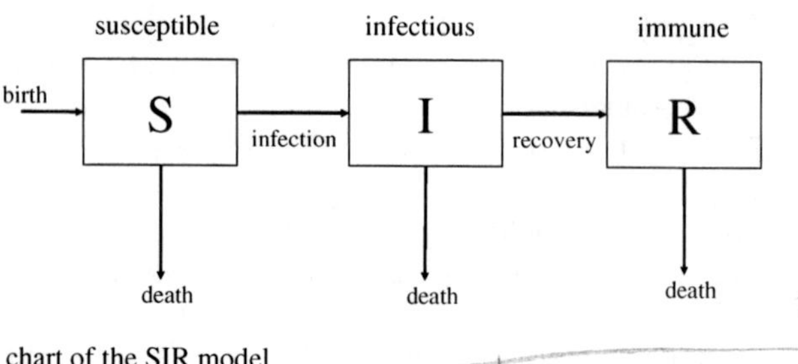

Fig. 12.5 Flow chart of the SIR model

Transitions between compartments are governed by rates, which in the simplest version of the model are assumed to be constant in time. The birth rate ν describes the recruitment of new susceptibles into the population, the death rate μ the loss of individuals due to a disease-unrelated background mortality, and γ denotes the recovery rate of infected individuals into immunity. The key element of the model is the term describing transmission of infection according to a rate β using a mass action term. The idea behind using a mass action term to describe transmission is that individuals of the population meet each other at random and each individual has the same probability per unit time to meet each other individual. Therefore, for a susceptible person the rate of meeting infected persons depends on their density or prevalence in the population, or in mathematical terms $\lambda = \beta I$, where λ is the so-called force of infection. The force of infection is a measure of the risk of a susceptible person to become infected per unit time. It depends on prevalence, either in an absolute sense on the number of infected people in the population, or in a relative sense on the fraction of infected people in the population. In the latter case we would get $\lambda = \beta I / N$ with N denoting the total population size. The parameter β is a composite parameter measuring the contact rate κ and the probability of transmission upon contact q, so $\beta = \kappa q$. The flow chart in Fig. 12.5 can be translated into a system of ordinary differential equations as follows:

$$\begin{aligned}\frac{dS}{dt} &= \nu - \beta S \frac{1}{N} - \mu S \\ \frac{dI}{dt} &= \beta S \frac{I}{N} - \gamma I - \mu I \\ \frac{dR}{dt} &= \gamma I - \mu R\end{aligned}$$

with $N = S+I+R$. For a full definition of the model the initial state of the system has to be specified, i.e. the numbers or fractions of the population in the states S, I, and R at time $t = 0$ have to be prescribed. Values for the parameters ν, μ, γ, and β have to be chosen either based on estimates from data or based on assumptions. Then standard numerical methods can be used to compute the time evolution of the system starting from the initial state.

Up to now the model describes disease transmission without any possible intervention. We now incorporate vaccination of newborns into this simple system to obtain some important insights into the effect of universal newborn vaccination. We denote the fraction of newborns that are vaccinated immediately after birth by p. Then instead of having a recruitment rate of ν the recruitment is now $(1\text{-}p)\nu$ into the susceptible compartment, while $p\nu$ is recruited directly into the immune compartment. In terms of model equations this leads to

$$\frac{dS}{dt} = \nu(1-p) - \beta S\frac{1}{N} - \mu S$$
$$\frac{dI}{dt} = \beta S\frac{I}{N} - \gamma I - \mu I$$
$$\frac{dR}{dt} = \nu p + \gamma I - \mu R$$

with $0 \leq p \leq 1$.

We will now derive some basic principles using this model as an example.

12.3 Basic Concepts: Reproduction Number, Final Size, Endemic Steady State, and Critical Vaccination Coverage

The most important concepts of epidemic models can be demonstrated using the SIR model. Let us first consider an infectious disease which spreads on a much faster time scale than the demographic process. Then, on the scale of disease transmission the birth rate ν and the death rate μ can be considered to be close to zero. When can the prevalence in the population increase? An increase in prevalence is equivalent with $dI/dt > 0$, which means that $\beta SI/N > \gamma I$. This leads to $\beta S/N > \gamma$ or equivalently to $\beta S/(\gamma N)>1$. In the situation that all individuals of the population are susceptible we have $S = N$; this means that an infectious disease can spread in a completely susceptible population if $\beta/\gamma>1$. The quantity $R_0 = \beta/\gamma$ is also known as the *basic reproduction number* and can in principle be determined for every infectious disease model and can be estimated for every infectious disease. In biological terms the basic reproduction number describes the number of secondary infections produced by one index case in a completely susceptible population during his entire infectious period (Diekmann et al. 1990; Diekmann and Heesterbeek 2000). *The effective reproduction number R* – as mentioned in Section 12.2– describes the number of secondary cases per index case in a situation where intervention measures are applied or where a part of the population has already been infected and is now immune.

If $R_0 > 1$ the infection can spread in the population, because on average every infected individual replaces himself by more than one new infected person. However, this process can only continue as long as there are sufficiently many susceptible individuals available. Once a larger fraction of the population has gone through the infection and has become immune, the probability of an infected person to meet a susceptible person decreases and with it the average number of secondary cases produced. If – as we assumed above – there is no birth into the population, no new susceptible individuals are coming in and the epidemic outbreak will invariably end. Analysis of the model shows, however, that the final size of the outbreak will never encompass the entire population, but there will always be a fraction of susceptible individuals left over after the outbreak has subsided. It can be shown that the final size A (attack rate in epidemiological terms) is related to the basic reproduction number by the implicit formula $A = 1 - \exp(-R_0 A)$. In other words, if the basic reproduction number of an infectious disease is known, the attack rate in a completely susceptible population can be derived.

The situation changes when we consider the system on a demographic time scale where births and deaths play a role. Assuming that ν and μ are positive, with the same arguments as above we get that $R_0 = \beta/(\gamma+\mu)$. Now if $R_0 > 1$ the system can develop into an equilibrium state where the supply of new susceptible persons by birth is balanced by the transmission process and on average every infected person produces one new infection. This so-called endemic equilibrium can be computed from the model equations by setting the left-hand sides to zero and solving for the variables S, I, and R in terms of the model parameters. First one obtains the steady state population size as $N^* = \nu/\mu$ (the superscript $*$ denotes the steady state value). The steady state values for the infection-related variables are then given by

$$S^* = \frac{(\gamma+\mu)\nu}{\beta\mu} = \frac{\nu}{\mu R_0}$$

$$I^* = \left(\frac{\nu}{\mu}\right)\left(\frac{\mu}{\gamma+\mu}\right)\left(1 - \frac{1}{R_0} - p\right)$$

$$R^* = \frac{\nu}{\mu} - S^* - I^*$$

Hence the fractions of the population that are susceptible, infected and recovered in an endemic steady state are given by

$$\frac{S^*}{N^*} = \frac{\gamma+\mu}{\beta} = \frac{1}{R_0}$$

$$\frac{I^*}{N^*} = \left(\frac{\mu}{\gamma+\mu}\right)\left(1 - \frac{1}{R_0} - p\right)$$

$$\frac{R^*}{N^*} = 1 - \frac{S^*}{N^*} - \frac{I^*}{N^*}$$

Note that the fraction of susceptible individuals S^*/N^* in the endemic steady state is independent of the vaccination coverage p. On the other hand, the prevalence of infection I^*/N^* depends on p: the prevalence decreases linearly with increasing vaccination coverage until the point of elimination is reached. This means we can compute the *critical vaccination coverage* p_c, i.e., the threshold coverage needed for elimination from $0 = 1 - 1 / R_0 - p_c$ as $p_c = 1 - 1 / R_0$. As we would expect intuitively, the larger the basic reproduction number, the higher the fraction of the population that has to be vaccinated in order to eliminate an infection from the population. However, it also follows that elimination can be reached without vaccinating everybody in the population. The reason is that with an increasing density of immune persons in the population, the risk for those who are not yet vaccinated to be exposed decreases. This effect – the indirect protection of susceptible individuals by increasing levels of immunity in the population – is known as *herd immunity*. Besides the positive effect of decreasing the risk of infection for non-vaccinated persons, herd immunity has the sometimes adverse effect of increasing the mean age at first infection in the population. This can lead to an increased incidence of adverse events following infection, if the coverage of vaccination is not sufficiently high.

For an infection such as smallpox with an estimated basic reproduction number of around 5, a coverage of 80% is needed for elimination, while for measles with a reproduction number of around 20 the coverage has to be at least 96%. This provides one explanation for the fact that it was possible to eradicate smallpox in the 1970 s whereas we are still a long way from measles eradication. There are some countries, however, that have been successful in eliminating measles based on a consistently high vaccination coverage (Peltola et al. 1997).

12.3.1 Advanced Models

Building on the basic ideas of the SIR framework, numerous types of mathematical models have been developed in the meanwhile, all incorporating more structure and details of the transmission process and infectious disease dynamics.

12.3.1.1 More Complex Compartmental Models

A first obvious extension is the inclusion of more disease-specific details into a model. Compartments describing a latent period, the vaccinated population, chronic and acute stages of infection, and many more have been described in the literature (Anderson and May 1991). Another important refinement of compartmental models is to incorporate heterogeneity of the population into the model, for example, by distinguishing between population subgroups with different behaviors or population subgroups with differences in susceptibility or geographically distinct populations. Heterogeneity in behavior was first introduced into models describing the spread of sexually transmitted infections by Hethcote and Yorke (Hethcote and Yorke 1994). Later, during the first decade of the HIV/AIDS pandemic, models were proposed that were able to describe population heterogeneity in sexual activity and mixing patterns between population subgroups of various sexual activity levels (Koopman et al. 1988). Models of this type are used frequently for assessing the effects of intervention on the spread of sexually transmitted infections. Age structure has also been modeled as a series of compartments with individuals passing from one compartment to the next according to an aging rate, but this requires a large number of additional compartments to be added to the model structure. This also shows the limitation of compartmental models: with increasing structure of the population the number of compartments increases rapidly and with it the necessity to define and parameterize the mixing between all the population subgroups in the model. The theory of how to define and compute the basic reproduction number in heterogeneous populations was developed by Diekmann et al. (1990). Geographically distinct population groups with interaction among each other have been investigated using the framework of meta-populations for analyzing the dynamics of childhood infections (Rohani et al. 1999).

12.3.1.2 Models with Continuous Age Structure

Age structure can best be described as a continuous variable, where age progresses with time. Mathematically this leads to models in the form of partial differential equations, where all variables of the model depend on time and age (Diekmann and Heesterbeek 2000). Analytically, partial differential equations are more difficult to handle than ordinary differential equations, but numerically solving an age-structured system of model equations is straightforward.

12.3.1.3 Stochastic Transmission Models

In a deterministic model based on a system of differential equations it is implicitly assumed that the numbers in the various compartments are sufficiently large such that stochastic effects can be neglected. In reality this is not always the case. For example, when analyzing epidemic outbreaks in small populations such as schools or small villages, typical stochastic events can occur such as extinction of the infection from the population or large stochastic fluctuations in the final size of the epidemic. In contrast to deterministic models, stochastic models are formulated in terms of integers with probabilities describing the transitions between states. This means that outcomes are given in terms of probability distributions such as the final size distribution. Questions of stochastic influences on infectious disease dynamics have been studied in various ways, starting with the Reed–Frost model for a discrete time transmission of infection up to a stochastic version of the SIR model introduced above (Bailey 1975; Becker 1989). Finally, stochastic models have been investigated using simulation techniques also known as Monte Carlo simulations. An important theoretical result from the analysis of stochastic models is the distinction between minor and major outbreaks for infectious diseases with $R_0 > 1$. While in a deterministic model a R_0 larger than unity always leads to an outbreak if the infection is introduced into an entirely susceptible population, in a stochastic model a certain fraction of introductions remain minor outbreaks with only a few secondary infections. This leads to a bimodal probability distribution of the final epidemic size following the introduction of one infectious index case. The peak for small outbreak sizes describes the situation that the infection dies out after only a few secondary infections, the peak for large outbreak sizes describes those outbreaks that take off and affect a large part of the population. The larger the basic reproduction number, the larger the fraction of major outbreaks in the susceptible population (Andersson and Britton 2000).

12.3.1.4 Network Models

Some aspects of contact between individuals cannot easily be modeled in compartmental models. In the context of the spread of sexually transmitted diseases models were developed that take the duration of partnerships into account, the so-called pair formation models (Hadeler et al. 1988). Extending those models to also include simultaneous long-term partnerships leads to the class of network models, where the network of contacts is described by a graph with nodes representing individuals and links representing their contacts (Keeling and Eames 2005). Different network structural properties have been related to the speed of spread of an epidemic through the population. In the so-called small world networks, most contacts between individuals are local, but some long-distance contacts ensure a rapid global spread of an epidemic (Watts and Strogatz 1998). Long-distance spread of infections is becoming increasingly important in a globalizing world with increasing mobility – as the example of the SARS epidemic in 2003 demonstrated. Recently the concept of scale-free networks where the number of links per node follows a power law distribution (i.e., the probability for a node to have k links is proportional to $k^{-\gamma}$ with a positive constant γ) was discussed in relation to the spread of epidemics. With respect to the spread of sexually transmitted diseases a network structure where some individuals have very many partners while the majority of people have only few might lead to great difficulties in controlling the disease by intervention (Liljeros et al. 2001). Network concepts have also been applied to study the spread of respiratory diseases (Meyers et al. 2003).

12.4 Use of Modeling for Public Health Policy

Mathematical models have been widely used to assess the effectiveness of vaccination strategies, to determine the best vaccination ages and target groups, and to estimate the effort needed to eliminate an infection from the population. More recently, mathematical modeling has supported contingency planning in preparation for a possible attack with smallpox virus (Ferguson et al. 2003) and in planning the public health response to an outbreak with a pandemic strain of influenza A (Ferguson et al. 2006). Other types of intervention measures have also been evaluated such as screening for asymptomatic infection with *Chlamydia trachomatis* (Kretzschmar et al. 2001), contact tracing (Eames and Keeling 2003), and antiviral treatment in the case of HIV. In the field of nosocomial infections and transmission of antibiotic-resistant pathogens modeling has been used to compare hospital-specific interventions such as cohorting of health workers, increased hygiene, and isolation of colonized patients (Grundmann and Hellriegel 2006). In health economic evaluations it has been recognized that dynamic transmission models are a necessary requisite for conducting good cost-effectiveness analyses for infectious disease control (Edmunds et al. 1999).

It is a large step from developing mathematical theory for the dynamics of infectious diseases to application in a concrete public health-relevant situation. The latter requires an intensive focusing on relevant data sources, clinical and microbiological knowledge to make a decision about how to design an appropriate model. Appropriate here means that the model uses the knowledge available, is able to answer the questions that are asked by policy makers, and is sufficiently simple so that its dynamics can be understood and interpreted. In the future it will be important to strengthen the link between advanced statistical methodology and mathematical modeling in order to further improve the performance of modeling as a public health tool.

12.5 Further Reading

One of the first comprehensive texts on epidemic modeling is Bailey (Bailey 1975). Bailey treats both deterministic and stochastic models and links them to data. A more recent, but also classic text for infectious disease modeling is Anderson and May (1991); however, it deals mainly with deterministic unstructured models. Its strength is a good link with data and discussion of public health relevant questions. In Diekmann and Heesterbeek (2000) the mathematical theory of deterministic modeling is laid out with many exercises for the reader. A focus of the book is the incorporation of population heterogeneity into epidemic modeling and a generalization of the basic reproduction number to heterogeneous populations. In Andersson and Britton (2000) an introduction to stochastic epidemic modeling is given. Becker (1989) describes advanced statistical methods for the analysis of infectious disease data taking the specific characteristics of these data into account. A recent text incorporating case studies from applications of epidemic modeling was published by Keeling and Rohani (2007).

References

Andersson H, Britton T (2000) Stochastic epidemic models and their statistical analysis. New York: Springer

Anderson RM, May RM (1991) Infectious disease of humans: dynamics and control. Oxford: Oxford University Press

Bailey NTG (1975) The mathematical theory of infectious diseases and its applications. 2nd ed. London: Griffin

Becker NG (1989) Analysis of infectious disease data. London: Chapman and Hall

Cauchemez S, Boelle PY, Thomas G, Valleron AJ (2006) Estimating in real time the efficacy of measures to control emerging communicable diseases. Am J Epidemiol; 164(6):591–7

Diekmann O, Heesterbeek JAP (2000) Mathematical epidemiology of infectious diseases. Chichester: Wiley

Diekmann O, Heesterbeek JA, Metz JA (1990) On the definition and the computation of the basic reproduction ratio R0 in models for infectious diseases in heterogeneous populations. J Math Biol; 28(4):365–82

Dietz K, Heesterbeek JA (2000) Bernoulli was ahead of modern epidemiology. Nature; 408(6812):513–4

Eames KT, Keeling MJ (2003) Contact tracing and disease control. Proc Biol Sci; 270(1533): 2565–71

Edmunds WJ, Medley GF, Nokes DJ (1999) Evaluating the cost-effectiveness of vaccination programmes: a dynamic perspective. Stat Med; 18(23):3263–82

Ferguson NM, Cummings DA, Fraser C, Cajka JC, Cooley PC, Burke DS (2006) Strategies for mitigating an influenza pandemic. Nature; 442(7101):448–52

Ferguson NM, Keeling MJ, Edmunds WJ, Gani R, Grenfell BT, Anderson RM, et al. (2003) Planning for smallpox outbreaks. Nature; 425(6959):681–5

Grundmann H, Hellriegel B (2006) Mathematical modelling: a tool for hospital infection control. Lancet Infect Dis; 6(1):39–45

Hadeler KP, Waldstatter R, Worz-Busekros A (1988) Models for pair formation in bisexual populations. J Math Biol; 26(6):635–49

Hamer WH (1906) Epidemic disease in England – the evidence of variability and persistency of type. Lancet; 1:733–39

Hethcote HW, Yorke JA (1984) Gonorrhea transmission dynamics and control. New York: Springer Verlag

Keeling MJ, Eames KT (2005) Networks and epidemic models. J R Soc Interface; 2(4):295–307

Keeling MJ, Rohani P (2007) Modeling infectious diseases in humans and animals. Princeton: Princeton University Press

Kermack WO, McKendrick AG (1991a) Contributions to the mathematical theory of epidemics–II. The problem of endemicity.1932. Bull Math Biol; 53(1–2):57–87

Kermack WO, McKendrick AG (1991b) Contributions to the mathematical theory of epidemics – I. 1927. Bull Math Biol; 53(1–2):33–55

Kermack WO, McKendrick AG (1991c) Contributions to the mathematical theory of epidemics–III. Further studies of the problem of endemicity.1933. Bull Math Biol; 53(1–2):89–118

Koopman J, Simon C, Jacquez J, Joseph J, Sattenspiel L, Park T (1988) Sexual partner selectiveness effects on homosexual HIV transmission dynamics. J Acquir Immune Defic Syndr; 1(5): 486–504

Kretzschmar M, Welte R, van den Hoek A, Postma MJ (2001) Comparative model-based analysis of screening programs for Chlamydia trachomatis infections. Am J Epidemiol; 153(1):90–101

Liljeros F, Edling CR, Amaral LA, Stanley HE, Aberg Y (2001) The web of human sexual contacts. Nature; 411(6840):907–8

Meyers LA, Newman ME, Martin M, Schrag S (2003) Applying network theory to epidemics: control measures for Mycoplasma pneumoniae outbreaks. Emerg Infect Dis; 9(2):204–10

Mills CE, Robins JM, Lipsitch M (2004) Transmissibility of 1918 pandemic influenza. Nature; 432(7019):904–6

Peltola H, Davidkin I, Valle M, Paunio M, Hovi T, Heinonen OP, et al. (1997) No measles in Finland. Lancet; 350(9088):1364–5

Rohani P, Earn DJ, Grenfell BT (1999) Opposite patterns of synchrony in sympatric disease metapopulations. Science; 286(5441):968–71

Watts DJ, Strogatz SH (1998) Collective dynamics of 'small-world' networks. Nature; 393(6684):440–2

Wallinga J, Teunis P (2004) Different epidemic curves for severe acute respiratory syndrome reveal similar impacts of control measures. Am J Epidemiol; 160(6):509–16

Chapter 13
Immunity to Infectious Diseases

Timo Ulrichs

13.1 History of Immunology

King Mithridates VI of Pontus (Black Sea region) who reigned from 132 to 63 BC and was known as a great enemy of the Roman Empire immunized himself against fungal toxins by administering small non-toxic amounts (he even wrote a book about toxins). As an autocratic ruler, he wanted to protect himself from assassination attempts by poisoned food and is nowadays considered the first known individual applying the principle of immunization. Besides the observation of immunization, the insight that some diseases are transmissible and that survival is often associated with protection from a secondary attack by the same disease forms the basis of immunology. Although in ancient times and the Middle Ages, its underlying mechanisms were still unknown, immunization with smallpox material for protection against this plague was very common in the Middle East and also in Europe and China.

In 1776, Edward Jenner applied this principle by vaccinating humans with the non-pathogenic cow pox (variolation) without understanding how the protection by vaccination functions. In the second half of the nineteenth century, great discoveries unveiled the basis of immunity. With his description of *Bacillus anthracis* as the etiologic agent of anthrax in 1876, Robert Koch (1843–1910) laid the ground for the understanding of the relationship between pathogen and infectious disease. His work was also the beginning of the concept of specific immunity. Louis Pasteur (1822–1895) attenuated pathogens for use as vaccines. Emil von Behring and Shibasaburo Kitasato showed that after immunization with bacterial toxins (like Mithridates did with fungal toxins) antibodies were formed in the serum of the vaccinees and laid the ground for the concept of humoral immunity. This concept was given its theoretical background by Paul Ehrlich's famous side chain theory describing the emergence of antibodies. Emil von Behring and Paul Ehrlich may be considered as founding fathers of the adapted immunity although their works

T. Ulrichs (✉)
Koch-Metschnikow-Forum, Luisenstr. 59, 10117 Berlin, Germany
e-mail: timo.ulrichs@bmg.bund.de

A. Krämer et al. (eds.), *Modern Infectious Disease Epidemiology*,
Statistics for Biology and Health, DOI 10.1007/978-0-387-93835-6_13,

were restricted to the humoral (antibody-mediated) immune response. In contrast to this model of immunity, Ilya Metchnikov described the principle of phagocytosis and phagocytosing cells like macrophages. He is the father of cellular immunity. The two concepts of immunity – specific humoral (antibodies) and unspecific cellular (macrophages) – were considered contradictory for a long time. In the second half of the twentieth century, new groundbreaking experiments could dissolve this contradiction and led to a comprehensive model of immunity.

In 2008, we celebrated the 100-year anniversary of the Nobel Prize award to Paul Ehrlich and Ilya Metchnikov. This is a good opportunity to commemorate their outstanding scientific work and at the same time to describe current problems in immunology.

In this chapter, a short definition of immunological terms is followed by the description of the immune response to tuberculosis, highlighting some aspects of regulation and interaction as well as their public health relevance.

13.2 Immunity

Immunization (like in Mithridates) leads to immunity. The underlying processes are called immune response. The immune response is ensured by specific organs, cells, and molecules (like antibodies) – these represent the immune system. An innate and an adapted immune response can be differentiated.

13.2.1 Innate Immunity

The innate immune response provides the early defense against invading pathogens. The innate response is unspecific, thus it cannot distinguish between different pathogens. But it can recognize surface patterns typical for pathogens and distinguish between own and foreign structures (a typical example of so-called pattern-recognition receptors are toll-like receptors [TLR], see below). This rough distinction allows a rapid response to invading pathogens. The *innate immune response* prepares and induces the adapted immune response (see below) and is mediated by the following cells and molecules:

- Granulocytes, monocytes, and macrophages phagocytize pathogens and kill them intracellularly
- Macrophages can also present pathogen material to specific T cells and thus activate the adapted immune response
- Natural killer cells eliminate virus-infected host cells

Important *humoral factors of the innate immune system* are the ones of the complement system that lyses bacteria and viruses upon activation in the blood system. Complement factors also bind to bacterial surfaces and improves phagocytosis (opsonization). Another humoral factor comprises interferons that inhibit intracellular replication of viruses.

13.2.2 Adaptive or Acquired Immunity

Adaptive immune response is highly specific and directed against specific foreign structures, the antigens. In contrast to the innate immune response, the adaptive immune response can develop a memory that allows a more specific and stronger reaction at a second contact with the same antigen. Adaptive immunity is mediated by *lymphocytes*.

B lymphocytes produce antigen-specific antibodies (see above). Antibodies can neutralize toxins, block virus attacks, and contribute to elimination of bacteria by several effector functions. They can only recognize and attack pathogens outside of cells. Thus, intracellular pathogens like intracellular viruses (measles, mumps, polio, etc.), protozoa, or mycobacteria (see below) are not targeted by antibodies.

This is done by *T lymphocytes* that specifically recognize infected cells. After activation, only the specific T cell clones grow and activate their effector functions, ranging from cytokine production to activate other immune cells to cytotoxic activity to kill the infected cell. A portion of the activated T lymphocytes develops into T memory cells. They allow a more specific and rapid immune response upon a second contact. This secondary response is also elicited after vaccination with specific antigens [in subunit (i.e., antigens, peptides, and proteins) or live vaccines]. Lymphocytes are also responsible for the regulation of the adapted immune response. Specialized regulatory T cells ensure that the acquired immune response is adapted in terms of specificity, strength, and duration. Effector functions are executed by T cells but also by cells from the innate immune response, especially from macrophages.

13.3 The Function of the Immune System – the Example of Tuberculosis

Infection with *Mycobacterium tuberculosis*, the etiologic agent of tuberculosis, leads to an intracellular infection, eliciting an adaptive immune response, mainly mediated by T cells. Tuberculosis is a good example of a well-coordinated reaction by different parts of the immune system. The various functions of the human immune system will be illustrated by the following description of the different phases of host–pathogen interaction.

From all individuals that become infected with *M. tuberculosis*, >90% successfully contain the infection by virtue of an efficient immune response during their life time, so that it remains clinically inapparent. A symptom of previous contact and subsequent infection with *M. tuberculosis* is the positive tuberculin skin reaction (distinct doses of tuberculin or purified protein derivative, PPD, are inoculated in the skin, induration is measured after 3–4 days). This is a *delayed-type hypersensitivity (DTH) reaction* which is caused by antigen-specific T lymphocytes which elicit an inflammatory response at the site of inoculation of specific antigens. The state of DTH indicates the existence of a specific immunity mostly involving antigen-specific T cells. Upon encounter of antigen presented by antigen-presenting cells (APC) these T cells produce inflammatory cytokines that attract monocytes to the site of reaction and activate them. DTH reactions are transient and vanish once the antigen has been destroyed by the activated monocytes.

A similar, though not fully identical reaction takes place at the site of mycobacterial persistence. However, because mycobacteria persist and are not readily destroyed, the antigenic depot sustains a granulomatous reaction at the site of bacterial implantation. Since the pathogen is inhaled in small droplets, the first contact of invading mycobacteria with the immune system is made with alveolar macrophages residing within lung alveoli which phagocytize the bacilli. T cells are recruited to the site of primary infection where the bacilli are contained, and they become activated by presentation of mycobacterial antigens. In an attempt to avoid direct confrontation with host effector mechanisms, *M. tuberculosis* successively retards its replication rate within the phagosomes of macrophages and transforms into a dormant state of low replication and strongly reduced metabolic activity.

This host–pathogen interaction has consequences on tuberculosis epidemiology: Approximately one-third of the world population, i.e., two billion people, is infected with the pathogen. A dynamic balance between the pathogen and the cellular immune response is established: *M. tuberculosis* is restricted to the primary site of infection by a coordinated immune response, but it cannot be cleared from the host. *M. tuberculosis* remains dormant until this labile balance between mycobacterial persistence and the immune response becomes disturbed. An impaired host response caused by a variety of reasons including aging, malnutrition, treatment with immunosuppressive drugs, or HIV infection reactivates the bacilli. The balance is tipped in favor of the pathogen: bacilli are spread to other sites in the lung or other organs and active tuberculosis develops (Fig.13.1).

The following parts of the immune system are involved in the containment of the pathogen:

Fig. 13.1 Balance between *M. tuberculosis* and the host immune system, (adapted from Ulrichs T and Kaufmann SHE (2002). Mycobacterial persistence and immunity. Front Biosci. 7: D458-D469) (**A**) *M. tuberculosis* is inhaled in droplets. After an incubation period of 4–12 weeks infected alveolar macrophages containing the pathogen either destroy their predators (a mechanism that has not yet been proven, but probably accounts for a small proportion, *left*) or they fail to contain the pathogen and die (*right*). In the first case, infection is abortive, in the second case, the pathogen spreads throughout the body and causes active disease. Given that the immune response and virulence of *M. tuberculosis* are balanced (*middle*), intracellular bacteria are contained by the macrophages, and the immune system isolates the primary site of infection by granuloma formation (primary lesion). In this third scenario, infection without clinical disease develops. (**B**) *M. tuberculosis* can persist in a dormant state for long periods of time. Any disturbance of the balance between host and pathogen after weakening of the cellular immune response (immunosuppression) causes endogenous exacerbation which leads to active (post primary) tuberculosis. Active tuberculosis can also be caused by exogenous reinfection

NOTE Diagram.

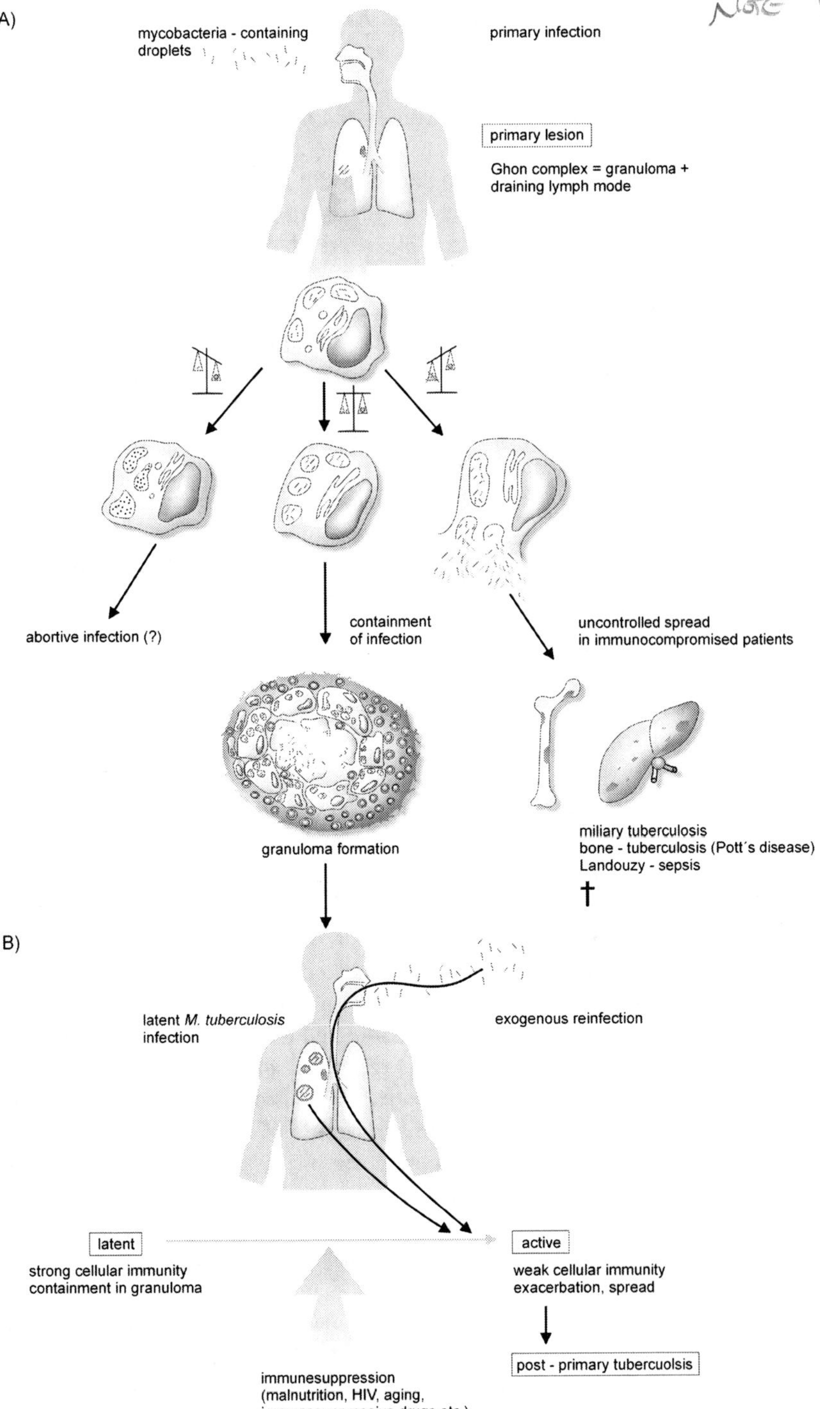

Fig. 13.1

13.3.1 The Early Phase of Immune Response: Innate Immune Defense

Phagocytosis of *M. tuberculosis* by *alveolar macrophages* is mediated by several host cell receptors. They include receptors recognizing surfactant proteins, complement proteins, or antibodies (IgG) bound to the mycobacterial surface, i.e., Fc receptors (FcR, receptors for the non-antigen-binding part of the antibody) and complement receptors (CR). Other receptors directly recognize certain molecules or patterns of the surface (pattern-recognition receptors, PRR, see above), like the macrophage mannose receptor (MMR) and CD14. Two members of the toll-like receptor (TLR) family are also involved in interactions between macrophages and mycobacteria. TLR-2 and TLR-4 interact with mycobacterial cell wall components, including lipoarabinomannan (LAM). The choice of the receptor used to enter the macrophage influences the cellular response: the entry of IgG-opsonized mycobacteria via FcR results in activation of macrophage antimicrobial systems (see below), whereas internalization via CR3 fails to activate effector mechanisms appropriately. Furthermore, internalized mycobacteria successfully inhibit intracellular attacks. Although the underlying mechanisms are still incompletely understood, arrest of the mycobacterial phagosome at an early stage is a major survival strategy of *M. tuberculosis* to avoid intracellular degradation. The infected macrophages contain their mycobacterial load and prevent it from spreading throughout the host organism.

13.3.2 Formation of the Human Tuberculous Granuloma

The confinement of mycobacteria to the site of infection is ensured by the formation of a granulomatous reaction. Granuloma formation is a specific immune response and represents a characteristic feature of tuberculosis which lead to its name (granuloma = tubercle, i.e., the anatomical description of small distinct nodules). The granuloma is formed by the recruitment of circulating mononuclear phagocytes and T cells to the site of infection where infected macrophages form the center of the cellular agglomeration. Infected macrophages differentiate into various forms ranging from tissue macrophages to epithelioid and multinucleated giant cells that result from the fusion of several infected cells. Recruited T cells secrete a variety of cytokines which activate infected cells to control their mycobacterial load or activate cytotoxic T cells. A characteristic feature of tuberculous granulomas is the formation of a caseotic center containing necrotic tissue, cell debris, and killed mycobacteria. Extracellular mycobacteria can be found within the zone between the necrotic center and the cellular wall of the granuloma. *M. tuberculosis* developed several strategies to survive in this hostile environment by adapting its metabolism to low oxygen content and switching to lipids as energy source as a highly abundant substrate in the caseous center of the granuloma. Activation of T cells and macrophages has to be tightly balanced to avoid any disruption of the integrity of the granuloma by excessive cytotoxic activity or apoptosis of infected cells which could promote dissemination of mycobacteria from a "productive" tuberculous lesion.

Except for the histological description of the human tuberculous granuloma little is known about the local interactions between immune cells within or neighboring the granuloma. Animal models insufficiently mimick the immune processes in the human host since mice and guinea pigs express different susceptibility to *M. tuberculosis* and subsequently display a different architecture of the forming granulomas.

13.3.3 Cell-Mediated Immunity Against M. tuberculosis During Later Phases of Infection

13.3.3.1 Cytokine Activation

In general, the immunocompetent human host controls mycobacterial infection efficiently. The cytokines *IFN-γ* and *TNF-α* play a key role in the establishment of an appropriate immune response. They activate macrophages to produce inducible nitric oxide synthase (iNOS) and to sustain pathways generating reactive nitrogen intermediates (RNI). In addition, oxidative effector molecules are generated. Although the oxidative and nitrosative stress reduces mycobacterial growth, it fails to eliminate the pathogen. One reason might be that *M. tuberculosis* resists host effector mechanisms by means of a peroxidase/phosphonitrite reductase system which also participates in intermediary metabolism. IFN-γ and iNOS are also crucial for containing the infection and keeping the balance between replication of *M. tuberculosis* and immune defense.

TNF-α plays a role in the containment of persistent *M. tuberculosis* organisms and in preventing them from reaching other regions of the lung or other organs. Encapsulation of the granuloma and formation of the fibrinous wall is primarily mediated by TNF-α. TNF-α, administered to mice depleted of $CD4^+$ T cells and latently infected with *M. bovis* BCG prevents recrudescence of infection. In mice, monoclonal antibodies against TNF-α cause reactivation of latent *M. tuberculosis* infection, suggesting that TNF-α prevents endogenous spreading of mycobacteria by modulating cytokine levels and limiting histopathology. Elevated levels of TNF-α, TGF-β, and IL-10 have been detected in sera and pleural fluids of patients with lung tuberculosis. In general, the risk of disturbing the delicate balance between pathogen and host seems to increase with decreasing levels of TNF-α. This is illustrated by the fact that reactivation of tuberculosis represents a major side effect of anti-TNF-α-antibody therapy of severe rheumatoid arthritis.

13.3.4 $CD4^+$ T cells

Substantial evidence emphasizes the major role of $CD4^+$ T cells in containing the disease at all stages. $CD4^+$ T cells control persistent mycobacteria contained within the granuloma. Depletion of $CD4^+$ T cells in the mouse model causes rapid reactivation of previously dormant *M. tuberculosis* organisms resulting in increased bacterial load and exacerbation to rapid-progressive tuberculosis. MHC class II knockout mice are more highly susceptible to *M. tuberculosis* infection than mice deficient for CD4$^+$ T cells. Endogenous reactivation of latent tuberculosis in the mouse model occurs despite normal levels of IFN-γ and iNOS, suggesting that CD4$^+$ T cells regulate the balance between *M. tuberculosis* and activated immune cells. CD4$^+$ but also CD8$^+$ T cells are found mainly in the periphery of intact granulomas, and a high total number of CD8$^+$ T cells are associated with the structural integrity of the granuloma, underlining their key role in containing infection. Lymphotoxin α3 (LTα3)-deficient mice fail to form intact granulomas and suffer from exacerbated tuberculosis, suggesting that production of LTα3 by CD4$^+$ T cells promote granuloma formation and its maintenance. Reduced numbers of CD4$^+$ T cells in HIV$^+$ patients have serious implications for reactivation of persistent *M. tuberculosis*, this phenomenon being largely responsible for the recent resurgence of *M. tuberculosis* and the increase of active disease especially in developing countries with high incidences of HIV infection, mainly in sub-Saharan Africa.

13.3.5 CD8$^+$ T cells

In addition to CD4$^+$ T cells, CD8$^+$ T cells also contribute to the successful immune response against *M. tuberculosis*. Experiments with mice deficient for β_2-microglobulin, an essential part of MHC class I and CD1 molecules, CD8$^+$, and the transporter-associated protein (TAP) revealed that these mice were all more susceptible to *M. tuberculosis* infection than their wild-type counterparts. At first sight, the involvement of antigen-specific CD8$^+$ T cells in the immune response against *M. tuberculosis* is surprising since the pathogen resides within phagosomes and has no direct contact with the MHC class I antigen processing machinery. Experiments with antigen model systems suggest that alternative MHC class I pathways exist permitting the processing of phagosomal antigens and allowing CD8$^+$ T cell activation. Additionally, *M. tuberculosis* induces apoptosis of host cells and formation of apoptotic blebs that can be internalized by bystander dendritic cells and presented to CD8$^+$ T cells in a cross presentation.

13.3.6 Unconventional T cells

Presentation of mycobacterial protein antigens via the MHC presentation system is supplemented by the presentation of lipid and glycolipid antigens by CD1 molecules. The CD1 family consists of antigen presenting molecules encoded by genes located outside of the MHC. The CD1 system is involved in activation of cell-mediated responses against mycobacterial infection: In mice, CD1d-restricted NKT cells are activated by mycobacterial cell wall components and involved in early granuloma formation. CD4$^+$ NKT cells produce IFN-γ in the early phase after infection of mice with BCG. However, it is unclear whether CD1d-restricted T cells play any significant role in the protective immune response to mycobacterial infection, since CD1D-deficient mice do not suffer from a higher susceptibility to TB.

Several mycobacterial lipid and glycolipid antigens have been identified that elicit a specific *CD1-restricted T cell* response. T cells recognizing CD1-restricted antigens have a broad range of functional effector mechanisms including cytotoxic activity. This suggests that the CD1 system is involved in cellular immune responses against infection with *M. tuberculosis* in the early and late phases of infection (Fig.13.2).

γδ T cells are involved in the rapid early phase of the immune response to mycobacteria. Human γδ T cells usually recognize pyrophosphate and alkylamine antigens. The antigen presenting molecule is still unknown (if it is required at all). Some γδ T cells recognize CD1c on infected cells. These recognition mechanisms could play a role in the early phase of the immune response following TB infection.

13.3.7 Implications of the Cell-Mediated Immune Response for the Outcome of Tuberculosis and Countermeasures

Dissecting the basic immunological processes underlying the interactions between *M. tuberculosis* and the host immune system allows a better understanding of epidemiologic developments of tuberculosis as well as developing strategies for prevention. From the acquired cellular immune response to *M. tuberculosis* infection the following conclusions can be deduced:

(1) The immune system is not able to completely eliminate the pathogen; thus, it has to do the next best thing and try to isolate the site of primary infection from the rest of the host.
(2) Although the main coordination of the immune response is performed by T lymphocytes, the innate immune system is crucial for the rapid early response. Since a coordinated transition from innate to adaptive immune response is required to contain the pathogen, the immune system activates unconventional cells like NKT cells and γδ T cells with effector functions of both innate and adaptive immunity.
(3) A delicate balance between host immune system and replication of the pathogen is established that can lead to lifelong peaceful coexistence. In 10% of the cases, the balance is disturbed, and *M. tuberculosis* can cause active tuberculosis.
(4) Several cellular systems ($CD4^+$, $CD8^+$ T cells, macrophages, unconventional T cells) are involved in the containment of the pathogen to the site of infection. Only a well-coordinated immune response can ensure the balance described above. A too weak response leads to reactivation of *M. tuberculosis* and exacerbation of the disease; a too strong activity (especially cytotoxic) leads to disruption of the granuloma integrity and outbreak opportunities for the pathogen.

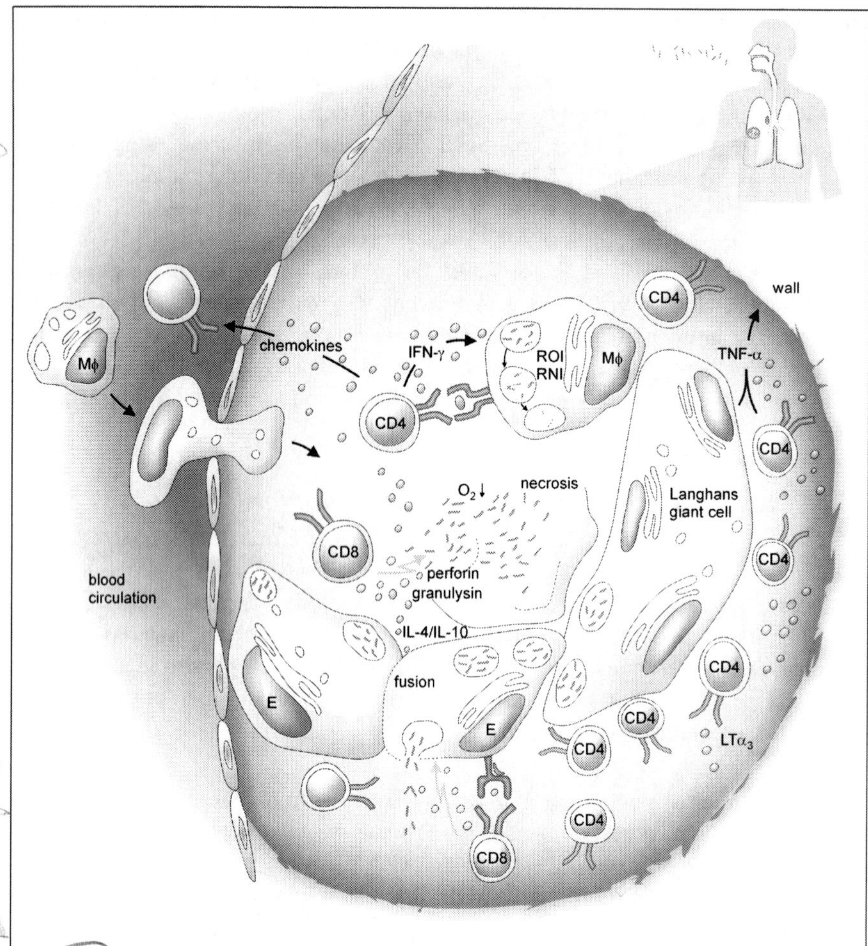

Fig. 13.2 Host response and granuloma formation, (adapted from Ulrichs and Kaufmann (2002). Mycobacterial persistence and immunity. Front Biosci. 7: D458–D469). The complex immune mechanisms that isolate the site of mycobacterial infection from the rest of the body still remain unknown. The following hypothetical picture can be drawn: alveolar macrophages (MF), epithelioid cells (E), or Langhans giant cells (generated by fusion of epithelioid cells) harboring intracellular mycobacteria form the center of the granuloma. They present antigens to T cells and activate them to produce a variety of cytokines and chemokines or to kill the infected cells and intracellular mycobacteria. Chemokines recruit additional cells from blood circulation to the site of primary infection. IFN-γ activates macrophages and other antigen presenting cells to kill the intracellular bacteria via reactive oxygen intermediates (ROI) or reactive nitrogen intermediates (RNI). $CD4^+$ T cells produce TNF-α and lymphotoxin α3 (LTα3) which are required for the formation of the wall surrounding the granuloma. In the center of the granuloma, cell detritus and low oxygen form a hostile environment for released mycobacteria. Activated $CD8^+$ T cells kill mycobacteria by means of granulysin and perforin. Killing of infected cells, however, needs to be controlled, in order to retain the integrity of the granuloma

13.3.8 Implications of the Immune Response for Vaccine Development

BCG is the most widely used vaccine worldwide. However, there is no effect of the vaccine in reducing prevalence and incidence of tuberculosis (the only proven effect of BCG is to reduce the risk of severe forms of childhood tuberculosis, such as tuberculous meningitis and miliar tuberculosis). Increasing numbers of multidrug-resistant tuberculosis and of HIV–TB coinfections make the development of a new vaccine very urgent.

Deduced from the immune response mechanisms against *M. tuberculosis* the following aspects concerning the development of a novel vaccine strategy have to be taken into consideration:

(1) In contrast to many vaccines (e.g., tetanus, measles), the new vaccine has to protect from the disease caused by an intracellular bacterium that does not elicit any significant antibody response. Therefore, antibody production, as Behring and Kitasato described it in their studies on immunization with bacterial toxins (e.g., against diphtheria), does not play a major role in the vaccine strategy (see also Chapter 14).
(2) To elicit a protective immune response, the cellular immune response must be activated by the vaccine. Since the regulatory processes among T cells and other cellular systems are not completely understood, it is difficult to define correlates of protection.
(3) Since a latent infection with a balance between host immune response and replication of *M. tuberculosis* inside the granuloma does not protect from exogenous reinfection, the new vaccine candidate has to activate the immune system better than the natural infection.
(4) Since one-third of the world population is already infected with the pathogen, the new vaccine should provide a postexposition prophylaxis to avoid exacerbation of the latent infection.
(5) To decrease tuberculosis numbers, both improved therapy regimens and better prevention strategies have to be implemented. Prevention can be achieved not only by a powerful vaccine, but also by public health measures (see Chapters 6 and 16).

13.3.9 Implications of the Immune Response for Public Health

In general, epidemiological and public health aspects of infectious disease can be better understood if the immunological and microbiological basis of the disease is known. Understanding immunity to infections as in the example of tuberculosis contributes to deducing reasonable countermeasures. Regarding tuberculosis in particular, the following immunological aspects might be considered in developing public health strategies for tuberculosis control (see Chapter 16):

(1) In 90% of all cases, the immune response is successful in permanent control of a latent tuberculosis infection. This implies that strengthening the immune system by fighting malnutrition, HIV, and bad hygienic environment contributes to decreasing tuberculosis numbers. However, these measures also contribute to reduce transmission of the pathogen and therefore might improve both immunity and public health.
(2) Tuberculosis is a poverty-related disease, therefore fighting poverty, improving hygienic and living conditions, and ensuring proper nutrition will also contribute to effective tuberculosis control.
(3) Tuberculosis primarily affects many autochthone people whose genetic background is unknown. Dissecting the genetic basis of a successful immune response might therefore contribute to direct recommendations for regional tuberculosis control.
(4) The immune response to *M. tuberculosis* is very complicated and still not completely understood. More efforts in basic research (immunology/microbiology) are necessary to develop better strategies in tuberculosis control.

Mithridates immunized himself successfully with low doses of toxins. At the end of his failed career he tried to commit suicide by poisoning himself. Because of his earlier immunization he failed. If we want to immunize humans against tuberculosis, we have to apply a different strategy. Immunization with a novel vaccine must be more effective than the immune response, elicited by a natural tuberculosis infection. Thus, we first have to completely understand the strategies of the pathogen and the regulation of the host immune response to develop efficient strategies. This cannot be done by one discipline alone; an interdisciplinary approach combining the fields of immunology, microbiology, and epidemiology would be the best option.

References

Abbas AK, Lichtman AH (2006–2007) Basic Immunology. Functions and Disorders of the Immune System; 2nd edition; Saunder Elsevier, Philadelphia; *good chapters on infection immunology*

Borrel A and Metchnikov M (1893) Tuberculose pulmonaire expérimentale. Ann Inst Pasteur; **8**: 594–625; *describes in detail the first animal experiments and the works of Ilya Metchnikov on macrophages in tuberculosis*

Janeway CA, Travers P, Walport M (2008) Immunobiology: The Immune System in Health and Disease. 7th edition; Lippincott William & Wilkins Philadelphia, London, Sydney, Hong Kong; *gold standard of immunology text book*

Nack W (1976) Bibliothek der alten Kulturen; Rom – Land und Volk der alten Römer; 2nd edition; Verlag Carl Ueberreuter; *for those who want to read more about Mithridates and his time*

Ulrichs T and Kaufmann SHE (2002) Mycobacterial persistence and immunity. Front Biosci; **7**: D458–D469; *contains definitions of latency, dormancy and persistence; source of the figures of this chapter*

Ulrichs T and Kaufmann SHE (2006) New insights into the function of granulomas in human tuberculosis. J Pathol; 208 (2):261–269; Wien (Vienna); *reviews the immune processes in granulomatous lesions*

Chapter 14
Principles and Practice of Vaccinology

Richard Pebody and Mirjam Kretzschmar

14.1 Introduction: Historical Background

Historically, infectious diseases have been a major cause of morbidity and mortality. Improved sanitation and living conditions are thought to have been major factors of the reduction in incidence of infectious diseases in the nineteenth and the early twentieth centuries in most industrialised countries. But the other public health intervention that has had the biggest impact on a global scale has been vaccination.

Smallpox has been known for centuries and reached plague proportions in the cities of Europe in the eighteenth century. It was widely feared and claimed the lives of at least five reigning monarchs. It was at the end of the eighteenth century that Jenner first introduced a vaccine against smallpox, *Vaccinia*. In 1956, the World Health Organization (WHO) selected smallpox for eradication (such that it was not circulating anywhere in the world). Following massive public health efforts, in 1982 the WHO officially declared the global eradication of smallpox 200 years after Jenner first developed the vaccine. The subsequent development of a variety of other vaccines during the twentieth century against various infectious diseases such as measles, diphtheria, pertussis and more recently hepatitis B has seen a dramatic reduction in their public health impact in both the developed and developing world (Table 14.1).

What does a vaccine aim to do? A vaccine aims to safely protect an individual/population from a specific infection. On a simplistic level, this is achieved by enhancing host immune defences by either mainly producing antibodies (which can neutralise toxins or block cell entry of bacteria or kill via complement fixation – an example is diphtheria vaccine which protects against the toxin), or by mainly producing cell-mediated immunity (e.g. BCG which results in a B and T cell response or activation of macrophages). For the former, antibody responses to vaccination can usually be measured and often a serological correlate of protection (against disease or infection) can be determined.

R. Pebody (✉)
Health Protection Agency, Communicable Disease Surveillance Centre, London, England
e-mail: richard.pebody@hpa.org.uk

A. Krämer et al. (eds.), *Modern Infectious Disease Epidemiology*,
Statistics for Biology and Health, DOI 10.1007/978-0-387-93835-6_14,

Table 14.1 The impact of the national vaccination programme in the United States. Impact of vaccination programme, United States

Disease	Pre-vaccine era[a]	Year	1998[b]	% change
Diphtheria	206,939	1921	1	−99.99
Measles	894,134	1941	89	−99.99
Mumps	152,209	1968	606	−99.60
Pertussis	265,269	1934	6,279	−97.63
Polio (wild)	21,269	1952	0	−100.00
Rubella	57,686	1969	345	−99.40
Congenital rubella syndrome	20000[c]	(1964–65)	6	−99.98
Tetanus	1560[c]	1948	34	−97.82
Invasive Hib disease	20000[c]	1948	51	−99.75
Total	1,639,066		7,411	−99.55
Vaccine adverse events	0		(10,236)5,522	

Source: Chen R. Vaccine risks: real, perceived and unknown. Vaccine 1999; 17(3): S41–46
[a]Maximum cases reported in pre-vaccine era and year
[b]Provisional
[c]Estimated because no national reporting in the prevaccine era

Vaccination can provide both *direct* (reduction of risk of infection in the vaccinated individual) and *indirect* protection (by vaccinating a certain proportion of the population, the circulation of the organism can be reduced, thus reducing the risk of infection for those in the population who remain unvaccinated), otherwise known as herd immunity. This indirect protection results in an increase in the period of time until individuals are infected, thus a lengthening of the inter-epidemic period, and thus an increase in the average age of infection. This phenomenon is often called the 'honeymoon' period (a period of reduced incidence, followed by disease recrudescence due to the accumulation of susceptibles over time) (see Chapter 12).

14.2 Pre-licensing Evaluation of Vaccine

The development of safe and effective vaccine is either undertaken by the private sector or National Public Health Institutes. This is through a series of clinical trials, known as phase I–III studies. These have to fulfil strict ethical guidelines, as originally outlined in the Helsinki Declaration. These clinical trials aim to determine if a vaccine is safe and effective in the target population against the endpoint of interest.

14.2.1 Phase I Studies

Researchers test the vaccine in a small population of healthy adult volunteers (usually tens of volunteers). The aim is to evaluate vaccine safety, determine possible dose ranges and identify any major side effects.

14.2.2 Phase II Studies

The vaccine is given to a larger group of volunteers (usually 200–1000 individuals) in the target group of interest. The aim is to further determine safety and tolerability, optimal dose and the immunogenicity of the vaccine (the ability to produce measurable antibody).

14.2.3 Phase III Studies

These are undertaken to further evaluate the safety of a vaccine (looking for less common adverse events) and optimal *vaccine efficacy* in the target population (usually thousands of persons). A variety of endpoints may be used in these trials, but the main focus is reducing cases (of infection or disease). The final formulation of the vaccine can also be developed.

But what is vaccine efficacy?

14.2.3.1 Vaccine Efficacy (VE)

Vaccine efficacy has been defined as the proportionate reduction in attack rate of disease in vaccinated (ARV) compared to unvaccinated (ARU) individuals relative to attack rate in unvaccinated:

$$\mathrm{VE} = (\mathrm{ARU} - \mathrm{ARV})/\mathrm{ARU}$$

$$\mathrm{VE} = 1 - (\mathrm{ARV}/\mathrm{ARU} = 1 - \text{Relative Risk})$$

This is otherwise known as the preventive fraction due to vaccination. Measurement of efficacy is usually undertaken through randomised, double blind-controlled clinical trials where the protective effect of the new vaccine is measured under idealised conditions and compared to either a placebo or control vaccine (usually current practice). This estimate is usually the gold standard. These are experiments where any potential biases and confounding should be minimised in the study design. The only difference (ideally) between the groups should be vaccine status. The studies are usually randomised on the individual and thus measure only the direct protective effect of the vaccine (these have also more recently been called phase IIIa studies). However, phase IIIb studies have been undertaken more recently. In these studies, communities or households are randomised to try to provide an estimate of the direct and indirect vaccine effect at the pre-licensure stage (Orenstein et al. 1985). Vaccine efficacy studies should be distinguished from vaccine effectiveness studies which are the measurement of VE, once a vaccine has been introduced into a routine programme.

Once the trials have been successfully completed the vaccine is submitted to the regulatory authorities for possible licensing – a process usually undertaken by each national government and other international agencies – in particular the FDA,

EMEA and WHO. Following their approval and introduction of a vaccine into a routine programme, phase IV studies are often undertaken to follow the safety and effectiveness of the vaccine.

14.3 Programme Implementation

Once a vaccine has passed through these stages and has been approved by the licensing authorities, it has to be decided whether or not the vaccine should be introduced into a national programme. Ideally national decision makers should evaluate a number of epidemiological, programmatic and economic factors that are often country specific.

14.3.1 Disease Burden in the Pre-vaccination Era

How high is the morbidity and mortality of the disease in a particular country? It is important to determine the impact (or burden) of the disease in question to enable governments to make informed decisions about the possible introduction of a new vaccine into a national immunisation programme and to be able to prioritise limited resources. A number of routine surveillance or statistical sources can potentially be used, including clinical notifications, hospitalisation episode statistics and death certificates (see Chapter 8). Special, time-limited epidemiological studies can also be established including enhanced surveillance programmes to estimate disease burden. For example, the World Health Organization has developed Rapid assessment tools to determine the disease burden due *to Haemophilus influenzae (HiB).* Another special type of study involves seroepidemiology. This is ascertaining the distribution of antibody positivity (as a marker of historical infection) in a population by age, sex, region and social group. This data can be used to determine the pre-vaccination epidemiology of an infection in a population, although there also needs to be knowledge of factors such as the length of protection and also a correlate of protection to enable interpretation of such data.

14.3.2 Effectiveness and Impact of Intervention

How much of the disease burden could potentially be prevented in terms of morbidity and or mortality by a particular intervention? Or how effective is the intervention that is available? The performance of a vaccine introduced into a public health programme is known as *vaccine effectiveness*, rather than vaccine efficacy (which is the performance of a vaccine under idealised conditions of a clinical vaccine trial). The latter can be derived either from phase IIIb studies or from phase IV studies that may have been undertaken in another geographical setting after the vaccine was licensed. The performance of a vaccine in terms of impact (percent reduction in disease incidences compared to incidences prior to introduction – which is a function of effectiveness, coverage and any herd effects) in real life may exceed expectation. For example, HiB conjugate vaccine was found to have a larger impact than expected compared to pre-licensure efficacy studies. This was due to the fact that the vaccine unexpectedly protected not only against disease, but also against infection (or carriage), and thus had a significant herd immunity effect.

14.3.3 Safety of Vaccine (Phase IV Studies)

Vaccine safety issues should be paramount in any decision to introduce a vaccine. Phase III studies, even if large, only detect common adverse events, which are usually mild. The rarer more serious potential adverse events may only become apparent after a vaccine is introduced on large scale in a national immunisation programme with post-licensure surveillance. However, experience from elsewhere may influence whether a vaccine is introduced into a particular national programme.

A rotavirus vaccine (Rotashield) was first licensed and introduced into the childhood immunisation schedule in the United States in the late 1990 s. It was only with post-licensure adverse event surveillance that an association between the vaccine and intestinal intussusception was detected. The vaccine was withdrawn from the US programme and was never introduced into routine use in Western Europe. Two other rotavirus vaccines have since been licensed following very large phase III trials; however, post-licensure surveillance has been critical to reassure that there is no elevated risk of intussusception following these vaccines.

14.3.4 Mathematical Modelling

Mathematical models have been described as "simplified descriptions of complex phenomena which are used to gain insights into the real world and thus guide vaccination policy" (Fine 1994). Based around a series of assumptions, they provide a theoretical framework and try to recreate reality. They can be used to make predictions of the impact of vaccination programmes including the indirect effects of vaccination. Furthermore, they can be used to compare the future risks and benefits of alternative vaccination strategies. For example, models have shown that theoretically a childhood rubella vaccination at low coverage could have a potentially perverse impact by increasing the mean age of infection and thus causing more infections in adult pregnant women than with no vaccine programme at all (Nokes, Anderson 1987). The model has now been validated by real life, with an outbreak of congenital rubella syndrome (CRS) in Greece following inadequate uptake over several years with the childhood measles–mumps–rubella (MMR) vaccination programme (Panagiotopoulos et al. 1999) (see Chapter 12).

14.3.5 Cost and Cost-Effectivenessof Intervention

Increasingly the economic cost (for the vaccine and the programme) and benefits (in terms of money (cost–benefit analysis), reduction in deaths/disease (cost-effectiveness analysis) or improvements of quality of life (cost–utility analysis) need to be evaluated for new vaccines (see Chapter 15).

Ideally, both the direct and indirect effects of a vaccine (herd immunity effect) should be taken into account. This requires the integration of economics with dynamic mathematical models.

Furthermore, the opportunity cost relative to other potential health interventions needs to be assessed, for example, should childhood rotavirus vaccination be introduced or improvements made in water quality in low income settings in order to reduce morbidity and mortality of infectious diarrhoea?

14.4 Vaccination Strategy

A national vaccination programme has to have clear objectives. The introduction of a vaccine may also be part of a regional or global strategy, for example, for smallpox eradication and measles elimination.

There are a number of alternative objectives:

Control, which is a reduction in morbidity and mortality in accordance with agreed targets and where continued intervention methods are required to maintain the reduction.

Elimination, where in a large geographical area, e.g. country or WHO region, endemic transmission of the infection has been stopped, and sustained transmission does not occur after an imported case, and where continued intervention measures are also required.

Eradication, which is the interruption of disease transmission worldwide, so that intervention methods may no longer be needed? An example of the last being the successful global eradication of smallpox.

14.4.1 Overall Strategy

To achieve these targets a variety of intervention strategies can be used. Broadly these can be classified as those delivered through the routine delivery system and supplemental mass campaigns, which are usually one-offs.

For the former, two approaches can be used: mass immunisation (usually vaccination of an entire birth cohort, e.g. for measles, mumps and rubella (MMR) vaccines, polio vaccine) or selective vaccination (where a particular group at higher risk of infection is targeted, e.g. adolescent girls with rubella vaccine or travellers with hepatitis A or rabies vaccine). In general, mass programmes can have both a direct and indirect effect, whereas selective programmes only have a direct effect, as circulation of the infection in the wider population is not interrupted. Thus an adolescent rubella vaccine programme can only make the epidemiological situation better whatever the coverage achieved.

14.4.2 Target Groups

Other decisions include the age at which vaccination should be delivered (factors of importance here include the age groups at highest risk of infection (and thus the time to have an effect, e.g. for an infant hepatitis B immunisation programme, where the group at highest risk may be adolescents through high-risk behaviour), and the age-specific efficacy of a vaccine. These two points are illustrated with measles infection. In highly endemic countries many infections occur under 12 months of age, however, live measles vaccine efficacy is much lower in this group, compared to older children. For a selective programme, it is important to identify the target groups with the highest risk of disease and ascertain that the vaccine is effective in these groups.

14.4.3 Number of Doses

The decision about the number of vaccine doses to be administered depends on how effective a vaccine is and what the aims of a programme are. For example, the measles virus is a highly infectious organism. The current vaccine has a primary vaccine failure rate of 5–10% when given at 12–15 months of age. Thus a single dose of measles vaccine even at extremely high coverage (95%), only protects 85–90% of vaccinees. Consequently, susceptibles accumulate over time (leading to the honeymoon phenomenon). For an elimination programme, this has to be prevented by the administration of a second dose (either routinely or as a mass campaign).

14.4.4 Type of Vaccine

Decisions may have to be made as well about what type of vaccine to administer. This may involve elements such as cost, effectiveness and side effect profile. A good example of this dilemma is the mumps vaccine, where there are several vaccine strains that vary considerably for each of these elements (Galazka et al. 1999). Jeryl Lynn is expensive, safe and effective; Urabe is cheaper, effective, but less safe; Rubini is the cheapest, but has poor effectiveness.

14.4.5 Delivery Setting

Finally, there is the question of what setting the vaccine programme is to be delivered to, and this depends on the health-care infrastructure. For example, for an adolescent HPV vaccine programme for girls, it may be more cost-effective to undertake a school-based programme rather than deliver the vaccine through primary health-care practitioners.

14.5 Post-licensing Evaluation

Once a programme is established, it is crucial to monitor it to ensure that it is meeting its original objectives and it is important that this evaluation is continuous. Furthermore, over time it may be necessary to adapt an intervention, as a country moves to a different level of control, e.g. to elimination or as problems emerge.

A number of process and outcome measures can be measured to see if programme targets are being reached or to detect unexpected events:

14.5.1 Vaccine Coverage

For assessment of vaccine coverage it is important that areas or groups with low vaccine coverage are rapidly identified, so that the appropriate targeted interventions can be implemented. There are three basic methods of measuring vaccine coverage, each with its own advantages and disadvantages. First, the *vaccine distribution* method: where the numerator is the number of vaccine doses distributed and the denominator the number of children of a defined age.

$$\text{Vaccine coverage} = \frac{\text{No. of vaccine doses}}{\text{No. children defined age}}$$

This method can potentially be very quick to identify major problems in a programme. However, it is only suitable for centrally distributed vaccines. Furthermore, in many settings vaccines are administered by both the public sector and the private sector. A further disadvantage is that no information is available about whether the vaccine was actually given, so no data on wasted doses, and of course no information on the vaccine recipients is available.

The second method is the *administrative method*. Here the numerator is the number of doses actually given and the denominator is the number of resident children/live births of a defined age. The advantage of this method is that data are available on primary and booster doses by age. The potential shortcomings are that good records are required and that population migration may not be reflected in the denominator. In fact a different data source may be used for the denominator (can result in numerator–denominator bias). It is also important to include all potential vaccinees in the denominator including those who may not be vaccinated because of potential contraindications. The registry method is a variation of this approach. All registered children are utilised together with their vaccination status, either locally or centrally.

The final method is the *sample population* method. Sampling can either be undertaken systematically or randomly using, for example, cluster sampling methodology. The advantage of this method is that it is efficient. One potential disadvantage is that pockets of low coverage may be missed (unless they are over sampled). In addition it is labour intensive.

So what is the best method to use? This should really be decided on the basis of the method of vaccine delivery, the organisation of vaccine delivery and health services, available resources and what recorded information is readily available.

14.5.2 Disease Surveillance

This is another indicator of programme performance. The maintenance or introduction of adequate surveillance systems for new and established vaccine programmes is essential to monitor disease and ensure targets are being met. Surveillance is required to describe the epidemiology of the disease post-vaccination, detect any increase and provide rapid understanding for any such increase in disease incidence above expected thresholds. This allows disease control measures to be modified quickly and in the most appropriate fashion (see also Chapter 8).

A variety of surveillance approaches can be used depending on the nature of the infection and the aims and stage of the control programme. Surveillance can be national (and attempt to detect all cases) or sentinel (where a number of sites are responsible for reporting).

The nature of the system changes with the level of control. Thus prior to the introduction of a programme, disease burden data is required. For measles infection when disease is still endemic (the early control phase), only aggregate reporting of clinical cases is appropriate, without laboratory confirmation of every suspected case, to avoid overburdening the system. Once the elimination phase is being reached, it is important that case definitions become more specific. As disease incidence of measles becomes lower, other causes of rash illness (such as rubella) are reported as suspected measles. Thus case-based reporting and laboratory confirmation of all cases become vital.

It is also important that information is collected on the vaccination status of cases, as this allows preliminary estimation of the vaccine effectiveness. This has been an integral part of the UK national surveillance system for HiB, meningococcal C and pneumococcal disease.

14.5.3 Outbreak Investigation (Particularly in Highly Vaccinated Populations)

An outbreak is an increase in the number of cases reported, with more expected compared to previous years. Investigation provides an opportunity to understand why cases have occurred and to take appropriate remedial steps (see Chapter 9).

The two main reasons for outbreaks in "vaccinated" populations is either failure to vaccinate or vaccine failure. Failure to vaccinate can be due to vaccine refusal on philosophical or religious grounds; it can relate to poor access to the healthcare system for marginalised populations or it can be post-honeymoon phenomena, where certain cohorts have not been targeted.

Vaccine failure has been divided into primary vaccine failure (which is a failure to seroconvert at the time of vaccine administration, e.g. measles vaccine) and secondary vaccine failure (which is waning of vaccine protection over time, e.g. polysaccharide pneumococcal vaccine). The possible reasons are explained in more depth below.

14.5.4 Serosurveillance

This provides a direct measure of the performance of a vaccination programme (unlike the measurement of coverage and disease incidence, which are more indirect), and measures the proportion of the population who are immune by age group, gender, region, etc. Immunity takes into account the historical vaccine coverage, vaccine effectiveness and natural infection.

A routine national serosurveillance programme involves the establishment of a serum bank. These need to be representative of the population of interest. Two methods of sampling can be undertaken: either population-based sampling (which may be unacceptable to a section of the population, resulting in a biased sample) or use of residual sera. These are samples that have been submitted to the laboratory for other purposes. Basic information should also be available on age, gender, region and date (see also Chapter 8).

England and Wales have a routine national serosurveillance programme. In 1994, it was ascertained that a significant number of susceptibles had accumulated over the previous 10–15 years following the introduction of single dose measles vaccine programme at less than 100% coverage. This had been enough to reduce circulating measles, and thus increase the mean age of infection, but not enough to provide direct protection to all children. A large measles epidemic was predicted – largely on children less than 16 years of age. Thus a national MR campaign was conducted targeted at school children (all those 5–16 years of age) that reduced susceptibility levels in the population at risk. Concurrently, a second dose of MMR was introduced as a booster at 3–5 years of age. Similar comparable national population-based serosurveys in a number of European countries can be used to monitor progress to WHO susceptibility targets. For example, those required to achieve measles elimination.

Serosurveillance can be used in combination with mathematical modelling to explore alternative intervention strategies.

One of the potential pitfalls of a serosurveillance programme is comparing serosurveys undertaken in different geographical areas. This is because, potentially, a wide variety of assays are in use, whose specificity and sensitivity can vary between centres. This can be minimised to some extent through the use of international standard sera (e.g. for measles), although these are lacking for other antigens (e.g. mumps) or through the use of external quality assurance panels of sera.

14.5.5 Adverse Event Surveillance

Once a vaccine has been introduced into a programme, there needs to be post-licensure monitoring, particularly for vaccine adverse events (phase IV studies). This is a crucial element. Although common reactions are likely to become evident during pre-licensing trials, rare reactions only become apparent once a vaccine has been brought into widespread routine use, hence the importance of post-licensing surveillance.

This surveillance can be a passive, where practitioners return reports to a national body. From Table 14.1 it is apparent that with the massive reduction in incidence of vaccine preventable infections, there is a rise in the number of reports of possible vaccine adverse events. This form of surveillance has the weakness of no case definition, incomplete reporting and unknown denominator. Furthermore, early childhood is a time for many mild illnesses and some can potentially be falsely attributed to almost universally administered vaccines, purely on a temporal association. However, the system can often pick up putative vaccine reactions, generating hypothesis that can then be formally investigated with an epidemiological study.

Special surveillance schemes have been used to test specific hypotheses and investigate possible vaccine-related adverse events. Several methods have been used. A more traditional case–control approach in the United States demonstrated an association between rotavirus vaccine and intussusception (Kramarz et al. 2001). The newer self-controlled case series approach demonstrated an association between mumps Urabe strain in the UK and encephalitis (Farrington et al. 1995). In this method, each case acts as its own control, thus effectively controlling for confounding.

14.5.6 Vaccine Effectiveness

Vaccine effectiveness is the protective effect of the vaccine under the ordinary conditions of the public health programme.

How are they measured? These estimates are usually based on observational studies, and it is particularly important to be aware of the potential for bias and confounding, which should be minimised in the study design and analysis. There are a number of potential pitfalls. These include

A. The case definition. With a non-specific case definition (i.e. clinical), it is more likely that a case is a false positive if vaccinated than if not. This can lead to an artificial reduction in vaccine effectiveness.

B. The method of case ascertainment. Case ascertainment must be independent of vaccination history. Two types of case finding can be used: population based and health-care provider based. The former tends to avoid the potential problem of differential use of health-care services, which may vary according to vaccination status, particularly for milder infections.
For example, in a suspected measles outbreak in a school, the school nurse conducted initial case finding. The attack rate according to vaccination status is given in Table 14.2. This gave a vaccine effectiveness of 60%. However, when case finding was conducted by directly contacting the parents, a large number of additional unvaccinated cases were detected who had not been in contact with the school medical services. This resulted in a much higher attack rate in the unvaccinated group and thus the overall vaccine effectiveness was elevated to 70%.

Table 14.2 Measles outbreak in a school: the effect of differential case finding

	School nurse case finding	Parental case finding
ARV	12% (22/183)	12% (22/182)
ARU	30% (95/317)	40% (126/316)
VE	60%	70%

C. Confounding. A confounder is a factor that is associated with both the exposure (vaccination in this instance) and also with the outcome (infection in this case). An example is age, as both infection and vaccination may vary with age. These confounders need to be controlled for either in the design or in the analysis using a stratified or a regression analysis approach.

A number of observational study approaches may be used to estimate vaccine effectiveness including

A. The screening method. This is the easiest. The "cover" or "rapid screening" method can provide a cheap, preliminary estimate of VE. The method involves comparing the proportion of cases vaccinated (PCV) with population vaccine coverage (PPV). These can be derived from routine surveillance data. The estimate is only approximate as usually there is no control for confounding although an adjustment for age can minimise this bias partially. The equation is given by

$$\mathrm{VE} = 1 - \frac{\mathrm{PCV}(1 - \mathrm{PPV})}{(1 - \mathrm{PCV})\mathrm{PPV}}$$

B. The case–control approach involves comparing cases with comparable controls (with no illness) and obtaining the vaccine history from both groups. Ideally the controls should be representative of the population from which the cases arose, but there is often a large potential for bias and confounding. The vaccine effectiveness is appropriately given by the following equation:

$$\mathrm{VE} \approx 1 - \mathrm{OR}$$

C. The cohort design involves comparing disease attack rates in vaccinated and unvaccinated groups who have been exposed in a closed setting, e.g. school or nursing home. If vaccination status changes during the outbreak then a person-time approach has to be used. A potential problem is the underlying assumption that the vaccinated and unvaccinated groups are equally exposed to infection but this is usually the case:

$$\mathrm{VE} = 1 - \mathrm{RR}$$

It should also be remembered that outbreaks will tend to occur in pockets of vaccine failures and as a consequence, vaccine effectiveness measured in outbreaks may not be representative of the total population experience. On the other hand they may reveal specific local problems and a low VE should prompt risk factor studies. These compare vaccinated cases and non-cases and are of particular relevance in outbreak settings, especially when the vaccine coverage is high. A number of reasons can be discovered for the outbreak including a breach of the cold chain, administration to a different target population, a change in the vaccine formulation or changes in the pathogen (antigenic switching).

14.5.7 Acceptability of Intervention

"Informed refusal must remain an acceptable choice in a free democracy, and the culture of informed consent, with both religious and philosophical exemption, must be maintained. The difficult balancing act will be in determining the right of the state to control an infectious disease and the right of the individual to choose."

For a new vaccine to succeed it is essential that it is considered acceptable by the various key stakeholders such as the public and the scientific community. It is possible to undertake special surveys examining knowledge and attitude of these populations. This has been undertaken regularly in the UK by the Department of Health to evaluate attitudes amongst various groups. An example is health-care workers on the safety of MMR vaccine. These studies are invaluable in developing communication and targeted health promotion strategies (Petrovic et al. 2001).

Public perception of adverse events can have devastating effects on a programme, as was seen with whole cell pertussis vaccine in many Western European countries. The putative association of encephalopathy with pertussis vaccine in the 1970 s led to a dramatic drop in coverage in a number of European countries and withdrawal of the vaccine in others (Fig. 14.1). This led to a resurgence of the disease and large outbreaks with significant morbidity and mortality. This has been called the natural history of a vaccine programme. A dramatic drop in disease incidence with introduction of a vaccine occurred, followed by an increase in reports of possible adverse

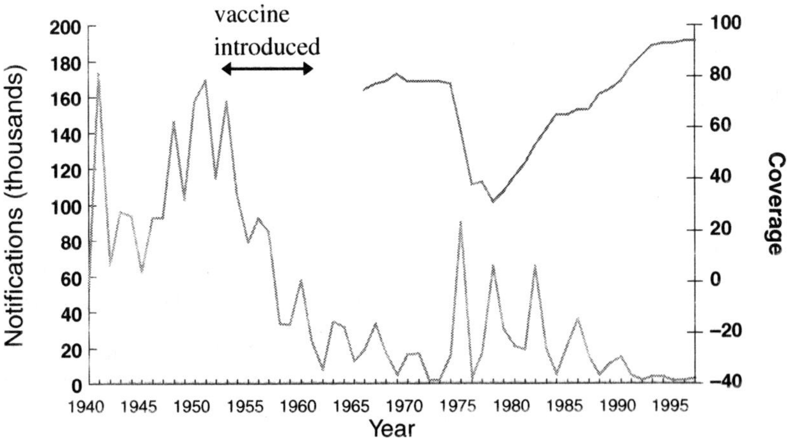

Fig. 14.1 We are keen to prevent a repeat of what happened with whooping cough where, after a study in the 1970s showed a very small risk of brain damage (<1 in 300,000) vaccine coverage dropped causing huge outbreaks in the 1970s and 1980s. Over time confidence was restored and diseases rates have dropped dramatically. Clearly if a true risk identified which out-ways the benefit of vaccination then the vaccine may need to be withdrawn or replaced (This recently occurred in the US when a risk of intussusception following Rotavirus vaccine was identified)

events. This can lead to a drop in confidence with the programme. The subsequent drop in coverage results in a recrudescence of disease, followed by an increase in coverage again. Eradication may eventually be reached, when the programme can potentially be ceased.

14.6 New Vaccines and Methods

A continuing challenge is to reduce the disease burden due to vaccine preventable infections in the developing world, where the establishment of routine vaccine delivery systems to the general population has proved a huge challenge in some areas.

This has led to the development of umbrella groups such as the Children's Vaccine Initiative (which includes UNICEF, WHO, NGOs, vaccine companies, the World Bank and funding groups such as the Rockefeller foundation) and more recently GAVI (the Global Alliance for Vaccines and Immunisations). Strategies for vaccine delivery of currently licensed vaccines, e.g. measles, need to be developed further to enable the entire world's population to have access to safe and effective vaccines. New vaccines have recently been licensed in some industrialised and middle income countries, e.g. rotavirus vaccine and pneumococcal conjugate vaccine. Their role and value in the developing world is being evaluated.

In summary, vaccination continues to provide an extremely important public health intervention. However, this chapter has shown that the implementation and evaluation of immunisation programmes is becoming an increasingly multi-disciplinary process, involving not only epidemiology, but also other bio-medical sciences such as mathematics and immunology. Furthermore, the role of qualitative methods such as sociology and anthropology are also becoming increasingly apparent.

References

Farrington P, Pugh S, Colville A, Flower A, Nash J, Morgan-Capner P, Rush M, Miller E (1995) A new method of active surveillance of adverse events from diphtheria/tetanus/pertussis and measles/mumps/rubella vaccines. Lancet; 345: 567–9

Fine P (1994) The contribution of modelling to vaccination policy. Vaccination and World Health. John Wiley & Sons Ltd., New York

Galazka AM, Robertson SE, Kraigher A (1999) Mumps and mumps vaccine: a global review. Bull World Health Organ; 77: 3–14

Kramarz P, France EK, Destefano F, Black SB, Shinefield H, Ward JI et al. (2001) Population based study of rotavirus vaccination and intussusception. Pediatr Infect Dis J; 20(4): 410–6

Nokes DJ, Anderson RM (1987) Rubella vaccination policy: a note of caution. Lancet; 1 (8547): 1441–2

Orenstein WA, Bernier RH, Dondero TJ, Hinman AR, Marks JS, Bart KJ, Sirotkin B (1985) Field evaluation of vaccine efficacy. Bull World Health Organ; 63(6): 1055–68

Panagiotopoulos T, Antoniadou I, Valassi-Adam E (1999) Increase in congenital rubella occurrence after immunisation in Greece: retrospective survey and systematic review. BMJ; 319: 1462–7

Petrovic M, Roberts R, Ramsay M (2001) Second dose of measles, mumps and rubella vaccine: questionnaire survey of health professionals. BMJ; 322: 82–5

Chapter 15
Health Economics of Infectious Diseases

Robert Welte, Reiner Leidl, Wolfgang Greiner, and Maarten Postma

15.1 Introduction

Due to technical innovations and demographic changes, many industrialized countries are facing problems in financing health-care costs. One way to guide decision makers in the allocation of their limited health-care budget is the use of economic evaluation. The economic evaluation of health technologies is a special discipline of health economics, which compares the technical efficiency of technologies in the health-care sector. The term technology covers everything from drugs to medical equipment to the design of intervention programs. Technical efficiency is achieved if with a minimum input (of resources) a given output is produced or if with a specific input a maximum of output (e.g., life years) is produced. Hence, technical efficiency considers both effectiveness and resource utilization. Only an effective technology can be efficient. Typically, in economic evaluations the incremental cost-effectiveness ratio (ICER) of a technology is estimated. The ICER is a measure for the technical efficiency of a technology and can be expressed, for example, as € 30,000 per life year gained (LYG) or US $ 15,000 per quality-adjusted life year (QALY) gained, reflecting the net costs (costs minus savings) of gaining one life year or QALY, respectively.

Several specific aspects characterize economic evaluations of infectious diseases. The main differentiating characteristic of infectious diseases is obviously their infectiousness. Hence, the prevention of an infection in one individual can decrease the infection risk of another individual. Next, many important infectious diseases occur at young ages, most notably during childhood which makes the measurement of quality of life (QoL) losses very difficult and raises questions about the estimation of the loss of future productivity. Furthermore, prevention programs against several infectious diseases require immediate investment of costs but render prevented

R. Welte (✉)
Helmholtz Zentrum München, German Research Center for Environmental Health (GmbH), Institute of Health Economics and Health Care Management (IGM), Ingolstädter Landstr. 1, 85764 Neuherberg, Germany
e-mail: robert.welte@helmholtz-muenchen.de

A. Krämer et al. (eds.), *Modern Infectious Disease Epidemiology*,
Statistics for Biology and Health, DOI 10.1007/978-0-387-93835-6_15,

sequelae and associated savings years later. Thus, the results of economic evaluations of prevention programs are often greatly influenced by the applied analysis horizon and the discount rates.

This chapter considers these special challenges, which are posed by the economic evaluation of infectious disease prevention. The main elements of economic evaluations are shortly described and the specific requirements of the prevention measures against infectious diseases are discussed. The cost-effectiveness analysis (CEA), which is the most common study type in the economic evaluation of infectious diseases, will be used as a case example.

15.2 Elements of Economic Evaluation with a Special Focus on Infectious Disease Prevention

15.2.1 Effectiveness

The effectiveness of a technology is one of the most important parameters for a CEA. Typically, effectiveness – aimed to reflect the drug's performance in real life conditions – differs from efficacy estimated from controlled studies, such as randomized clinical trials. Effectiveness may generally be plausibly approximated from efficacy estimates by accounting for possible non-compliance, non-adherence, and non-persistence. In the case of infectious diseases this approximation is, however, more difficult. As infectious diseases are transmissible, the direct aversion of an infectious disease in one person might also lead to the indirect aversion of the disease in other persons. These indirect protection effects can occur if an intervention, such as vaccination, reduces the force of infection in the population. The force of infection has been defined as the rate at which susceptibles acquire infection (Edmunds et al. 1999). As a consequence, incidence decreases beyond the immediate effect of the intervention under study. The overall effectiveness of a prevention measure against an infectious disease is made up of the direct effectiveness (the vaccinated person is protected) and the indirect effectiveness (the risk of non-vaccinated persons becoming infected is decreased). Hence, the overall effectiveness cannot be derived from a randomized clinical trial alone – instead it is necessary to look at the population level. Of course, the exact relative size of the indirect effect depends on the specific infectious disease and intervention under study.

There are two ways of obtaining the overall, i.e., direct and indirect effectiveness of an infectious disease prevention measure:

Retrospective data analysis: The disease incidence or prevalence before and after the intervention is analyzed. For instance, De Wals et al. calculated retrospectively the overall effectiveness of meningococcal C vaccination in Quebec in 1992–1993 (De Wals et al. 2001). Similarly, Ramsey et al. estimated the overall effectiveness for meningococcal serogroup C conjugate vaccination in England retrospectively (Ramsay et al. 2003).

Prospective simulation using mathematical modeling (see Section 15.3)**:** This is the typical method of estimating the overall effectiveness of introducing a new prevention intervention. For parameterization and validation of the model retrospective data are typically used. A good example is the meningococcal C simulation model by Trotter et al. which estimates the effectiveness of serogroup C meningococcal C vaccination in the UK (Trotter et al. 2005).

To generate indirect protection effects, the pathogen and technology must meet the following conditions: (a) the pathogen is mainly transmitted between humans and (b) the intervention influences the spread of the pathogen in the population (Welte 2007). Examples for which the first condition is not fulfilled are rabies or tetanus. Interventions targeting only a part of a population which contributes marginally to the spread of the infection in the population do not fulfill the second condition, e.g., hepatitis B vaccination as travel prophylaxis of probably predominantly monogamous individuals in Germany. This intervention will not result in substantial indirect protection effects, as hepatitis B in Germany is mostly spread via sexual contacts with multiple partners.

Typically, indirect protection effects represent positive externalities of the intervention. The protection of one individual simultaneously reduces the risk of other individuals to become infected, and thus extends the benefit beyond the treated individual. As such, indirect protection often leads to an improved cost-effectiveness of the intervention. Examples are shown in Tables 15.1 and 15.2

Table 15.1 Examples of the impact of indirect protection effects on the cost-effectiveness of vaccination programs

Pathogen	Vaccination program	Country	Cost-effectiveness ratio		Reference
			With indirect protection effects	Without indirect protection effects	
Hepatitis A virus	Routine childhood	USA	Cost saving	US$ 228,000/LYG	Armstrong et al. (2007)
Human papillomavirus 6,11,16,18	Routine girls	USA	US$ 3,906/QALY	US$ 8,137/QALY	Chesson et al. (2008)
Influenza virus	Working population	ESP	Cost saving	€ 76/influenza case avoided	Pradas-Velasco et al. (2008)
Meningococcus C	Routine childhood	UK	£ 8713/LYG	£ 44,639/LYG	Trotter and Edmunds (2006)
Bordetella pertussis	Routine adolescents	USA	20%*: US$ 6253/LYG	5%*: US$ 187,081/LYG	Caro et al. (2005)
Streptococcus pneumonia	Routine childhood	GER	€ 164/LYG	€ 100,636/LYG	Lloyd et al. (2008)
	Routine childhood	NL	€ 15,600/LYG	€ 58,700/LYG	Hubben et al. (2007)
	Routine childhood	UK	£ 4360/LYG	£ 33,687/LYG	McIntosh et al. (2005)
	Routine childhood	USA	$ 7500/LYG	$ 112,000/LYG	Ray et al. (2006)

* Caro et al did not show the results with and without indirect protection effects, instead, they showed them with 20% (baseline) and 5% indirect protection effects

Table 15.2 The impact of indirect protection effects on the cost-effectiveness of screening programs using genital *Chlamydia trachomatis* infections as case example (Welte et al. 2005a)

	Cost-effectiveness ratio of screening	Incremental cost-effectiveness ratio for extending the screening to	
	Females aged 15–24 years (baseline)	Females aged 15–29 years	Females aged 15–34 years
With indirect protection effects	Cost saving	Cost saving*	Cost saving*
Without indirect protection effects	US $ 700/MOA	US $ 1800/MOA	US $ 2520/MOA

* Both strategies strictly dominate screening females aged 15–24 years, i.e., they render more MOAs and savings
MOA = Major outcome averted

Sometimes, these effects can cause a less attractive ICER, as have been shown for meningococcal C conjugate vaccination in the Netherlands: The ICER for routine childhood vaccination at ages 2 + 3 + 4 months (three vaccine doses in total) versus at 14 months (one vaccine dose) strongly increased when the likely indirect protection effects of the catch-up vaccination program (all persons aged 14 months to 18 years) was considered. These indirect protection effects lowered the number of avoidable meningococcal cases in the age group 0–14 months and thus reduced the health benefit of vaccinating during the first year of life versus at the beginning of the second year of life (Welte et al. 2004c).

Moreover, in some cases indirect protection effects can also turn out as negative externalities if an age shift occurs or if the exposure of immune persons to the pathogen is important for boosting their immunity:

Age shift of infection: The indirect protection effect of a mass infant vaccination program can result in a shift of the age at infection. Vaccination of most infants against a childhood disease reduces the force of infection in the population considerably. Thus, non-immunized individuals have a decreased infection risk and therefore tend to be older when they get infected. For diseases, which are more severe in adulthood than in childhood, such as polio, hepatitis A virus, mumps, rubella, and varicella, this age shift might lead to additional health problems and thus to a worsening of the economic attractiveness of a vaccination program. For instance, after the implementation of infant vaccination against rubella in Greece an age shift was observed that resulted in an increase of congenital rubella (Panagiotopoulos et al. 1999). On the other hand, for diseases which are less severe in adulthood than in childhood, this age shift leads to an improved cost-effectiveness of the vaccination program. Examples are pertussis and hepatitis B vaccination: Pertussis is less severe in older children and adults than in infants and a higher age of infection with hepatitis B virus results in fewer chronic infections (Welte 2007).

Reduction in boosting of immunity. The indirect protection effect may decrease the exposure of immune persons to the pathogen yielding to a reduction in the rate of reactivation and boosting of immunity. This has been observed for varicella zoster (Brisson and Edmunds 2002; Thomas et al. 2002) and its negative influence on the economic attractiveness of routine infant varicella vaccination has been simulated for Canada, England and Wales, and the USA (Brisson and Edmunds 2002; Brisson and Edmunds 2003; Goldman 2005). Modeling results show that in the short and medium term (35–50 years) after the introduction of a mass infant varicella vaccination program, herpes zoster would increase in the population. However, in the long term (50–70 years), as the immunized children aged further, a decrease of herpes zoster was predicted (Thomas et al. 2002). So far, there is mixed evidence in the USA whether the incidence of zoster has increased or not since the introduction of universal varicella vaccination (Heininger and Seward 2006). The time period since vaccination is still too short to really obtain practical evidence of the accurateness of the simulated results.

Currently, vaccination and screening programs are the primary prevention measures against infectious diseases. For vaccination programs, indirect protection effects are commonly labeled herd immunity effects and have been frequently defined as the indirect protection of non-immune individuals by the presence and proximity of immune individuals (Fine 1993). Typically, a vaccinated person leaves the susceptible pool of the population as most vaccinations result in protection from the infectious pathogen for several years. Herd immunity also implies that full vaccination coverage is not required to achieve elimination of an infectious disease in a population. Based on the concept of herd immunity, the critical level of vaccination in a population for elimination of infection has been estimated for various infectious diseases, such as measles (coverage of about 83–94%), pertussis (92–94%), and rubella (83–85%) (Fine 1993).

For screening programs, indirect protection effects have been less investigated than for vaccination programs. Screening programs for sexually transmitted diseases (STDs) lead to the identification and subsequent treatment of asymptomatic infected persons. After eradication of the pathogen the body is usually not immune against reinfection and the individual is susceptible again. Examples are genital infections with *Chlamydia trachomatis* and *Neisseria gonorrhoeae*. Thus, STD screening programs differ from vaccination programs with respect to the susceptibility to a disease. This difference might influence the impact of an intervention on the spread of disease and thus on the force of infection.

Besides these indirect protection effects, the effectiveness of an infectious disease prevention programs can also be influenced by cross protection, waning immunity, serotype replacement, and development of treatment resistance:

Cross protection may occur, with the vaccine providing protection beyond the serotypes explicitly included in the vaccine, as has been recently shown for human papillomavirus vaccines (Herrero et al. 2009). Clearly, cross protection will improve the effectiveness and cost-effectiveness of the respective vaccines.

Waning immunity, i.e., decreasing vaccine-induced immunity over time, has been observed for many vaccines, e.g., diphtheria, pertussis, or tetanus vaccines. It may result in the necessity of booster vaccine shots and a worsening of the cost-effectiveness of the vaccination program.

Serotype replacement means that the virus or bacteria serotype(s), contained in the vaccine, is (are) replaced by other types not covered in the vaccine. In case the replacing type is pathogenic, the (cost)effectiveness of vaccination against the specific disease will decrease. This has been observed in Alaska after the introduction of routine infant pneumococcal vaccination in 2001. At first the invasive pneumococcal disease rate decreased but subsequently increased due to serotype replacement (Singleton et al. 2007).

Development of treatment resistance: Another problem in the optimizing of strategies against infectious disease may emerge over time in cases where effective treatment exists for infected persons, but its broad, intensive, and long-term use nourishes the development of treatment-resistant strains of the infective agent. The treatment of one generation of susceptibles may increase the risks of a next generation of susceptibles for whom effective treatment may no longer be available. Tuberculosis is an example of a disease incurring problems of this type (Maartens and Wilkinson 2007).

15.2.2 Comparator and Cost-Effectiveness ratio

In an economic evaluation, the costs and effects of the investigated technology are compared with costs and effects of the most common or best available technology. Thus, the incremental costs and effects are evaluated and typically integrated into the ICER. If no intervention is the most plausible comparator the comparator is "no intervention" and hence the incremental costs and effects compared to "no intervention" are calculated. The resulting cost-effectiveness ratio (CER) is often called the average cost-effectiveness ratio (ACER) or also the ICER versus "no intervention" (Welte et al. 2004c). Commonly, the results of an economic evaluation are shown in the cost-effectiveness plane (Fig. 15.1). It shows the incremental costs (ΔC) and effects (ΔE) per patient. The slope of a straight line from the origin through the coordinates of a technology (e.g., point A for technology A) gives the ICER for technology A.

The difference between the ICER and ACER is at the heart of health economics. A small example may help illustrate the difference between the ACER and ICER further. Let us assume two technologies F and G for averting a disease. Technology F costs € 1000 and leads to 5 LYGs, technology G costs € 1800 and renders 6 LYGs. The ACER of technology F is € 1000/ 5 LYGs = € 200 per LYG, the ACER of technology G is € 300 per LYG. However, the ICER of technology G versus technology F is (€ 1800–€ 1000)/(6 LYGs – 5 LYGs) = € 800 per LYG.

The ACER has become a rather uncommon measure in the economic evaluation of therapeutics, as effective treatments are usually available for the respective diseases. Yet, in the field of vaccination and screening programs the ACER is still often encountered as there is generally no implemented screening or vaccination program for comparison. Nevertheless, even in cases, where the relevant alternative is really "no intervention", the ICER can still be important for identifying the best vaccination strategy. An example is meningococcal C conjugate vaccination in the Netherlands. First the ACER of universal childhood vaccination at 14 months was estimated to be € 1900 per LYG. Subsequently, the ICER of different possible

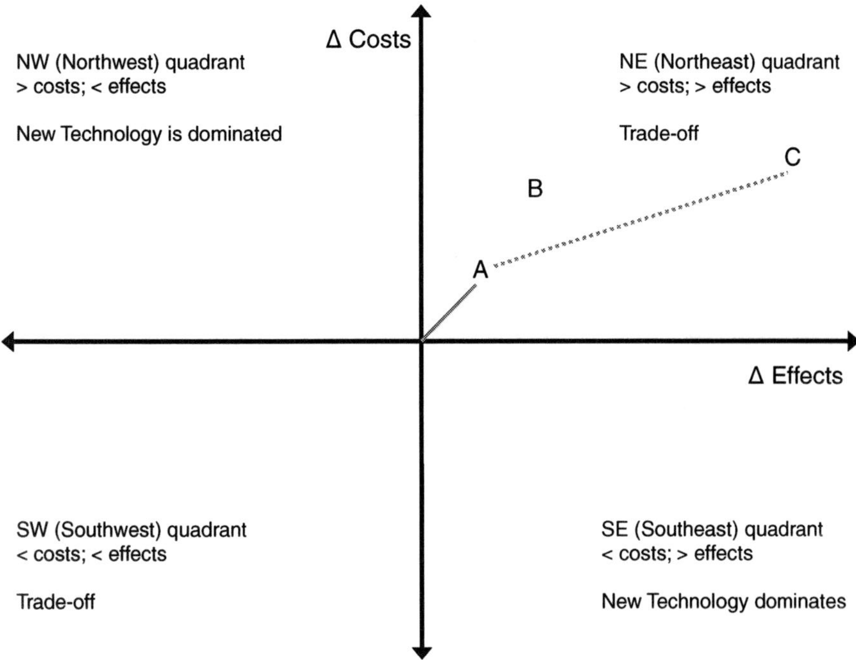

Fig. 15.1 The cost-effectiveness plane

vaccination strategies was calculated, e.g., each additional LYG by vaccination at 2, 3, and 4 months versus vaccination at 14 months was estimated to incrementally cost about € 147,000 (Welte et al. 2004c).

Consistent application of the ICER concept may reveal cases of so-called dominance. One strategy can be dominated by another strategy, either by strict or extended dominance. A strategy is strictly dominated when it is both less effective and more costly than another strategy, i.e., it lies in the northwest quadrant of the cost-effectiveness plane (Fig. 15.1). A strategy is extended dominated when it is both less effective and more costly than a linear combination of two other strategies with which it is mutually exclusive (Gold et al. 1996; Postma et al. 2008). This can be graphically illustrated by plotting the incremental costs and effects of different technologies (using the same comparator) on a cost-effectiveness plane. In Fig. 15.1, technology B is extended dominated by A and C (see dotted line). Examples of dominance are chlamydial and HIV screening as well as pneumococcal vaccination: In the Netherlands chlamydial screening every 10 years only was extended dominated by a combination of one–off screening and screening every 5 years (de Vries et al. 2008). Universal HIV screening among pregnant women in Chicago results in a decreased number of HIV-infected newborns and also cost savings, i.e., it strictly dominates no screening (Immergluck et al. 2000). Similarly, universal childhood vaccination with the pneumococcal conjugate vaccine in Germany renders health gains and cost savings (Claes et al. 2009).

15.2.3 Perspective

The perspective determines which costs (and effects) are relevant and should be considered in an economic assessment. For prevention measures against infectious diseases, commonly both the societal and the health-care payer perspective are taken. Typically, the former leads to a more attractive CER than the latter. However, this is not always the case and hence should be checked for each strategy individually (Welte 2007). For diseases causing relevant absenteeism, sometimes also the perspective of an employer is applied, e.g., for influenza vaccination (Postma et al. 2005). While the productivity loss is relevant to the employer it is often not of interest to the health-care payer. Oppositely, the direct medical costs are not always important to the employer, whereas they clearly are for the health-care payer. For the societal perspective, which is recommended in most guidelines for economic evaluation, the cost of all resource consumption is relevant, no matter who causes or pays for it.

15.2.4 Costs

Costs in economic evaluations are usually divided into direct and productivity costs.

Direct costs are the valued resource consumptions of tangible goods and services actually delivered to address the consequences of a disease (e.g., acute medical care) or to prevent the disease (e.g., vaccination). They are often distinguished into direct medical (e.g., hospital visit, vaccine) and non-medical (e.g., transport cost to the hospital) costs.

Productivity costs (also called indirect costs) are the value of productive services not performed. They can be caused by a disease (e.g., absenteeism, early retirement, and mortality) or a technology (e.g., taking time off to receive a vaccine shot). Productivity costs occur in both the paid and unpaid work sector. Those in the paid work sector can be defined as all work activities that contribute to the gross domestic product (GDP), while unpaid work is not recognized in the classical system of national accounts. Unpaid work mainly consists of household work, caring for family and non-family members (informal care), maintenance of transport, consumer items and homes, and engagement for society (work in an honorary position and voluntary work) (Welte et al. 2004b).

In economic evaluations of prevention measures against infectious disease, productivity costs frequently represent one of the major categories of averted costs as infectious diseases often occur in young children (childhood diseases) and can lead to severe life-long sequelae or even death. Typical examples are infant vaccination programs. In particular, productivity costs make up 54% of the estimated cost savings for pneumococcal conjugate vaccination in the USA (Welte 2007). Productivity costs are typically either measured with the human capital approach or the friction cost method.

The *human capital approach* is the standard approach for estimating productivity costs and can be used for assessing the productivity costs due to paid and unpaid work loss. It estimates the maximum potential loss of production as a consequence of disease or death. In particular, the full extent of output that a person cannot produce due to a disease is assessed. For long-term work absence, the present value of the future net product has to be calculated with discounting (Welte et al. 2004b).

The *friction cost method* can also be applied to estimate the actual loss of paid work. It assumes that the paid work of any long-term absent person can be undertaken by a previously unemployed person. The time span required to find and train a replacement worker is defined as the friction time. For any work absence longer than the friction time, only the friction time is taken into account for the calculation of the production loss. It is further assumed that during work absence, about 80 % of the production of a person will be lost, as the other 20 % is assumed to be taken over by colleagues or made up for by the sick person after recovery. The value of lost production plus the costs for finding and training a replacement worker plus the costs of the negative medium-term macro-economic consequences of absence and disability render the friction costs, i.e., the productivity costs based on the friction cost method (Koopmanschap et al. 1995; Koopmanschap and Rutten 1996).

If the infectious disease causes only short-term work loss (work-loss time shorter than the friction time), the two methods render rather similar results for the paid work sector. Uncomplicated cases of diarrhea are one example of this. Otherwise, results may differ substantially, especially for diseases that cause mortality and inability to work, such as meningococcal disease. With the human capital approach, the productivity costs of a child's death are valued at the present value of the future net product of an average child at the same age, rendering considerable productivity costs. The same event is valued at € 0 with the friction cost method. The strong impact of the measurement method has been demonstrated for a routine childhood meningococcal vaccination program in the Netherlands: Applying the human capital approach instead of the friction cost method decreased the costs per life year gained by almost 700% and was identified as the most sensitive assumption in the model (Welte et al. 2004c).

Health technologies typically lead to a net decrease of productivity costs, i.e., the productivity loss caused by a disease is exceeded by the productivity gains attributable to preventing the disease. However, this cannot be taken for granted and should be checked for each technology case by case. A CEA for a meningococcal vaccination catch-up program in the Netherlands rendered higher productivity costs than productivity savings (Welte et al. 2004c).

Childhood diseases often result in parental work loss which in turn can influence the cost-effectiveness of prevention measures. The respective productivity costs are typically included in the CEA of childhood vaccination programs, such as for meningococcus (Welte et al. 2004c), pneumococcus (Hubben et al. 2007), rotavirus (Jit and Edmunds 2007), and varicella (Brisson and Edmunds 2002).

15.2.5 Effects

The effects of a technology can be measured in natural clinical (e.g., prevented deaths, LYGs, or major outcomes averted (MOAs) for *C. trachomatis*) and non-clinical (e.g., avoided work-loss days) outcomes or in combined outcomes such as

QALYs. For the measurement of QoL there are several disease-specific and some generic instruments. They can be grouped into profile and index instruments. The former describe single dimensions of QoL with values for each dimension, while in the latter all QoL dimensions are summarized in a single value using a specific algorithm. This single value represents a QoL weight, which can then be used for calculating QALYs (see below). Many authors consider the QoL weight a utility if it is being measured by methods with an axiomatic base in utility theory – as for example, the standard gamble method. Examples of index instruments are the EQ-5D of the EuroQol group, the Health-Utility-Index Mark III (HUI Mark III), and the Quality of Well-Being Scale. Specific health profiles include the Medical Outcome Study 36 – Item Short Form Health Survey (SF-36). Methods exist to map the SF-36 results into a single value or QoL weight (Brazier et al. 2002; Brazier et al. 2007).

While the LYG only considers mortality, the QALY takes both morbidity and mortality into account. For the calculation of QALYs, the time a person spends in a specific health status is multiplied with the QoL weight that ranges from 0 (death) to 1 (perfect health). One QALY equals 1 year in perfect health. There are two different theories of the QALY: The welfarist theory interprets the QALY as a representation of individual utility over health. The extra-welfarist approach sees the QALY as a measure of health as a social desideratum, i.e., as a measure of social good in health policy (Brazier et al. 2007). For the determination of QALY weights different methods can be applied, of which the standard gamble method, the time trade-off method, and the visual analogue or rating scale method are common (Berger et al. 2003). As the application of these methods is very resource consuming, index instruments such as the EQ-5D are used more often. For each possible health status indicated by these instruments (e.g., 243 possible health states for the EQ-5D) there are already QALY weights for several countries available (Greiner et al. 2003). For example, the EQ-5D QoL-weights have been estimated using the time trade-off method in the UK, Germany, Denmark, Japan, Spain, Zimbabwe, and the USA (Szende et al. 2006).

Besides the QALY there is the DALY (disability-adjusted life year) which is also a combined measure of morbidity and mortality. In the DALY approach each health state is assigned a disability weighting on a scale from 0 (perfect health) to 1 (death). Furthermore, while QoL weights in the QALY are based on preferences of either the general public or the patients, the disability weights in the DALY are person trade-off scores elicited from a panel of health experts. Unlike QALYs, DALYs are age-weighted in order to take into account welfare interdependence, i.e., individuals support others during adulthood while they are supported by others during infancy and at an advanced age (Robberstad 2005; Drummond et al. 2005). The World Health Bank introduced DALYs to measure the global burden of disease in 1993 (Robberstad 2005) and the World Health Organization recommends the use of DALYs for CEAs (WHO 2003). While in developed countries the QALY is the health effect of choice for CEA, DALYs are primarily used in developing countries. From the standpoint of economic theory, the preferences of those affected, as used in the QALY approach, and not those of experts are preferable. The weighting of QoL by DALYs may provide a substitute in population-oriented approaches where a data basis for QALYs is lacking.

Many infectious diseases occur in childhood. The measurement of QoL in children, especially of infants and toddlers, is very difficult as almost all generic index instruments have been developed for the QoL measurement of adults. Parents or doctors have often been used as proxies for indirectly estimating the QoL of children. Recently, new instruments have been specifically developed for children, such as the EQ-5D-Y (for children between 8 and 14 years), the KIDSCREEN (8–18 years), or the KINDL-R (4–16 years), which directly measure the QoL of children (Ravens-Sieberer et al. 2006). At the time being the value of all these instruments designed for the use in children cannot be considered as utilities. Therefore, the development of QoL measurement in children and especially very young children (before school age) can be considered to be still in its infancy. The QoL loss due to childhood diseases may not be limited to the affected children but may also impact their caregivers. For example, a recent study estimating the cost-effectiveness of rotavirus vaccination in England and Wales applied QALY losses for a child and two caregivers for each episode of rotavirus gastroenteritis (Jit and Edmunds 2007). It should be noted that taking into account the caregivers' QoL loss is rarely seen in economic evaluations.

The prevention of a disease leads not only to the utility gain by the avoided disease itself but also to a gain due to utility-in-anticipation. In the case of a vaccination program, the latter is the utility yielded immediately after vaccination due to the risk reduction until the time the infectious disease was expected (Drummond et al. 2007). Obviously, the utility-in-anticipation depends on the severity of the disease, the risk of non-immunized persons getting the disease, and the effectiveness of the vaccination. It is typically not considered in economic evaluations.

15.2.6 Time Horizon

The time horizon of an analysis determines how long the costs and effects of an intervention shall be measured. It is usually assumed that the current method of diagnosis and treatment will remain the same during the assessed time period in an economic evaluation. Clearly, new diagnostics and treatments can be expected to be introduced in the near future. Hence, a longer analysis horizon increases the uncertainty of the results. In general, the time horizon of an economic evaluation should be long enough to capture all relevant costs and effects of the investigated technology and the identical time horizon should be applied for both costs and effects. For interventions aimed at infectious diseases, this time span may vary from very short to very long. Medications to treat uncomplicated cases of common cold or diarrhea are examples for which a short time frame may apply. On the other hand, vaccination programs in childhood against hepatitis B or in adolescents against cervical cancer require a life-long span. If the aim of an intervention is eradication, the time horizon might even be longer to allow the model sufficient time to achieve the new steady-state of eradication. The Viral Hepatitis Prevention Board suggested in its consensus statement that the analysis horizon for economic evaluation of vaccination programs should not be less than the time required for the decrease in incidence to stop and for the ICER to plateau, i.e., a new epidemiological equilibrium has been reached. It postulated that the necessary time span may roughly range from 1 to 100 years, depending on the intervention and the disease (Beutels et al. 2002). Given the potential long time spans investigated, one should be aware of the following issue: The actual payments and the health gains obtained per period may deviate significantly from the ICER that is calculated over the whole time span. In populations with long-term dynamic factors beyond those integrated in the model framework the estimated ICER may never be achieved.

The analysis horizon has a strong impact on the economic attractiveness of interventions when they lead to a decreased force of infection or even to the eradication of a disease in a population. Prolonging the analysis horizon will lead to the avoidance of more negative health outcomes and associated costs compared to the "no intervention" scenario and hence to a better cost-effectiveness (Welte et al. 2000).

15.2.7 Discounting

Individuals have a positive time preference for money, i.e., they would choose to get a specific amount of money rather today than tomorrow, irrespective of the presence of inflation. In order to adjust for this positive time preference, future costs are discounted to their current present net value. Thus, the further in the future the costs occur, the lower is their present value. Typically, costs are discounted on a yearly basis and exponentially, i.e., at a constant rate. The respective equation for discounting is

$$\text{Present value} = (\text{Future cost at year } t)/(1 + \text{discount rate})^t$$

There are two main theoretical approaches for estimating the discount rate for future costs of health technologies:

(a) Social rate of time preference approach: It measures the willingness of the society to forgo consumption today to enable greater consumption in the future. It can be estimated by the rate on a risk-free investment (e.g., long-term government bonds) adjusted for inflation.

(b) Social opportunity cost approach: It takes into account that public investments can displace private investments or consumption. It uses the real rate of return forgone to society in the private sector which can be empirically estimated by calculating a weighted average of discount rates of those sectors of the economy that contribute resources to the investigated health technologies (Drummond et al. 2005).

Internationally, there is no consensus on which discount rate should be used for costs and different guidelines ask for different discount rates (e.g., 5% in Canada, 4% in the Netherlands, and 3% in the USA). There is even less clear evidence on whether and how health effects should be discounted. Currently, there is an ongoing scientific debate whether the same discount rate should be applied for costs and for effects or whether differential discounting should be applied. At this time, almost all guidelines ask for equal discounting of costs and effects. However, the

Belgium and Dutch guidelines request differential discounting with 3% (Belgium) and 4% (Dutch) for costs and 1.5% for effects. Common arguments for using the same discount rate for costs and effects are as follows:

- Economic theory implies that in a perfectly competitive, risk-free, tax-free world in which all commodities (including something called "health") are perfectly divisible – so that individual decision makers could precisely adapt their consumption of goods and services over time – there would be but one discount rate (Gold et al. 1996).
- Consistency argument contends that using different discount rates for costs and effects can lead to inconsistent reasoning. Example: Intervention K costs € 10,000 this year and renders 1 QALY this year, Intervention L costs € 10,000 in 10 years and renders 1 QALY in year 10. Using the same discount rate for costs and effects would lead to the same CER and hence would give the same priority to both interventions. On the other side, applying different discount rates for costs and effects would render different CERs (Brouwer et al. 2005; Claxton et al. 2006).
- Keeler and Cretin paradox: A higher discount rate for costs than effects would result in a better CER the later the technology is implemented. Hence, it might lead to an eternal delay of the introduction of investigated technologies (Brouwer et al. 2005; Claxton et al. 2006).

Typical arguments for using different discount rates are as follows:

- Time preference might be different for effects.
- The world is not perfectly competitive, risk-free, and tax-free (Gold et al. 1996) and neither is health perfectly divisible nor is it a fully tradable good.
- The monetary valuation of health effects might change over time, invalidating the consistency argument (Brouwer et al. 2005; Gravelle et al. 2007).
- Keeler and Cretin paradox is usually not relevant for decision makers as the typical decision is not when but whether a medical technology should be implemented (Brouwer et al. 2005; Cairns 2001).
- The problem of double discounting of QALYs if calculated from time trade-off-based preferences. In the time trade-off method, the preferences already include discounting (MacKeigan 2003).
- Inter-generational discounting: Discounting effects gained in the future gives more weight to the current generation compared to the future one (Cairns 2001). This argument is especially relevant for infectious disease prevention. From any program that aims at the eradication of a disease, future generations will strongly benefit – but this benefit is basically discounted away. For example, smallpox was a major threat to people until its successful eradication and all current and future populations have an obvious benefit from the successful eradication campaign.

Finally, we note that for both money and health the functional form for discounting is questioned. In particular the time preference might not be linear considering different time periods. For instance, hyperbolic discounting has been suggested as an alternative for the linear relationship described above.

Discounting can have a profound impact on the results of economic evaluation. It always has an influence if there is a differential timing of costs (and effects), e.g., investment costs occur now while the health effects and associated savings with a technology occur later.

The impact of discounting strongly depends on two factors:

(a) The time interval between the investment (e.g., vaccination) and the health effect (e.g., averted death). As the interval increases, the impact of discounting becomes more profound. This is the case for most prevention programs against infectious diseases. For example, cervical cancers may occur on average at ages 35–55 years while HPV vaccination might take place at 12 years of age.
(b) The exact rate of discounting applied: The higher the discount rate, the less the future is valued and thus the less the future health effect and associated savings are valued. The impact of the discount rate can be easily seen in Fig. 15.2. At a discount rate of 5% the present value of any savings or effects occurring after more than 50 or 100 years is less than 10 or 1% of the future value, respectively. As a result, discounting leads to a restriction of the time horizon.

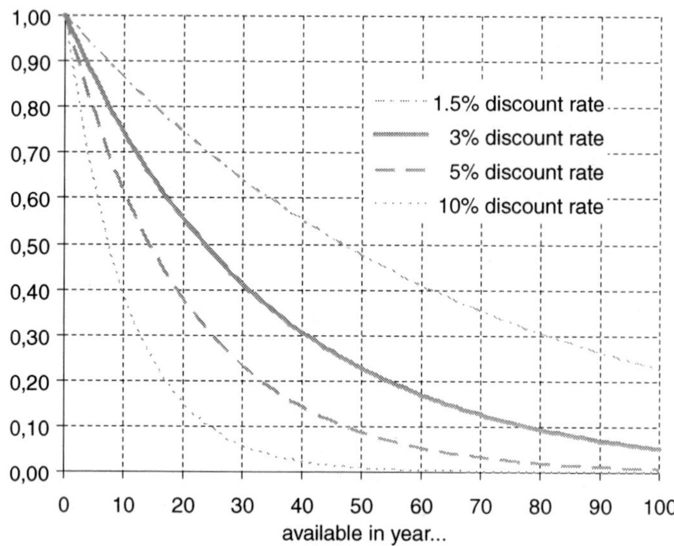

Fig. 15.2 Present value of € 1 or 1 life year

The question has been raised whether a different discounting method should be applied for prevention measures for infectious diseases. Bos et al. propose that the timing of the risk reduction and not the timing of the avoided morbidity or mortality should be incorporated in the discounting (Bos et al. 2005). This would lead to more attractive CERs for prevention measures as the benefit would be valued from the time of risk reduction and not from the later time of exposure. However, instead of trying to address this topic by changing the discounting procedure, it could also be addressed using the utility-in-anticipation concept (see above) (Drummond et al. 2007).

15.2.8 Uncertainty

In an economic evaluation, first the base case or baseline analysis is performed (Gold et al. 1996). The most likely values are used as model input parameters to yield the main results. Second, the sensitivity analysis is conducted to assess the robustness of the results, i.e., what is the probability that the results are correct or that the outcomes are robust when changes in parameters are made? Different types of uncertainty are commonly distinguished:

- *Parameter uncertainty:* What is the true value of an input parameter, whereby the available information on the parameter is merely conceived as one possibility out of a broader set (a random draw from a distribution)?
- *Methodological uncertainty:* Are the appropriate methods used, e.g., what is the correct perspective and discount rate, what approach should be used for measurement of productivity costs, which time horizon should be applied?
- *Model (or structural) uncertainty:* Has the right model been designed, have the right relations been specified, and have the right modeling assumptions been made?

Uncertainty can be reduced through collecting more data. This is, however, not the case with variability, e.g., the variation of patient outcomes such as QoL. Variability has also been called first-order uncertainty while parameter uncertainty has also been defined as second-order uncertainty. In the sensitivity analysis, parameter and methodological uncertainty and sometimes also model uncertainty are explored but not variability. There are two main approaches for conducting a sensitivity analysis, as specified in Sections 15.2.8.1 and 15.2.8.2.

15.2.8.1 Deterministic Sensitivity Analysis

In deterministic sensitivity analysis alternative values for the point estimates of key parameters are explored and compared to those values used in the base case analysis.

- Univariate sensitivity analysis involves the variation of one input parameter at a time. This is a relatively simple but very important method to identify the most important model input parameters as well as the influence of the applied methodology. Typically, the results are presented as a tornado diagram, showing the most sensitive parameters at the top and the least at the bottom.
- Multivariate sensitivity analysis involves the variation of several parameter at a time, e.g., all parameters are set to the advantage or to the disadvantage of the investigated technology leading to a best and worst case scenario, respectively.

15.2.8.2 Probabilistic Sensitivity Analysis (PSA)

Instead of using point estimates probability distributions can be assigned to the specified ranges for the key parameters, i.e., probabilities, costs and effects to represent uncertainty. Multiple samples are drawn at random from these distributions, e.g., by Monte Carlo simulation, to generate an empirical distribution of the CER. If probability distributions are used for all uncertain input parameters, the model is called a full probabilistic model.

Typically, the results are presented as a scatter plot on the cost-effectiveness plane where each point presents one simulation. Subsequently, the results can be summarized in a cost-effectiveness acceptability curve (CEAC) where the horizontal axis represents the maximum willingness to pay and the vertical axis the probability that the technology is cost-effective (Fig. 15.3). The CEAC is derived from the joint uncertainty of incremental costs and effects of the investigated technology. It shows the probability that an intervention is more cost-effective than its comparator. Thus, the CEAC can provide a decision maker with the probability that, if the intervention is funded or reimbursed, this will be the correct decision. Moreover, the curve contains additional information: The 50% probability point on the CEAC corresponds to the median CER. Note that this median will only correspond to the mean-based CER when the CER is distributed symmetrically. The CEAC cuts the vertical axis at the probability that the investigated intervention is cost saving. When the curve is monotonically increasing, the (1–2*X*)% cost-effectiveness confidence interval can be obtained by cutting *X*% from either end of the vertical axis and using the curve to map these values on the horizontal axis. Using this approach, the 95% confidence interval in Fig. 15.3 can be determined as € 10,000–50,000 per QALY.

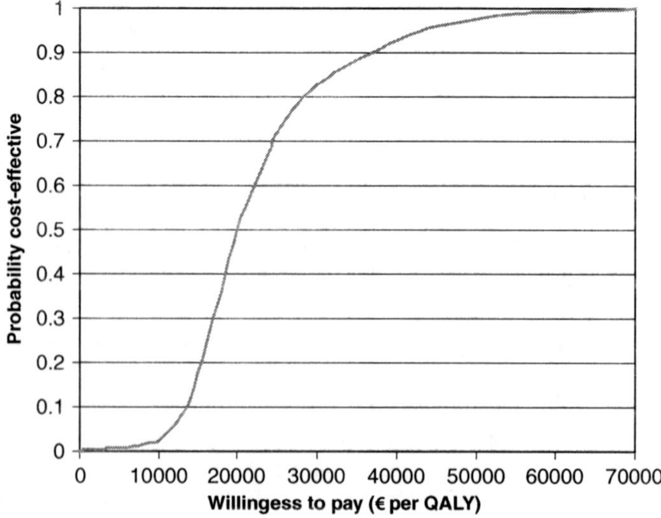

Fig. 15.3 Example of a cost-effectiveness acceptability curve

The CEAC in Fig. 15.3 represents only one of many shapes the CEAC can take; i.e., a monotonically increasing form is not the only possibility (Fenwick 2004).

While the PSA is the state of the art method for assessing overall parameter uncertainty, it is not suitable for assessing model or methodological uncertainty and hence its confidence interval omits the latter two uncertainties.

To account for methodological uncertainty the univariate sensitivity analysis is still the method of choice. Often, a combination of the PSA and univariate sensitivity analysis is applied: Running a PSA one time with the baseline estimates and subsequently with upper and lower values. For example, in the baseline PSA, a 3% discount rate might be applied and then a discount rate of 0 or 5% is used. In order to check model uncertainty, different models or parts of models need to be compared, as has been recently done for HPV vaccination (Chesson et al. 2008).

The evaluation of prevention measures against infectious diseases has to cope with two additional uncertainties: Fluctuating incidences (e.g., meningococcal or pneumococcal disease) and the disease transmission dynamics. Both represent very sensitive parameters for CEA and especially the latter is tricky to include in a PSA, given the already time- and computing consuming character of analyzing dynamic disease transmission models. PSA itself further adds to the huge time and computing requirements for such models. Furthermore the (appropriate) consideration of indirect protection effects, the perspective, the approach for productivity cost measurement, and the applied discount rate, i.e., the model and methodological assumptions, often have a great impact on the cost-effectiveness. For instance, a recent case study with varicella vaccination showed that a combination of model choice (in- or exclusion of zoster) and perspective (health-care payer or societal) can lead to the exact opposite conclusions: Either vaccination is almost certain to dominate the current strategy of no vaccination and vice versa (Brisson and Edmunds 2006). For vaccination programs where benefits occur in the medium-to-long term, e.g., hepatitis B and cervical cancer, the discount rate is typically one of the most sensitive model parameters.

15.2.9 Transferability

Not every country can perform an economic evaluation for each technology due to resource restrictions. Therefore, the assessment of the transferability of CEA results from one country to another country is often requested by decision makers. Currently, there are checklists (Boulenger et al. 2005; Welte et al. 2004a) and also a decision chart (Welte et al. 2004a) available for this assessment. The transfer of study results between countries is difficult but it is even more difficult to transfer prevention measures against infectious diseases due to possible differences in disease transmission. Nevertheless, transferring the health economic model or at least parts of it has been shown to be very efficient and helpful (Welte et al. 2004a). Making a model available via the Internet seems to be a promising way to help decision makers and researchers to adjust a model. Examples are the cost-effectiveness models used for the report "Vaccines for the 21st century" by the

Institute of Medicine (Institute of Medicine 2000), "Socrates (Screening Optimally for Chlamydia: Resource Allocation, Testing and Evaluation Software)," "Fluaid," "Flusurge" and "Fluworkloss" by the Centers for Disease Control and Prevention (CDC), "Quickflu" by the University of Tübingen or the pneumococcal conjugate vaccine cost-effectiveness model by the University of Groningen (Hubben et al. 2007).

15.3 Modeling

Models are an important tool for the economic evaluation of infectious diseases. The intervention's influence on the force of infection and the indirect protection effects can only be simulated using models (Ferguson et al. 2003). Furthermore, modeling is also required to combine the data and results from different sources and to predict the impact of different intervention strategies. Models are also necessary to extrapolate from short-term results to the long-term and to determine the effectiveness in the real world. Often they are used to estimate the uncertainty of the results and sometimes to transfer the results to other settings (Welte 2007). Finally, it has also been shown that highly flexible models are needed to support decision makers when deciding about a new vaccination program (Welte et al. 2005b).

15.3.1 Common Models for Economic Evaluation

In economic evaluations, most often decision tree or Markov models are applied. If diseases include different disease states and movements between them, Markov models are suitable, otherwise decision trees can be applied.

In a decision tree, the strategies to be compared are represented by the primary branches rising from the initial decision node. Each strategy branch has a series of probability nodes that reflect uncertain events. Payoffs such as costs, utilities, life years, QALYs are entered at terminal nodes. The decision tree is averaged out and rolled back to derive the expected value for each strategy. The expected value equals the sum of products of the path probabilities multiplied by the payoffs. Figure 15.4 shows a simple decision tree: Against a specific disease a healthy individual can either be vaccinated or not. Without the vaccination, he has a risk of 20% of falling sick. Vaccination halves this risk to 10%. The probability of staying healthy equals 1 minus the probability of falling sick. The vaccination costs € 200 while the treatment of the disease costs € 10,000. The expected costs of the vaccination strategy are € $200 \times 0.9 +$ € $10{,}200 \times 0.1 =$ € 1200. Similarly, the expected costs of the no vaccination strategy are € $0 \times 0.8 +$ € $10{,}000 \times 0.2 =$ € 2000. Thus, the expected costs of the vaccination strategy are € 800 less than the one of the no vaccination strategy.

The Markov model is the model of choice for representing random processes that evolve over time and is suited for calculating long-term outcomes. It is especially useful for modeling chronic diseases such as Hepatitis B or HIV. It leads to a simplification of "bushy" decision trees. For creation of a Markov model, the disease states

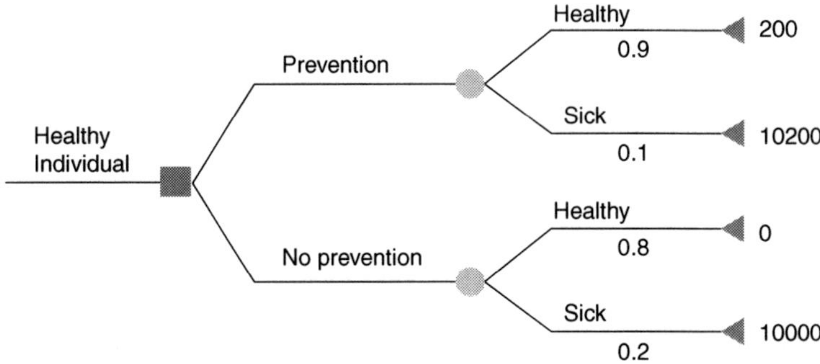

Fig. 15.4 Example of a decision tree

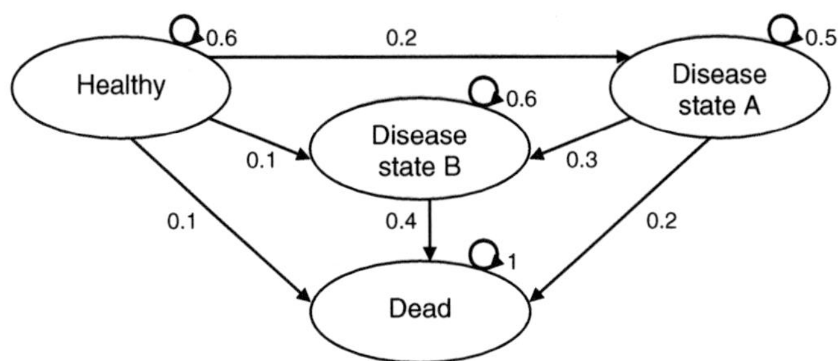

Fig. 15.5 Example of a Markov model

Table 15.3 Matrix of the transition probabilities per cycle

Health state	Healthy	Disease state A	Disease state B	Dead	Total
Healthy	0.6	0.2	0.1	0.1	1
Disease state A	0	0.5	0.3	0.2	1
Disease state B	0	0	0.6	0.4	1
Dead	0	0	0	1	1

are divided into distinct health states and absorbing states (e.g., death). Transition probabilities are assigned for movement between states over a discrete time period (=Markov cycle). Payoffs are attached to the states and transitions in the model and the model is run over a large number of cycles to obtain the long-term costs and effects. A simple Markov model is shown in Fig. 15.5, representing four health states – Healthy, Disease state A, Disease state B, and Dead. The arrows present the different possible pathways while the numbers show the assigned transition probabilities. For example, a healthy person can either stay healthy (probability = 0.6), move to Disease state A (0.2) or B (0.1), or can die (0.1). A person in Disease state A can either stay there or move on to Disease state B or die. A person in Disease state B can either stay there or die. The respective probabilities are also given in Table 15.3.

They are not depending on the states a patient might have experienced before entering this health state. Thus, a Markov model is without memory which has also been described as the Markovian assumption. However, by adding more health states or by using multidimensional transition probability matrices "memory" can be added (Briggs et al. 2007).

Decision trees and Markov models are the two basic models commonly used in the economic evaluation of all types of health-care technologies. Typically, they are analyzed as cohort models. However, there are also other models that can be applied, such as mathematical models using sets of differential equations or discrete-event simulation models. In fact, a whole taxonomy of model structures has been developed for health economic modeling which takes into account the level of aggregation by which the disease problem is analyzed (from individual to cohort level) and the degree of interaction that is being considered between individuals in a model (Brennan et al. 2006). In the case of infectious diseases, models are in addition differentiated by the way how they consider indirect protection effects.

Over the last years, the use of modeling in the economic evaluation of medical technologies has significantly benefited from discussion on a standardized, transparent documentation and motivation of the approaches used, the data used for model parameters, and the consistency checks to be conducted for improved model validity (Philips et al. 2006).

15.3.2 Approaches to Consider Indirect Protection Effects

For modeling health economics in infectious disease prevention, it is important to note whether indirect protection effects are included in the model or not. In particular, two types of models can be distinguished that differ with respect to considering the force of infection:

15.3.2.1 Static Models

Static models assume a constant force of infection. To include indirect protection effects, the increased effectiveness of the treatment is superimposed upon the core model. For example, if one knows from epidemiological studies that a herd immunity effect of 50% was observed in a specific age group then this percentage is directly put into the model. Thus, one can use this model nicely to simulate the cost-effectiveness of prevention programs in the past. However, they are less suitable for assessing the cost-effectiveness of current or future interventions due to the following reasons:

(a) They can only be used for an initial approximation of the expected herd immunity effects, e.g., based on observations for similar infections and types of vaccines.
(b) They are not able to simulate the potential absolute age shift caused by the indirect protection effects of mass infant vaccination programs.

(c) They are not an appropriate tool for CEAs of prevention measures that influence the force of infection but do not lead to a smaller number of susceptible individuals (i.e., successfully treated persons can be reinfected). In these cases, the transmission dynamics are far too complex to approximate them with a static model as has been demonstrated for chlamydial screening (Welte et al. 2005a). Whether net costs or net savings were simulated when including older women into the screening program depended, respectively, on whether only a portion (static model) or all indirect protection effects (dynamic model) were included into the analysis (Table 15.2). Hence, by taking into account the full indirect protection effect the authors identified a different optimal screening strategy, which rendered more savings and more health effects. Similarly, only by using a dynamic model the ICER of repeated chlamydial screening at various time intervals can be assessed (de Vries et al. 2008).

15.3.2.2 Dynamic Models

Dynamic models simulate the changes in the force of infection, i.e., they model the dynamic transmission of the infectious pathogen in the population. As a result, they are population and not cohort models. Often, a Markov model or decision tree is used for the progression of disease and is subsequently being coupled with a transmission model.

There are different types of dynamic models, based on their level of complexity included. They span from rather simple SIR or SIS models to highly sophisticated and complex individual-based models. The choice of model strongly depends on the type of disease, population, and intervention (Ferguson et al. 2003).

All dynamic models share one major challenge. Unlike static models they require detailed information about transmission routes and infectiveness, are more complex, and more difficult to understand. Thus, they take much more time and resources to build. Furthermore, because of the added information needs, there is more uncertainty surrounding the results. However, as stated above, for many situations they represent the only way to obtain meaningful results.

15.4 Supporting Decision Making

In the field of infectious diseases the cost-effectiveness of prevention measures has been investigated since several years. A special focus has been the evaluation of large-scale measures such as vaccination and screening programs due to their typical substantial budget impact. The cost-effectiveness of vaccination programs has even been systematically investigated in some countries such as the Netherlands (Van der Zeijst et al. 2000) and the USA (Institute of Medicine 2000). Currently, economic evaluations are done on a regular basis for new vaccines in several countries as they are requested by the national authorities to support decision making.

Economic evaluations can have a major impact on decision making in infectious disease prevention as has been demonstrated for meningococcal C conjugate vaccination: A study investigated the role economic evaluation played in the decision process to introduce this vaccine into either the routine childhood vaccination schedule, as a mass vaccination "catch-up" campaign, or not at all for 21 developed countries. Economic evaluations for meningococcal C conjugate vaccination were identified for Australia, Canada (Quebec), The Netherlands, Portugal, Switzerland, and the UK. In all except the UK the economic evaluation had an important role in the decision-making process, especially with respect to the vaccination strategy (Welte et al. 2005b).

A further example is the assessment of the pneumococcal conjugate vaccine in the Netherlands: At the time of its initial cost-effectiveness analysis there was not enough evidence to simulate any indirect protection effects and hence they were not included. The results rendered an unfavorable CER which was one of the major reasons why it was not included in the routine vaccination schedule in 2002 (Bos et al. 2003). However, the vaccine showed surprisingly strong indirect protection effects in countries where the vaccine was included in the routine vaccination program, such as the USA. Based on these new findings, the CEA was repeated, this time including indirect protection effects. The results showed that the program would be cost-effective and this analysis supported the subsequent decision to introduce the vaccine in the Dutch routine childhood vaccination program in 2006 (Hubben et al. 2007).

Which cost-effectiveness threshold should be applied, e.g., until which CER should a technology be considered cost-effective? This is one of the questions regularly raised by decision makers (Welte et al. 2005b). Table 15.4 gives an overview of different values often used or cited.

Most thresholds lack a theoretical foundation. The most frequently used threshold by health economists seems to be US $ 50.000 per QALY or LYG, which has been often applied after 1996 (Grosse 2008). The WHO advice is unique by recommending thresholds that are depending on the economic power of countries. The gross domestic product (GDP) per capita is suggested as reference point. For the Netherlands and the UK, there are different thresholds published.

It should be noted that cost-effectiveness is never the only reason for implementing a new technology or not. For instance, the medical need, public anxiety, the availability of other treatment options, the budget impact, and budget constraints are all typical factors that are also often taken into consideration.

15.5 Conclusions

The economic evaluation of prevention measures against infectious diseases is typically more complex and difficult than for other technologies. Especially the simulation of disease transmission represents a major challenge for each new pathogen. Neglecting the externalities and hence the indirect protection effects of prevention measures can lead to wrong results and conclusions. The additional parameters needed for the disease transmission also contribute an additional complexity in the sensitivity analysis. Furthermore, as prevention programs typically require initial investments but will render health effects and resource savings in the future, the

Table 15.4 International thresholds for cost-effectiveness

Organization/group	Cost-effectiveness thresholds	Reference
Australia*	Costs per LYG < AU $ 42,000 – 76,000 (costs per LYG < AU $ 42,000: reimbursement likely, costs per LYG > AU $ 76,000 reimbursement unlikely)	George et al. (2001)
The Netherlands	Costs < € 20.000 per QALY or LYG: cost-effective* Costs < € 80.000 per QALY: cost-effective**	Welte et al. (2004c); Raad voor de Volksgezondheid & Zorg (2007)
UK National Institute of Clinical Evidence (NICE)*	Costs per QALY < £ 20,000–30,000: cost-effective Costs per QALY < £ 45,000: cost-effective	Devlin and Parkin (2004); Appleby and Devlin, Parkin (2007)
US Institute of Medicine (IOM)**	Saves money and QALYs: most favorable Costs per QALY < US $ 10,000: more favorable Costs per QALY > US $ 10,000 and < 100.000: favorable Costs per QALY > US $ 100,000: less favorable	Institute of Medicine (2000)
World Health Organization (WHO)**	Costs per DALY < GDP per capita: highly cost-effective Costs per DALY = 1x – 3x GDP per capita: cost-effective Costs per DALY > 3x GDP per capita: not cost-effective	WHO (2008)
International and especially US decision analysts**	Costs per QALY or LYG < US $ 50.000: cost-effective	Grosse (2008)
US and British health economists**	Costs per LYG < US $ 60.000: cost-effective	Newhouse (1998)

* Thresholds derived from past decisions
** Officially stated thresholds
LYG = Life year gained
QALY = Quality-adjusted life year
GDP = Gross domestic product

choice of the discount rate for costs and effects as well as the time horizon are of high importance. Finally, the approach for measuring the productivity costs has often a strong impact on the results.

15.6 Looking to the Future

Due to the better understanding of disease transmissions and the availability of epidemiological models and sophisticated software, dynamic models are likely to become the standard in the economic evaluation of infectious diseases. The QoL measurement in children will progress further and so will the transferability of models. Finally, more countries are likely to use the tool "economic evaluation" for supporting decision making. Improved standardization and transparency in the modeling approaches may support the future assessment and appraisal of the economic evidence on intervention into infectious disease. In result, the effectiveness and cost-effectiveness of health care in this field may be further promoted.

References

Appleby J, Devlin N, Parkin D (2007) NICE's cost effectiveness threshold. BMJ 335:358–359

Armstrong GL, Billah K, Rein DB et al. (2007) The economics of routine childhood Hepatitis A immunization in the United States: the impact of herd immunity. Pediatrics 119:e22–e29

Berger ML, Bingefors K, Hedblom E, Pashos CL, Torrance G (2003) Health care cost, quality, and outcomes: ISPOR book of terms. ISPOR, Lawrenceville, NJ

Beutels P, Edmunds WJ, Antonanzas F et al. (2002) Economic evaluation of vaccination programmes: a consensus statement focusing on viral hepatitis. Pharmacoeconomics 20:1–7

Bos JM, Postma MJ, Annemans L (2005) Discounting health effects in pharmacoeconomic evaluations: current controversies. Pharmacoeconomics 23:639–649

Bos JM, Rumke H, Welte R et al. (2003) Epidemiologic impact and cost-effectiveness of universal infant vaccination with a 7-valent conjugated pneumococcal vaccine in the Netherlands. Clin Ther 25:2614–30

Boulenger S, Nixon J, Drummond M et al. (2005) Can economic evaluations be made more transferable? Eur J Health Econ 6:334–346

Brazier J, Ratcliffe J, Salomon JA, Tsuchiya A (2007) Measuring and valuing health benefits for economic evaluation. Oxford University Press, Oxford

Brazier J, Roberts J, Deverill M (2002) The estimation of a preference-based measure of health from the SF-36. J Health Econ 21:271–292

Brennan A, Chick SE, Davies R (2006) A taxonomy of model structures for economic evaluation of health technologies. Health Econ 15:1295–1310

Briggs A, Claxton K, Sculpher M (2007) Decision modelling for health economic evaluation. Oxford University Press, Oxford

Brisson M, Edmunds WJ (2002) The cost-effectiveness of varicella vaccination in Canada. Vaccine 20:1113–25

Brisson M, Edmunds WJ (2003) Varicella vaccination in England and Wales: cost-utility analysis. Arch Dis Child 88:862–9

Brisson M, Edmunds WJ (2006) Impact of model, methodological, and parameter uncertainty in the economic analysis of vaccination programs. Med Decis Making 26:434–446

Brouwer WB, Niessen LW, Postma MJ et al. (2005) Need for differential discounting of costs and health effects in cost effectiveness analyses. BMJ 331:446–448

Cairns J (2001) Discounting in economic evaluation. In: Drummond M, McGuire A (eds): Economic evaluation in health care. Merging theory with practice. Oxford University Press, New York

Caro JJ, Getsios D, El-Hadi W et al. (2005) Pertussis immunization of adolescents in the United States: an economic evaluation. Pediatr Infect Dis J 24:S75–S82

Chesson HW, Ekwueme DU, Saraiya M et al. (2008) Cost-effectiveness of human papillomavirus vaccination in the United States. Emerg Infect Dis 14:244–251

Claes C, Reinert RR, von der Schulenburg JM (2009) Cost effectiveness analysis of heptavalent pneumococcal conjugate vaccine in Germany considering herd immunity effects. Eur J Health Econ 10:25–38

Claxton K, Sculpher M, Culyer A et al. (2006) Discounting and cost-effectiveness in NICE – stepping back to sort out a confusion. Health Econ 15:1–4

Devlin N, Parkin D (2004) Does NICE have a cost-effectiveness threshold and what other factors influence its decisions? A binary choice analysis. Health Econ 13:437–452

de Vries R, van Bergen JE, de Jong-van den Berg LT et al. (2008) Cost-utility of repeated screening for *Chlamydia trachomatis*. Value Health 11:272–274

De Wals P, De Serres G, Niyonsenga T (2001) Effectiveness of a mass immunization campaign against serogroup C meningococcal disease in Quebec. JAMA 285:177–81

Drummond M, Chevat C, Lothgren M (2007) Do we fully understand the economic value of vaccines? Vaccine 25:5945–5957

Drummond M, Sculpher MJ, Torrance GW, O'Brien BJ, Stoddart GL (2005) Methods for the economic evaluation of health care programmes, 3rd edn, revised. Oxford University Press, Oxford

Edmunds WJ, Medley GF, Nokes DJ (1999) Evaluating the cost-effectiveness of vaccination programmes: a dynamic perspective. Stat Med 18:3263–3282

Fenwick E, O'Brien BJ, Briggs A (2004) Cost-effectiveness acceptability curves–facts, fallacies and frequently asked questions. Health Econ 13:405–415

Ferguson NM, Keeling MJ, Edmunds WJ et al. (2003) Planning for smallpox outbreaks. Nature 425:681–685

Fine PE (1993) Herd immunity: history, theory, practice. Epidemiol Rev 15:265–302

George B, Harris A, Mitchell A (2001) Cost-effectiveness analysis and the consistency of decision making: evidence from pharmaceutical reimbursement in Australia (1991 to 1996). Pharmacoeconomics 19:1103–1109

Gold MR, Siegel JE, Russel LB, Weinstein MC (1996) Cost-effectiveness in health and medicine. Oxford University Press, Oxford

Goldman GS (2005) Cost-benefit analysis of universal varicella vaccination in the U.S. taking into account the closely related herpes-zoster epidemiology. Vaccine 23:3349–3355

Gravelle H, Brouwer W, Niessen L et al. (2007) Discounting in economic evaluations: stepping forward towards optimal decision rules. Health Econ 16:307–317

Greiner W, Weijnen T, Nieuwenhuizen M et al. (2003) A single European currency for EQ-5D health states. Results from a six-country study. Eur J Health Econ 4:222–231

Grosse SD (2008) Assessing cost-effectiveness in healthcare: history of the $50,000 per QALY threshold. Expert Rev Pharmacoeconomics Outcomes Res 8:165–178

Heininger U, Seward JF (2006) Varicella. Lancet 368:1365–1376

Herrero R (2009) Human papillomavirus (HPV) vaccines: limited cross-protection against additional HPV types. J Infect Dis 199:919–922

Hubben GA, Bos JM, Glynn DM et al. (2007) Enhanced decision support for policy makers using a web interface to health-economic models–illustrated with a cost-effectiveness analysis of nation-wide infant vaccination with the 7-valent pneumococcal conjugate vaccine in the Netherlands. Vaccine 25:3669–3678

Immergluck LC, Cull WL, Schwartz A et al. (2000) Cost-effectiveness of universal compared with voluntary screening for human immunodeficiency virus among pregnant women in Chicago. Pediatrics 105:E54

Institute of Medicine. Committee to study priorities for vaccine development (2000) Vaccines for the 21st century: a tool for decisionmaking. National Academy Press, Washigton, DC

Jit M, Edmunds WJ (2007) Evaluating rotavirus vaccination in England and Wales. Part II. The potential cost-effectiveness of vaccination. Vaccine 25:3971–3979

Koopmanschap MA, Rutten FF, Van Ineveld BM et al. (1995) The friction cost method for measuring indirect costs of disease. J Health Econ 14:171–89

Koopmanschap MA, Rutten FF (1996) A practical guide for calculating indirect costs of disease. Pharmacoeconomics 10:460–466

Lloyd A, Patel N, Scott DA et al. (2008) Cost-effectiveness of heptavalent conjugate pneumococcal vaccine (Prevenar) in Germany: considering a high-risk population and herd immunity effects. Eur J Health Econ 9:7–15

Maartens G, Wilkinson RJ (2007) Tuberculosis. Lancet 370:2030–2043

MacKeigan LD, Gafni A, O'Brien BJ (2003) Double discounting of QALYs. Health Econ 12: 165–169

McIntosh ED, Conway P, Willingham J et al. (2005) Pneumococcal pneumonia in the UK – how herd immunity affects the cost-effectiveness of 7-valent pneumococcal conjugate vaccine (PCV). Vaccine 23:1739–1745

Newhouse JP (1998) US and UK health economics: two disciplines separated by a common language? Health Econ 7 Suppl 1:S79–S92

Panagiotopoulos T, Antoniadou I, Valassi-Adam E (1999) Increase in congenital rubella occurrence after immunisation in Greece: retrospective survey and systematic review. BMJ 319:1462–1467

Philips Z, Bojke L, Sculpher M et al. (2006) Good practice guidelines for decision-analytic modelling in health technology assessment: a review and consolidation of quality assessment. Pharmacoeconomics 24:355–371

Postma MJ, de Vries R, Welte R et al. (2008) Health economic methodology illustrated with recent work on Chlamydia screening: the concept of extended dominance. Sex Transm Infect 84: 152–154

Postma MJ, Jansema P, Scheijbeler HW et al. (2005) Scenarios on costs and savings of influenza treatment and prevention for Dutch healthy working adults. Vaccine 23:5365–5371

Pradas-Velasco R, Antonanzas-Villar F, Martinez-Zarate MP (2008) Dynamic modelling of infectious diseases: an application to the economic evaluation of influenza vaccination. Pharmacoeconomics 26:45–56

Raad voor de Volksgezondheid & Zorg (2007) Rechtvaardige en duurzame zorg. Raad voor de Volksgezondheid & Zorg, Den Haag

Ramsay ME, Andrews NJ, Trotter CL et al. (2003) Herd immunity from meningococcal serogroup C conjugate vaccination in England: database analysis. BMJ 326:365–6

Ravens-Sieberer U, Erhart M, Wille N et al. (2006) Generic health-related quality-of-life assessment in children and adolescents: methodological considerations. Pharmacoeconomics 24:1199–1220

Ray GT, Whitney CG, Fireman BH et al. (2006) Cost-effectiveness of pneumococcal conjugate vaccine: evidence from the first 5 years of use in the United States incorporating herd effects. Pediatr Infect Dis J 25:494–501

Robberstad B (2005) QALYs vs DALYs vs LYs gained: What are the differences, and what difference do they make for health care priority setting? Norsk Epidemiologi 15:183–191

Singleton RJ, Hennessy TW, Bulkow LR et al. (2007) Invasive pneumococcal disease caused by nonvaccine serotypes among alaska native children with high levels of 7-valent pneumococcal conjugate vaccine coverage. JAMA 297:1784–1792

Szende A, Oppe M, Devlin N (2006) EQ-5D value sets: inventory, comparative review and user guide. Springer, Dordrecht

Thomas SL, Wheeler JG, Hall AJ (2002) Contacts with varicella or with children and protection against herpes zoster in adults: a case-control study. Lancet 360:678–82

Trotter CL, Gay NJ, Edmunds WJ (2005) Dynamic models of meningococcal carriage, disease, and the impact of serogroup C conjugate vaccination. Am J Epidemiol 162:89–100

Trotter CL, Edmunds WJ (2006) Reassessing the cost-effectiveness of meningococcal serogroup C conjugate (MCC) vaccines using a transmission dynamic model. Med Decis Making 26:38–47

Van der Zeijst BAM, Dijkman MI, Kramers PGN, Luytjes W, Rumke HC, Welte R (2000) Naar een vaccinatieprogramma voor Nederland in de 21ste eeuw. RIVM report 000 001 001. National Institute for Public Health and the Environment, Bilthoven

Welte R (2007) Methodological advances in the economic evaluation of infectious disease prevention. Peter Lang, Frankfurt am Main

Welte R, Feenstra T, Jager H et al. (2004a) A decision chart for assessing and improving the transferability of economic evaluation results between countries. Pharmacoeconomics 22: 857–876

Welte R, König HH, Jager JC, Leidl R (2004b) Assessment of the indirect costs of injecting drug use: which methods should be employed? In: Jager J, Limburg W, Kretzschmar M, Postma

M, Wiessing L (eds): Hepatitis C and injecting drug use: impact, costs and policy options. European Monitoring Centre for Drugs and Drug Addiction (EMCDDA) Scientific Monograph, Lisbon

Welte R, van den Dobbelsteen G, Bos JM et al. (2004c) Economic evaluation of meningococcal serogroup C conjugate vaccination programmes in The Netherlands and its impact on decision-making. Vaccine 23:470–479

Welte R, Kretzschmar M, Leidl R et al. (2000) Cost-effectiveness of screening programs for *Chlamydia trachomatis*: a population-based dynamic approach. Sex Transm Dis 27:518–529

Welte R, Postma M, Leidl R et al. (2005a) Costs and effects of chlamydial screening: dynamic versus static modeling. Sex Transm Dis 32:474–483.

Welte R, Trotter CL, Edmunds WJ et al. (2005b) The role of economic evaluation in vaccine decision making: focus on meningococcal group C conjugate vaccine. Pharmacoeconomics 23:855–874.

World Health Organization (2003) WHO guide to cost-effectiveness analysis. World Health Organization, Geneva

World Health Organization (2008) Choosing Interventions that are Cost Effective (WHO Choice). http://www.who.int/choice/costs/CER_thresholds/en/index.html (2008). Accessed 10 March 2008

Part III
Epidemiology of Particular Infectious Diseases

Chapter 16
Airborne Transmission: Influenza and Tuberculosis

Timo Ulrichs

16.1 Influenza

Seasonal influenza occurs in waves and can vary in strength. It affects all age groups, but mainly little children and the elderly. In Germany, about 10,000 people die each year from seasonal influenza, mostly elderly people. The death rate is associated with the influenza strain: H3N2 subtype causes a higher death toll than H1N1. Children play an important role in spread and transmission dynamics during an influenza wave (winter holidays may delay the peak of an influenza wave).

Avian influenza virus subtypes reside in their reservoir of wild birds; some of them may also replicate in pigs and horses. The subtypes H5 and H7 can develop into highly pathogenic avian influenza viruses (HPAIV) by insertional mutations, causing avian influenza epidemics among poultry. In the last few years, some outbreaks of H5N1 in poultry in Europe have been described.

As a zoonotic disease, avian influenza can also affect humans. Since 1997, direct transmissions of HPAIV from poultry to humans have been described. Since December 2003, H5N1 epidemics dramatically spread in Asia; human cases mainly occurred in countries with severe avian influenza among poultry and with close contacts between animals and the human population. A first wave (2003–2005) mainly affected Viet Nam, Thailand and Cambodia, whereas from 2005 the focus moved to Indonesia, China and newly affected countries like Turkey, Iraq, Djibouti, Azerbaidzhan and Egypt. In 2007, in addition Nigeria, Laos, Myanmar and finally Pakistan reported human cases. Among all cases confirmed by WHO, H5N1-affected humans mainly belonged to the age group of 10 to 29-year-olds. From 2003 to April 2009, WHO reported 421 human cases, of which 257 died. Among the dead, nearly 50% were reported in Indonesia (for a general overview see Chapter 3).

Novel influenza: As this book is in the finalization process, a new influenza virus evolved derived from avian, swine and human pathogenic viruses called novel virus

T. Ulrichs (✉)
Koch-Metschnikow-Forum, Luisenstr. 59, 10117 Berlin
e-mail: timo.ulrichs@bmg.bund.de

A. Krämer et al. (eds.), *Modern Infectious Disease Epidemiology*,
Statistics for Biology and Health, DOI 10.1007/978-0-387-93835-6_16,

(A/H1N1; so-called swine influenza). The first cases were reported in Mexico and Northern America. The virus rapidly spread to other countries, mainly in Europe.

For containment, surveillance and monitoring of this influenza disease, the instruments and measures described in the forthcoming chapters (especially Section 16.1.2) were activated.

16.1.1 Pandemic Influenza

The most important influenza pandemic occurred in 1918. The Spanish flu caused an estimated death toll of about 20–50 million people, dying from infection with the influenza virus subtype H1N1 – more than all deaths caused by the First World War, 1914–1918. The mortality rates of the Asian flu in 1957 and the Hong Kong flu 1968 (1 million deaths each) were less severe. All three influenza pandemics of the twentieth century consisted of at least two waves: a weaker one followed by a strong wave after 4–6 months, eventually followed by a third wave. It has been shown for the USA that children played a major role in the early spread of the waves (see also Chapter 6). In the UK, high rates of serological conversion were noticed during the three waves of the Spanish flu in 1918. This suggests that infection during a previous wave does not protect from reinfection in the following one. Morbidity rates were estimated with 5.9 and 4%, respectively. Mortality increased during the Spanish flu from 0.7% to 3.3 and 2.7%. Morbidity rates during the later pandemics in 1957 and 1968 were much higher (up to 30%).

In the Spanish flu, most of the victims were young; in the later pandemics of the twentieth century, more and more older people were affected, but young age groups were still at a higher risk. This could be explained by either an acquired long-term immunity (see Chapter 13) or by the hypothesis that the immune response in younger individuals is usually stronger and that collateral damage of a strong immune response causes disease and death, e.g. by destroying lung tissue.

Coping with the consequences of a pandemic may lead to a breakdown of the health-care system. Therefore it is crucial to estimate potential consequences of a new pandemic. Mathematical models estimate the potential effects of a new influenza pandemic. Modelling tries to predict effects of a new pandemic, but also of countermeasures (see below). The following applications of modelling may help pandemic preparedness planning:

- calculation of a potential curve of the pandemic wave(s);
- possibility of regional spread under certain conditions;
- epidemiological and economic effects of a pandemic;
- effects of pharmaceutical (drugs, vaccines) and non-pharmaceutical countermeasures (school closures, cancellation of mass events; potentially delaying effects by limitations to (air) travel);
- real-time modelling, simulating the time during a pandemic when more and more information about epidemiology and consequences become available.

16.1.2 Pandemic Preparedness Planning

WHO prepared a global influenza preparedness plan and also provided checklists for national pandemic preparedness plans. The following pandemic response strategies are essential and currently discussed in international councils and workshops:

- antiviral drug use strategies and prioritization;
- prepandemic vaccine strategy and prioritization;
- pandemic vaccine prioritization;
- community mitigation strategies;
- respiratory protection strategies (face masks);
- border measures;
- preparedness exercises.

Antiviral medication: Stockpiling antivirals as strategic first response makes sense because modelling has shown that consequent therapy of affected individuals results in effective containment of the virus spread. Many countries stockpiled antivirals, ranging from amounts for 3–17% of the population (Canada, Italy, Mexico) to 20–25% (Japan, UK, USA, Germany) and to 67% (France). Currently it is also considered to increase the stockpiles, not only for therapy but also for prophylaxis, i.e. use of antivirals in exposed individuals to prevent the disease.

Prepandemic vaccines: Vaccine candidates with new adjuvants may stimulate a better immune response because of a greater cross-immunogenicity against related influenza vaccines. The new adjuvants may allow the usage of less antigen for each vaccine dose. According to studies in the USA, stockpiling of prepandemic vaccines may be possible up to 30 months. Many countries consider prepandemic vaccine stockpiling for their medical personnel and first responders [i.e. health-care workers, police and fire departments, critical infrastructure (e.g. farmers)].

Pandemic influenza vaccine: Experience with prepandemic vaccine development provides the basis for the development of better pandemic vaccines, especially concerning their formulations, the processes of licensing and manufacturing experiences. However, a pandemic vaccine will not be produced in time during the first wave, but be available during the second in increasing portions. Therefore, strategies of prioritization are necessary. In Germany, the whole population will be vaccinated according to age groups, starting with the youngest.

Community mitigation strategies: Social distancing measures are the core strategy in this context. Also, closing schools, cancelling public gatherings and voluntary isolation of ill persons and quarantine of their families are currently discussed as countermeasures. For this, a good educational programme on social distancing in workplaces and the community is required.

Respiratory protection: Although there is a general agreement that influenza viruses are spread by respiratory secretions, there is only limited scientific evidence that face masks or respirators really contribute to protection during a pandemic.

Border measures: Countermeasures in the field of isolating the own country from potential outbreak sites worldwide range from closing borders completely to selected limitation of air travel (i.e. reducing the number of flights, screen travellers upon arrival, quarantine-exposed individuals). In addition, recommendations and warnings have been prepared for potential travel to affected countries.

Pandemic preparedness exercises: These are crucial to test preparedness and suitability of the national and international planning. Exercises include table-top exercises and command post exercises and have already been conducted in many countries. According to the pandemic influenza working group of the Global Health Security Action Group (members are Canada, European Commission, France, Germany, Italy, Japan, Mexico, UK, USA, WHO) the main lessons learned from these exercises are the following:

- rapidly define pandemic severity and risk groups;
- maintain and communicate situational awareness;
- define communication channels in advance;
- provide regular and credible updates;
- additional planning and exercises are needed.

For a general overview of public health measures, see also Chapter 4.

16.2 Tuberculosis

Tuberculosis has been one of the most threatening health problems since antiquity. It was formerly called "consumption" or "phthisis". In contrast to other dreadful diseases like cholera or plague, it is, on the person level, chronic, and on the population level, endemic. It is used to be put into the category of "social" diseases because social risk factors are particularly pronounced; for early and contemporary work in this domain, see Chapter 6.

Even in the twenty-first century, tuberculosis remains one of the three big killers worldwide – together with HIV/AIDS and malaria. Tuberculosis is still the bacterial disease caused by a single pathogen responsible for the highest number of deaths. It threatens the socio-economic basis of many high-burden countries. In sub-Saharan Africa, the tuberculosis problem is aggravated by HIV coinfection. In Central Asia and Eastern Europe, tuberculosis is becoming more and more difficult to treat because of the emergence of multidrug resistance. On 22 October 2007, a Ministerial Forum on Tuberculosis "All Against Tuberculosis" was organized by the WHO Euro Office and the German Federal Ministry of Health in Berlin. The delegates and ministers from the 53 countries of the WHO–Euro region (ranging from Portugal to Kamchatka, including Central Asia) adopted the so-called Berlin Declaration on Tuberculosis. This declaration identifies the most imminent problems of tuberculosis control in WHO–Euro and puts forward strategic solutions. Therefore, and because the regional problems stand pars pro toto for the global TB problem, the following description of the epidemiology of tuberculosis will focus on public health aspects of tuberculosis in the WHO–Euro region.

16.2.1 Current Situation

The 18 priority countries for TB control in the region are Armenia, Azerbaijan, Belarus, Estonia, Georgia, Kazakhstan, Kyrgyzstan, Latvia, Lithuania, the Republic of Moldova, the Russian Federation, Tajikistan, Turkmenistan, Ukraine and Uzbekistan in the Eastern part of the region, and Bulgaria, Romania and Turkey in Central Europe.

Tuberculosis control in the Russian Federation and in other successor states of the former Soviet Union faces several specific problems requiring adapted approaches in the fields of infection epidemiology and public health. Prevalence and incidence of tuberculosis strongly increased in the years after the disintegration of the former Soviet Union into the Russian Federation and the other successor states and has now stabilized at a high level. (Figures 16.1 and 16.3; according to WHO estimates, Russia is on position 11, according to estimated burden of disease 2007, see WHO TB Report 2009). The percentage of multidrug-resistant strains of *Mycobacterium tuberculosis* is increasing dramatically; the number of resistances per clinical isolate is also increasing. The tuberculosis control systems in these countries are still based on the old Soviet system. After introduction of the WHO-recommended tuberculosis control programme (DOTS, see below), several forms of tuberculosis control exist in parallel in their public health systems. Thus, the quality of epidemiological

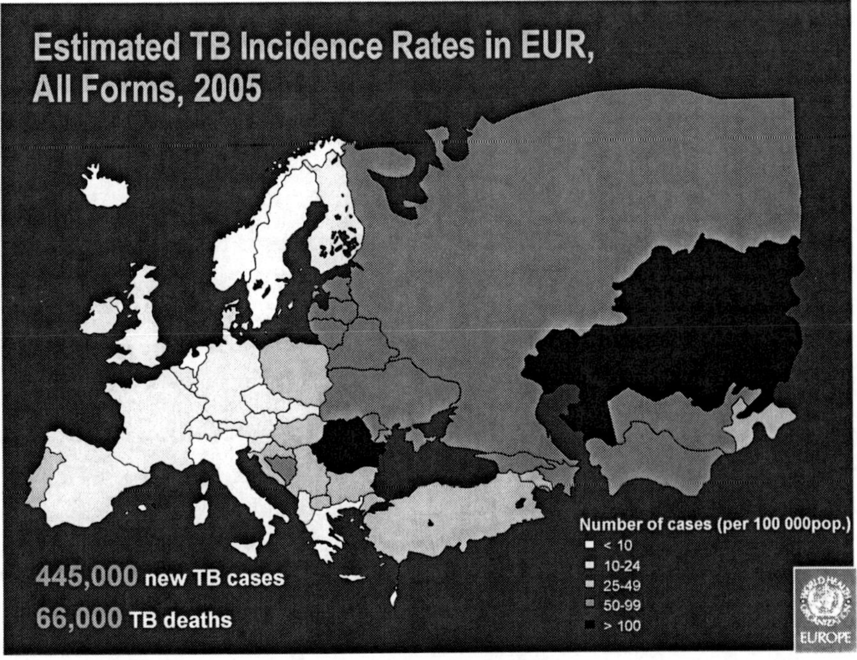

Fig. 16.1 Estimated TB-incidence rates in the WHO Euro region (EUR) (kindly provided by WHO Euro)

data concerning prevalence and incidence of tuberculosis and concerning microbiological data and public health issues are insecure and heterogeneous (for more information about surveillance systems see Chapter 8).

16.2.2 Increase in Tuberculosis Case Numbers

Tuberculosis in Russia and in the successor states of the former Soviet Union is becoming more and more a serious public health problem, not only affecting the health of individuals, but also endangering the stability of whole countries regarding economic and political issues.

At the end of the 1990 s, a dramatic increase in tuberculosis cases in the Russian Federation was noticed: an increase in new cases by 7.5% and in the death rate by 11% in the time between 1991 and 1998 (in 1999, Russia reported 124,000 new cases and 30,000 TB deaths; WHO TB Report 2000). In 1991, 34 existing cases per 100,000 inhabitants were reported, in 1994 already 48 and in 1998 76. Currently, the TB case numbers have stabilized on a high level: According to WHO annual report 2006, the prevalence in all of Russia was 160/100,000 inhabitants; the incidence was estimated with 110/100,000 inhabitants (WHO TB Report 2009, Fig. 16.1). There are strong differences between the regions in the Western and Eastern (Siberian) parts of Russia and Central Asia: Eastern parts of Russia and Central Asia suffer from high incidence rates whereas the European part of Russia reports decreasing numbers (Fig. 16.2).

For this dramatic re-emergence of tuberculosis, several reasons are currently being discussed (see also Chapter 3):

1. One consequence of the fall of the Soviet Union was the breakdown of the system of drug supply and health-care coverage. The coverage with antituberculotic drugs was insufficient, resulting in inadequate treatment of tuberculosis patients. Funding of the national tuberculosis control programme was subsequently reduced in the years after 1991. Consequences were a decrease in quality of diagnostics and in clinical care of tuberculosis patients.
2. The second reason for the increase in tuberculosis case numbers could be found in a decrease of the socio-economic level in Russia in the 1990s. Transmission and susceptibility of tuberculosis increased, facilitated by a high turnover of working places and by a high unemployment rate, increasing social insecurity and decreasing social coherence. In addition, a dramatic decrease in life expectancy in Russia and an increasing problem of alcoholism and malnutrition starting from the middle of the 1980s accompanied the problem of tuberculosis. This crisis in the middle of the 1990s still has effects on TB prevalences at present.
3. Finally, since 1991 an increased turnover in Russian prisons could have contributed to a faster spread of *M. tuberculosis* within the civil society than during Soviet times. In addition, there was a particular increase in multidrug-resistant

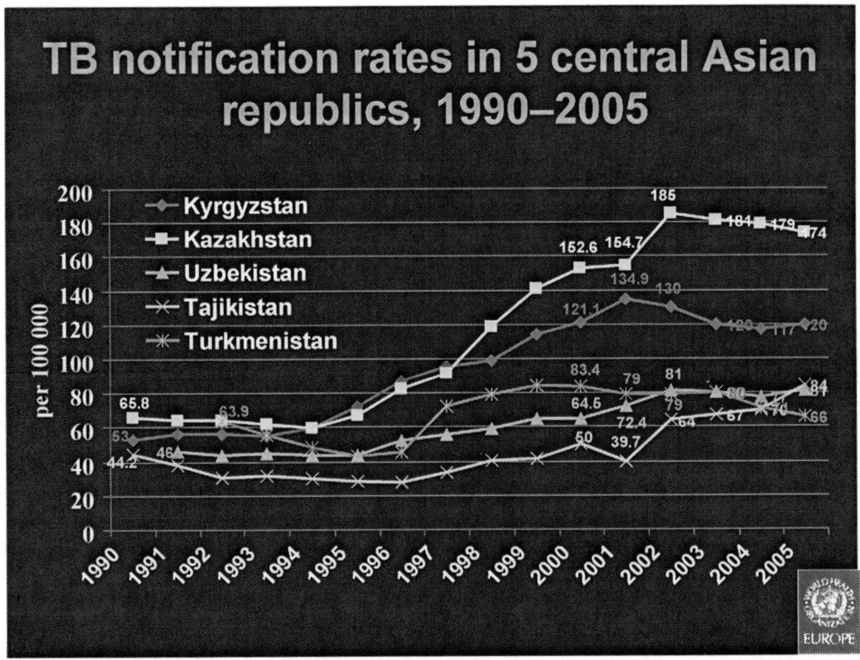

Fig. 16.2 TB notification rates in the five central Asian Republics, 1990–2005 (kindly provided by WHO Euro)

strains of *M. tuberculosis* among prison inmates due to inadequate therapy schemes. Problematic hygienic conditions and overcrowded prisons contribute to a rapid spread of the pathogen among prison inmates. Prisoners with high and those with low sentences are often put together, aggravating the secondary spread among the civil population.

16.2.3 Increase of the Rate of Multidrug-Resistant Strains of M. tuberculosis

The global incidence of multidrug-resistant (MDR) tuberculosis cases was approximately 500,000 cases in 2007, equalling 5.4% of all new cases worldwide. There are 27 countries worldwide (among them 15 in the WHO Euro region) accounting for 85% of all such cases. In WHO–Euro region, Eastern Europe (especially Russia and the successor states of the former Soviet Union) has approximately 10–15% of MDR cases, other regions in WHO–Europe report between 1 and 4%. Even the MDR rate among previously treated tuberculosis patients is highest in Eastern Europe (WHO TB Report 2009); the other regions have rates between 6 and 29%.

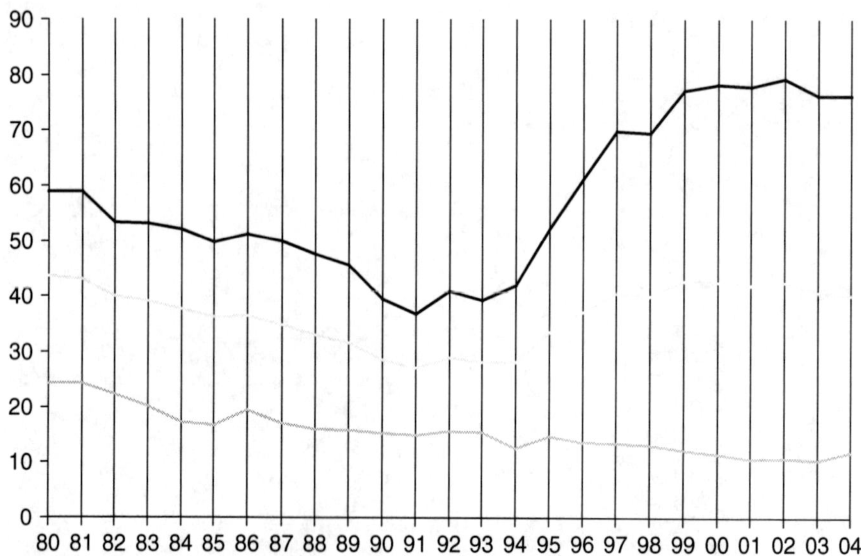

Fig. 16.3 TB notification rate in the WHO Euro region (annual TB cases per 100,000 population; *lower curve*: EU countries [EU of 25]; Eastern European countries; *upper curve*: all 53 member states of the WHO Euro region)

Per definitionem, a multidrug-resistant strain contains at least resistances against two first-line drugs, namely rifampin and isoniazide. Most of the clinical isolates in Eastern Europe contain much more. Some fulfil the criteria of an extensively multidrug-resistant strain (XDR). In the Russian Federation, MDR rates differ massively between the different regions. Available data are inadequate for a comprehensive epidemiological study. The virulent strain *M. tuberculosis* Beijing is very frequently found among MDR strains. Its rapid spread from Southeast Asia via Russia to Eastern Europe is accompanied by an increase in MDR rates in these regions (for immunological and genetic predisposition to attract different strains of *M. tuberculosis*, see Chapter 13).

16.2.4 Implementation of the DOTS System in Russia

In order to fight emergence of multidrug resistance and to improve tuberculosis control globally, WHO initiated the DOTS programme (directly observed therapy, short course). Since 1995, DOTS programmes are being performed in many countries, supported by World Bank and by the US Centers for Disease Control. Generally, the DOTS strategy comprises five aspects (see also Chapter 8):

- Continuing political support of the programme in countries affected by tuberculosis

- Quality-controlled microbiological tuberculosis diagnostics
- Standardized short-course therapy (2 months intensive therapy with combination of four drugs, 4 months therapy with combination of two drugs) under adequate conditions of outpatient and hospital patient care
- Free access to quality-controlled antituberculotic drugs (first-line drugs)
- Adequate documentation to monitor therapy outcomes and epidemiological data.

While the WHO tuberculosis report 2009 (Global tuberculosis control – surveillance, planning, financing – WHO report on tuberculosis 2009, see below) reports that the DOTS programme is now officially implemented in all of the 89 regions, the case notification by DOTS varies largely between the different Russian regions and oblasts.

Some regions in Russia have already reported remarkable success in consequent implementation of DOTS and in the number of tuberculosis rates, especially Tomsk oblast (oblast is an administrative division). Some oblasts exclusively diagnose and treat tuberculosis according to DOTS recommendations, others have DOTS programme and the conventional tuberculosis control system in parallel; some only refer to the conventional system.

In Prikaz No. 50, the Russian Ministry of Health specified the system of case notification and tuberculosis surveillance in Russia. However, because of the different levels of DOTS implementation and sticking to the conventional Soviet system of tuberculosis control, problems raise concerning interpretation of epidemiological data (see also Chapter 8).

16.2.5 Policy Considerations of WHO

The Global Plan to Stop TB, 2006–2015 identified sub-Saharan Africa and Eastern Europe as the only two WHO regions in the world where it will be very difficult to achieve the TB targets under Millennium Development Goal 6 (reduction of tuberculosis prevalence by 50% in 2015, compared to the numbers of 1990). According to this document, WHO Euro outlines the main directions for effectively increasing access to quality diagnosis and treatment of TB. According to WHO, the expansion of high-quality TB diagnostic and treatment services in Eastern Europe is limited by the following obstacles in the countries of the former Soviet Union:

- lack of political will
- weak public health infrastructure, insufficient integration of TB control programmes into general health services
- inadequate engagement of the full range of care providers
- poorly developed human resource capacity and
- lack of involvement of people with TB and communities

It is urgent that the Stop TB Strategy should be fully implemented on a broad scale. In this context, a big step forward is the adoption of the Berlin Declaration from October 2007.

As pointed out above, *multidrug resistance* is the main cause of the low success rates in TB treatment in the WHO Euro region and the main constraint on achieving the TB control targets by 2015. Thus, WHO focuses on strengthening laboratory diagnosis and treatment for a much larger number of MDR-TB patients.

In Eastern Europe, prisons are important breeding grounds for TB, and especially MDR-TB. TB diagnostic and treatment services of the same standard as those available to the general community should be established as part of the penal system reform and through close collaboration between the justice, internal affairs and health ministries.

During the last years, *HIV* has spread rapidly in Eastern Europe, particularly among intravenous drug users. WHO recommends an effective coordination between TB and HIV/AIDS control programmes, and collaborative interventions must be implemented to ensure a continuum of care for patients. WHO–Euro region is now at a critical point of HIV/AIDS development: Consequent containment of HIV and opportunistic infections like tuberculosis could save the countries from catastrophic developments like in some countries of sub-Saharan Africa where every fourth is already infected with HIV (see Chapter 18)

The *Stop TB Strategy* and the Global Plan to Stop TB 2006–2015 were launched in January 2006 and should be translated into a medium-term strategic plan, in view of the specific needs and resources of Eastern European countries. The Berlin Declaration on Tuberculosis provides the main strategy for WHO Euro; the newly founded *Stop TB Partnership for Europe* will provide an organizational framework for bi- and multilateral joint projects in tuberculosis control.

Many of the scientific collaborative projects with Eastern European partners are organized and done by the Koch-Metchnikov-Forum (website: www.KMForum.eu).

16.2.6 Public Health Relevance

As mentioned above, the fight against tuberculosis is based on the Stop TB Strategy, which also includes a passage dedicated to "contribute to health system strengthening", acknowledging that effective and sustainable TB control relies on the strength of the general health system (see Chapter 4).

Many successor states of the former Soviet Union and other Eastern European states are currently rebuilding their health-care system. This provides a good opportunity for making TB control more effective. However, according to WHO global experiences over the past decades some types of health system reforms (mainly the complete reconstructions in some Eastern European countries) may even worsen the situation of tuberculosis control, if they are not carried out with due concern for the importance of specific disease control functions. Therefore, WHO prefers well-designed TB control strategies strengthening the general health system, for example, by improving laboratory networks, drug distribution systems and human resource capacity, and by providing quality services integrated into primary health care. A prerequisite for this is that TB control activities should be coordinated and harmonized with wider efforts to strengthen the health system. To achieve this goal, a well-coordinated action by high- and low-burden countries is required under the auspices of WHO.

Many health-care reforms performed in countries of the WHO–Euro region comprise the following tasks:

- ensuring leadership and governance in the health sector
- ensuring sustainable financing and the priority development of delivery of primary health care
- establishing services for disadvantaged populations
- motivating and retaining health staff
- promoting evidence-based care.

It is difficult to quantify financial and organizational efforts for improving health-care systems to enable them to provide efficient tools for prevention and therapy of tuberculosis. However, in many countries in Europe, effective implementation of appropriate tools in health-care services is not possible without substantial national and international funding for an efficient tuberculosis control. At the same time, highly centralized, vertical TB control programmes inherited from the Soviet system are difficult to integrate with the general health services because of insufficient funding, irrational allocation of available resources, poorly developed primary health-care services and, often, psychological resistance on the part of TB specialists. National TB programmes are an important part of health systems and can contribute substantially to health system strengthening by integrating functioning control structures into the health-care system, making use of their experiences and international integration and partnerships. Furthermore, an international network of external quality control is necessary for the diagnostic laboratory work, therapy regimens and strategies as well as for public health measures. A good example of quality control in diagnostics is the system of national and supranational reference centres for TB diagnostics (Ridderhof et al., 2007).

16.2.6.1 Health System Strengthening

National TB Programmes are an important tool for strengthening national health-care systems as a whole in high-burden countries; these programmes need to be implemented according to WHO guidelines. Harmonization between TB control efforts and budgeting processes is crucial to ensure long-term success. Furthermore, investments in laboratory infrastructure and training of health professionals are also a prerequisite for applying public health measures in TB control. WHO especially furthers initiatives of public–public and public–private partnerships, and community-based care, in response to specific health-care system barriers.

References

Influenza

Ferguson NM, Cummings DAT, Fraser C, Cajka JC et al. (2006) Strategies for mitigating an influenza pandemic. Nature; 442(7101):448–52; *critical discussion on counter-measures in case of a pandemic*

National Pandemic Preparedness Plan Germany (in German). www.rki.de (latest access: May 2009)

Nguyen-Van-Tam JS, Hampson AW (2003) The epidemiology and clinical impact of pandemic influenza. Vaccine 21: 1762–8; *good overview of the epidemiology of influenza*

Nicholson KG, Webster RG, Hay AJ (eds.) (1998) Textbook of influenza. 1st edition, Blackwell Scientific Publications, Oxford

WHO Global Influenza PreparednessPlan, http://www.who.int/csr/disease/influenza/pandemic/en/, (latest access: May 2009); published in 2005; *update in progress*, planned for May 2009.

Tuberculosis

Atun RA, Samyshkin YA, Drobniewski F, Skuratova NM, Gusarova G, Kuznetsov SI, Fedorin IM, Coker RJ (2005) Barriers to sustainable tuberculosis control in the Russian Federation health system. Bull World Health Organ.; 83(3):217–23

Coker RJ, Atun RA, McKee M (2004) Health-care system frailties and public health control of communicable disease on the European Union's new eastern border. Lancet 363(9418):1389–92; *review on the occasion of the enlargement of the EU in May 2004*

Kaufmann SHE, Hahn H (editors) (2002) Mycobacteria and TB, 1st edition (update in preparation); Karger Verlag; *combines epidemiological aspects with basic research in tuberculosis*

Ridderhof JC, van Deun A, Man Kam K, Narayanan PR, Aziz MA (2007) Roles of laboratories and laboratory systems in effective tuberculosis programmes. Bulletin of the World Health Organization 85 (5): A-419; *detailed overview about the WHO system of the supranational reference laboratory network.*

Rom WN, Garay SM, (editors) (2004) Tuberculosis. 2nd edition; Lippincott, Williams & Wilkins; *good chapters on infection epidemiology*

WHO Tuberculosis Report 2007 (2007). Global tuberculosis control – surveillance, planning, financing – WHO report on tuberculosis 2007. http://www.who.int/tb/publications/global_report/2009/en/index.html (latest access: May 2009; *excellent annual overview of the current development in TB numbers*)

WHO Fact Sheet EUTB/02 (2007). Epidemiology of tuberculosis in Europe; *updated on the occasion of Ministerial Forum on Tuberculosis, state-of-the-art of evaluation of TB epidemiology*

Chapter 17
Infectious Childhood Diarrhea in Developing Countries

Charles P. Larson, Lars Henning, Stephen Luby, and ASG Faruque

17.1 Introduction

Diarrhea in young children is a killer illness. While considerable progress has been made over the past two decades in the prevention and treatment of diarrhea in children under 5 years of age, childhood diarrhea remains one of the leading causes of preventable mortality and disease burden throughout the developing world. Worldwide, between 1.5 and 2.0 million children die annually from diarrhea-related illnesses and over 95% of these children live in underdeveloped countries. In developing countries childhood diarrhea accounts for approximately 15–20% of all under-5 deaths (Morris et al. 2003).

Childhood diarrhea is defined as the passage of three or more loose or watery stools over a 24-h period. Diarrheal illnesses are commonly sub-grouped by the character of the stool and duration of illness. These include secretory (watery), dysentery (bloody, mucoid), prolonged (greater than 7 days), and persistent (greater than 14 days) diarrhea.

17.2 Morbidity and Mortality

Children under 5 years of age living in unhygienic environments with frequent exposure to fecal contamination will average three to four episodes of diarrhea per year. This estimate has not changed since the early 1990s (Keusch et al. 2006). The occurrence of diarrhea will vary widely by geographic location, availability of safe water, and the age of the child, with the peak incidence being between 6 and 24 months of age. In contrast to the stagnant morbidity rates, mortality has fallen from nearly 5 million deaths in 1980 to less than 2 million by 2005, although this may have reached a plateau since the late 1990s (Snyder and Merson 1982; Morris et al. 2003;

C.P. Larson (✉)
International Centre for Diarrhea Disease Research, Bangladesh (ICDDR,B), Dhaka, Bangladesh; Centre for International Child Health, British Columbia Children's Hospital and Department of Pediatrics, University of British Columbia, Vancouver, Canada
e-mail: clarson@icddrb.org

A. Krämer et al. (eds.), *Modern Infectious Disease Epidemiology*, Statistics for Biology and Health, DOI 10.1007/978-0-387-93835-6_17,

Jones et al. 2003). About 5% of acute diarrhea episodes will evolve into persistent childhood diarrhea. This is much more likely to occur in malnourished children (Ochoa et al. 2004)

17.2.1 Etiologic Agents

Infectious childhood diarrhea can be due to bacterial, viral, protozoa, or helminthic organisms. Because many of these agents can be carried by asymptomatic children, their presence in the stool of a sick child may or may not explain the child's illness. Due to logistical, financial, and technical constraints, most of the time diarrhea is diagnosed on the basis of clinical symptoms and no etiologic agent is ever identified.

17.2.2 Bacterial Agents

Escherichia coli: Five pathogenic *E. coli* strains have been identified, which in total account for 10–20% of diarrheal episodes.

1. Enterotoxigenic *E. coli* (ETEC): ETEC is a common cause of childhood diarrhea, in particular in South Asia, where it may account for up to one-fifth of all cases (Qadri et al. 2005). It is also an important contributor to traveler's diarrhea, as it is frequently found and rapidly multiplies in contaminated food. The presentation is typically the acute onset of watery diarrhea, with or without fever.
2. Enteropathogenic *E. coli* (EPEC) (also known as Shiga toxin-producing *E. coli*): EPEC is an important contributor to diarrhea in sub-Saharan Africa, in particular in infants under 1 year of age. The typical presentation is acute watery diarrhea with vomiting (Donnenberg and Whittam 2001).
3. Enterohemorrhagic *E. coli* (EHEC): Although less common, EHEC can cause acute, severe bloody diarrhea episodes and life-threatening illness. Humans acquire this infection from the spread of animal feces into the environment (Beutin 2006). Two important complications of EHEC are hemolytic uremic syndrome and severe hemorrhagic colitis.
4. Enteroinvasive *E. coli* (EIEC): Affecting children of any age, EIEC presents with acute bloody, mucoid diarrhea
5. Enteroaggregative *E. coli* (EAEC): This is the least common of the pathogenic *E. coli* strains. It presents with acute watery diarrhea and is more prone to lead to persistent childhood diarrhea (Weintraub 2007).

Salmonella: Over 2,000 pathogenic *Salmonella* serotypes have been identified. At ICDDR,B *Salmonella* is found to occur in all age groups, but accounts for less than 5% of diarrhea illnesses (Fig. 17.1). Episodes present with the acute onset of fever, nausea, vomiting, and watery diarrhea. *Salmonella* Typhi, an important *Salmonella* serogroup, is characterized by a relatively brief episode of diarrhea (or none) and general malaise followed by fever that persists from one to several weeks. Non-typhoid salmonella infections are becoming increasingly common in crowded, urban slum environments. These organisms rapidly develop resistance to antibiotics (Su et al. 2004).

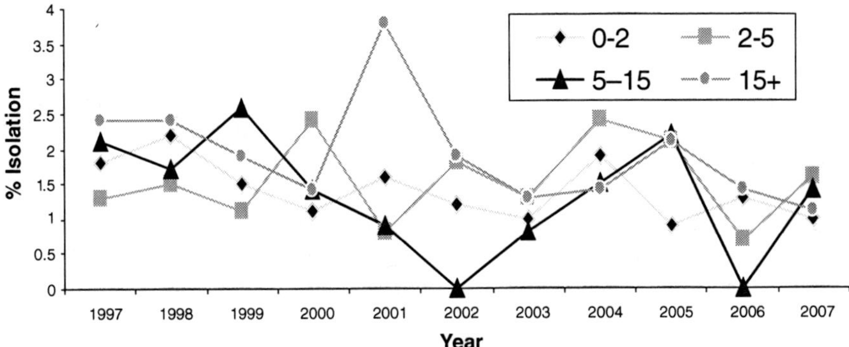

Fig. 17.1 Isolation of Salmonella by age group, 1997–2007. Source: International Centre for Diarrhea Disease Research, Bangladesh – Dhaka Hospital Surveillance

Shigella: This agent typically occurs in children between 2 and 5 years of age, suggesting that immunity is conferred after that (Tayler et al. 1986). It is this age group that accounts for the majority of fatal cases. *Shigella* will account for between 5 and 10% of hospitalized cases (Fig. 17.2). Clinically, *Shigella* diarrhea presents with visible blood in the stools. Four pathogenic species have been identified, each including several serotypes. *Shigella* spp. are of increased public health concern because of the low infectious dose required to cause illness (as few as 10 bacteria). This creates tremendous potential for outbreaks whenever sanitation or hygiene is compromised. In developing countries *Shigella* infection is an important contributor to overall mortality rates (Kotloff et al. 1999).

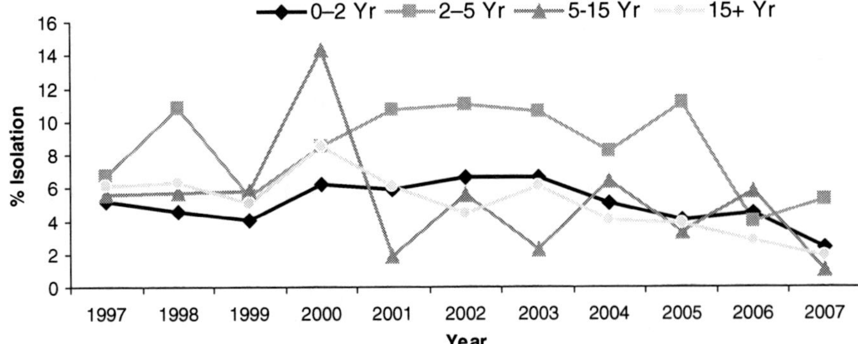

Fig. 17.2 Isolation of Shigella by age group, 1997–2007. Source: International Centre for Diarrhea Disease Research, Bangladesh – Dhaka Hospital Surveillance

1. *S. flexneri*: This is the most common species in developing countries. It presents with acute onset, bloody diarrhea. *S. flexneri* presents a greatest public health burden because it is endemic and is the leading cause of the dysentery in developing countries.
2. *S. boydii*: This is a relatively uncommon cause of diarrhea in developing countries.
3. *S. dysenteriae*: This strain accounts for periodic epidemics of severe, bloody diarrhea (shigellosis). This is the most virulent *Shigella* illness and can rapidly develop resistance to antimicrobials. *S. dysenteriae* serotype 1 is associated with epidemic shigellosis, a highly lethal illness that rapidly spreads within infected populations.
4. *S. sonnei*: This is most commonly found in developed countries. The ratio of *S. sonnei* to *S. flexneri* can be interpreted as an index of a population's level of development, in particular with respect to sanitation and hygiene practices.

Campylobacter: Occurring most commonly in children 6–24 months of age, this agent can cause either watery or bloody diarrhea. Campylobacter enteritis is attributable to two strains, *C. jejuni* and *C. coli*. Children can be asymptomatic carriers of *Campylobacter* organisms. *Campylobacter* infections have taken on added significance because of its increased virulence among HIV-infected individuals, often leading to death. Important uncommon sequela of *Campylobacter* infection is Guillain–Barre syndrome. Common sources include chickens, domestic animals, and water (Coker et al. 2002).

Vibrio cholerae: There are several distinct serogroups, serotypes, and biotypes of *V. cholerae*. Only two serogroups, *V. cholerae* 01 (classical and El Tor biotypes) and 0139, are toxin producing and cause illness in humans. In clinical practice this differentiation is not relevant, as the treatment is the same. Cholera is most commonly associated with the ingestion of contaminated water, but can also be found in contaminated food. As opposed to *Shigella*, large doses of cholera organisms must be ingested to cause symptomatic illness. During cholera outbreaks in non-endemic areas, children and adults both contract the disease. However, because adults are more mobile and have more risk exposures outside the home, they are typically infected more often than children. In endemic areas the situation is reversed. Most adults in an endemic area have been previously exposed to cholera conferring some degree of immunity, thus children over the age of 2 years have higher rates of infection. In such populations an increased proportion of cholera cases in children under the age of 5 years is an early marker of a cholera outbreak (Sack et al. 2004). Infants and toddlers usually do not ingest enough organisms to lead to symptomatic illness. For reasons that are not clear, strains of O139 have tended to have higher rates in adults than children. Because of the required high ingested dose ($\sim 10^6$), contaminated water is the primary source of infections. Improved water sanitation is crucial to containment of cholera in endemic regions and will prevent cholera outbreaks (as in contrast to shigellosis where personal hygiene plays a pivotal role). In cholera endemic locations, such as Bangladesh, as many as 50% of hospital admissions will be due to cholera (Fig. 17.3).

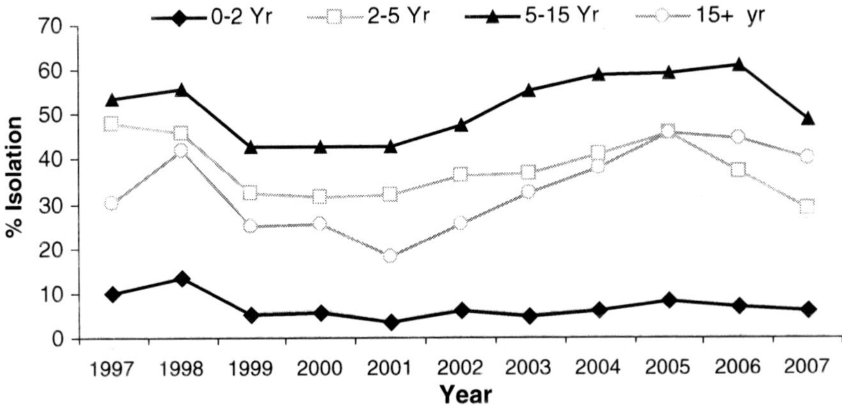

Fig. 17.3 Isolation of V. Cholerae 01 by Age Group, 1997–2007. Source: International Centre for Diarrhea Disease Research, Bangladesh – Dhaka Hospital Surveillance

17.2.3 Viral Agents

Rotavirus: With the notable exception of cholera in a few endemic countries, rotavirus is the most common cause of severe, dehydrating diarrhea in infants and young children in developing countries, accounting for several hundred thousand preventable deaths per year (Leung et al. 2005; Tanaka et al. 2007). In Dhaka over 50% of children under 2 years of age admitted for diarrhea have a rotavirus infection (Fig. 17.4). Rotavirus is a ubiquitous, highly contagious organism that infects nearly all children by the age of 3. Group A serotype strains 1–4 account for the large majority of rotavirus diarrhea, however, this varies by region, with additional group A serotypes having an important role. The clinical presentation is typically the acute onset of fever, vomiting, and watery diarrhea. Rotavirus infections lead to a disproportionate number of severe episodes and increased likelihood of hospitalization (Glass et al. 2003).

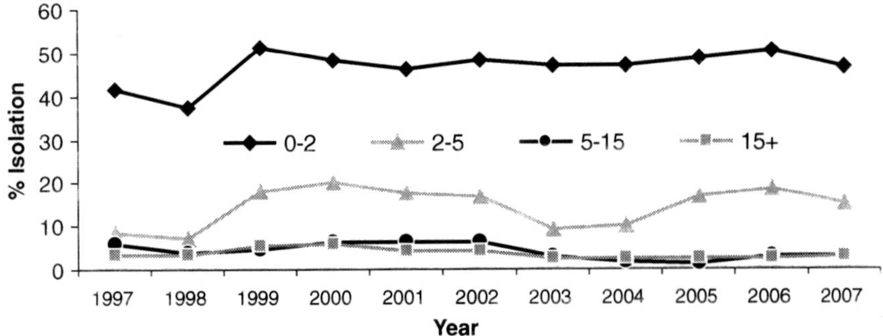

Fig. 17.4 Isolation of Rotavirus by age group, 1997–2007. Source: International Centre for Diarrhea Disease Research, Bangladesh – Dhaka Hospital Surveillance

Other much less common viral etiologic agents include human caliciviruses and adenoviruses. The former includes the Norwalk virus that can account for large outbreaks affecting all age groups.

17.2.4 Protozoa

Giardia lamblia: This parasite has a wide range of hosts, including birds, domestic and wild animals, and humans. For this reason it is one of the most common parasitic infections in the world. Humans typically become infected through ingestion of fecally contaminated water (Ali and Hill 2003). Infected children can present with acute or persistent histories of diarrhea, but may also be asymptomatic or only detected because of their malnutrition. *Giardia lamblia* and *Cryptosporidium parvum* cause malabsorptive diarrhea by breaking down the epithelial barrier of the intestine (Savioli et al. 2006).

Cryptosporidium parvum: This parasite was initially considered to be a diarrhea pathogen limited to animals, but is now recognized as an important cause of diarrhea in humans worldwide. *Cryptosporidium* infection has been reported to account for over 20% of hospital diarrhea admissions in reports out of Africa and Central America. HIV-infected children are at greatly increased risk for cryptosporidia infection and subsequent death (Fayer et al. 2000; Gatei et al. 2006).

Entamoeba histolytica: Two entamoeba species infect humans; *E. histolytica* and *E. dispar*. The latter is non-pathogenic, but indistinguishable from the former by microscopic examination of stools (Staufer and Ravdin 2003). In recent years it has become apparent that *E. histolytica* infections are a far more important contributor to diarrhea in children than had previously been recognized. With newer PCR diagnostic capabilities, it is estimated that nearly half of all children in sanitation compromised environments will become infected with *E. histolytica*, but only about 20% will become symptomatic, usually with diarrhea (Huque et al. 2002).

Cyclospora cayetanensis: This parasite is found in the tropics and subtropics, with humans being the only known host. It is most frequently a cause of diarrhea in children, in particular if HIV infected. *C. cayetanensis* has been responsible for large outbreaks of diarrhea in developed and developing countries. A specific high-risk group is raspberry pickers. For reasons probably related to climatic change, it is a highly seasonal disease, but the seasons vary by region (Eberhard and Arrowood 2002).

17.3 Risk Factors for Childhood Diarrhea

17.3.1 Malnutrition

Malnutrition has been estimated to be an underlying factor in over 60% of childhood diarrhea deaths (Caulfield et al. 2004). This is a two-way causal pathway. Diarrhea episodes lead to decreased energy intake and the disproportionate loss of essential micronutrients. Equally important, malnutrition leads to increased vulnerability to infection, including diarrhea as a result of micronutrient deficiencies, intestinal malabsorption, the breakdown of mucosal barriers to infection, and immune system dysfunction (Brown 2003). While controversial at the time, this concept of dual causality was laid out by Scrimshaw nearly 40 years ago (Scrimshaw et al. 1968). The improved understanding of the associations between nutrition and diarrhea has led to profound changes in the approach to diarrhea illness management. Instead of "starving" diarrhea, it is now universally accepted that, with the exception of severe cases or repeated vomiting, children with diarrhea should be fed. This includes continued breastfeeding and/or resumption of normal energy intake (Brown 1994).

17.3.2 Sanitation and Hygiene

Contaminated food: Foodborne infection is a common cause of diarrhea throughout the developing world. Common etiologic agents found in food vary by region. They include *Salmonella*, *Campylobacter*, ETEC or EHEC, and cholera. The most frequent food sources include raw milk, eggs and poultry, other meats, and seafood.

Contaminated water: Intervention studies demonstrate that pathogen contaminated drinking water is an important exposure that causes diarrhea. In settings where diarrhea is a leading cause of death, effective removal of microbiological contaminants from drinking water typically reduces diarrhea incidence by 29–39% (Clasen et al. 2007; Fewtrell et al. 2005; Arnold and Colford 2007). Moreover, when water that is contaminated with fecal pathogens is used to prepare food, the food becomes contaminated. If ambient temperatures are conducive, the concentration of pathogenic bacteria can increase exponentially in contaminated food.

17.4 Illness Management

17.4.1 Acute Watery Diarrhea

The large majority of childhood diarrhea episodes can be managed in the home, with or without the advice of a local health provider. The home management of diarrhea is based upon four basic principles: (1) oral rehydration, (2) appropriate energy intake, (3) zinc supplementation for 10–14 days, and (4) early health facility referral if not improving. Due to the changing antibiotic resistance patterns, the use of antibiotics without health provider information is not advised. Common criteria for admission to a health facility are high fever, fast breathing (0–2 months: >60/min, 2–12: > 50/min, 12–60 months: >40/min), lethargy, convulsions, persistent vomiting, and abdominal distension. As soon as a patient is rehydrated and can maintain oral hydration level, assuming no further complications, they can be discharged and can return to home management of their illness. In a resource-limited settings it is not feasible to keep patients in hospital until the diarrhea episode is completely resolved.

Rehydration: Dehydration is a dangerous and often deadly consequence of diarrhea in young children. Considering the risks of intravenous therapy, with the exception of severe, ongoing fluid loss, oral rehydration is the treatment of choice and equally effective (Hartling et al. 2006; Bellemare et al. 2004). In general, the aim is to correct the dehydration over 6 h in infants or over 3 h in children greater than 12 months of age. In addition, there is the need to compensate for ongoing fluid loss (5 ml/kg/stool).

Intravenous fluids: IV fluids are required only in cases of severe dehydration or specific circumstances such as severe vomiting, unconsciousness, ileus, glucose malabsorption, or high volume stool output (more than 10 ml/kg/h). Most often it is possible to quickly switch to Oral Rehydration Solution (ORS) after initially correcting the severe dehydration with IV fluids. In infants 30% of the fluid correction should be given in 30 min and the remaining 70% in the next 5–6 h. Older children can receive 30% of the required fluid in the first 30 min and the remaining 70% in the following 2–3 h. Severe cholera-related dehydration must be aggressively combated, with the risk of fluid overload and heart failure being minimal. By switching to oral rehydration solution as soon as possible these and other risks are further minimized and patients are more quickly ready for discharge.

Oral rehydration solution (ORS) /oral rehydration therapy (ORT) : One of the most significant medical discoveries of the twentieth century was the development of a rehydration solution that could be given orally. Oral rehydration therapies (ORT) have contributed more than any other single intervention by reducing diarrhea-related deaths in children by more than half. ORS is a specially formulated mixture of water with salts and carbohydrate. Although it is a simple mixture, it is actually based on a scientific understanding of the rather complex process of the absorption of salts and water from the intestine. In spite of its remarkable effectiveness, overall rates of use still remain under 50%. This is in part explained by the fact that the originally marketed oral rehydration solution (ORS) did not reduce stool volume (Victora et al. 2000). This led to the testing of a modified ORS with reduced sodium and glucose content (hypo-osmolar ORS). This modified ORS formulation has been demonstrated to reduce stool output, decrease vomiting, and lessen the necessity of IV rehydration (Hanh et al. 2001; Murphy et al. 2004). An easy way to estimate the amount of ORS to be given is one teaspoonful of ORS per kg of loose stool. The risk of fluid overload is practically impossible and only a theoretical concern. Much more common is the occurrence of hypernatremia because of inappropriate dilution of the ORS.

The search for an improved ORS with a higher glucose content (to increase the sodium-carrying capacity), while still having a low osmolarity, led to the development of starch-based solutions, e.g., rice or barley ORT. The advantage of cereal-based ORTs are their higher content of glucose but in a polymeric form that does not add to its osmolarity. ORS and cereal-based ORTs can be purchased in prepackaged sachets or they can be made at home. The latter requires careful instruction and follow-up monitoring, but is an excellent alternative where the supply of sachets is difficult to maintain. Other home-made oral rehydration therapies include sugar–salt solution and soups (e.g., chicken rice soup) that provide salts and carbohydrates.

Although these home-based fluids do not contain potassium or base, they are very useful for diarrheal illnesses that are not severe.

Appropriate energy intake: As already mentioned, do not "starve the diarrhea." No special food is required in cases of uncomplicated diarrhea. Infants should be breastfed and older children should be offered the normal family diet. Following more severe or prolonged episodes, children should be fed at least one extra meal per day for 2 weeks to recover from any nutritional deficit they may have acquired during their illness.

Zinc treatment: Several efficacy studies of zinc as a treatment for childhood diarrhea have demonstrated both curative and preventive benefits to children under 5 years of age. This includes decreased duration or severity of an acute or persistent diarrheal illness episode and decreased likelihood of a repeat episode (Bhutta et al. 2000; Fontaine 2001). In a community-based, effectiveness study conducted in Matlab, Bangladesh, zinc treatment of under-5 children with an acute diarrheal episode resulted in decreased duration of the illness, decreased repeat episodes of diarrhea, and an estimated 50% reduction in non-injury mortality (Baqui et al. 2002). Based on the weight of this evidence, the WHO/UNICEF guidelines for the treatment of childhood diarrhea have been modified to include zinc treatment of any diarrheal illness episode in children under 5 years of age (WHO/UNICEF 2004).

Antibiotics: WHO/UNICEF diarrhea management guidelines limit the use of antibiotics to dysentery (bloody diarrhea), typhoid fever, and cholera. Agents most commonly responsible for bloody diarrhea include *Shigella,* ETEC, and EIEC. Due to overuse and misuse, widespread antibiotic resistance is now a common occurrence throughout the developing world. Antimicrobial resistance patterns vary by region and pose a potentially catastrophic scenario where resistance to all conventional antibiotics might occur. This is particularly the case for epidemic shigellosis. Cholera is a self-limiting disease and antibiotic treatment only shortens the duration of the illness, not its severity. If adequate fluid replacement therapy is provided, the effect of antibiotic treatment is minimal on an individual level, but will play an important role during cholera outbreaks because it leads to the earlier discharge of less severe cases.

Antihelminthics: Helminths are a relatively uncommon cause of diarrhea in children. In the absence of laboratory confirmation of a helminthic etiologic agent antihelminthics are not recommended as a treatment.

Probiotics/Lactobacillus therapy: Generically, probiotics refer to non-pathogenic bacterial or fungal organisms colonized in the bowel that are believed to have beneficial health effects. Orally administered lactobacillus, usually in the form of yogurt, has for many decades been a commonly administered home remedy for diarrhea in many societies. The mechanisms explaining why probiotics improve diarrheal illness outcomes are not well understood. Competition with pathogenic organisms for mucosal receptor sites, thus preventing their adhesion and growth, has been observed (Neeser et al. 2000). Meta-analyses of randomized trials estimate that lactobacillus therapy can reduce the frequency of diarrhea and the duration of an illness by about 1 day (Van Niel et al. 2002; Huang et al. 2002). Probiotics have not been sufficiently tested for effectiveness and impact in developing country populations and, therefore, are not currently recommended.

Antidiarrheal agents: It has to be clearly stated that antidiarrheal agents do not play any role in the treatment of diarrhea and can lead to severe complications, such as intestinal perforation. Antidiarrheal agents are not recommended by WHO for the management of childhood diarrhea (WHO/UNICEF 2004). A Cochrane Collaboration systematic review of antidiarrheals for use in developing countries is currently being conducted (Dalby-Payne et al. 2007).

Antiemetic agents: There is modest evidence that antiemetics, such as ondansetron, shorten the duration of vomiting in children with acute gastroenteritis. Less vomiting, however, leads to increased fluid or toxin retention that, in turn, increases the volume of diarrhea (Alhashimi et al. 2007).

17.4.2 Persistent Childhood Diarrhea (PCD)

The likelihood of an acute case of diarrhea advancing to PCD (greater than 14 days) varies widely by region and location, with published proportions ranging from less than 1% to greater than 20%. As improvements in the treatment of ACD occur, in particular the use of ORS, the proportion of PCD cases seen in health facilities will increase (Victora et al. 2000). The case fatality rate for PCD is approximately 50%. With improvements in the prevention of ACD, PCD accounts for over 50% of all childhood diarrhea deaths (Black 1993). Because of their increased likelihood in persistent illnesses, parasitic infections such as *Giardia lamblia* and *E. histolytica* need to be ruled out. In addition, sources of repeated inoculation, such as contaminated water holding systems or stored food, should be considered.

Resource-deprived health systems do not have the capacity to treat children in health facilities over extended periods of time. Therefore, management of PCD often requires caretaker education in order to manage their child at home. Once the child's hydration status is stabilized, the principal element in home management is nutrition. This includes replacement and ongoing maintenance of energy and micronutrient requirements. This should include zinc supplementation, which has been demonstrated to prevent the occurrence of PCD, but also to shorten in its duration once it has occurred (Bhutta et al. 2000; Rahman et al. 2001).

17.4.3 Diagnostic Tests

Most diagnoses of diarrhea disease can be based only on clinical symptoms. In some cases it might be necessary to confirm the diagnosis in the laboratory. The laboratory diagnosis consists of sample collection which is usually followed by macroscopic and microscopic observations. In addition, culture for growth and isolation, biochemical characterization, immunodiagnostics, and antibiograms can add valuable information, but needs a more sophisticated setup which is not always found in developing countries. A rapid dip stick is now available for detecting cholera. This dip stick can be used on a representative sample of specimens to confirm *V. cholerae* as the cause of the outbreak and the test results are available in only 5 min. Then, a sample of the positive samples can be sent to reference laboratory for confirmation by culture and antibiotic sensitivities.

Communication between laboratories and public health professionals is very important because of their interdependency. In some cases, an outbreak will be suspected by clinical suspicion, which then needs laboratory confirmation. In other cases the laboratory may notice an increase in a certain type of specimen, which needs a clinical correlation. In either case good bilateral communication is necessary. Finally, the laboratory can provide data on changing antimicrobial sensitivities, which can occur during the same outbreak, and which can directly affect treatment efficacy.

17.4.4 Early Referral

Most diarrheal episodes can be treated at home or after a short stay in a outpatient clinic. Mothers/caretakers should be educated about early danger signs and told to seek health advice if their child does not improve. Danger signs include, but are not restricted, increase in temperature, becoming lethargic, convulsions, increased vomiting, abdominal distention, turning blue, loss of appetite, and fast breathing. Additional considerations for referral are the age of the child, especially those under 12 months of age, infants not breastfed, and those who are malnourished.

Integrated approaches to child health care that combine preventive with curative care also serve to detect children early in their illness and avoid missed opportunities. This is the aim of integrated management of child illness (IMCI) programs that are currently being introduced at the community level within most developing countries. Health workers are trained to identify children with diarrhea and refer those who require facility-based care.

17.4.5 Nutritional Therapy and Rehabilitation

Appropriate energy intake is essential for speedy recovery and the prevention of hypoglycemia. The latter in shigellosis is one of most important risk factors for mortality (always ask the mother/caretaker when she last breastfed or fed her infant/child). Severely malnourished children need special attention and may require referral to nutritional rehabilitation. Rehabilitation includes micronutrient supplementation, including vitamin A and zinc, as well as specialized diets (Ahmed et al. 1999). Based on standardized protocols, subsequent morbidity and mortality can be decreased substantially.

17.5 Prevention

In nearly all instances, diarrhea is the result of fecal organisms eventually being orally ingested (fecal–oral transmission). With the exception of vaccines, all appropriate, developing country public health interventions will require behavior change.

These behaviors will require effective knowledge transfer to households and communities, the provision of the necessary skills, and the elimination of environmental and social barriers to diarrhea prevention practices. For this to occur, supportive policies and systems need to be in place, backed up by sustained commitment and financing. With these in place, breastfeeding, safe water, and improved sanitation and hygiene can be expected to reduce the incidence of childhood diarrhea by over two-thirds (Fewtrell et al. 2005).

17.5.1 Exclusive Breastfeeding

Exclusive breastfeeding (EBF) is defined as the oral intake of only breast milk. In population with inadequate amounts of micronutrients in the diet, micronutrient supplements are also included. EBF is recommended for the first 6 months of life and should be continued throughout any diarrhea illness unless unable to feed or experiencing severe vomiting (WHO/UNICEF 2004). EBF is associated with large reductions in diarrhea morbidity and morality (Bhandari et al. 2003). It has been estimated that EBF will lead to a six-fold reduction in the likelihood of diarrhea mortality during infancy (WHO Collaborative Study Team 2000). If a mother is known to be HIV positive, the preferred options are antiretroviral treatment or affordable, safe replacement feedings (DeCock et al. 2000; WHO 2003). Mixed breastfeeding has been shown to lead to increased HIV transmission and early introduction of solid foods and animal milk should be avoided (Coovadia et al. 2007).

17.5.2 Safe Water

About 1.1 billion people lack reliable access to safe water and about 2.2 million die of waterborne diseases each year (Bartram et al. 2001). Centralized water treatment systems are the source of choice, but for most of those living in developing countries this is not available or, where it is, highly unreliable. This implies that if households and communities in low-income settings value safe water, they need to take steps themselves. A variety of fairly low cost point-of-use disinfection technologies are highly effective in improving the microbiological quality of water and reducing diarrheal disease (Mintz et al. 2001; Sobsey 2002). Chemical disinfection with chlorine (hypochlorite) is effective against bacterial contamination, but leaves consumers vulnerable to viruses and parasites (e.g., *E. histolytica*). Solar (thermal) disinfection is another bactericidal choice, but must raise water temperatures above 45°C. These technologies remove more pathogens if combined with filtration. Safe water storage is also essential. The quality of drinking water can significantly decline after its collection and disinfection (Write et al. 2004). Placing disinfected water in contaminated bottles or other storage devices will lead to re-infection, in particular if the water has only been boiled or thermally treated. The central limitation to wider use of point-of-use water treatment is that it requires substantial investment of time, money and effort by vulnerable, low-income households. To date, the population level benefits of these interventions have been modest (Luby et al. 2008).

17.5.3 Sanitation and Hygiene

In a variety of low-income settings behavior change programs targeting handwashing with soap have resulted in an average 47% reduction in the number of diarrheal episodes (Curtis and Cairncross 2003). Importantly, such notable reductions in diarrhea incidence have occurred even when water remains contaminated and sanitary infrastructure is poor.

Community-wide improvements in sanitation are more difficult to study than household level improvements in drinking water quality and handwashing behavior. As a consequence, there is much less rigorous scientific data on the benefit of improvements in sanitation in diarrhea prevention, compared to the available data for improving water quality and handwashing promotion. However, as pathogens in human feces are the causative agent for most diarrheal disease, disposal of feces in a manner that prevents contamination of the drinking water and food supplies is a logical step in preventing diarrhea. Moreover, the available evidence suggests that improvements in sanitation reduce the incidence of diarrheal disease (Barreto 2007).

17.5.4 Vaccines

Rotavirus: Two effective live virus vaccines are available against rotavirus (Vesikari et al. 2006; 2006 Glass et al. Ruiz-Palacios et al. 2006). Both are over 85% effective in reducing the incidence of severe rotavirus gastroenteritis in settings where they have been tested. An earlier live rotavirus vaccine was removed from the market after postlicensing data demonstrated a rise in the incidence of intussusception with its use. The current vaccines have no effect on the incidence of intussusception. Their effectiveness in settings of poor nutrition and poor sanitation, settings where live enteric vaccines have performed sub-optimally is currently under study.

Cholera: Two oral cholera vaccines are available. WC/rBS includes whole killed *V. cholerae* O1 cells combined with a recombinant B subunit of cholera toxin. Two doses of vaccine provide more than 85% protection against cholera for 6 months among persons over 2 years of age, and 50% protection after 3 years (Clemens et al. 1990). CVD103-HgR is a live vaccine that has been effective when given to adults in the United States (Tacket et al. 1992), but is not yet proven to provide protection to populations living in cholera endemic areas. Cholera vaccines are not yet used routinely in cholera endemic settings.

There are a number of enteric vaccines under development, including those providing protection against *Shigella* and *E. coli* organisms, but none of them are yet available.

17.5.5 Micronutrients

Vitamin A: Cod liver oil, high in vitamin, has for several decades been associated with reduced infectious disease severity and mortality in children under 5 years of age. Several vitamin A supplementation trials for the prevention of childhood infections were carried out in the early 1990s. These were found to reduce all-cause deaths, deaths due to diarrhea, and overall infectious disease burden (Beaton et al. 1993; Ghana 1993). The results from subsequent randomized trials that focus more specifically on diarrhea have been inconsistent. A randomized trial in a peri-urban, relatively poor population of children less than 2 years of age found vitamin A supplementation resulted in over a 25% increase in diarrhea occurrence (Long et al. 2006). A recent meta-analysis of vitamin A supplementation found no overall consistent protection from vitamin A supplementation (Grotto et al. 2003). Vitamin A supplementation given every 6 months continues to be recommended because of its effect on reducing overall mortality in children under 5 years of age. It is not effective as a treatment of diarrhea (Fischer Walker and Black 2007)

Zinc: Zinc deficiency has been found to be widespread among children in developing countries, including Latin America, Africa, the Middle East, and South and East Asia (Shrimpton 1993; Black et al. 2008). Facility and population-based studies have consistently observed an association between zinc deficiency and infectious disease morbidity (Srinivas et al. 1988; Bahl et al. 1998). Based on estimates of the impact of zinc deficiency on diarrheal disease alone, it is estimated that correction of this deficiency could save over 450,000 under-5 deaths annually (Black et al. 2003; Jones et al. 2003). Over the past decade several randomized trials have been carried out to determine the efficacy of zinc provided as a daily supplement. These investigations have consistently demonstrated reductions in the occurrence of acute and persistent childhood diarrhea (Sazawal et al. 1997; Bhandari et al. 2002; Penny et al. 2004; Bhutta et al. 2008). In addition to its treatment effects, zinc given either as a 10 to 14-day treatment or on a daily basis has also been demonstrated to prevent future episodes of acute diarrhea episodes (15–20% reduction), the likelihood of an acute episode becoming persistent (25–30% reduction), and prevent non-injury deaths (as high as a 50% reduction, but lower estimates in children under 12 months of age) (Aggarwal et al. 2007; Bhutta et al. 2000; Fontaine 2001). It has been estimated that the combined scale up of zinc treatment and supplementation could prevent up to 750,000 deaths in children under 5 years of age.

17.6 Conclusion

Childhood diarrhea remains an important disease priority in the developing world, accounting for 15–25% of all under-5 mortality. Diarrhea is unique in that it is easy to detect and, with few exceptions, can be managed in the home with low technology interventions. The challenge facing health professionals is not the identification of new “magic bullets,” but in the more widespread scale up of proven preventive and treatment interventions, such as exclusive breastfeeding, handwashing, safe water,

ORS, and zinc supplementation. These interventions must be supported by health policies and programs that will facilitate and sustain their introduction into public and private health-care systems.

References

Aggarwal R, Sentz J, Millar MA (2007) Role of zinc administration in prevention of childhood diarrhea and respiratory illnesses: a metaanalysis. Pediatrics 119:1120–1130

Ahmed T, Ali M, Ullah MM, Choudhury IA, Haque ME, Salam MA, Rabbani GH,Suskind RM, Fuchs GJ (1999) Mortality in severely malnourished children with diarrhea and use of a standardised management protocol. Lancet 353:1919–1922

Alhashimi D, Alhashimi H, Fedorowicz Z (2007) Antiemetics for reducing vomiting related to acute gastroenteritis in children and adolescents. Cochrane database of systematic reviews (online); (2):CD 005506.

Ali SA, Hill DR (2003) Giardia intestinalis. Curr Opin Infect Dis 16(5):453–460

Arnold BF, Colford JM Jr (2007) Treating water with chlorine at point-of-use to improve water quality and reduce child diarrhea in developing countries: a systematic review and meta-analysis. Am J Trop Med Hyg 76, 354–364

Bahl R, Bhandari N, Hambidge KM, Bhan MK (1998) Plasma zinc as a predictor of diarrhea and respiratory morbidity in children in an urban slum setting. Am J Clin Nutr 68:414S–417S

Barreto ML, Genser B, Strina A, et al. (2007) Effect of city-wide sanitation programme on reduction in rate of childhood diarrhea in northeast Brazil: assessment by two cohort studies. Lancet 370:1622–1628

Bartram ME, Lochery P, Wegelin M (2001) Not just a drop in the bucket: Expanding access to point-of-use water treatment systems: Expanding access to point-of-use water treatment systems. Am J Pub Health 91:1565–1570

Baqui AH, Black RE, Arifeen SE, Yunus M, Chakraboty J, Ahmed S, Vaughan JP (2002) Effect of zinc supplementation started during diarrhea on morbidity and mortality in Bangladeshi children: community randomised trial. BMJ 325:1059

Beaton GH, Martorell R, L'Abbe KA, et al. (1993) Effectiveness of vitamin A supplementation in the control of young child mortality in developing countries. ACC/SCN Geneva, Switzerland

Bellemare S, Hartling L, Wlebe N, Russell K, Craig WR, McConnell D, Klassen TP (2004) Oral rehydration versus intravenous therapy for treating dehydration due to gastroenteritis in children: a meta-analysis of randomized controlled trials. BMC Med 2:11

Beutin L (2006) Emerging enterohaemorrhagic Escherichia coli, causes and effects of the rise of a human pathogen. J Veterinary Med 53:299–305

Bhandari N, Bahl R, Taneja S, Strand T, Molbak K, Ulvik RJ, et al. (2002) Substantial reduction in severe diarrheal morbidity by daily zinc supplementation in young north Indian children. Pediatrics 109:e86

Bhandari N, Bahl R, Mazumdar S, Marinez J, Black RE, Bahl MK (2003) Infant feeding Study Group: Effect of community-based promotion of exclusive breastfeeding on diarrheal illness and growth. A cluster randomized trial. Lancet 361:1418–1423

Bhutta ZA, Bird SM, Black RE, et al. (2000) Therapeutic effects of oral zinc in acute and persistent diarrhea in children in developing countries: pooled analysis of randomized controlled trials. Am J Clin Nutr 72:1516–1522

Bhutta ZA, Ahmed T, Black RE, et al. (2008) What works? Interventions for maternal and child health undernutrition and child survival. Lancet online publication January 17

Black RE.(1993) Persistent diarrhea in children of developing countries Pediatr Inf Dis J 12: 751–761

Black RE, Morris S, Bryce J (2003) Where and why are 10 million children dying every year? Lancet 361:2226–34

Black RE, Allen LH, Bhutta ZA, et al. (2008) Maternal and child undernutrition: global and regional exposures and health consequences Lancet 371(9608):243–260

Brown KH (1994) Dietary management of acute diarrheal disease: contemporary scientific issues. J Nutrition 124:1455S–1460S

Brown KH (2003) Diarrhea and malnutrition. J Nutr 133:328S–332S

Caulfield LE, de Onis M, Blossner M, Black RE (2004) Undernutrition as an underlying cause of child deaths associated with diarrhea, pneumonia, malaria, and measles. Am J Clin Nutr 80:193–198

Classen T, Schmidt WP, Rabie T, Roberts I, Cairncross S (2007) Interventions to improve water quality for preventing diarrhea: systematic review and meta-analysis.BMJ 334:782

Clemens JD, Sack DA, Harris JR, et al. (1990). Field trial of oral cholera vaccines in Bangladesh: results from three-year follow-up. Lancet 335:270–273.

Coker AO, Isokpehi RD, Thomas BN, Amisu KO, Obi CL (2002) Human campylobacteriosis in developing countries. Emerg Inf Dis 8:237–243

Coovadia HM, Rollins NC, Bland RM, Little K, Coutsoudis A, Bennish ML, Newell ML (2007) Mother-to-child transmission of HIV-1 infection during exclusive breastfeeding in the first 6 months of life: an intervention cohort study. Lancet 369:1107–1116

Curtis V, Cairncross S (2003) Effect of washing hands with soap on diarrhea risk in the community: a systematic review. Lancet Infect Dis 3:275–281

Dalby-Payne JR; Morris, AM, Elliott EJ (2004) Antimotility drugs for managing acute diarrhea in children. The Cochrane Library, Issue 2, 2004. Chichester, UK: John Wiley & Sons, Ltd.

DeCock KM, Fowler ME, Mercier M, et al. (2000) Prevention of mother to child transmission in resource poor countries: translating research into policy and practice. JAMA 283:1175–1182.

Donnenberg MS, Whittam TS (2001). Pathogenesis and evolution of virulence in enteropathogenic and enterohemorrhagic *Escherichia coli*. J Clin Invest 107:539–548

Eberhard ML, Arrowood MJ (2002) Cyclospora spp. Curr Opin Infec Dis 15:519–522

Fayer R, Morgan U, Upton SI (2000) Epidemiology of cryptosporidium transmission, detection and identification. Int J Parasitol 30:1305–1322

Fewtrell L, Kaufmann RB, Kay D, Enanoria W, Holler L, Colford JM (2005) Water, sanitation, and hygiene interventions to reduce diarrhea in less developed countries: a systematic review and meta-analysis. Lancet Infect Dis 5:1253–1258

Fischer Walker CL, Black RE (2007) Micronutrients and diarrheal disease. Clin Infect Dis 45 (Suppl 1):S73–S77

Fontaine O (2001) Effect of zinc supplementation on clinical course of acute diarrhea. J Health Popul Nutr 19(4):339–346

Gatei W, Wamae CN, Mbae C, et al. (2006) Cryptosporidiosis: prevalence, genotype analysis, and symptoms associated with infections in children in Kenya. Am J Trop Med Hyg 75:78–82

Ghana VAST Study Team (1993) Vitamin A supplementation in northern Ghana: effects on clinic attendance, hospital admissions, and child mortality. Lancet 342:7–12

Glass RI, Bresee J, Parashar U (2003) The global burden of dehydrating disease. In: MJ Farthing and D Mahalanabis, Editors. The Control of Food and Fluid Intake in Health and Disease Vol 51, Vevey Nestec Ltd. And Lippincott Williams & Wilkins, Philadelpphia, pp 17–30

Glass RI, Parashar UD, Bresee JS et al. (2006) Rotavirus vaccines: current prospects and future challenges. Lancet 368:323–332.

Grotto I, Mmouni M, Gdelevich M, Mmouni D (2003) Vitamin A supplementation and childhood morbidity from diarrhea and respiratory infections: a meta-analysis. J Pediatr 142:297–304

Hanh SK, Kim J, Garner P (2001) Reduced osmolarity oral rehydration solution for treating dehydration due to diarrhea in children: a systematic review. BMJ 323:81–85

Hartling L, Bellemare S, Wlebe N, Russell K, Klassen TP, Craig W (2006) Oral versus intravenous rehydration for treating dehydration due to gastroenteritis in children. Cochrane Data Base Syst Rev CD004390

Huang JS, Bousvaros A, Lee JW, Diaz A, Davidson EJ (2002) Efficacy of probiotic use in acute diarrhea in children. Dig Dis Sci 47:2625–2634

Huque R, Duggal P, Ali IM, et al. (2002) Innate and acquired resistance to amebiasis in Bangladeshi children. J Infect Dis; 86:547–552

Jones G, Steketee RW, Black RE, Bhtta ZA, Morris SS, Bellagio Child Survival Study Group(2003) How many child deaths can we prevent this year? Lancet 362:65–71

Keusch GT, Fontaine O, Bhargawi A, et al. (2006) Diarrheal Diseases. In: Jamison DT, Breman JG, Measham AR, Alleyne G, Claeson M eds. Disease control priorities in developing countries. 2nd ed. World Bank, Washington, DC

Kotloff KL, Winickoff JP, Ivanoff B, Clemens JD, Sweidlow DL, Sansonetti PJ, et al. (1999) Global burden of shigella infections: implications for vaccine development and implementation of control strategies. Bull WHO 77:651–666

Leung AK, Keller JD, Davies HD (2005) Rotavirus gastroenteritis. Adv Ther 22:476–487

Long KZ, Montoya Y, Hertzmark E, Santos JI, Rosado JI (2006) A double-blind, randomized trial, clinical trial of the effect of vitamin A and zinc supplementation on diarrheal disease and respiratory tract infections in children in Mexico City, Mexico. Am J Clin Nutr 83: 693–700

Luby SP, Mendoza C, Keswick B, Chiller TM, Hoekstra RM (2008) Difficulties in bringing point-of-use water treatment to scale in rural Guatemala. Am J Trop Med Hyg 78(3):382–387.

Mintz E, Barteram J, Lochery P, Wegflin M (2001) Not just a drop in the bucket: expanding access to point-of-use water treatment systems. Am J Public Health 91:1565–1570

Morris S, Black RE, Tomaskoviv L (2003) Predicting the distribution of under-five deaths by cause in countries without adequate vital registration systems. Int J Epidemiol 32:1041–1051

Murphy C, Hahn B, Volmink J (2004) Reduced osmolarity oral rehydration solution for treating cholera. Cochrane Data Base Rev CD003754

Neeser JR, Granato D, Rouvet M et al. (2000) *Lactobacillus johnsonii* La1 shares carbohydrate-binding specificities with several enteropathogenic bacteria. Glycobiology 10:1193–1199

Ochoa TJ, Salazar-Lindo E, Cleary TG (2004) Management of children with infection-associated persistent diarrhea. Semin Pediatr Infect Dis 15:229–236.

Qadri F, Svennerholm AM, Faruque AS, Sack RB (2005). Enterotoxigenic Escherichia coli in developing countries: epidemiology, microbiology, clinical features, treatment, and prevention. Clin Microbiol Rev 18:465–483

Penny ME, Marin RM, Duran A, Peerson JM, Lanata CF, Lonnerdal B, et al. 2004). Randomized controlled trial of the effect of daily supplementation with zinc or multiple micronutrients on the morbidity, growth, and micronutrient status of young Peruvian children. Am J Clin Nutr 79:457–465

Rahman MM, Vermund SH, Wahed MA, Fuchs GJ, Baqui AH, Alverez JO (2001). Simultaneous zinc and vitamin A supplementation in Bangladeshi children: a randomized double blind controlled trial. BMJ 323:314–318

Ruiz-Placacios GM, Perez-Schael L, Velazquez FR et al. (2006) Safety and efficacy of an attenuated vaccine against severe rotavirus gastroenteritis. N Engl J Med, 354:11–12

Sack DA, Sack RB, Nair B, Siddique AK (2004) Cholera. Lancet 363:223–233

Savioli L, Smith H, Thompson A (2006) *Giardia* and *Cryptosporidium* join the "neglected diseases initiative". Trends Parasitol 22:203–208

Sazawal S, BLack RE, Bhan MK, Jalla S, Sinha A Bhandari N (1997) Efficacy of zinc supplementation in reducing the incidence and prevalence of acute diarrhea – a community-based, double-blind, controlled trial. Am J Clin Nutr 66:413–418

Scrimshaw NS, Taylor CE, Gordon AJE. (1968) Interactions of nutrition and infection. WHO monograph series no. 57. World Health Organization, Geneva, Switzerland

Srinivas U, Braconier JH, Jeppsson B, Abdulla M, Akesson B, Ockerman PA (1988) Trace element alterations in infectious diseases. Scand J Clin Lab Invest 48:495–500

Shrimpton R (1993) Zinc deficiency – is it widespread but under-recognized? I: Subcommittee on Nutrition News. Vol 9, United Nations Administrative Committee on Coordination, Geneva

Snyder JD, Merson MH (1982) The magnitude of the global problem of acute diarrheal disease: a review of active surveillance data. Bull WHO 60:604–613

Sobsey MD (2002) Managing Water in the Home: Accelerated Health Gains from Improved Water Supply, Geneva, World Health Organization

Stauffer W, Ravdin JI (2003) Entamoeba histolytica: an update. Curr Opin Infect Dis 16(5): 479–485

Su LH, Chiu CH, Chu C, Ou JT (2004) Antimicrobial resistance in nontyphoid Salmonella serotypes: a global challenge. Clin Inf Dis 39:546–551

Tacket CO, Losonsky G, Nataro JP et al. (1992) Onset and duration of protective immunity in challenged volunteers after vaccination with live oral cholera vaccine CVD 103-HgR. J Infect Dis 166:837–841

Tanaka G, Faruque ASG, Luby SP, et al. (2007) Deaths from rotavirus disease in Bangladeshi children: estimates from hospital-based surveillance. Pediatr Inf Dis J 26:1014–1018

Taylor DN, Echeverria P, Pal T, Sethabutr O, Saiborisuth S, Sricharmorn S, Rowe B, Cross J (1986) The role of *Shigella* spp., enteroinvasive *Escherichia coli*, and other enteropathogens as causes of childhood dysentery in Thailand. J Inf Dis 153(6):1132–1138

Van Niel CW, Feudtner C, Garrison MM, Christakis DA (2002) Lactobacillus therapy for acute infectious diarrhea in children: a meta-analysis. Pediatrics 109:678–684

Vesikari T, Matson DO, Dennehy P, et al. (2006) Safety and efficacy of a pentavalent human-bovine (WC3) reassortant rotavirus vaccine. N Engl J Med 354, 23–33

Victora CG, Bryce J, Fontaine O, Monasch R (2000) Reducing deaths from diarrhea through oral rehydration therapy. Bull WHO 78:1246–1255

Weintraub A (2007) Enteroaggregative Escherichia coli: epidemiology, virulence and detection. J Med Microbiol 56:4–8

WHO Collaborative Study Team (2000) Effect of breastfeeding on infant and child mortality due to infectious diseases in less developed countries: a pooled analysis. Lancet, 355:451–455

WHO (2003) HIV and Breastfeeding – a Framework for Priority Action. Geneva: WHO

WHO/UNICEF (2004) Joint Statement on Clinical Management of Acute Diarrhea. WHO/FHC/CAH/04.7. Geneva: WHO; New York: UNICEF

Write J, Gundry S, Conroy R (2004) Household drinking water in developing countries: a systematic review of microbiological contamination between source and point-of-use. Trop Med Int Health 9:106–117

Chapter 18
Bloodborne and Sexual Transmission: HIV/AIDS

Charlotte van den Berg, Karen Lindenburg, and Roel Coutinho

18.1 HIV-1 Pandemic

In 2007, approximately 33 million people were estimated to be living with human immunodeficiency virus (HIV)-1 worldwide. An estimated 2.5 million became newly infected with HIV-1 that year, while an estimated 2.1 million died of AIDS. This means that everyday almost 6,850 people are newly infected with HIV-1, and over 5,750 die from AIDS, mostly because of inadequate access to HIV-1 prevention and treatment services. In the 27 years since the first cases of AIDS were described, approximately 20 million people have died from AIDS.

HIV-1 infection predominantly strikes young, sexually active adults, and children. This has an important impact on the social and economical situation in countries with a high HIV-1-prevalence, because this way the people who can make the largest contribution to the social structures and economical vitality in a region are lost through illness or death.

Worldwide most new HIV-1 infections are transmitted heterosexually or from mother to child. Depending on the geographic region, a sizeable proportion of new HIV-1 infections are attributable to other risk factors like male homosexual contact or injecting drug use.

18.1.1 Sub-Saharan Africa

Sub-Saharan Africa is the region with the largest burden of the AIDS epidemic, more than two thirds of all HIV-1-positive people live in this region and about three quarters of all AIDS deaths in 2007 occurred in sub-Saharan Africa. Approximately 1.7 million people were newly infected with HIV-1 in 2007, bringing the total number of HIV-1-infected individuals in the region to 22.5 million. The HIV-1 epidemic

K. Lindenburg (✉)
Cluster Infectious Diseases, Public Health Service of Amsterdam, Amsterdam, The Netherlands
e-mail: klindenburg@ggd.amsterdam.nl

**CB and KL contributed equally to this chapter*

A. Krämer et al. (eds.), *Modern Infectious Disease Epidemiology*,
Statistics for Biology and Health, DOI 10.1007/978-0-387-93835-6_18,

in sub-Saharan Africa is mainly driven by heterosexually transmitted infections. Therefore, and unlike HIV-1 epidemics in other parts of the world, the majority of people living with HIV-1 in sub-Saharan Africa (61%) are women.

Southern Africa is the most gravely affected region of sub-Saharan Africa. In 2005, national adult HIV-1 prevalence exceeded 15% in 8 countries (Botswana, Lesotho, Mozambique, Namibia, South Africa, Swaziland, Zambia, and Zimbabwe). In studies among women attending antenatal care in South Africa, prevalences as high as 30% have been reported. In most countries in southern Africa the epidemics seem to be plateauing (UNAIDS 2008).

18.1.2 Europe and North America

The World Health Organization (WHO) calculated that in 2007 there were an estimated 740,000 people living with HIV-1 or AIDS in Western and Central Europe. The largest proportion of new HIV-1 diagnoses is heterosexually acquired, mainly in migrants and immigrants from high endemic countries. In Western Europe in 2007, approximately 30% of new HIV-1 diagnoses were among men having sex with men (MSM). Only 6% was attributable to injecting drug use. Between 1999 and 2006 the number of new HIV-1 diagnoses attributed to unsafe sex between men nearly doubled, while those attributed to injecting drug use declined in the same period. In Spain and Portugal, countries where injecting drug use is more prevalent than in the rest of Western Europe, the majority of new HIV-1 infections occurs through the use of contaminated equipment by injecting drug users (IDU). There has been an increase in the number of new HIV-1 diagnoses in Western Europe since 2002, opposed to a relatively stable number of new HIV-1 infections each year in North America. This discrepancy is probably partly explained by an increase in HIV-1 testing resulting from a change in HIV-1 testing policy in Europe. As many as 30% of people infected with HIV-1 in Europe may be unaware of their HIV-1-status. People who are unaware of their HIV-1-status cannot benefit from treatment and care and may transmit HIV-1 to others. Almost universal access to effective antiretroviral treatment (ART) has helped to keep the number of AIDS-related deaths in these regions comparatively low.

Like in Western Europe, the most important risk factor for HIV-1 is unsafe sex between men in the United States and Canada. Furthermore, racial and ethnic minorities have a higher HIV-1 prevalence (UNAIDS 2008; EuroHIV 2007).

18.1.3 Former Soviet Union and Central Asia

Approximately 150,000 people were newly infected with HIV-1 in 2007, bringing the number of people living with HIV-1 in Eastern Europe and Central Asia to approximately 1.6 million people. This is a 1.5-fold increase compared to the situation in 2001. The majority (90%) of the new infections were in two countries: the Russian Federation and Ukraine. Also in Azerbaijan, Georgia, Kazakhstan, Kyrgyzstan, the Republic of Moldova, Tajikistan, and Uzbekistan the annual numbers of newly reported HIV-1 diagnoses are rising. The driving force behind the epidemic in Eastern Europe and Central Asia is injecting drug use; nearly two thirds of the new HIV-1 infections could be attributed to this route of transmission. In the Baltic States (Estonia, Latvia, and Lithuania), where the epidemics appear to have stabilized, injecting drug use is also the most-reported mode of HIV-1 transmission (UNAIDS 2008).

18.1.4 Southeast Asia

In Southeast Asia the HIV-1 epidemic is widespread and behaves differently in different countries. In some countries HIV-1 prevalence is declining (i.e., Cambodia, Myanmar, and Thailand), while in others (e.g., Indonesia) the epidemic is increasing.

In China, injecting drug use has been the most important driving force behind the HIV-1 epidemic; however, heterosexual transmission is an increasingly important issue. The Chinese Ministry of Health and UNAIDS estimated that half of new HIV-1 infections were due to injecting drug use, and half to unprotected sex. One of the problems China is facing is the overlap between injecting drug use and commercial sex work, with many female IDUs selling sex and many male IDUs buying sex, often without using condoms. In the larger Chinese cities, the HIV-1 epidemic among MSM is also rising, with some studies reporting a HIV-1 prevalence of 1.5–4.6% (UNAIDS 2008; Liu et al. 2006).

18.1.5 Other Areas of the World

No region of the world has remained untouched by the HIV pandemic. In Asia, besides Southeast Asia, the main mode of acquisition is through injecting drug use, and the prevalence in the general population remains low. The available epidemiological data for the Middle Eastern and North-African region is limited. It is estimated that there are 380,000 people living with HIV-1 in this region.

In the Caribbean the prevalence of HIV-1 in adults is estimated to be 1.0%; the main mode of transmission is through unprotected sexual intercourse. In Central and South America the HIV-1 epidemic remained stable in the past years with higher HIV-1 prevalence in high-risk populations, i.e., MSM and commercial sex workers.

About three quarters of the people living with HIV/AIDS in Oceania live in Papua New Guinea, where the HIV-1 prevalence in adults is 1.8%. In Australia and New Zealand the most new HIV-1 infections occur in MSM (UNAIDS 2008).

18.2 HIV Pathogenesis

18.2.1 Virology

18.2.1.1 HIV-1

The probable origin of HIV-1 in humans is the introduction of simian immunodeficiency virus (SIVcpz) from chimpanzees (*Pan troglodytes*) in the human population, while HIV-2 has originated from SIVsm in sooty mangabeys (*Cercocebus atys*). The worldwide pandemic is caused by HIV-1. Based on molecular epidemiological models it is estimated that HIV-1 was introduced in the human population in the mid-20th century. Phylogenetic analyses have shown that there must have been at least three distinct introductions of HIV-1 in the human population. These three introductions – originating from different three SIVcpz subtypes – gave rise to the three HIV-1 lineages: M-, N-, and O-group (Main, non-M-non-O, and Outlier group). Within the M-group nine subtypes exist (named A through K). HIV-1 viruses from the M-group are most widespread and have originated from a *lentivirus* found in *Pan troglodytes troglodytes*. Individuals infected with viruses from the O-group originate mainly from Cameroon, Gabon, and Equatorial Guinea and the viruses have originated from a *lentivirus* in a distinct Chimpanzee subspecies, *Pan troglodytes schweinfurthii*. Group N was most recently discovered and it has spread the least, it has been documented in individuals from Cameroon. This virus is a mosaic of SIVcpz and HIV-1-related sequences, indicating a recombination event in an ancestral chimpanzee host. The clinical course of infection with diverse subtypes is similar.

18.2.1.2 HIV-1 Lifecycle

When a cell is infected with two different HIV-1 subtypes, the viruses can swap parts of their genetic material (i.e., recombination). When the resultant virus recombinant is found in one individual, this new virus is called a unique recombinant form. When recombinant forms are found in at least three individuals that cannot be epidemiologically linked to each other, this recombinant form is called a circulating recombinant form (CRF). In some parts of the world, these CRF contribute substantially to the epidemic (e.g., in Thailand AE-CRF).

HIV-1 infected individuals can be infected with another HIV-1 virus after their initial infection, so-called superinfection.

HIV-1 is a retrovirus and belongs to the family of lentiviruses. When HIV-1 enters the human body via mucosal membranes (e.g., sexual transmission) or via direct injection in the bloodstream (e.g., injecting drug use, blood transfusion), it binds to a CD4 receptor and a coreceptor on the cell surface. The virus undergoes a conformational change and fuses with the cell membrane. The HIV-1 RNA is released into the cell. Next, HIV-1 reverse transcriptase transcribes single-stranded HIV-1 RNA into double-stranded HIV-1 DNA. This HIV-1 DNA is then transported to the cell nucleus, where it is integrated in the host DNA, this is called a provirus. The provirus can remain inactive in the host DNA for years without producing new HIV-1 copies. The formation of new HIV-1 copies starts when (host) RNA polymerase transcribes the provirus into HIV-1 RNA and messenger RNA (mRNA). The HIV-1 enzyme protease cuts the long chains of HIV-1 proteins into smaller individual proteins. Once these proteins and HIV-1 RNA come together, new HIV-1 particles are formed. These newly formed HIV-1 particles bud out of the cell, and while doing that they also use some of the cell membrane as their envelope. This envelope is heavily covered with so-called glycoproteins, necessary for binding to CD4 and other cell surface receptors. The newly formed viruses can now move further and infect other cells (Geretti 2006; Coakley et al. 2005; Kanki et al. 1997).

18.2.1.3 HIV-2

HIV-2 has approximately 60% genetic homology with HIV-1, but is transmitted at a lower rate and the clinical course is much more benign. However, progression to AIDS does occur and some patients will require therapy. HIV-2 is more or less geographically restricted to West Africa, and HIV-2 infected people in other regions of the world are mostly epidemiologically linked to this region. The genomic arrangement of HIV-2 is indistinguishable from SIVsm, the two viruses are phylogenetically closely related and the sooty mangabey natural habitat coincides with the epicenter of the HIV-2 epidemic. The prevalence of SIVsm is high in wild-living sooty mangabeys. Close contact between humans and sooty mangabeys is common because the monkeys are hunted for food and they are kept as pets. It has been proposed that at least six independent transmissions of SIVsm to humans have taken place (Myers et al. 1992; Stebbing and Moyle 2003; AIDSinfo 2008; Peeters 2000).

18.2.2 Immunology

HIV-1 uses two different types of receptors for attachment to target cells and viral entry. First the envelope protein gp120 attaches to the CD4 molecule expressed mainly on the surface of helper T lymphocytes and macrophages. Viral binding to CD4 is crucial, but for viral entry also coreceptors are needed. Interaction between CD4 and gp120 increases the affinity of virus for coreceptor molecules. The two most important HIV-1 coreceptors, CCR5 and CXCR4, are differentially expressed on subpopulations of CD4-expressing cells. Viruses differ in ability to attach to different coreceptors and can be defined by coreceptor use. The coreceptor usage of a HIV-1 virus is determined by genetic variation in HIV-1 envelope domains. Host genetic polymorphisms or deletions within the gene coding for CCR5 diminish or abrogate viral binding to the coreceptor, which leads to a lower susceptibility to infection and slower disease progression in such persons (e.g., CCR5Δ32 deletion) (Coakley et al. 2005).

In the first weeks after HIV-1 infection, there is a massive depletion of $CD4^+/CCR5^+$ memory T cells in all mucosal surfaces. Normally, the largest pool of memory $CD4^+$ T cells in the body resides in submucosal areas. This depletion is caused by target cell infection and virus-induced apoptosis. In the acute phase of HIV-1 infection, HIV-1 viremia can reach very high levels of more than 1×10^6 HIV-1-RNA copies/mL.

After approximately 6 months the plasma HIV-1-RNA concentration stabilizes, and this more or less stable level is called the viral setpoint. This viral setpoint is one of the strongest predictors of the time of progression to AIDS, independent of age at time of infection. Although the rate of progression from infection to AIDS is multifactorially determined, individuals with a higher viral setpoint typically have a faster progression to AIDS than individuals with a lower viral setpoint. There is a strong correlation between the height of the viral setpoint and the amount of immune activation, as measured by immune activation markers like CD38 and HLA-DR or proliferation markers like Ki67. Individuals with a high viral load have higher levels of immune activation.

The CD4 decline eventually leading to AIDS is attributed to the chronic immune activation that is caused by the high amount of virus present in the blood. This idea is supported by studies showing that in patients that are treated with highly active antiretroviral therapy (HAART) the activation status of $CD4^+$ T cells normalizes while the CD4 count has not yet returned to normal levels.

18.3 HIV-1 Transmission

18.3.1 Sexual Transmission

Although HIV-1 has been isolated from many body fluids of HIV-1 infected individuals, the virus is only transmitted through contaminated blood and blood products, semen, vaginal fluids, and breast milk. Worldwide, most HIV-1 infections are transmitted sexually. The probability of sexual transmission is a function of infectivity, susceptibility, and type of sexual practice. These factors are closely interconnected, with each individual factor influenced by several aspects. HIV-1 blood plasma viral load (BPVL) is the strongest predictor of sexual HIV-1 transmission with higher BPVL associated with an increased infectivity, probably through increased genital HIV-1 viral loads (Chan 2006). High BPVL is observed during primary HIV-1 infection and advanced HIV-1 disease. The risk for HIV-1 transmission is calculated to increase by 8–10 times during primary HIV-1 infection (Wawer et al. 2005).

In Table 18.1, risks of HIV-1 transmission per exposure to a known HIV-1 positive source are presented (Eurosurveillance 2004). For sexual transmission, receptive partners are at greater risk for HIV-1 acquisition through unprotected sex compared with insertive partners. The odds ratio (OR) for male to female HIV-1 transmission is 2–3 times higher than the OR for female to male transmission. The

Table 18.1 HIV-1 transmission risk per exposure to a known HIV-1 positive source (Almeda et al. 2004)

Type of exposure	Risk of HIV-1 transmission per exposure (%)
Receptive oral sex	0– 0.04
Insertive vaginal sex	≤ 0.1
Insertive anal sex	≤ 0.1
Receptive vaginal sex	0.01– 0.15
Receptive anal sex	≤ 3
Accidental needlestick	0.2–0.4
IDU sharing needle	0.7
Transfusion	90–100

larger anatomical surface area of the vagina, with a higher number of HIV-1 susceptible cells, might be a biological explanation for this difference. Unprotected receptive anal intercourse with a known HIV-1 positive partner is associated with the highest sexual transmission risk. Rectal mucosa is easily ruptured, providing an entry point for HIV-1 and the lymphoid tissue of the gut wall contains many lymphocytes which are targets for HIV-1. Risk for HIV-1 transmission for women during unsafe receptive vaginal intercourse varies between 0.01 and 0.2% per coitus for serodiscordant couples. For oral-genital sexual contacts the risk of HIV-1 transmission is thought to be very low. Transmission risks are shown in Table 18.1 and discussed in Chapter 7.

Sexually transmitted infections (STI) increase both the infectiousness of HIV-1 infected individuals as well the susceptibility for HIV-1 acquisition of those uninfected. Genital tract inflammation increases the genital shedding of HIV-1, most likely as the result of locally released cytokines as well as leakage of HIV-1 from the blood plasma. The number of activated target cells for HIV-1 ($CD4^+$ T cells and macrophages) may be increased by several bacterial and viral STI, leading to an increased susceptibility. In addition, STI can cause (micro) ulcerations that may bleed, thereby increasing both the infectiousness of and the susceptibility to HIV-1.

The most common ulcerative genital disease worldwide, caused by Herpes simplex virus type 2 (HSV-2), is associated with 4.5 times increased infectivity and susceptibility for HIV-1 infection (Wald and Link 2002; Corey et al. 2004). Recent acquisition of HSV-2, compared with prevalent HSV-2 infection, carries a higher risk of HIV-1 transmission, while asymptomatic and symptomatic HSV-2 infection carry almost the same probability of acquiring HIV-1 per coital act. Most HSV-2 reactivations are subclinical, but mucosal damage and lymphocytosis occur during this phase as shown by microscopy. HIV-1 is associated with an increased rate of reactivation of HSV-2, with the rate of reactivation correlated to CD4+ T-cell count and HIV-1 BPVL (Schacker et al. 1998). Non-ulcerative STI, like gonorrhea and *Chlamydia trachomatis* infection can increase both infectivity and susceptibility to HIV transmission. Additionally, several other factors influence sexual HIV-1 transmission. Systemic illnesses, opportunistic infections, as well as recent vaccinations may increase the HIV-1 BPVL, increasing HIV-1 infectivity (Chan 2006). Nonspecific urethritis is associated with increased susceptibility for HIV-1. Cervicitis, pelvic inflammatory disease, and bacterial vaginosis, associated with low concentrations of hydrogen peroxide-producing lactobacilli, appear to increase the risk of HIV-1 acquisition (Fig. 18.1).

18.3.2 Blood and Blood Products

IDU are at risk for HIV-1 infection through sharing of needles and syringes and borrowing and lending of other paraphernalia. The risk for HIV-1 transmission through the sharing of needles and syringes is approximately 0.7% (Eurosurveillance 2004)

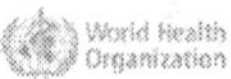

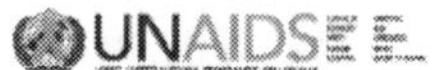

Adults and children estimated to be living with HIV, 2007

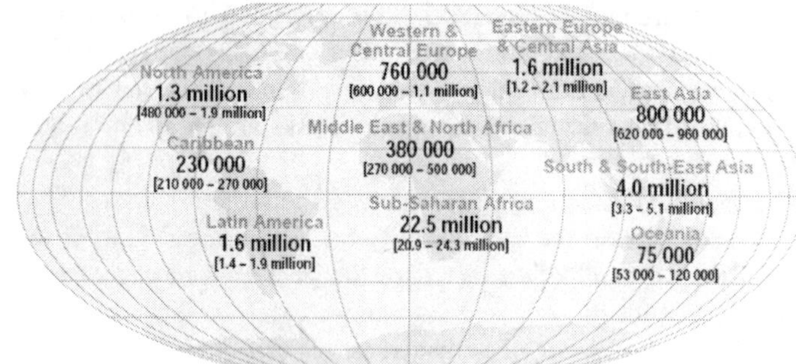

Total: 33.2 (30.6 – 36.1) million

Fig. 18.1 Worldwide distribution of HIV-1 infections. Reproduced with kind permission from UNAIDS (www.unaids.org)

per act. Increased inoculum size is associated with an increased risk of HIV-1 transmission.

Transfusion of HIV-1 infected blood and blood products carries a 90–100% chance of HIV-1 transmission. In the early 1980s, before the implementation of safe methods to make blood products, many hemophiliacs were infected with HIV-1.

18.3.3 Mother-to-Child Transmission

Worldwide, mother-to-child transmission (MTCT) is the primary mode of HIV-1 acquisition among children. HIV-1 transmission can occur during pregnancy, labor, or breast-feeding. In non-breast-feeding women, the estimated risk of HIV-1 MTCT is between 15 and 25%, while this risk varies between 25 and 40% in breast-feeding populations (Dao et al. 2007). High maternal HIV-1 BPVL and preterm delivery are risk factors for HIV-1 transmission. Vaginal delivery carries an increased risk of MTCT, compared to elective caesarean section (before labor and before ruptured membranes). HIV-1 transmission through breast-feeding accounts for about 33–50% of all HIV-1 MTCT in resource-limited settings where breast-feeding into the second year of life is the norm. Some studies have suggested that the highest risk of breast milk transmission is in the immediate neonatal period but it is difficult to differentiate between early breast milk transmission and intrapartum transmission. However, two studies showed a high risk of HIV-1 transmission in the first weeks of life through breast-feeding, compared to those who gave formula from birth. In breast milk of infected women HIV-1 viral load was found to be highest immediately after delivery. The risk of HIV-1 transmission per month of breast-feeding was calculated to be 0.6–0.7% in the first year of life and 0.3% in the second year in a study in Malawi. However, a recent meta-analysis showed a more constant risk of about 0.9% per month after the first month of life. Risk factors associated with postnatal HIV-1 transmission include higher HIV-1 viral load in plasma and in milk, decreased maternal CD4$^+$ T-cell count, mastitis or breast milk stasis, oral thrush of the baby, and longer duration of breast-feeding. Additionally, breast- and formula-feeding combined, versus exclusive breast-feeding, is associated with a higher HIV-1 transmission. This might be explained by intestinal mucosal damage or immune activation, providing a port of entry for HIV-1.

18.4 HIV-1 Disease Progression

18.4.1 Natural History

HIV-1 infects CD4$^+$ T lymphocytes, thereby destroying and harming important players in the immune reaction against foreign pathogens. The natural history of HIV-1 infection can be divided in three phases: acute 'primary' HIV-1 infection, the chronic phase of infection, and the last stage: AIDS (acquired immunodeficiency syndrome).

The primary HIV-1 infection can take up to 6 months. During this phase, most patients remain asymptomatic, approximately one-third of patients suffer from a-specific flu-like symptoms. During acute HIV-1 infection, the number of HIV-1 copies in plasma is usually very high and there is frequently a simultaneous drop in CD4$^+$ T-cell count.

After acute infection, infected persons remain asymptomatic for years during chronic infection. During this period however, the CD4$^+$ T-cell count continues to decrease gradually. The median time without treatment from acute infection to the AIDS is 8–10 years, but this varies widely between individuals (Collaborative Group on AIDS incubation and HIV survival 2000).

Host genetic factors play a role in susceptibility to HIV-1 infection and are the main determinants of the time from infection to development of AIDS. Since HIV-1 uses CCR5 as coreceptor for host cell entry, a normal structure of this molecule is required for infection. People with a certain genetic variation of their CCR5-molecule have a truncated form of this molecule (CCR5Δ32), and are less vulnerable to infection after exposure. While some individuals develop AIDS fast, approximately 5% of HIV-1 infected individuals are so-called long-term non-progressors and can take more than 20 years to progress to AIDS. One of the major host genetic factors associated with long-term non-progression are the human leukocyte antigens (HLA) B27 and HLA B57, molecules involved in presenting antigens to the immune system.

It has been suggested that geographic factors and behavior influences the rate of progression to AIDS. However, the overall time span is the same for all individuals and is not dependent on demographic factors (e.g., where one lives: tropics or

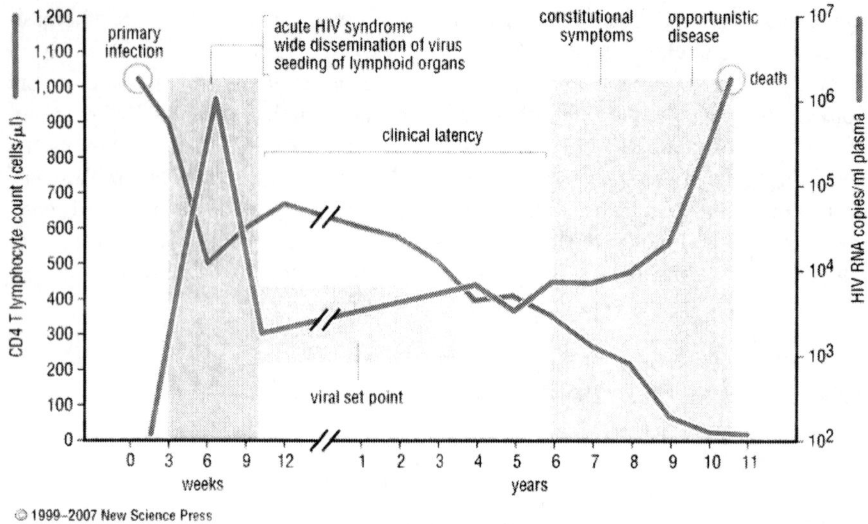

Fig. 18.2 The natural history of HIV [(reproduced with permission from Immunity by AL DeFranco, RM Locksley and M Robertson (New Science Press, London, 2007)]

western world) or on acquisition route (e.g., how one contracted HIV-1: injecting drug use, unsafe homosexual, or heterosexual contact). Age does influence the rate of progression to AIDS, older individuals progress faster to AIDS than do younger individuals (Pezzotti et al. 1996) (Fig. 18.2).

18.4.2 Opportunistic Infections and Coinfections

As the immune system deteriorates during the course of HIV-1 infection, infections with other micro-organisms or viruses that do not necessarily cause illness in immunocompetent hosts, can cause severe morbidity and mortality. Opportunistic and coinfections with other micro-organisms or viruses in HIV-1 infected individuals cause a great increase of HIV-1-related morbidity and mortality. Some micro-organisms share geographic regions or routes of transmission. When the $CD4^+$ T-cell count drops below 200 $CD4^+$ T cells/mL, the risk of opportunistic infections increases dramatically. Also cancers in which a viral pathogenesis is involved (e.g., human herpes virus 8 (HHV-8) in Kaposi's sarcoma, Epstein–Barr virus in Burkitt lymphoma) have a higher incidence in HIV-1 infected individuals.

18.4.2.1 Tuberculosis

Tuberculosis (TB) is caused by infection with *Mycobacterium tuberculosis*. After infection with *M. tuberculosis* some persons develop disease early, while in others it causes latent infection and is not infectious for the surrounding. When active TB develops, the mycobacterium can be transmitted to other people. HIV-1 infection is the strongest risk factor for the development of active TB. TB is an aggressive opportunistic infection that arises at higher median CD4 counts than other opportunistic infections. HIV-1 also increases the risk of rapid TB progression after infection or re-infection with TB. TB is the leading cause of death among HIV-1-infected persons and may accelerate the course of HIV-1 infection, increasing the HIV-1 load in some patients (Corbett et al. 2003; Corbett et al. 2006).

18.4.2.2 Hepatitis C Virus

Hepatitis C virus (HCV) was first identified in 1989. HCV is mainly transmitted parenterally, and therefore HIV-1-HCV coinfection is common in individuals that are exposed to infected blood (e.g., IDU, recipients of blood transfusion before screening was introduced). Acute HCV is usually asymptomatic and progresses to chronic HCV viremia in 60–80% of individuals. After decades of chronic HCV infection liver cirrhosis develops in a third of individuals. Of these 1–5% per year develop hepatocellular carcinoma (primary liver cell cancer). There is no prophylactic or therapeutic vaccination against HCV available.

HIV-1/HCV coinfection is associated with a faster progression to liver cirrhosis and with lower success rates of anti-HCV treatment. Furthermore, HIV-1/HCV coinfection leads to higher mortality, even if HIV-1 is treated with HAART. The effect of HCV coinfection on HIV-1 disease progression is not clear (Shepard et al. 2005; Alter 2006; Koziel and Peters 2007).

18.4.2.3 Hepatitis B Virus

Hepatitis B virus (HBV) accounts for an estimated 370 million chronic infection worldwide, an estimated 2–4 million HIV-1-infected persons have chronic HBV coinfection. Vaccination against HBV is possible. The rate of HBV viral persistence after acute infection depends on the age at HBV infection. Immunocompetent adults clear HBV in more than 90% of infections, while children infected in the perinatal period or during childhood clear only in approximately 10% of infections. In adult HIV-1 infected individuals that are acutely infected with HBV, 20% develop chronic HBV infection. As with HCV infection, HIV-1/HBV coinfection increases the progression to cirrhosis, and death from liver disease, especially in patients with a low $CD4^+$ cell count or concomitant alcohol use (Alter 2006; Koziel and Peters 2007).

18.5 Prevention

Models have predicted that strong global commitment for the expansion of HIV-1 prevention programs might avert 28 million new HIV-1 infections through 2015 (Stover et al. 2006). Prevention methods are focused on decreasing risk behavior, infectivity, and susceptibility for HIV-1.

18.5.1 Behavioral Interventions

Behavioral interventions aim to reduce sexual and drug use-related risk behavior. Male condoms are cheap and effective in preventing HIV-1 and other STI. Female condoms have these same features, but are hardly used because of impracticalities. Many countries have adopted the ABC approach, sequentially advising sexual abstinence, being faithful, and Condom use. Reduction of the presence of STI on population level might affect the HIV-1 epidemic but its effectiveness on population levels depends on factors like the stage of the HIV-1 epidemic and sexual networks. Many approaches to prevent STI have been implemented and have proven to effectively lower the prevalence of some major STI in many parts of the world. However, the effectiveness of these programs to reduce HIV-1 incidence remains unproven.

Needle exchange and methadone maintenance programs have been found to decrease drug use-related risk behavior. However, the coverage of such programs for drug users is still very low.

18.5.2 Prophylactic Antiretroviral Interventions to Prevent MTCT

In their landmark study, the Paediatric AIDS Clinical Trial Group found that by treating women and their infants with the antiretroviral agent zidovudine, the HIV-1 transmission risk was reduced from 25 to 8% (Ellerbrock et al. 1991). Additionally, several trials were conducted to evaluate the effect of short-course antiretroviral therapy (ART) regimens on MTCT, comparing different agents and regimens. Overall, combining several ART agents proved to be more effective as did longer duration of prophylactic ART. In developed countries where women have access to HAART the risk of HIV-1 transmission from mother to child can be reduced to 1–2%.

An important clinical study, the HIV-1 NET 012 trial showed that, in breast-feeding populations, a single dose of nevirapine (NVP) at labor onset and a single dose of NVP to newborns reduced the risk of HIV-1 transmission by nearly 50% at approximately 6–8 weeks after birth compared to a short course of zidovudine. In Africa, this shortest possible ART regimen has greatly reduced the risk of intrapartum HIV-1 transmission (Guay et al. 1999). However, the efficacy of prophylaxis against MTCT diminishes gradually with continued breast-feeding after the prophylaxis has stopped. The long half-life of NVP might have a protective effect on early breast milk HIV-1-transmission, thereby possibly preventing MTCT during the first weeks of life (Fowler and Newell 2002). On the other hand, the prolonged presence of this single drug promotes the development of drug resistance by HIV-1. This risk is strongly related to higher maternal plasma RNA levels and lower CD4 counts at the time of exposure (Eshleman et al. 2001). The proportion of viral variants with NVP resistance declines over time, but low levels of resistant virus can be detected for more than 1 year after exposure (Dao et al. 2007). The clinical significance of this resistance remains unclear. Studies have shown that previous exposure to a single-dose NVP (SD-NVP) did not reduce the efficacy of SD-NVP in subsequent pregnancies. In addition, studies did not find a significant difference in virological response to NVP-based regimens among women who began treatment more than 6 months after SD-NVP, while initiating treatment less than 6 months after SD-NVP was associated with worse virological response in two studies.

The 2006 WHO guidelines regarding the use of ART for prevention of MTCT in resource-limited countries aim to optimize access to high-quality services. It calls for the best MTCT interventions where feasible, at least some effective MTCT interventions at all levels of the health system, and worldwide maximization of populations reached. The key principle in the 2006 WHO guidelines is the evaluation of pregnant women for their personal ART need; ART should be provided if necessary and continued indefinitely after delivery. This requires adequate infrastructure and manpower for CD4+ T-cell testing. While choosing ART regimens maternal health status and possible detrimental effects of drug exposure to fetal organ development should be evaluated. For women who are not eligible for ART, the WHO recommends AZT starting at 28 weeks of gestation (or as soon as feasible thereafter), intrapartum SD-NVP, and a single dose of NVP combined with 1 week of AZT for the infant. Where access to ART is limited, at least the SD-NVP should be made available to mothers and infants. However, this most simple regime is not widely accessible. It is estimated that currently <10% of HIV-1-infected women in sub-Saharan Africa receive ART during pregnancy or delivery. Even in settings where SD-NVP is available, uptake has been limited due to infrequent HIV-1 testing (not offered or not accepted), inconsistent supplies, inadequate numbers of staff, and reluctance of women to disclose their status. As a result, only half of eligible women receive NVP in settings where PMTCT programs are in place. In contrast, in developed countries, with the implementation of universal prenatal HIV-1 testing, using a combination of several ART agents and elective caesarean delivery when indicated, overall MTCT rates have dropped to about 1–2% (Dao et al. 2007; Fowler et al. 2007; Cooper et al. 2002; Luzuriaga and Sullivan 2005).

A key factor limiting the scaling up of MTCT programs is the lack of knowledge of HIV-1 serostatus. For that reason, several countries have recently adopted the opting-out approach in which certain risk groups attending health facilities are informed that a HIV-1 test is routinely performed, unless individuals specifically refuse.

18.5.3 Formula Feeding

The WHO recommends exclusive breast-feeding for HIV-1-infected women for the first 6 months of their baby's life, unless replacement feeding is 'acceptable, feasible, affordable, sustainable, and safe for mother and child.' In many parts of the world these criteria cannot be met, but if so, avoidance of all breast-feeding by HIV-1-infected women is recommended. The benefits of breast-feeding in settings with poor hygiene, unsafe water and lack of affordable substitutes for breast milk, and the related child morbidity and mortality thereof, have to be balanced against the risk of postnatal HIV-1 transmission.

18.5.4 Caesarean Deliveries

Early observational studies showed conflicting results on the preventive effect of caesarean delivery, through which exposure to blood and genital secretions in the birth canal is reduced, on MTCT. In 1998, elective caesarean delivery was demonstrated to reduce HIV-1 transmission by 50–80% in both a European randomized trial, dependent on the timing of the procedure, as well as on a meta-analysis (Fowler et al. 2007). In the USA this led to the recommendation that all women with HIV-1 viral loads >1000 copies/mL should be counseled on the benefits of elective caesarean delivery, which should be performed at 38 completed weeks of gestation. In America and Europe this has led to an increase in the proportion of HIV-1-infected women having caesarean deliveries. In developing countries there are limited data suggesting that the risks of postpartum morbidity or mortality among HIV-1-infected women who have caesarean deliveries are increased (Jamieson et al. 2007). The benefits of caesarean delivery in these settings need to be weighed against potential increases in maternal and infant morbidity and mortality and the costs related to this procedure. Whether caesarean delivery is beneficial in the era of HAART among women with undetectable viral load, remains unanswered; a report from the European Collaborative Study did not find a statistically significant protective effect of caesarean delivery in multivariate analyses (Luzuriaga and Sullivan 2005).

18.5.5 Male Circumcision

Over the years, several epidemiological studies have suggested the protective effect of male circumcision on HIV-1-acquisition. However, early studies could not control for potential confounding factors and results were conflicting. Since 2005, three randomized controlled field trials have been stopped after interim analyses on the recommendation of the Data Safety and Monitoring Boards (DSMB), when strong reductions (51–60%) in HIV-1-acquisition were observed among those circumcised (Auvert et al. 2005; Bailey et al. 2007; Gray et al. 2007). This reduction might be explained by several biological mechanisms. The inner mucosa of the foreskin is less keratinized and has a higher density of HIV-1 target cells (Langerhans cells and dendritic cells) than external skin mucosa, rendering the foreskin more susceptible for HIV-1 infection. The foreskin may be damaged by epithelial lesions during sexual intercourse, providing an entry point for HIV-1. Whether male circumcision will be implemented on larger scales will be influenced by social factors, and cultural and religious acceptability of this prevention method relative to the availability and acceptance of other prevention methods. Increased sexual high-risk behavior by circumcised men may negatively influence HIV-1-incidence and prevention messages should focus on this aspect. Studies are currently undertaken to look into the long-term effects of male circumcision, measuring HIV-1-incidence and post-intervention risk behavior.

18.5.6 Microbicides

Women are at risk for HIV-1 infection mainly through heterosexual transmission and often have no control over condom use by their sexual partners based on cultural, social, or economic inequalities. The development of topical agents which could be applied vaginally or rectally, aiming to prevent transmission of HIV-1 and/or other STI, so-called microbicides, could empower women and influence the HIV-1 epidemic. Over the years, advances in investment and product development have occurred. A major obstacle in the development of effective microbicides is the absence of an in vivo biomarker associated with protection. Agents in development focus on direct inactivation of HIV-1 through HIV-1 membrane disruption or the decrease of vaginal acidity, which has been associated with limited HIV-1 viral proliferation. Others agents target HIV-1 viral replication and HIV-1 or host-cell structures, thereby inhibiting HIV-1 entry. Several drugs that are currently used for systemic HIV-1 treatment might qualify for microbicidal use. However, issues on the possible development and transmission of drug resistant virus need to be resolved. Effective microbicides will probably contain several agents, targeting different steps of HIV-1 replication and entry. Ideally, microbicides should be non-immunogenic, provide long-lasting and broad protection through simple dosing regimens while being easily manufactured and distributed. Safety in microbicide development is of great concern with one of the first microbicides (cellulose sulfate) tested showing increased HIV-1 transmission through the induction of local inflammation. For this reason, two phase III trials with cellulose sulfate were ended prematurely. A recently completed phase III trial testing the efficacy of Carraguard found this product to be safe for vaginal use. However, Carraguard was not shown to be effective against HIV-1 transmission. Results from additional phase III trials are expected in 2009 (http://www.microbicide.org). Whether effective microbicides can be developed remains a topic of scientific debate.

18.5.7 HIV-1 Vaccines

The only solution to halt the HIV-1 pandemic may be a safe, broadly protective vaccine. Development is hindered by the lack of a good animal model for HIV-1, the great genetic variability of HIV-1, and the lack of clear correlates of protection against HIV-1 infection. Additionally, HIV-1 epitopes are hidden by protective structural carbohydrates that cover the antigens on the virus's surface and specific molecule configurations. Prophylactic vaccines are aimed at preventing HIV-1 infection. In contrast, therapeutic vaccines are designed to alter HIV-1 disease progression by lowering the level of viral replication and immune deterioration. Partially effective vaccines might render individuals less infectious which could reduce transmission probabilities. Overall, scientists believe that a vaccine that induces both strong humoral and cellular immune responses might provide the most promising agent to prevent or control HIV-1 infection. Several types of vaccines have been studied: envelope-based subunit vaccines, containing recombinant parts of HIV-1 envelope proteins; DNA vaccines; and recombinant vector vaccines, where HIV-1 genetic material is placed into harmless viruses expressing these genes to present pieces of HIV-1 to the immune system. Live attenuated HIV-1 vaccines are currently not being investigated for use in humans because of safety concerns. Since 1987 numerous HIV-1 vaccine products have entered clinical trials, including four phase III trials. Major setbacks in HIV-1 vaccine development occurred when the first phase III trial with Aidsvax, a single subunit vaccine, proved to be ineffective. Currently ongoing phase III vaccine trials consist of a prime-boost combination including a recombinant vector vaccine and a subunit, aiming to provoke both cellular and humoral immune responses (www.iavi.org). Disappointing results with clinical trials using the recombinant adenovirus type 5 (rAd5) vector developed by Merck were observed. Despite the potential of this vaccine to induce robust and durable cell mediated HIV-1 immune response no evidence of protection was found. Disturbingly, persons with high preexisting antibodies against adenovirus 5 were found to have an increased HIV incidence. These findings raise doubts about the possible future development of an effective HIV-1 vaccine.

18.5.8 PEP

Post-exposure prophylaxis (PEP), the provision of ART to prevent HIV-1 infection after risk situations have occurred, has become the standard of care in many developed countries for health-care workers who are accidentally exposed to an HIV-1 infected source. When the HIV-1 serostatus of the source is unknown, an individual risk assessment should be made when considering PEP, including evaluation of the risk group of the source and the type of exposure. PEP should be initiated within 72 hours after the incident and consists of 1 month of HAART. Over the years, only small observational studies have found PEP use to be protective and cost-effective for occupational exposure with a high risk of HIV-1 transmission (Pinkerton et al. 1997). However, a randomized controlled clinical trial to study PEP is neither feasible nor ethical. Guidelines for PEP after non-occupational exposure, like unprotected sex and unsafe drug use are of more recent date (European and American guidelines). Like for occupational accidents, PEP should be prescribed when the source is known to be HIV-1-infected and/or the type of exposure contains a high risk for transmission, i.e., receptive anal sex and deep injuries with fresh blood during needle stick exposures, and otherwise considered on a case-by-case basis. The efficacy of PEP for non-occupational exposure has not been shown. Subjects receiving PEP should be followed up for 6 months and checked for other infectious diseases like hepatitis B and hepatitis C.

18.5.9 PREP

Pre-exposure prophylaxis (PREP) is the use of ART before HIV-1 exposure, aiming to prevent infection in HIV-1 negative individuals. Animal studies have shown some protection through PREP. For years, PREP was thought to be unfeasible since no drug was available for the long-term use in healthy individuals, but the licensing of tenofovir (TDF) changed that situation. The only completed study to date, performed in Ghana, showed that TDF was safe but did not find a statistically significant protective effect. Currently, four clinical trials are conducted worldwide, evaluating the safety and efficacy of PREP regimens and results are expected in 2008. Three additional studies are planned (www.prepwatch.org). The effects of future (partially) protective PREP regimens might be counteracted, however, by simultaneous increases in sexual risk behavior.

18.6 Highly Active Antiretroviral Therapy

18.6.1 ART Classes

The HIV-1 replicative life cycle has different phases which form the potential targets for antiretroviral therapy (ART). ART can be divided into five main classes and the US Food and Drug Administration (FDA) had approved 31 compounds, including 6 combination products, by the end of 2007. The nucleoside reverse transcriptase inhibitors (NRTIs) and non-nucleoside reverse transcriptase inhibitors (NNRTIs) limit the effect of the viral reverse transcriptase, blocking the transcription of viral RNA into DNA. Protease inhibitors (PI) block the enzyme protease and prevent new infectious particles from being formed. The first fusion inhibitor was marketed in 2003, a new ART class that prevents merging of the viral membrane with the membrane of $CD4^+$ T cells, thus preventing HIV-1 entry. In 2007, products of two new classes of ART received approval by the FDA. First, an entry inhibitor, which blocks the chemokine receptor CCR5 which HIV-1 uses as a coreceptor to bind and enter $CD4^+$ T cells. This product needs to be injected twice daily and is reserved for treatment of drug-experienced patients since it can help overcome drug resistance. Second, an integrase inhibitor, which prevents viral DNA to be integrated into the DNA of host cell. Currently, there is one multi-class combination product on the market, combining an NNRTI with two NRTIs.

18.6.2 HAART

The goal of ART is to decrease HIV-1-related morbidity and mortality. The clinical effectiveness of ART has improved markedly with the introduction of HAART in 1996. HAART combines three ART agents, generally including at least one NNRTI or PI. The rationale for combining several agents is provided by the high genetic variability of HIV-1. The virus has an extremely high rate of viral turnover. During transcription, the viral enzyme reverse transcriptase has a high mutation rate and

HIV-1 has the capacity to recombine. These factors lead to a great diversity of HIV-1 (quasi) species in chronically infected individuals.

HAART aims to reduce and sustain HIV-1 plasma viral load below levels of detectability of current ultra sensitive viral load assays (<50 copies/mL). The likelihood of accumulation of drug-resistance mutations is thus minimalized. The inhibition of viral replication results in a partial reconstitution of the immune system in most patients, thereby reducing the risk of clinical disease progression and death. Even those with more advanced HIV-1 disease and low $CD4^+$ T-cell counts who initiate HAART can achieve substantial increases in $CD4^+$ T-cell counts, leading to clinical benefit (Weller and Williams 2001). However, current HAART regimens do not clear HIV-1 infection and HIV-1 establishes latent infection in resting memory CD4+ T cells, monocytes, macrophages, and perhaps other cells. These cells can harbor infectious HIV-1 for decades. Therefore, lifelong treatment is needed.

Limited data are available, but treatment for HIV-2 mirrors treatment approaches of HIV-1. However, currently available NNRTIs are ineffective in treating HIV-2, therefore the use of a protease inhibitor with two NRTIs to treat HIV-2 infection is recommended.

18.6.3 Side Effects

Between 25 and 50% of patients discontinue their initial HAART regimen because of treatment failure or non-compliance within the first year of therapy. All ART can have a wide range of both short-term and long-term adverse effects. Gastrointestinal side effects like nausea and diarrhea, occurring early on and sometimes continuously throughout the use of many ARTs can negatively effect adherence. Other frequently observed effects are fatigue, headaches, nightmares, and more serious adverse events like anemia, peripheral neuropathy, hepatotoxicity, and hypersensitivity reactions. NRTIs can disrupt mitochondrial function causing hyperlactatemia, hepatic steatosis, and lactic acidosis, which may lead to death. PI-based regimens sometimes cause diabetes mellitus type 2 and insulin resistance. Lipodystrophy, defined as a metabolic syndrome including fat redistribution, hyperlipidemia, and insulin resistance or diabetes mellitus, is caused by PIs and some NRTIs. Lipodystrophy includes fat loss in face, limbs and buttocks, together with fat accumulation in abdomen, breasts, and over the dorsocervical spine. ART is associated with dyslipidemia and especially in the presence of other risk factors, like smoking, the risk for cardiovascular disease in HAART receiving subjects might be increased. The pathogenesis of lipodystrophy, insulin resistance, and dyslipidemia are still unclear. Treatment for dyslipidemia, diabetes, and insulin resistance should be prescribed according to national guidelines.

Individuals initiating HAART may experience a worsening of preexisting medical conditions through the restoration of antigen specific immune response through HAART. This immune reconstitution syndrome is more often seen among individuals initiating therapy with a low $CD4^+$ T-cell count (Montessori et al. 2004; French 2007).

18.6.4 Adherence

Inadequate adherence remains an important reason for poor treatment outcome in HIV-1 disease. Adherence is influenced by several factors among which are the frequently observed side effects during HAART regimens, pill burden, dosing frequency, food requirements, mental health, substance abuse, and social or psychological barriers to adherence. In the past several years, progress has been made in that convenient regimens with few or no food restrictions, decreased pill burden and dosing, and one-pill once-daily regimens have become available, which may improve adherence. It is suggested that very high adherence rates (defined as the number of doses taken divided by the number of doses prescribed) of >95% to PI-based regimens are needed to prevent treatment failure (Paterson et al. 2000). Some studies have demonstrated that adherence in resource-limited countries is as high as in the industrialized world. Whether population-based introduction of (HA)ART will confirm these results remains to be proven.

18.6.5 Drug Resistance

The most common reason for treatment failure is the emergence of drug resistance, limiting future treatment options. Drug-resistant HIV-1 is transmissible and in developed countries with broad access to HAART, HIV-1 resistance can be found in up to 10–20% of newly infected individuals. Several western world guidelines recommend resistance testing before the initiation of the first HAART regimen. In resource-limited countries with low access to (HA)ART the prevalence of drug resistance remains low (Gilks et al. 2006).

18.6.6 Structured Treatment Interruptions

The rationale for structured treatment interruptions during the course of HAART is that the immune system, if exposed to low levels of viral replication, might be stimulated to control HIV-1. Besides, structured treatment interruptions might add to the quality of life of HIV-1-infected individuals, reduce treatment costs, and reduce (long-term) side effects. The largest structured treatment interruptions study so far was closed early because of both increased HIV-1 and non-HIV-1-related illnesses in the treatment interruption arm. At this point, except for reasons of treatment intolerance, structured treatment interruptions are discouraged (el-Sadr et al. 2006).

18.6.7 Global Perspectives of HAART

Combination therapy is becoming more widely available throughout the world, including in resource-limited countries. Over the years, several international organizations provoked price reductions through the adaptation of international laws on patents, the introduction of generic products, and the creation of relief funds. Depending on the regimen, prices of most first-line ART products dropped between

37 and 53% between 2003 and 2006 in low and middle-income countries. Currently, the cheapest form of HAART is between 132 and 148 dollars/person/per year. However, this exceeds the health-care budget per person in many developing countries. In 2003, the WHO issued their '3 by 5'-slogan aiming to provide 3 million persons with ART in 2005. In 2006 a campaign for universal access to ART by 2010 was launched. However, UNAIDS reported that globally only 24% of people who needed HIV-1 treatment had access to it by mid-2006. HIV-1-diagnostic and treatment evaluation assays are often not available in resource-limited countries and the WHO has created guidelines for simplified treatment initiation and follow-up centered around the four 'S-es': when to Start drug treatment, Substitute for toxicity, Switch after treatment failure, and Stop criteria (Gilks et al. 2006).

In 2006, almost 700,000 people received ART for the first time. By December 2006 it was estimated that approximately 2 million people living with HIV-1/AIDS in low- and middle-income countries were receiving treatment, this being approximately 28% of the close to 7 million people in need (www.who.com). In sub-Saharan Africa an estimated 1.3 million persons are taking ART while this number was 100,000 three years earlier.

18.7 Conclusion

In the 28 years that have passed since the start of the HIV-1 epidemic, HIV-1 has had a devastating effect on global morbidity and mortality. This has greatly impacted the socio-economical situation in many parts of the world. So far, despite many efforts and attempts to develop effective prevention methods (e.g., vaccination, risk behavior reduction strategies, microbicides), these have not been shown to be successful. Recently, studies on the effect of circumcision have demonstrated promising results in decreasing HIV-1 transmission. However, population-wide implementation of this prevention method might have unforeseen counteractive effects, when risk behavior or HIV-1 infectivity is increased.

Alarmingly, in recent years most industrialized countries have reported increased sexual risk behavior and HIV-1 incidence especially among MSM. This trend could fuel the HIV-1 transmission in regions where the HIV-1 epidemic was thought to be under control.

Through effective HAART regimens and subsequently lowered mortality, the total pool of HIV-1 infected individuals will grow. Extended survival in combination with the fact that prevention methods do not seem to have the desired impact on the spread of HIV-1 suggest that the HIV-1 pandemic is likely to increase worldwide, despite the progress that has been made in raising international funds and making HAART available for more people, especially in sub-Saharan Africa.

References

AIDSinfo (2008) HIV-1 LifeCycle. www.aidsinfo.nih.gov/contentfiles/HIVLifeCycle_FS_en.pdf

Almeda J, Casabona J, Simon B, Gerard M, Rey D, Puro V et al. (2004) Proposed recommendations for the management of HIV post-exposure prophylaxis after sexual, injecting drug or other exposures in Europe. Euro Surveillance : Bulletin Europeen sur les Maladies Transmissibles = European Communicable Disease Bulletin; 9(6):35–40

Alter MJ (2006) Epidemiology of viral hepatitis and HIV co-infection. J Hepatol; 44(1 Suppl): S6–S9

Auvert B, Taljaard D, Lagarde E, Sobngwi-Tambekou J, Sitta R, Puren A (2005) Randomized, controlled intervention trial of male circumcision for reduction of HIV infection risk: the ANRS 1265 Trial. PLoS Medicine/Public Library of Science; 2(11):e298

Bailey RC, Moses S, Parker CB, Agot K, Maclean I, Krieger JN et al. (2007) Male circumcision for HIV prevention in young men in Kisumu, Kenya: a randomised controlled trial. Lancet; 369(9562):643–656

Chan DJ (2006) Fatal attraction: sex, sexually transmitted infections and HIV-1. Int J STD AIDS; 17(10):643–651

Coakley E, Petropoulos CJ, Whitcomb JM (2005) Assessing chemokine co-receptor usage in HIV. Curr Opin Infect Dis; 18(1):9–15

Collaborative Group on AIDS incubation and HIV survival including the CASCADE EU Concerted Action(2000) Time from HIV-1 seroconversion to AIDS and death before widespread use of highly-active antiretroviral therapy: a collaborative re-analysis. Lancet; 355:1131–1137

Cooper ER, Charurat M, Mofenson L, Hanson IC, Pitt J, Diaz C et al. (2002) Combination antiretroviral strategies for the treatment of pregnant HIV-1-infected women and prevention of perinatal HIV-1 transmission. J Acquir Immune Defic Syndr; 29(5):484–494

Corey L, Wald A, Celum CL, Quinn TC (2004) The effects of herpes simplex virus-2 on HIV-1 acquisition and transmission: a review of two overlapping epidemics. J Acquir Immune Defic Syndr; 35(5):435–445

Corbett EL, Marston B, Churchyard GJ, De Cock KM (2006) Tuberculosis in sub-Saharan Africa: opportunities, challenges, and change in the era of antiretroviral treatment. Lancet; 367(9514):926–937

Corbett EL, Watt CJ, Walker N, Maher D, Williams BG, Raviglione MC et al. (2003) The growing burden of tuberculosis: global trends and interactions with the HIV epidemic. Arch Intern Med; 163(9):1009–1021

Dao H, Mofenson LM, Ekpini R, Gilks CF, Barnhart M, Bolu O et al. (2007) International recommendations on antiretroviral drugs for treatment of HIV-infected women and prevention of mother-to-child HIV transmission in resource-limited settings: 2006 update. Am J Obstet Gynecol; 197(3 Suppl):S42–S55

Ellerbrock TV, Bush TJ, Chamberland ME, Oxtoby MJ (1991) Epidemiology of women with AIDS in the United States. 1981 through 1990 A comparison with heterosexual men with AIDS. JAMA; 265(22):2971–2975

el-Sadr WM, Lundgren JD, Neaton JD, Gordin F, AbramsD, Arduino RC et al. (2006) CD4+ count-guided interruption of antiretroviral treatment. N Engl J Med; 355(22): 2283–2296

Eshleman SH, Mracna M, Guay LA, Deseyve M, Cunningham S, Mirochnick M et al. (2001) Selection and fading of resistance mutations in women and infants receiving nevirapine to prevent HIV-1 vertical transmission (HIVNET 012). AIDS; 15(15):1951–1957

EuroHIV (2007) HIV/AIDS Surveillance in Europe. End-year report 2006.Saint-Maurice: Institut de veille sanitaire

Fowler MG, Lampe MA, Jamieson DJ, Kourtis AP, Rogers MF (2007) Reducing the risk of mother-to-child human immunodeficiency virus transmission: past successes, current progress and challenges, and future directions. Am J Obstet Gynecol; 197(3 Suppl):S3–S9

Fowler MG, Newell ML (2002) Breast-feeding and HIV-1 transmission in resource-limited settings. J Acquir Immune Defic Syndr; 30(2):230–239

French MA (2007) Disorders of immune reconstitution in patients with HIV infection responding to antiretroviral therapy. Curr HIV/AIDS Rep; 4(1):16–21

Gilks CF, Crowley S, Ekpini R, Gove S, Perriens J, Souteyrand Y et al. (2006) The WHO public-health approach to antiretroviral treatment against HIV in resource-limited settings. Lancet; 368(9534):505–510

Gray RH, Kigozi G, Serwadda D, Makumbi F, Watya S, Nalugoda F et al. (2007) Male circumcision for HIV prevention in men in Rakai, Uganda: a randomised trial. Lancet; 369(9562):657–666

Guay LA, Musoke P, Fleming T, Bagenda D, Allen M, Nakabiito C et al. (1999) Intrapartum and neonatal single-dose nevirapine compared with zidovudine for prevention of mother-to-child transmission of HIV-1 in Kampala, Uganda: HIVNET 012 randomised trial. Lancet; 354(9181):795–802

Geretti AM (2006) HIV-1 subtypes: epidemiology and significance for HIV management. Curr Opin Infect Dis; 19(1):1–7

Jamieson DJ, Read JS, Kourtis AP, Durant TM, Lampe MA, Dominguez KL (2007) Cesarean delivery for HIV-infected women: recommendations and controversies. Am J Obstet Gynecol; 197(3 Suppl):S96–S100

Kanki PJ, Peeters M, Gueye-Ndiaye A (1997) Virology of HIV-1 and HIV-2: implications for Africa. AIDS; 11 Suppl B:S33–S42

Koziel MJ, Peters MG (2007) Viral hepatitis in HIV infection. N Engl J Med 2007; 356(14): 1445–1454

Liu Z, Lian Z, Zhao C (2006) Drug use and HIV/AIDS in China. Drug Alcohol Rev; 25(2): 173–175

Luzuriaga K, Sullivan JL (2005) Prevention of mother-to-child transmission of HIV infection. Clin Infect Dis; 40(3):466–467

Montessori V, Press N, Harris M, Akagi L, Montaner JS (2004) Adverse effects of antiretroviral therapy for HIV infection. Can Med Assoc J; 170(2):229–238

Myers G, MacInnes K, Korber B (1992) The emergence of simian/human immunodeficiency viruses. AIDS Res Hum Retroviruses; 8(3):373–386

Paterson DL, Swindells S, Mohr J, Brester M, Vergis EN, Squier C et al. (2000) Adherence to protease inhibitor therapy and outcomes in patients with HIV infection. Ann Intern Med; 133(1):21–30

Pezzotti P, Phillips AN, Dorrucci M, Lepri AC, Galai N, Vlahov D et al. (1996) Category of exposure to HIV and age in the progression to AIDS: longitudinal study of 1199 people with known dates of seroconversion. HIV Italian Seroconversion Study Group. BMJ; 313(7057): 583–586

Pinkerton SD, Holtgrave DR, Pinkerton HJ (1997) Cost-effectiveness of chemoprophylaxis after occupational exposure to HIV. Arch Intern Med; 157(17):1972–1980

Peeters M (2000) Recombinant HIV-1 Sequences: their role in global epidemic. In: Kuiken C FBHBE, editor. HIV-1 Sequence Compendium. Theoretical Biology and Biophysics Group, Los Alamos National Laboratory: Los Alamos: 39–54

Schacker T, Zeh J, Hu HL, Hill E, Corey L (1998) Frequency of symptomatic and asymptomatic herpes simplex virus type 2 reactivations among human immunodeficiency virus-infected men. J Infect Dis; 178(6):1616–1622

Shepard CW, Finelli L, Alter MJ (2005) Global epidemiology of hepatitis C virus infection. Lancet Infect Dis; 5(9):558–567

Stebbing J, Moyle G (2003) The clades of HIV: their origins and clinical significance. AIDS Rev; 5(4):205–213

Stover J, Bertozzi S, Gutierrez JP, Walker N, Stanecki KA, Greener R et al. (2006) The global impact of scaling up HIV/AIDS prevention programs in low- and middle-income countries. Science; 311(5766):1474–1476

UNAIDS (2008) AIDS epidemic update : December 2007

Wald A, Link K (2002) Risk of human immunodeficiency virus infection in herpes simplex virus type 2-seropositive persons: a meta-analysis. J Infect Dis; 185(1):45–52

Wawer MJ, Gray RH, Sewankambo NK, Serwadda D, Li X, Laeyendecker O et al. (2005) Rates of HIV-1 transmission per coital act, by stage of HIV-1 infection, in Rakai, Uganda. J Infect Dis; 191(9):1403–1409

Weller IV, Williams IG (2001) ABC of AIDS. Antiretroviral drugs. BMJ; 322(7299):1410–1412

Chapter 19
Blood Borne and Sexual Transmission: Hepatitis B and C

Freke Zuure, Susan Hahné, Thijs van de Laar, Maria Prins, and Jim van Steenbergen

19.1 Introduction

Although the routes of transmission and infectivity differ, the three blood borne infections with most impact on public health are caused by viruses that can cause chronic asymptomatic infections. Human immunodeficiency virus (HIV) is discussed in Chapter 3. Here we discuss hepatitis B virus (HBV) and hepatitis C virus (HCV). HBV and HCV are grouped together for certain similarities (both causing hepatitis, hence the name, both caused by a virus, and both can lead to chronic asymptomatic infections and liver disease) but the differences are prominent enough to warrant separate presentations. Some of the main similarities and differences are listed in Table 19.1. Other hepatitis viruses include hepatitis A virus and hepatitis E virus that are both feco-orally transmitted. The hepatitis D virus, commonly called deltavirus, occurs only as a superinfection in persons with active HBV infection. Without laboratory testing, different causes of hepatitis cannot be distinguished.

Table 19.1 Main similarities and differences between HBV and HCV

		HBV	HCV
Efficiency of transmission	blood borne	++++	+++
	sexual	+++	+/–
	perinatal	+++	+
	through intact mucosa (not sexual)	++	–
progress to chronic infection	adults	5–10%	75%
	neonates of HBeAg positive mothers	90%	
	neonates of antiHBe positive mothers	<30%	
% icteric acute infection (in adults)		5–10%	minority
Treatment success rate for chronic infection		30%	42–80%
Vaccination available		Yes	No

F. Zuure (✉)
Cluster Infectious Diseases, Public Health Service of Amsterdam, Amsterdam, Netherlands
e-mail: fzuure@ggd.amsterdam.nl

A. Krämer et al. (eds.), *Modern Infectious Disease Epidemiology*,
Statistics for Biology and Health, DOI 10.1007/978-0-387-93835-6_19,

19.1.1 Prevalence

A single blood borne exposure (e.g., through a needle stick injury) to HBV leads to acute infection in an estimated 3–30% of cases and exposure to HCV in 1–10% of cases as compared to HIV where the proportion of infections is 0.3%. Sexually, HBV is transmitted ten times more effectively than HIV (Kingsley et al. 1990). For HBV countries are classified as areas of low, middle, and high endemicity, whereas the distribution of HCV equally shows regional variations but these are more focal. In areas of low endemicity for HBV import through migration is the major contributor to prevalence. For HCV in low-endemic countries, injecting drug use (IDU) is the major mode of HCV transmission, and migration contributes to a lesser extent to HCV prevalence.

For both HBV and HCV, the overall prevalence can be ascertained by population-based sero-epidemiological studies. Data of donor screening is often used to estimate the overall prevalence. However, as high-risk groups are excluded from donating blood and donor inclusion criteria differ across countries, this data refers to a highly selected subpopulation. Some countries have antenatal screening for HBV in order to identify newborns at increased risk. Although pregnant women are a selected subpopulation as well, this screening may provide a more representative source. Incidence data on reported acute infections are of limited value for assessing the prevalence as most HBV and practically all HCV infections in the acute phase are asymptomatic and therefore undiagnosed. Moreover, using the long-term sequelae of HBV and HCV (i.e., liver cirrhosis, fibrosis, and carcinoma) based on clinical data to estimate the prevalence is difficult as the results of serological tests are often not included in morbidity and mortality registries.

These factors hinder efforts in determining HBV and HCV prevalence. However, for both infections valid data are needed as they should guide public health measures, either directed at specific high-risk groups (e.g., screening and early treatment) or the population (e.g., universal vaccination against HBV).

19.1.2 Prevention

As for most blood borne infections, undiagnosed individuals are a reservoir and a predominant source of new infections. Primary prevention of HBV and HCV is therefore directed at hygienic precautions in all percutaneous procedures and, for HBV, at promoting condom use and less risky sexual behavior. As there is a safe and effective vaccine available against HBV, vaccination is the most important public health measure in primary prevention. There is no vaccine available that prevents HCV infection. For both HBV and HCV, early diagnosis (only established through blood tests) and treatment of infectious individuals reduce the background prevalence of chronic infections and thus contribute to primary prevention. Concomitant source and contact tracing has additional benefits in the case of the 30% symptomatic acute HBV infections (identifying asymptomatic sources and preventing new symptomatic infections), but has limited value in HCV where new infections often go undiagnosed and infection is identified long after exposure.

Whilst treatment of HBV and HCV previously relied only on immune modulation, in the last decade new antivirals have been developed against both viruses. Treatment success has increased and will further increase when new and combined antiviral drugs become available.

In this chapter, we will describe the public health importance of these two silent killers HBV and HCV, which annually cause more deaths than HIV in high-income countries. We clarify the main epidemiological methods and obstacles in public health prevention and control of these infections.

19.2 Hepatitis B

19.2.1 Epidemiology

19.2.1.1 Global Patterns and Transmission Routes

HBV is of major public health importance due to its high burden of disease and its preventability. An estimated 360 million people worldwide have chronic HBV infection, and 600,000 deaths occur each year due to HBV-related liver disease or hepatocellular carcinoma (Shepard et al. 2006). HBV is transmitted by percutaneous or permucosal exposure to blood or body fluids from infected persons. Transmission usually takes place either through sexual contact, blood contact, or perinatally. Perinatal transmission is highly efficient (the major route in Southeast Asia), with the highest risk in children born to HBeAg positive mothers (Beasley et al. 1977). HBV is also transmitted within households to young children through close non-sexual contact (the major route in Africa) (Davis et al. 1989).

Since the age of HBV acquisition is inversely associated with the risk of becoming chronically infected, infections acquired in infancy or childhood contribute disproportionally to the pool of chronic carriers. The lifetime infection risk varies dramatically between 0.4% in Western Europe to 90% in East Asia, and is usually described in three groups (Fig. 19.1) (Shepard et al. 2006).

19.2.1.2 Risk Groups

The prevalence of HBV in a country is associated with its predominant transmission modes and the duration and quality of its vaccination strategy. In countries with high prevalence (HBsAg seroprevalence $\geq$8%), most infections are acquired perinatally or in early childhood (Shepard et al. 2006). In these countries, health-care associated HBV transmission is also frequent (Hauri et al. 2004). In low prevalence countries (HBsAg seroprevalence <2%) most infections are acquired through adult risk behavior including IDU and male homosexual contact (Hahné et al. 2004). Other groups with increased risk for acquiring HBV include infants born to infectious mothers, health-care workers, children with developmental disabilities, patients undergoing hemodialysis, and close contacts of infected people. Long-term travelers to endemic areas are generally also advised to be vaccinated (Salisbury et al. 2006).

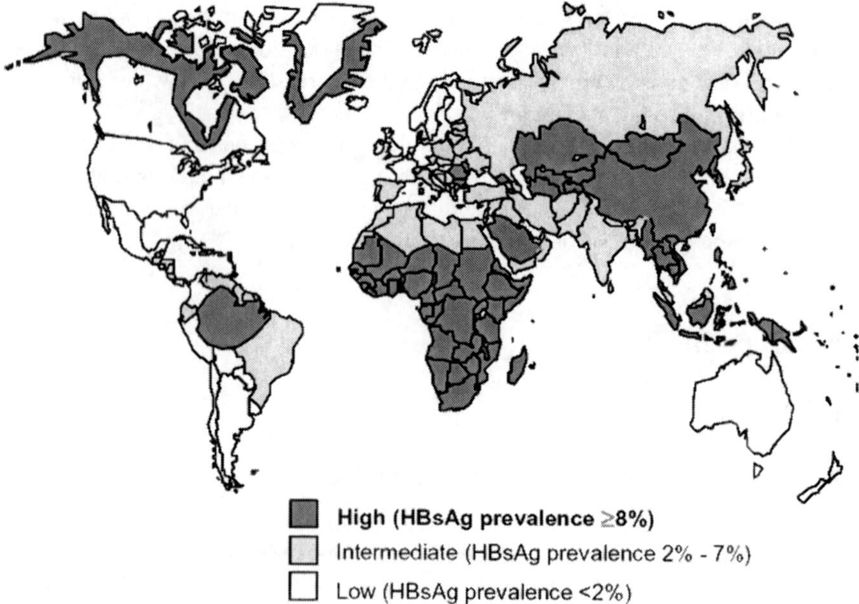

Fig. 19.1 Geographical distribution of HBV endemicity. Source: World Health Organization (2001) Introduction of hepatitis B vaccine into childhood immunization services, Geneva, WHO, WHO/V&B/01.31

Within low prevalence countries, one can distinguish subgroups with relatively high prevalence and incidence, with associated transmission patterns including frequent perinatal and household transmission (Aweis et al. 2001; Hahné et al. 2003; Hurie et al. 1992). These subgroups can be indigenous or arise through migration from endemic areas. For public health management of HBV, it is important that surveillance distinguishes between transmission occurring within a country (local transmission) and infections imported by immigration of carriers (imported infections). Whereas the former can be influenced by a country's vaccination policy, the latter cannot.

19.2.2 Molecular Epidemiology

Hepatitis B virus belongs to the family of hepadnaviridae. It has a small double-stranded circular DNA genome of around 3200 base pairs, which encodes seven viral proteins. HBV is an unusual DNA virus as it replicates through an RNA intermediate which is transcribed back into cDNA using reverse transcriptase. This process is prone to errors, leading to a higher than usual mutation rate for DNA viruses and to diversification of the virus. However, as over half of the genome consists of overlapping open reading frames; most errors result in viruses with reduced fitness. The diversification does allow tracking of virus transmission. In addition, it also has consequences for the prevention, diagnostic methods, natural history, and treatment of HBV infections (Echevarria and Avellon 2006; Lok and McMahon 2007).

The earliest grouping of HBV types made was based on variants of its surface protein (HBsAg), determined by the antigens present in the HBsAg (Courouce et al. 1976). Antigen a is common to all known HBsAg subtypes. Since it is the main epitope recognized by neutralizing antibodies arising through infection or vaccination, vaccine protection is not subtype specific. Next to a, there are two pairs of mutually exclusive antigens (d/y and w/r), whereby w can exist in four forms (1–4). This results in subtypes such as "adw4" and "ayr."

Subsequent to the description of HBsAg subtypes, eight genotypes (A–H) have been identified based on genome sequencing of HBV strains (Norder et al. 2004). The genotype grouping does not overlap with the HBsAg subtype grouping, although some correlations can be found. Within genotypes A, B, C, D, and F, but not (yet) in E, G, and H, subgenotypes have been identified. The occurrence of the HBsAg- and geno(sub)types varies geographically, which allows tracking virus transmission and population movement between regions (Echevarria and Avellon 2006; Norder et al. 2004).

Within almost all groups of hepatitis B virus (sub)types, mutants have been described according to where the mutation has occurred (pre-Core, Core, HBsAg). These mutations can have important implications for public health: They can interfere with the effectiveness of (passive and active) immunization and treatment, and can also affect the sensitivity of diagnostic assays (Echevarria and Avellon 2006). For example, a viable one point mutation in the pre-core region results in virus that cannot produce a particular protein that is traditionally used as a marker for viral load (the HBe protein). This can result in infectious individuals at risk of severe disease being missed (Omata et al. 1991). Although this is a diagnostic challenge, its public health impact has (so far) been limited.

Surveillance of HBV's diversity and its implications is therefore a key component of the public health response to HBV.

In addition to the study of subgroups of HBV and their characteristics, the relatedness of individual viruses can be studied in more detail using phylogenetics (see Chapter 7). The phylogenetic resolution depends on the length and specific part of the HBV genome that is sequenced (Boot et al. 2008). Phylogenetic analyses that integrate epidemiological information (such as risk behavior, country of origin) have become a powerful tool to assess the intensity of HBV transmission within and between high-risk groups (van Steenbergen et al. 2002), to identify outbreaks (Fisker et al. 2006), and to evaluate the effectiveness of vaccination programs (van Houdt et al. 2007).

Recent molecular epidemiological analysis suggests that in the Netherlands men who have sex with men (MSM) are the predominant high-risk group, with ongoing local transmission reflected by the very close relatedness of genotype A strains from MSM. In contrast, among heterosexually acquired HBV, sequences show a wide variation suggesting that they result from multiple introductions (by chronic carriers that moved from endemic areas and, to a lesser extent, by returning travelers) rather than from sustained transmission in a core-group of high-risk individuals. Based partly on these findings, it was decided, in the Netherlands, to intensify vaccination of MSM but to cease the free vaccination offer for heterosexuals with high rates of partner change. HBV transmission among heterosexuals may be prevented more effectively by screening (some groups of) immigrants and vaccination of their contacts. Since treatment of HBV has improved, secondary prevention is becoming more important (Hutton et al. 2007), not only to prevent morbidity for the individual patient but also to eliminate the patient as a source for others.

19.2.3 Clinical Course

19.2.3.1 Diagnostics

The immune reaction determines the clinical course of HBV infection. An inadequate, but persistent, immune response can lead to chronic infection. Testing of antibodies against hepatitis B proteins (anti-HBc, anti-HBs, anti-HBe) and antigens (HBsAg, HBeAg) are thus the means of diagnosing the stage of hepatitis B infection. Table 19.2 presents the most common course of occurrence of antigens and antibodies after infection. Additional testing of liver enzymes, with liver biopsy for histological classification, if justified, is required for clinical follow-up in chronic infection. HBV-DNA by PCR can quantify the viral load and classify infectiousness and therapeutical effect.

19.2.3.2 Immunological Reactions

There are important clinical differences (with epidemiological consequences) between acute and chronic HBV infection. Acute infection can lead to acute (infectious) disease, lasting several weeks or months. Acute hepatitis B in adults is usually self-limiting, but 5–10% of infections become chronic. In neonates acute infections usually are asymptomatic but the majority become chronic. Chronic infections cause the major burden of disease (and are a constant source of infection for others–"the reservoir"-) due to the increased risk of liver cirrhosis and hepatocellular carcinoma after decades of chronic infection. There are various categories of chronic infection, with corresponding long-term risk differences. To better understand the disease process, four phases of infection are distinguished that consequently occur in all infected individuals, while the length of stay in each phase is highly variable (Lok 2002).

Phase 1: immuno-tolerant phase: "incubation period". Tolerance with low immune response resulting in HBV replication (circulating viral proteins – antigens HBsAg, HBeAg and high viral load HBV-DNA, but normal liver function tests – "transaminases") and antibodies against the HBcore protein (anti-HBc).

Table 19.2 Serological findings in HBV infection (adapted with permission, National Hepatitis Centre, Netherlands). N.a. = not applicable

	Phase 1	Phase 2	Phase 3	Phase 4		Prolonged phase 1	Prolonged phase 2	Prolonged phase 3	Not infected
	Late in incubation period	Acute hepatitis B	Late acute hepatitis B	Recent hepatitis B	Ever hepatitis B	Chronic active hepatitis B		Chronic inactive hepatitis B	After successful vaccination
Time since infection	2–12 Weeks	2–4 months	3–6 months	<1 year	<1 year	HBeAg pos >6 months	HBeAg neg >6 months	>6 months	N.a.
ALAT	Normal	Increased	Normal/ increased	Normal	Normal	Increased	Increased	Normal	Normal
HBsAg	+	+	+	–	–	+	+	+	–
HBeAg	+/–	+	–	–	–	+	–	–	–
IgM-anti-HBc	–	++	++	+	–	–(+)	–(+)	–	–
Total anti-HBc	–	+	++	++	++	++	++	++	–
Anti-HBe	–	–	+	+	+	–	+	+	–
Anti-HBs	–	–	+/–	++	+	–	–	–	++
HBV-DNA	+	+	+/–	–	–	+	+	+/–	–
Infectiousness	+	++	+	–	–	++	++	+	–
Symptoms	–	+	+/–	–	–	+/–	+/–	–	–

Phase 2: immuno-active phase: "symptomatic disease". Enhanced immune response, leading to inflammation of liver cells (decreased viral load (HBV-DNA), increased transaminases). Over time, seroconversion of the viral e-antigen (HBeAg) to antibodies to the viral e-antigen (anti-HBe) might occur. Many years in phase 2 can show periods of increased immune activity, with symptomatic disease, and lead to serious liver damage.

Phase 3: inactive phase. Persistent anti-HBe, low HBV-DNA, normal transaminases. Occasionally, HBsAg seroconversion to low anti-HBs levels. However, persistent HBV-DNA in liver cells might result in liver cirrhosis and hepatocellular carcinoma (HCC). HBV-DNA integrates in liver cell-DNA and might disturb regulatory mechanisms in cell division and multiplication. There is no evidence that viral factors are important in development of chronic sequelae (as in HCV), but host factors (chronic necrosis, inflammation, and regeneration of liver cells) and external (e.g., smoking) factors contribute to HCC as is the case in HCV.

Phase 4: immune phase. High levels of anti-HBs and anti-HBc, absence of HBV-DNA. This is the preferred endpoint of infection: lifelong immunity. It is not excluded that HBV-DNA is integrated in the DNA of certain liver cells, but this does not lead to any chronic sequelae, unless there is a serious immunosuppression for other reasons (e.g., after organ transplant).

Adults most commonly proceed in a short (few months) time from phase 1–2 and 3–4 (asymptomatic, or with mild or seldom serious symptoms), resulting in complete recovery with lifelong immunity. In contrast, infected new born children might stay in phase 1 for many years and slowly progress over the years from phase 2 to 3 when, after several decades, serious liver disease might lead to early death (never reaching phase 4).

19.2.3.3 Clinical Spectrum

The incubation period (phase 1) varies depending on the host's immunity, transmission route, and inoculum size. Symptoms are a sign of entering phase 2, and,if occurring, start 6 weeks to 6 months after exposure. Only one-third of infected adults, and an even smaller proportion of children, develops an icteric phase. Rarely, acute symptomatic HBV infection leads to fulminant liver failure (1%) and death (0.1%). HBV clearance is age dependent (Edmunds et al. 1993). Over 95% of adults spontaneously and completely recover (phase 4). However, in 95% of cases infection at birth leads to persistent infection (phase 3), as compared to 30% for those infected at age 0–6 years. Persons with persistent infection are at increased risk of developing cirrhosis and HCC over the ensuing decades.

The liver-related mortality rate for chronically infected HBV patients is estimated at around 1/1000 person years. In HIV co-infected individuals, the risk of HBV chronicity and liver-related mortality is increased (Thio et al. 2002).

19.2.3.4 Therapy

Acute hepatitis B is a self-limiting disease. However, in the rare cases of fulminant liver failure antiviral therapy might be beneficial (Tillmann et al. 2006) and ultimately liver transplantation is the only life saving treatment option (still an important reason for liver transplantation in the Western world).

Treatment of chronic hepatitis B is indicated if the viral load is high (HBV-DNA >10^5 IU/ml) and if there are also signs of disturbance of liver function (elevated transaminases –ALAT-) or the presence of liver inflammation and or fibrosis. Present treatment options include immune modulation with interferon alfa, peginterferon alfa, and direct antiviral treatment with nucleoside analogues (such as lamivudine, adefovir, entecavir, or telbivudine) (European Association for the Study of the Liver 2009).

Pegylated interferon alfa during 12 months leads to sustained viral response in 35% of patients and complete cure in 7% (Buster et al. 2008). However, inconvenient administration (subcutaneous) and frequent side effects hamper wider use. Antiviral nucleoside analogues can be given for prolonged periods: one year of treatment leads to reduction in viral load, lowering of transaminases, and improvement of the liver histology in almost all patients. After discontinuation of antiviral therapy the viral load might increase to pre-treatment values. Antiviral treatment can only pave the way for the patient's immune reaction; complete cure relies on the patient's immune system.

A serious drawback of long-term use of antivirals (especially lamivudine, but also adefovir and telbivudine) is the occurrence of viral resistance. Resistance against the newer entecavir is at present limited, but the follow-up period is still short.

19.2.4 Prevention and Control

19.2.4.1 Hygienic Precautions

For blood borne pathogens, hygienic precautions in the health-care setting are essential for control. This includes avoiding the use of contaminated instruments, universal precautions for invasive procedures, and screening of blood products, tissue and organs. Health-care workers and the public should be educated. Outside health care, the use of contaminated instruments by tattoo, piercing, nail studios, and IDU should be avoided, e.g., by offering needle exchange programs for IDUs. For prevention of sexual transmission condom use is effective.

19.2.4.2 HBV Notification and Post-exposure Prophylaxis

In areas of low endemicity notification remains important for HBV control. For reported patients, serological markers are evaluated and source and contacts are traced and vaccinated if susceptible. Needle stick injuries and other percutaneous and permucosal exposures, including sexual exposures, always warrant risk assessment for immediate post-exposure prophylaxis (with HBV vaccine and possibly hepatitis B immune globulin (HBIg)).

19.2.4.3 Universal HBV Vaccination

HBV vaccine (available since 1982) is safe and >95% effective in preventing HBV infection, and is thus the first vaccine against a virus that also causes human cancer. In 1992, the World Health Organization (WHO) called for all countries to implement universal vaccination, and 151 of 192 member states complied (Shepard et al. 2006). In areas with very low prevalence, the cost-effectiveness of universal vaccination is still under debate. Irrespective of universal immunization, selective targeted vaccination for those at highest risk remains important for the coming decades. Universal vaccination in high and medium incidence countries has led to a considerable reduction in prevalence, morbidity, and mortality (Ni et al. 2007; Bonanni et al. 2003). Costs are the major barrier for vaccine introduction in developing countries. Fortunately, the Global Alliance for Vaccines and Immunization (a coalition between public and private institutions) and the Global Fund for Children's Vaccines is making HBV vaccine available for 74 low-income countries (Lavanchy 2004).

19.2.4.4 Selective Targeted HBV Vaccination

Low prevalence areas usually target only groups at increased risk for free vaccination: medical risk groups, babies of chronically infected women (requiring antenatal screening and subsequent administration of HBIg at birth, followed by HBV vaccine), IDUs, MSM, and heterosexuals with multiple partners (Salisbury et al. 2006). However, the vaccination coverage in these groups is often low, even among employees at increased risk for HBV that are obliged to be vaccinated, such as health-care workers (Ndiaye et al. 2005).

Travelers of low prevalence areas going to intermediate or high endemicity areas are also advised to have HBV vaccination depending on duration of stay and additional risk factors.

The impact of selective vaccination on the epidemiology of HBV in low incidence countries appears at present to be limited. In the UK and The Netherlands, transmission is ongoing in IDUs and MSM, respectively (Sutton et al. 2006a; van Houdt et al. 2007). This can be explained by low vaccination coverage, increase in the size and changes in behavior of high-risk populations, and enhanced testing and subsequent reporting of (anicteric) infections that previously went undetected. To better assess the effectiveness of selective vaccination, additional methods including behavioral and molecular surveillance are therefore needed. The impact of selective adult vaccination on the burden of disease is limited, as newly acquired infections in adulthood progress to chronic infection only in a minority of cases (5%) and the current disease burden mainly originates from chronic carriers who immigrated from higher prevalence countries.

19.2.5 Modeling

For HBV, mathematical models have broadly three aims: to study the epidemiology of HBV, to guide public health interventions, and to predict the future burden of disease.

Since the adverse health outcomes of HBV infection mostly take place years after infection, Markov models are used to estimate the effect of HBV screening (Hutton et al. 2007) and treatment of chronic HBV (Takeda et al. 2007).

Obtaining insight into the epidemiology of HBV and its determinants is complex since infection is often asymptomatic. Since the risk of acquiring chronic infection is age dependent and the average age of infection is influenced by the prevalence of carriage, a positive feedback mechanism exists. Mathematical models have been highly instrumental in explaining the extreme differences in levels of HBV endemicity between countries and populations (Medley et al. 2001). Models are also needed for estimating transmission parameters (e.g., the force of infection or basic reproductive ratio) from (sero)prevalence data obtained through surveys (Sutton et al. 2006a; Coleman et al. 1998). These quantities provide information about the prevention effort needed to eliminate the virus and the population groups best targeted by prevention measures.

For HBV, as for many other communicable diseases, interventions such as vaccination and treatment not only reduce the risk of infection and disease in the vaccinated or treated individual, but also in his or her close contacts. A comprehensive assessment of the impact of vaccination and treatment therefore requires that these indirect effects are quantified and taken into account. To do so, dynamic models have been used that simulate the transmission of HBV in a population given determinants such as age, sexual risk behavior, and vaccination coverage. These models have been used to inform decision making on the introduction of public health interventions by assessing the (cost)-effectiveness of HBV vaccination (Williams et al. 1996). Dynamic models have also been used to assess the short- and long-term impact of public health interventions subsequent to implementation, for example, the impact of high-risk group vaccination on the prevalence of chronic infections among MSM (Xiridou et al. 2008). These studies can provide realistic expectations of when the impact of a vaccination program can be expected, and to what extent, e.g., given different levels of sexual risk behavior in MSM. Lastly, dynamic models can guide intervention programs so that maximum impact is achieved. This can result in recommendations to prioritize vaccination of those with the highest levels of risk behavior or new IDUs (Sutton et al. 2006b; Sutton et al. 2006a).

As for other diseases, mathematical modeling has also been used to predict the future burden of disease due to chronic HBV infection (Goldstein et al. 2005). These estimates are relevant to demonstrate potential impact of vaccination, and also for health-care planning. As described in Chapter 12 mathematical models also have their limitations, and surveillance and (molecular) epidemiological studies remain important tools for generating data to support and validate models.

19.3 Hepatitis C

19.3.1 Epidemiology

19.3.1.1 Transmission Routes

HCV was first identified in 1989. It was the most common cause of post-transfusion non-A–non-B hepatitis, as it was especially recognized among individuals who had received contaminated blood products. In 1991, the first commercial HCV antibody test became available, leading to a dramatic decrease in the incidence of transfusion-acquired HCV in countries that introduced screening of donor blood (Memon and Memon 2002).

19.3.1.2 Global Pattern

HCV has infected an estimated 2.2% of the world's population (The Global Burden of Hepatitis C Working Group 2004). The reported prevalence rates vary greatly per country. A serious limitation is the lack of reliable population-based studies. Overall, WHO estimates that the African and Eastern Mediterranean regions have the highest HCV prevalence, but for many countries reliable population-based studies are lacking (The Global Burden of Hepatitis C Working Group 2004). The world's highest HCV prevalence has been reported in Egypt, as a result of mainly intravenous administered therapy against schistosomiasis. From the 1920s till the 1980s multiple doses of therapeutic injections were administered in mass settings without sufficient sterilization of re-used injection materials, leading to a HCV prevalence of 15–20% in the general Egyptian population (Frank et al. 2000). Although in high-income countries health-care associated HCV transmission incidentally occurs, its contribution to the overall prevalence in these countries is low (Thompson et al. 2009). In contrast, in median- and low-income countries non-sterile injection practices, lack of HCV screening of donor blood, and other iatrogenic routes of transmission still account for significant HCV transmission and serve as a bridge to the general population (Madhava et al. 2002).

19.3.1.3 Risk Groups

IDUs are at high risk of HCV infection (prevalence 31–98%) (Memon and Memon 2002). Other risk groups for HCV infection are recipients of blood products before 1992 [i.e., hemophilia patients, prevalence ~70% (Posthouwer et al. 2005)]; hemodialysis patients [prevalence 3–23% (Fissel et al. 2004)]; non-injection drug users (prevalence 2–35%), although the causal pathway to infection in the latter group remains unclear (Scheinmann et al. 2007); people who experienced a needle stick injury and health-care professionals dealing with blood and blood products (prevalence unknown) (Gerberding 1995); household contacts of HCV-infected individuals (possible transmission through the shared use of toothbrushes, razors, etc., prevalence 0–11% (Memon and Memon 2002)); and children born to HCV-infected mothers, with transmission rates of ~4%, increasing in maternal HCV/HIV co-infection to ~20% (Yeung et al. 2001). In contrast to HIV and HBV, so far no specific measures are available to prevent mother-to-child transmission for HCV. Mode of delivery and breastfeeding do not influence transmission rates significantly (Yeung et al. 2001).

Other activities that may cause blood–blood contact have been described as routes of HCV infection, such as tattooing, body piercing, and cultural/religious practices (e.g., scarification, circumcision, acupuncture). However, results are inconsistent and it is uncertain whether these risk factors make any measurable contribution to overall HCV transmission (Alter 2007).

Even in the presence of HIV co-infection, HCV is rarely transmitted by heterosexual intercourse (Vandelli et al. 2004). Since 2000, however, HCV emerges among HIV-infected MSM (Giraudon et al. 2007; van de Laar et al. 2009). Phylogenetic analyses showed clusters of MSM-specific HCV strains, indicating a sexual route of HCV transmission. Based on mainly case studies, it has been suggested that sexually acquired HCV is associated with HIV infection, the presence of ulcerative sexually transmitted diseases, sexual techniques causing mucosal damage, and sex under the influence of non-injecting drugs (Danta et al. 2007; van de Laar et al. 2009).

19.3.2 Virology and Molecular Epidemiology

19.3.2.1 Virology

HCV is a single-stranded RNA virus, whose host range is confined to humans and closely related primates. It primarily targets hepatocytes. Due to its similarities in genome organization, structure and replication to a large group of vector borne diseases (e.g., yellow fever) and animal pestiviruses, HCV was added to the family of Flaviviridae. The viral genome codes for one single polyprotein, which is processed into three structural proteins and seven non-structural proteins that code for the viral enzymes (Simmonds 2001). The high viral turnover and the error-prone replication process result in rapid evolution of HCV within an infected host. The swarm of highly similar viral variants that develop within one host is called quasispecies and probably provide the mechanism by which HCV evades host immune surveillance and establishes and maintains chronic infection (Gale and Foy 2005) (Fig. 19.2).

19.3.2.2 Molecular Epidemiology

The high genetic variability of the HCV genome has led to a classification of the virus into seven major genotypes (1–7) which except for genotypes 5 and 7 are each further divided into more than 80 related subtypes (a, b, c,. . .) (Simmonds et al. 2005; Murphy et al. 2007). Genotypes have 65–70% similarity on the nucleotide level, subtypes 75–80%, and within a subtype sequence variability is below 10% (Simmonds et al. 2005). As HCV genotype distribution depends on geographic area,

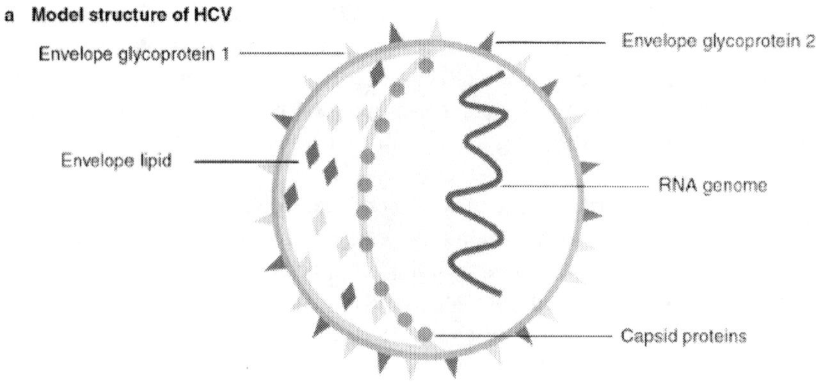

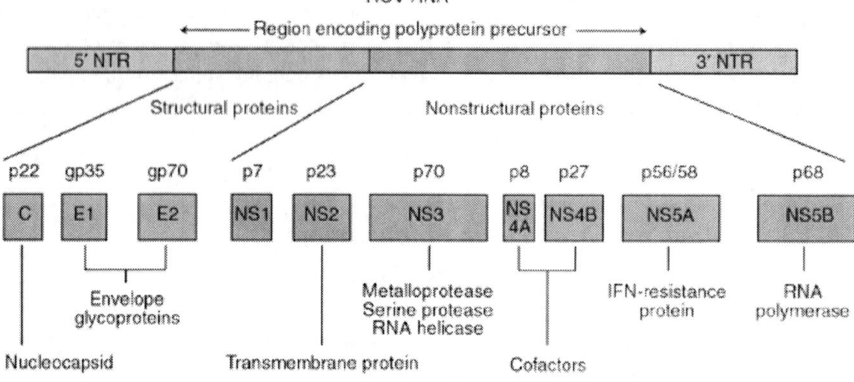

Fig. 19.2 HCV model structure and genome organization. Reproduced from reference Anzola and Burgos 2003 with permission from the author

mode of transmission, and varies over time, it provides clues about the historical origin and the spread of the virus. Some HCV subtypes are found globally due to a swift spread in the 20th century through needle sharing among IDUs (types 1a and 3a) or contaminated blood products (types 1b, 2a, and 2b). These genotypes represent the majority of infections in Europe and Northern America. In contrast, the presence of numerous and highly diverse subtypes in Western/Central Africa and the Middle East (genotypes 1, 2, and 4) as well as Southeast Asia (genotypes 3 and 6) suggest that these genotypes originate from these areas where they have been endemic for a long time (Simmonds 2001).

Evolutionary relationships among genes and organisms can be illustrated by a phylogenetic tree, comparable to a pedigree showing which genes or organisms are most closely related. As the degree of diversity (or similarity) among HCV viral variants provides information on the likelihood that strains were acquired in the same transmission network, phylogenetic analysis can be used to investigate the spread of HCV. The high similarity of HCV isolates observed among MSM in Europe revealed a large transmission network of HIV-infected MSM in which HCV transmission was linked to high-risk sexual behavior (van de Laar et al. 2009). In contrast, the degree of diversity among HCV and HIV isolates obtained from children attending a hospital in Benghazi, Libya showed that four different HIV and HCV outbreaks in this hospital were due to a long-standing infection-control problem instead of the arrival of a foreign medical staff, who were found guilty in 2004 of deliberately infecting 426 children with HIV. Based on inferred nucleotide evolutionary rates, the date of origin of the four outbreaks proved to vary between 1985 and 1997, which is before the arrival of the foreign staff (de Oliveira et al. 2006).

19.3.2.3 HCV Superinfection and Reinfection

Molecular typing techniques have confirmed that both HCV reinfection and superinfection with a homologous or a heterologous HCV strain occur, suggesting that neither virological clearance nor ongoing HCV chronic infection provides full protection against new HCV infections (Blackard and Sherman 2007). Evidence for partial HCV protective immunity derives largely from chimpanzee studies. Chimpanzees that previously cleared HCV and subsequently were rechallenged with homologous HCV strains, generally show lower levels of HCV viremia and self-limited infection (Bassett et al. 2001). In humans, the presence of such partial protective immunity remains controversial. IDUs from Baltimore who spontaneously cleared their HCV infection were found to be less likely to develop new episodes of HCV viremia compared to IDUs without previous infection (Mehta et al. 2002). No such protection, however, was observed among a cohort of young Australian IDUs (Micallef et al. 2007). Moreover, as the generation of a recombinant virus requires that a cell must be infected simultaneously with two or more distinct HCV strains, the recent documentation of recombinant HCV strains is de facto evidence that dual HCV infections also occur (Kalinina et al. 2004). The reported frequency of such HCV superinfection in active IDUs varies between 0 and 20% (Herring et al. 2004; Dove et al. 2005). The true incidence, however, is hard to establish as current laboratory methodologies make characterization of superinfection cumbersome (Blackard and Sherman 2007).

19.3.2.4 Diagnostics

Standard HCV testing includes screening for HCV antibodies using an anti-HCV EIA confirmed by immunoblot. In a clinical setting, a positive HCV antibody test will be directly followed by RNA testing to establish the presence of ongoing infection. In order to diagnose the widest span of viral variants, HCV-RNA tests are generally based on the highly conserved 5′ untranslated region (UTR) of the HCV genome. Genotyping on the other hand requires viral heterogeneity, reference regions globally used for genotyping are structural proteins core/E1 and the non-structural NS5B protein that codes for the RNA polymerase (Simmonds et al. 2005).

The time between the infection and the appearance of HCV antibodies is estimated to be approximately 60 days (Busch 2001). Hence, the presence of active HCV-RNA in HCV antibody negative individuals indicates acute infection. However, prolonged seroconversion windows or complete failure to mount or maintain HCV antibodies have been observed among immunosuppressed individuals, e.g., those co-infected with HIV (Chamie et al. 2007). Once HCV antibody positive, current lab techniques are unable to provide information on the moment HCV was acquired. Loss of HCV antibodies (HCV seroreversion) has been described, but mainly among individuals that were able to clear the virus (Lannote et al. 1998).

19.3.3 Clinical Course of Infection

In the majority of cases acute HCV is asymptomatic. Less than one-third of individuals with an acute HCV infection experiences mostly mild and aspecific symptoms such as loss of appetite, fatigue and flu-like symptoms, and occasionally jaundice (Hoofnagle 2002). Natural viral clearance of HCV only occurs in a minority (~25%) of patients (Micallef et al. 2006). Chronic infection is defined as the persistence of HCV-RNA for more than 6 months after infection. As the onset of the infection and the development of cirrhosis in chronically infected patients usually are asymptomatic, diagnosis often occurs late, limiting efforts to determine natural history of HCV (Seeff 2002). Depending on the study design and population, a large variation in progression rate has been found. Approximately 20 years after the onset of chronic infection, HCV leads to liver cirrhosis in 6–25% of patients, of whom per year 1–4% develop hepatocellular carcinoma (Seeff 2002; Sweeting et al. 2006; Patel et al. 2006). Next to viral factors, host and external factors such as male sex, older age at the time of infection, HBV or HIV-1 co-infection, and alcohol intake might accelerate disease progression (Seeff 2002; Patel et al. 2006). Some of these factors are also associated with viral persistence after acute infection and therapy outcome. New non-invasive methods have been developed that can be used for clinical decision making, including combined serological markers and liver scan techniques to establish the degree of fibrosis. However, until now liver histology is still considered to be the most reliable method to stage and grade the severity of liver disease (Patel et al. 2006).

19.3.3.1 Therapy

Recently, important advances in the treatment of chronic HCV infection have been made. Currently, the recommended therapy consists of the use of a modified form (pegylated) of interferon alpha (protein with immunomodularity and antiviral properties) in combination with ribavirin (a nucleoside analogue with antiviral activity). In the absence of HIV co-infection, HCV treatment duration is usually 24–48 weeks, depending on the HCV genotype. The aim of the treatment is to eradicate viral RNA and to reach a sustained virological response (SVR) , which is the absence of HCV-RNA at 24 weeks after the end of treatment (National Institutes of Health Consensus Development Conference Statement 2002). The most important predictor of SVR, which occurs in 42–80% of the cases, is HCV genotype (Weigand et al. 2007). Genotypes 1 and 4 are difficult-to-treat genotypes, with approximately 50% of treated patients achieving SVR, compared to an SVR up to 90% in patients with genotypes 2 and 3. Other predictors of therapeutic outcome that influence treatment duration include rapid viral response (RVR) (undetectable HCV-RNA levels at week 4) and early viral responses (EVR) ($\leq$2 log decrease in viral load during the first 12 weeks) and low HCV-RNA level prior to treatment (Weigand et al. 2007).

All patients should be considered for treatment. However, patients with mild disease activity can be given the option of deferring therapy (Patel et al. 2006). Despite this, a high number of IDU still has limited access to HCV antiviral treatment, as cost-effectiveness of HCV treatment in this population is often questioned. Those successfully treated are at risk of HCV reinfection when sharing of injection equipment is continued (Micallef et al. 2007). Moreover, low treatment adherence with ongoing risk behavior, as well as the possibility of HCV superinfection at the start of treatment might negatively affect HCV treatment outcome itself (Blackard and Sherman 2007). However, recent studies suggest that when HCV care is integrated with methadone provision drug users can be successfully treated (Novick and Kreek 2008).

Approximately 10–14% of all patients discontinue treatment because of serious side effects (National Institutes of Health Consensus Development Conference Statement 2002). Some others experience viral relapses after the end of treatment. Currently new therapeutic concepts are being developed which directly target HCV-RNA and viral enzymes, or influence host–virus interactions (Takkenberg et al. 2008). Despite toxicity issues and rapid selection of resistance, which did restrain some of the initial enthusiasm, several of these new compounds are very promising and are expected to be registered within the next 3 years. Future treatment of chronic HCV infection will probably be more effective and shorter, and consist of a combination of peginterferon, ribavirin together with one or more new drugs (Takkenberg et al. 2008).

19.3.4 Prevention and Control

19.3.4.1 Prevention of Further Spread of HCV

In contrast to HBV, for HCV there is no vaccine available, nor are there drugs for post-exposure prophylaxis or prevention of mother-to-child-transmission. Prevention relies completely on precautionary measures preventing further spread, which are similar to those taken for HBV (e.g., hygienic measures, screening of donor blood). As effective treatment is available, creating awareness and stimulating testing behavior among HCV risk groups is of major importance.

As IDUs are at high risk of HIV and HCV due to the reuse and sharing of needles and/or injecting paraphernalia, in high-income countries many HIV harm reduction programs have been targeted at this population. These include needle exchange programs, social care, opioid replacement therapy (mainly methadone and buprenorphine), or a combination of these. Many interventions have shown to be cost-effective since they have reduced HIV prevalence (Wright and Tompkins 2006). Studies evaluating the effect of separate harm reduction programs on HCV incidence or prevalence show inconsistent results. Van den Berg et al. suggested that a combined comprehensive approach is effective (van den Berg et al. 2007).

Improvement of blood transfusion safety and health-care conditions are the main factors that will contribute to the control of HCV transmission in low- and medium-income countries.

19.3.4.2 Identifying Undiagnosed HCV Infections

Mass population screening for HCV in low prevalence countries is considered to be inappropriate as its cost-effectiveness is poor. Several targeted screening programs have been carried out aimed at risk groups for HCV infection. Screening policies are based on various considerations, including the prevalence of risk behavior (i.e., injecting drugs) or exposure (blood transfusion before HCV screening of donor blood started) in the population, the prevalence of HCV among those with the risk profile, and the need for persons with a recognized exposure to be evaluated for HCV (Alter 2002). Tracing HCV-infected individuals can lead to individual lifestyle adjustments (improving HCV prognosis), treatment, and prevention of further transmission (e.g., to household contacts).

As HCV had spread among individuals who received blood products before the introduction of the first HCV antibody test in 1991, various high-income countries introduced look-back programs in which recipients of blood from HCV-infected donors were notified and motivated for testing. As in other look-back programs, the Canadian HCV look-back experience successfully identified previously undiagnosed HCV-infected patients, but the costs were high and the yield relatively low (Bowker et al. 2004). Other interventions aimed at identifying undiagnosed HCV-infected individuals used targeted screening programs based on risk factors (Sypsa et al. 2001; Mallette et al. 2007), which may prove to be a more cost-effective screening policy. HCV information campaigns have been initiated in various high-income countries including Australia, the UK, the USA, and Canada, but data on the results of these campaigns have not been published so far.

Many medium- and low-income countries lack an active policy for identifying HCV-infected individuals or for raising awareness, as other health or economic problems have more urgency.

19.3.5 Modeling

Mathematical models have been used to reconstruct the spread of HCV. For example, using molecular evolutionary analysis and a logistic growth model (see Chapter 12) it has been estimated that the spread of HCV genotype 1 in Japan in the 1930s took place before widespread dissemination of HCV in the United States in the 1960s when IDU and transfusion of unscreened blood (products) were widespread (Tanaka et al. 2002). A coalescent approach estimated that the timing of the HCV epidemic in Egypt was between 1930 and 1950 (Pybus et al. 2003), whereas a back calculation model estimated that the epidemic exploded in 1970 in line with the massive use of parenteral anti-schistosomiasis treatment in this period (Deuffic-Burban et al. 2006). The discrepancy in the estimation of the timing of the epidemic might be due to the different methods applied and the assumptions made. It is hard to conclude which estimate is most likely because no serological data are available for that time period.

Because of the relatively long time from infection to disease outcome, Markov and other mathematical models (including forward projection models) have been developed to predict the future epidemic and burden of disease and to evaluate the effect of interventions. Based on these models it has been estimated that, for various medium- to high-income countries, HCV-related morbidity and mortality will at least double in the next two decades (Sypsa et al. 2005; Deuffic-Burban et al. 2006), and will exceed the number of deaths from HIV. The improvements of HCV therapy are too recent and the identification of infected individuals for treatment is too low to reverse the increase in mortality (Deuffic-Burban et al. 2007). Models have also been helpful in planning and evaluating the effect of interventions aimed at preventing new HCV infections. They have suggested that because of the high reproductive rate of HCV compared to HIV comprehensive harm reduction programs must complement syringe exchange to successfully prevent HCV. The interventions should also be sustained for many years to reduce HCV infections (Vickerman et al. 2007).

19.4 Conclusions

There are overlaps and differences in the (efficiency of) transmission routes of HBV and HCV. Although blood–blood transmissibility is higher for HBV than HCV, the higher rate of chronicity for HCV has resulted in a large number of chronic carriers for both viruses. These chronic infections have an increased risk for serious liver disease decades after initial infection and have therefore a significant impact on public health. Presently, in high-income countries, more people die from HBV and HCV than from HIV.

For HBV, effective public health intervention to prevent new infections is feasible with a safe and effective vaccine. Universal childhood vaccination can eradicate hepatitis B. However, this will not prevent serious liver disease and early death in the coming decades for the 350 millions that are already chronically infected with

HBV. In the absence of a vaccine against HCV, HCV prevention relies completely on precautionary measures preventing its further spread.

For both HBV and HCV, molecular epidemiology and mathematical modeling have greatly contributed in clarifying routes of transmission, and in predicting the (impact of interventions on the) future burden of disease.

Besides development of public health interventions, future challenge exists of unraveling the specific mechanisms of spontaneous viral clearance, super-/co-infection, and viral resistance, and of gaining insight into determinants predicting therapy success. Further efforts will focus on advances in therapy which now show encouraging results for HCV in preclinical studies.

For both HBV and HCV, identification of asymptomatic chronically infected individuals is extremely important. In affluent societies effective (expensive) treatment is available for both, to improve individual long-term outcome. Additionally, effective treatment will eliminate the reservoir for new infections. Development of new drugs has to keep pace with inevitable development of viral resistance. Through various donor organizations universal HBV vaccination is made available in most low-income countries. Now, efforts should be made so that treatment is also available in developing countries where most of the burden of disease due to hepatitis B and C occurs. Infected individuals can take precautionary measures to prevent further spread (e.g., wound care, using condoms), and susceptible (household) contacts of HBV-infected individuals should be vaccinated. As the majority of acute HBV and HCV infections go unnoticed, educating the public about (differences in) the often mixed-up hepatitis viruses and their nature is of great importance to enhance awareness and facilitate early identification.

References

Alter MJ (2002) Prevention of spread of hepatitis C. Hepatology; 36(5):593–598

Alter MJ (2007) Epidemiology of hepatitis C virus infection. World J Gastroenterol; 13(17): 2436–2441

Anzola M, Burgos JJ (2003) Hepatocellular carcinoma: molecular interactions between hepatitis C virus and p53 in hepatocarcinogenesis. Expert Rev Mol Med; 5(28):1–16

Aweis D, Cooper CD, Brabin B, Beeching N (2001) Serological evidence for Hepatitis B infection in the Somali population of Liverpool. Arch Dis Child; 84 (suppl I):A62

Bassett SE, Guerra B, Brasky K, Miskovsky E, Houghton M, Klimpel GR et al. (2001) Protective immune response to hepatitis C virus in chimpanzees rechallenged following clearance of primary infection. Hepatology; 33(6):1479–1487

Beasley RP, Trepo C, Stevens CE, Szmuness W (1977) The e antigen and vertical transmission of hepatitis B surface antigen. Am J Epidemiol; 105(2):94–98

Blackard JT, Sherman KE (2007) Hepatitis C virus coinfection and superinfection. J Infect Dis; 195(4):519–524

Bonanni P, Pesavento G, Bechini A, Tiscione E, Mannelli F, Benucci C et al. (2003) Impact of universal vaccination programmes on the epidemiology of hepatitis B: 10 years of experience in Italy. Vaccine; 21(7–8):685–691

Boot HJ, Cremer J, Koedijk F, Ballegooijen M, Op de Coul ELM (2008) Improved tracing of hepatitis B virus transmission chains by phylogenetic analysis based on C region sequences. J Med Virol; 80:233–241

Bowker SL, Smith LJ, Rosychuk RJ, Preiksaitis JK (2004) A review of general hepatitis C virus lookbacks in Canada. Vox Sang; 86(1):21–27

Busch MP (2001) Closing the window on viral transmission in blood transfusion. In: Stramer SL, ed. Blood safety in the new millennium. American Association of Blood Banks:Betehsda, MD; 33–54

Buster EH, Flink HJ, Cakaloglu Y, Simon K, Trojan J, Tabak F et al. (2008)Sustained HBeAg and HBsAg loss after long-term follow-up of HBeAg-positive patients treated with peginterferon alpha-2b. Gastroenterology; 135(2):459–467

Chamie G, Bonacini M, Bangsberg DR, Stapleton JT, Hall C, Overton ET et al. (2007) Factors associated with seronegative chronic hepatitis C virus infection in HIV infection. Clin Infect Dis; 44(4):577–583

Coleman PJ, McQuillan GM, Moyer LA, Lambert SB, Margolis HS (1998) Incidence of hepatitis B virus infection in the United States, 1976–1994: estimates from the National Health and Nutrition Examination Surveys. J Infect Dis; 178(4):954–959

Courouce AM, Drouet J, Muller JY (1976) Australia antigen subtypes identification. Results. Bibl Haematol; 42:89–127

Danta M, Brown D, Bhagani S, Pybus OG, Sabin CA, Nelson M et al. (2007) Recent epidemic of acute hepatitis C virus in HIV-positive men who have sex with men linked to high-risk sexual behaviours. AIDS; 21(8):983–991

Davis LG, Weber DJ, Lemon SM (1989) Horizontal transmission of hepatitis B virus. Lancet; 1(8643):889–893

de Oliveira T, Pybus OG, Rambaut A, Salemi M, Cassol S, Ciccozzi M et al. (2006) Molecular epidemiology: HIV-1 and HCV sequences from Libyan outbreak. Nature; 444(7121): 836–837

Deuffic-Burban S, Mohamed MK, Larouze B, Carrat F, Valleron AJ (2006) Expected increase in hepatitis C-related mortality in Egypt due to pre-2000 infections. J Hepatol; 44(3):455–461

Deuffic-Burban S, Poynard T, Sulkowski MS, Wong JB (2007) Estimating the future health burden of chronic hepatitis C and human immunodeficiency virus infections in the United States. J Viral Hepat; 14(2):107–115

Dove L, Phung Y, Bzowej N, Kim M, Monto A, Wright TL (2005) Viral evolution of hepatitis C in injection drug users. J Viral Hepat; 12(6):574–583

Echevarria JM, Avellon A (2006) Hepatitis B virus genetic diversity. J Med Virol; 78 (Suppl 1):S36–S42

Edmunds WJ, Medley GF, Nokes DJ, Hall AJ, Whittle HC (1993) The influence of age on the development of the hepatitis B carrier state. Proc R Soc Lond B Biol Sci; 253(1337): 197–201

European Association for the Study of the Liver (2009) EASL clinical practice guidelines: management of chronic hepatitis B. J Hepatol; 50:227–242

Fisker N, Carlsen NL, Kolmos HJ, Tonning-Sorensen L, Host A, Christensen PB (2006) Identifying a hepatitis B outbreak by molecular surveillance: a case study. BMJ; 332(7537):343–345

Fissell RB, Bragg-Gresham JL, Woods JD, Jadoul M, Gillespie B, Hedderwick SA et al. (2004) Patterns of hepatitis C prevalence and seroconversion in hemodialysis units from three continents: the DOPPS. Kidney Int; 65(6):2335–2342

Frank C, Mohamed MK, Strickland GT, Lavanchy D, Arthur RR, Magder LS et al. (2000) The role of parenteral antischistosomal therapy in the spread of hepatitis C virus in Egypt. Lancet; 355(9207):887–891

Gale M, Jr., Foy EM (2005) Evasion of intracellular host defence by hepatitis C virus. Nature; 436(7053):939–945

Gerberding JL (1995) Management of occupational exposures to blood-borne viruses. N Engl J Med; 332(7):444–451

Giraudon I, Ruf M, Maguire H, Charlett A, Ncube F, Turner J et al. (2007).Increase in newly acquired hepatitis C in HIV positive men who have sex with men across London and Brighton, 2002–2006. Is this an outbreak? Sex Transm Infect 84(2):111–115

Goldstein ST, Zhou F, Hadler SC, Bell BP, Mast EE, Margolis HS (2005) A mathematical model to estimate global hepatitis B disease burden and vaccination impact. Int J Epidemiol; 34(6): 1329–1339

Hahné S, Ramsay M, Balogun K, Edmunds WJ, Mortimer P (2004) Incidence and routes of transmission of hepatitis B virus in England and Wales, 1995–2000: Implications for immunisation policy. J Clin Virol; 29:211–220

Hahné S, Ramsay M, Soldan K, Balogun K, Mortimer P (2003) Hepatitis B incidence among South Asian children in England and Wales: implications for immunisation policy. Arch Dis Child; 88:1082–1083

Hauri AM, Armstrong GL, Hutin YJ (2004) The global burden of disease attributable to contaminated injections given in health care settings. Int J STD AIDS; 15(1):7–16

Herring BL, Page-Shafer K, Tobler LH, Delwart EL (2004) Frequent hepatitis C virus superinfection in injection drug users. J Infect Dis; 190(8):1396–1403

Hoofnagle JH (2002) Course and outcome of hepatitis C. Hepatology; 36(5):521–529

Hurie MB, Mast EE, Davis JP (1992) Horizontal transmission of hepatitis B virus infection to United States- born children of Hmong refugees. Pediatrics; 89(2):269–273

Hutton DW, Tan D, So SK, Brandeau ML (2007) Cost-effectiveness of screening and vaccinating Asian and Pacific Islander adults for hepatitis B. Ann Intern Med; 147(7):460–469

Kalinina O, Norder H, Magnius LO (2004) Full-length open reading frame of a recombinant hepatitis C virus strain from St Petersburg: proposed mechanism for its formation. J Gen Virol; 85(7):1853–1857

Kingsley LA, Rinaldo CR Jr., Lyter DW, Valdiserri RO, Belle SH, Ho M (1990) Sexual transmission efficiency of hepatitis B virus and human immunodeficiency virus among homosexual men. JAMA; 264(2):230–234

Lanotte P, Dubois F, Le PS, Guerois C, Fimbel B, Bacq Y et al. (1998) The kinetics of antibodies against hepatitis C virus may predict viral clearance in exposed hemophiliacs. J Infect Dis; 178(2):556–559

Lavanchy D (2004) Hepatitis B virus epidemiology, disease burden, treatment, and current and emerging prevention and control measures. J Viral Hepat; 11(2):97–107

Lok AS (2002) Chronic hepatitis B. N Engl J Med; 346(22):1682–1683

Lok AS, McMahon BJ (2007) Chronic hepatitis B. Hepatology; 45(2):507–539

Madhava V, Burgess C, Drucker E (2002) Epidemiology of chronic hepatitis C virus infection in sub-Saharan Africa. Lancet Infect Dis; 2(5):293–302

Mallette C, Flynn MA, Promrat K (2007) Outcome of screening for hepatitis C virus infection based on risk factors. Am J Gastroenterol 103(1):131–137

Memon MI, Memon MA (2002) Hepatitis C: an epidemiological review. J Viral Hepat; 9(2): 84–100

Medley GF, Lindop NA, Edmunds WJ, Nokes DJ (2001) Hepatitis-B virus endemicity: heterogeneity, catastrophic dynamics and control. Nat Med; 7(5):619–624

Mehta SH, Cox A, Hoover DR, Wang XH, Mao Q, Ray S et al. (2002) Protection against persistence of hepatitis C. Lancet; 359(9316):1478–1483

Micallef JM, Kaldor JM, Dore GJ (2006) Spontaneous viral clearance following acute hepatitis C infection: a systematic review of longitudinal studies. J Viral Hepat; 13(1):34–41

Micallef JM, Macdonald V, Jauncey M, Amin J, Rawlinson W, van Beek I et al. (2007) High incidence of hepatitis C virus reinfection within a cohort of injecting drug users. J Viral Hepat; 14(6):413–418

Murphy DG, Willems B, Deschenes M, Hilzenrat N, Mousseau R, Sabbah S (2007) Use of sequence analysis of the NS5B region for routine genotyping of hepatitis C virus with reference to C/E1 and 5′ untranslated region sequences. J Clin Microbiol; 45(4):1102–1112

National Institutes of Health Consensus Development Conference Statement (2002) Management of hepatitis C: 2002-June 10–12, 2002. Hepatology; 36(5 Suppl 1):S3–20

Ndiaye SM, Hopkins DP, Shefer AM, Hinman AR, Briss PA, Rodewald L et al. (2005) Interventions to improve influenza, pneumococcal polysaccharide, and hepatitis B vaccination coverage among high-risk adults: a systematic review. Am J Prev Med; 28(5 Suppl):248–279

Ni YH, Huang LM, Chang MH, Yen CJ, Lu CY, You SL et al. (2007) Two decades of universal hepatitis B vaccination in Taiwan: impact and implication for future strategies. Gastroenterology; 132(4):1287–1293

Norder H, Courouce AM, Coursaget P, Echevarria JM, Lee SD, Mushahwar IK et al. (2004) Genetic diversity of hepatitis B virus strains derived worldwide: genotypes, subgenotypes, and HBsAg subtypes. Intervirology; 47(6):289–309

Novick DM, Kreek MJ (2008) Critical issues in the treatment of hepatitis C virus infection in methadone maintenance patients. Addiction; 103(6):905–918

Omata M, Ehata T, Yokosuka O, Hosoda K, Ohto M (1991) Mutations in the precore region of hepatitis B virus DNA in patients with fulminant and severe hepatitis. N Engl J Med; 324(24):1699–1704

Patel K, Muir AJ, McHutchison JG (2006) Diagnosis and treatment of chronic hepatitis C infection. BMJ; 332(7548):1013–1017

Posthouwer D, Plug I, van der Bom JG, Fischer K, Rosendaal FR, Mauser-Bunschoten EP (2005) Hepatitis C infection among Dutch haemophilia patients: a nationwide cross-sectional study of prevalence and antiviral treatment. Haemophilia; 11(3):270–275

Pybus OG, Drummond AJ, Nakano T, Robertson BH, Rambaut A (2003) The epidemiology and iatrogenic transmission of hepatitis C virus in Egypt: a Bayesian coalescent approach. Mol Biol Evol; 20(3):381–387

Salisbury D, Ramsay M, Noakes Keds. (2006) Immunisation against infectious disease. HMSO: London

Scheinmann R, Hagan H, Lelutiu-Weinberger C, Stern R, Des Jaklais D, Flom PL et al. (2007) Non-injection drug use and Hepatitis C Virus: a systematic review. Drug and Alcohol Dependence; 89(1):1–12

Seeff LB (2002) Natural history of chronic hepatitis C. Hepatology; 36(5):S35–S36

Shepard CW, Simard EP, Finelli L, Fiore AE, Bell BP (2006) Hepatitis B virus infection: epidemiology and vaccination. Epidemiol Rev; 28:112–125

Simmonds P (2001) The origin and evolution of hepatitis viruses in humans. J Gen Virol; 82(Pt 4):693–712

Simmonds P, Bukh J, Combet C, Deleage G, Enomoto N, Feinstone S et al. (2005) Consensus proposals for a unified system of nomenclature of hepatitis C virus genotypes. Hepatology; 42(4):962–973

Sutton AJ, Gay NJ, Edmunds WJ (2006b) Modelling the impact of prison vaccination on hepatitis B transmission within the injecting drug user population of England and Wales. Vaccine; 24(13):2377–2386

Sutton AJ, Gay NJ, Edmunds WJ, Hope VD, Gill ON, Hickman M (2006a) Modelling the force of infection for hepatitis B and hepatitis C in injecting drug users in England and Wales. BMC Infect Dis; 6:93

Sweeting MJ, de Angelis D, Neal KR, Ramsay ME, Irving WL, Wright M et al. (2006) Estimated progression rates in three United Kingdom hepatitis C cohorts differed according to method of recruitment. J Clin Epidemiol; 59(2):144–152

Sypsa V, Hadjipaschali E, Hatzakis A (2001) Prevalence, risk factors and evaluation of a screening strategy for chronic hepatitis C and B virus infections in healthy company employees. Eur J Epidemiol; 17(8):721–728

Sypsa V, Touloumi G, Papatheodoridis GV, Tassopoulos NC, Ketikoglou I, Vafiadis I et al. (2005) Future trends of HCV-related cirrhosis and hepatocellular carcinoma under the currently available treatments. J Viral Hepat; 12(5):543–550

Takeda A, Jones J, Shepherd J, Davidson P, Price A (2007) A systematic review and economic evaluation of adefovir dipivoxil and pegylated interferon-alpha-2a for the treatment of chronic hepatitis B. J Viral Hepat; 14(2):75–88

Takkenberg B, de Bruijne J, Weegink C, Jansen P, Reesink H (2008) Novel therapies in hepatitis B and C. Curr Gastroenterol Rep; 10(1):81–90

Tanaka Y, Hanada K, Mizokami M, Yeo AE, Shih JW, Gojobori T et al. (2002) Inaugural Article: A comparison of the molecular clock of hepatitis C virus in the United States and Japan predicts that hepatocellular carcinoma incidence in the United States will increase over the next two decades. Proc Natl Acad Sci USA; 99(24):15584–15589

The Global Burden Of Hepatitis C Working Group (2004) Global burden of disease (GBD) for hepatitis C. J Clin Pharmacol; 44(1):20–29

Thio CL, Seaberg EC, Skolasky R, Jr., Phair J, Visscher B, Munoz A et al. (2002) HIV-1, hepatitis B virus, and risk of liver-related mortality in the Multicenter Cohort Study (MACS). Lancet; 360(9349):1921–1926

Thompson ND, Perz JF, Moorman AC, Holmberg SD (2009) Nonhospital health care-associated hepatitis B and C virus transmission: United States, 1998–2008. Ann Intern Med; 150(1):33–39

Tillmann HL, Hadem J, Leifeld L, Zachou K, Canbay A, Eisenbach C et al. (2006) Safety and efficacy of lamivudine in patients with severe acute or fulminant hepatitis B, a multicenter experience. J Viral Hepat; 13(4):256–263

van de Laar TJ, Pybus OG, Bruisten SM, Brown D, Nelson M, Bhagani S et al. (2009) Evidence of a large, international HCV transmission network in HIV-positive men who have sex with men. Gastroenterology 136(5):1609–1617

Vandelli C, Renzo F, Romano L, Tisminetzky S, De Palma M, Stroffolini T et al. (2004) Lack of evidence of sexual transmission of hepatitis C among monogamous couples: results of a 10-year prospective follow-up study. Am J Gastroenterol; 99(5):855–859

van den Berg C, Smit C, van Brussel G, Coutinho R, Prins M (2007) Full participation in harm reduction programmes is associated with decreased risk for human immunodeficiency virus and hepatitis C virus: evidence from the Amsterdam Cohort Studies among drug users. Addiction; 102(9):1454–1462

van Houdt R, Bruisten SM, Koedijk FD, Dukers NH, op de Coul EL, Mostert MC et al. (2007) Molecular epidemiology of acute hepatitis B in the Netherlands in 2004: nationwide survey. J Med Virol; 79(7):895–901

van Houdt R, Koedijk FDH, Bruisten SM, op de Coul EL, Heijnen MLA, Waldhober Q, et al. (2009) Hepatitis B vaccination targeted toward behavioral-risk groups in the Netherlands: does it work? Vaccine 27(27):3530–3535

van Steenbergen JE, Niesters HGM, Op de Coul ELM, van Doornum GJJ, Osterhaus ADME, Leentvaar-Kuijpers A et al. (2002) Molecular epidemiology of Hepatitis B Virus in Amsterdam 1992–1997. J Med Virol; 66:159–165

Vickerman P, Hickman M, Judd A (2007) Modelling the impact on Hepatitis C transmission of reducing syringe sharing: London case study. Int J Epidemiol; 36(2):396–405

Weigand K, Stremmel W, Encke J (2007) Treatment of hepatitis C virus infection. World J Gastroenterol; 13(13):1897–1905

Williams JR, Nokes DJ, Medley GF, Anderson RM (1996). The transmission dynamics of hepatitis B in the UK: a mathematical model for evaluating costs and effectiveness of immunization programmes. Epidemiol Infect; 116(1):71–89

Wright NM, Tompkins CN (2006) A review of the evidence for the effectiveness of primary prevention interventions for hepatitis C among injecting drug users. Harm Reduct J; 3:27

Xiridou M, Wallinga J, Dukers-Muijers N, Coutinho R (2008) Hepatitis B vaccination and changes in sexual risk behaviour among men who have sex with men in Amsterdam. Epidemiol Infect; 137(4):504–512

Yeung LT, King SM, Roberts EA (2001) Mother-to-infant transmission of hepatitis C virus. Hepatology; 34(2):223–229

Chapter 20
Sexual Transmission: *Chlamydia trachomatis*

Robert E. Johnson and Stuart M. Berman

20.1 Introduction

20.1.1 Basic Biology

Chlamydia trachomatis is an obligate intracellular Gram negative bacterium, which infects mucosal epithelial cells (Schachter and Stephens 2008). *Chlamydia* display a unique two-stage life cycle consisting of an infectious stage and a replicative stage. During the infectious stage the organism assumes a metabolically inactive form, the elementary body, which can survive in the host extracellular environment. Upon entry into a host cell the elementary body transforms within a host cell vacuole into a metabolically active, replicating form, the reticulate body. Over a period of approximately 36–72 hours of growth and replication, the reticulate bodies transform into infectious elementary bodies, which are extruded from the cell and repeat the cycle by infecting additional cells of the same or a second host.

A serotyping scheme, based on antibodies to the *C. trachomatis'* major outer membrane protein, permits the division of *C. trachomatis* strains into serovars (Schachter and Stephens 2008). Strains belonging to serovars A–C, the trachoma biovar, infect conjunctival epithelium, which can progress to the disease trachoma. The subject of this chapter is the group of *Chlamydia trachomatis* strains that causes sexually transmitted genital mucosal infections, the most common bacterial sexually transmitted disease. Characteristic of such strains is a predilection for asymptomatic infection. A principal focus for concern, and a focus of this chapter, is preventing ascending reproductive tract infection in women resulting in clinical pelvic inflammatory disease (PID) and, with or without symptomatic PID, sequelae that include tubal factor infertility, ectopic pregnancy, and chronic pelvic pain. An increasing number of countries are implementing national chlamydia screening programs that are motivated by apparent prior success with such

R.E. Johnson (✉)
Centers for Disease Control and Prevention, Atlanta, GA, USA
e-mail: rej1@cdc.gov

A. Krämer et al. (eds.), *Modern Infectious Disease Epidemiology*,
Statistics for Biology and Health, DOI 10.1007/978-0-387-93835-6_20,

programs for gonorrhea and randomized controlled trials that demonstrate reduction of PID among screened women. Recent observational studies of chlamydial natural history and the introduction of population chlamydial prevalence and sexual behavior surveys and dynamic models of transmission within virtual populations have helped to quantify and explain varying chlamydial prevalence. These studies have also raised questions about chlamydial pathogenesis and immunity and the impact of screening programs. Addressing these questions will require continued studies of pathogenesis and immunity and better evaluation of public health programs by improved measurement of the intensity of interventions and better and less invasive methods to detect onset of tubal disease. The remainder of this chapter is devoted to heterosexually transmitted infections with genital biovar strains, which are widely distributed in developed as well as developing countries. We focus on *C. trachomatis* infection in North American and northern European countries that are developing early diagnosis and treatment interventions.

20.1.2 Overview of Natural History of C. trachomatis Infection

Heterosexual vaginal or penile exposure to genital biovar *C. trachomatis* strains results most commonly in endocervical and male urethral infections, respectively. Symptoms, including vaginal and penile discharge and dysuria, can develop due to an inflammatory response at the site of infection, but many *C. trachomatis* infections are asymptomatic. Ascending reproductive tract infection resulting in epididymitis occurs in a small minority of men and responds to treatment so that sequelae such as infertility are rare. Ascending reproductive tract infection occurs in a larger minority of women resulting in salpingitis or, more generally, pelvic inflammatory disease (PID). PID may be associated with acute lower abdominal symptoms, but commonly occurs with minimal or no symptoms. In either case, sequelae of PID include infertility, ectopic pregnancy, and chronic pelvic pain. The natural history and epidemiology of uncomplicated male and female *C. trachomatis* infections and of PID will be discussed below. Additional manifestations of *C. trachomatis* infection, which will not be further discussed, include an uncommon reactive arthritis and transmission from mother to baby at delivery followed by neonatal conjunctivitis and infant pneumonia, which are not sight or life threatening, but are associated with substantial morbidity.

20.2 Descriptive Epidemiology of *C. trachomatis* Infection

20.2.1 Prevalence of C. trachomatis Infection

National or community population probability surveys that include testing for *C. trachomatis* infection provide prevalence estimates not susceptible to the selection bias inherent in case reporting and health care provider-based testing. In the United States (the USA) (Datta et al. 2007) and the United Kingdom (the UK) (Fenton et al. 2001) surveys, C. *trachomatis* prevalence was highest among sexually active adolescent girls and the youngest adult women. Prevalence was not markedly lower among men, but peak prevalence among men occurs a few years later than among women. In the USA, prevalence was highest among females aged 14–19 (4.6%, 95% CI 3.7–5.8%) and among males aged 20–29 (3.2%, 95% CI 2.4–4.3%) (Datta et al. 2007).

In such surveys, *C. trachomatis* prevalence has been weakly to moderately associated with socioeconomic status, although socioeconomic status is difficult to assess in adolescents and young adults (Datta et al. 2007; Fenton et al. 2001; van Bergen et al. 2005). In the USA, *C. trachomatis* prevalence has been more strongly associated with race ethnicity than socioeconomic status. In a US survey of young adults, ages 18–26, prevalence of *C. trachomatis* infection among black women (14.0%, 95% CI 11.3–17.2%) and men (11.1%, 95% CI 8.5–14.4%) was substantially higher than among white women (2.5%, 95% CI 1.9–3.3%) and men (1.4%, 95% CI 0.9–2.0%) (Miller et al. 2004). Where assessed, *C. trachomatis* prevalence was lower among married individuals (Datta et al. 2007; Fenton et al. 2001).

20.2.2 Disease Burden Attributable to C. trachomatis Infection

It has been difficult to determine what proportion of PID and its sequelae are attributable to *C. trachomatis* infection. Detecting tubal inflammation and scarring and determining whether infertility, ectopic pregnancy, or chronic pelvic pain is attributable to such disease requires invasive diagnostic procedures. Serologic tests to detect untreated prior *C. trachomatis* infection are subject to errors of sensitivity and specificity. Other sexually transmitted organisms, in particular *Neisseria gonorrhoeae*, but also, possibly, *Mycoplasma genitalium*, as well as enteric and anaerobic gram negative organisms commonly found in the vagina contribute to the occurrence of PID. Parsing out the contribution of *C. trachomatis* from these other contributors to clinical and subclinical PID and subsequent sequelae has been difficult and only partly successful.

20.2.2.1 Pelvic Inflammatory Disease

Most cases of PID are managed in ambulatory settings and few countries or communities can determine frequencies of ambulatory cases of PID. The US Centers for Disease Control and Prevention has tracked physician diagnoses of PID utilizing national surveys of hospital discharges, visits to hospital emergency rooms and outpatient clinics, and visits to office-based practitioners (Sutton et al. 2005).

During 1995–2001, the average estimated annual rate of hospital discharges and ambulatory visits for acute and unspecified PID in the USA was highest for age group 25–29 with a discharge rate of 1.1 (95%, CI 0.9–1.3%) per 1,000 women and an ambulatory visit rate of 19.0 (95%, CI 12.0–26.0%) per 1,000 women. In a retrospective cohort study, Low et al. (2006) selected female residents of Uppsala, Sweden, that were between 15 and 24 years of age between 1985 and 1989 and conducted a record search through 1999 for in-hospital, and for the last 6 years of that interval, for hospital outpatient diagnoses of PID. Although non-hospital ambulatory cases of PID were missed, the study provided a unique cumulative incidence minimum estimate, 3.9% (95%, CI 3.7–4.0%) of females by age 35.

The proportion of PID that is caused by *C. trachomatis* is not well defined. The overall cervical isolation rate was 29% with a range of 5–51% in a compilation of studies published between 1975 and 1995 (Paavonen et al. 2008). More recently, an English study conducted during 2000–2002, using nucleic acid amplification testing of endocervical or urine specimens, detected *C. trachomatis* in 12% of 140 outpatient PID cases (Simms et al. 2006). A large US study detected *C. trachomatis* by PCR or *N. gonorrhoeae* by culture testing of endocervical specimens in 40% of patients who were eligible for out-of-hospital care (Ness et al. 2002). The relatively low specificity of outpatient clinical diagnosis of PID (Jacobson and Westrom 1969; Simms et al. 2003) contributes a substantial negative bias to estimates of *C. trachomatis* prevalence among patients with outpatient-diagnosed PID.

Subclinical PID caused by *C. trachomatis* appears to be a significant problem. Although these cases impose no burden with respect to acute disease, they may be very important, since the majority of women presenting with tubal infertility or ectopic pregnancy occur among women with no prior history of PID (reviewed in Wiesenfeld and Cates 2008).

20.2.2.2 Sequelae of PID

In 2002, a US household probability survey estimated that 7.4% of married or cohabiting US women were infertile (Stephen and Chandra 2006). No population survey has included the invasive diagnostic procedures required to identify tubal disease as the cause of infertility. However, in 2006, 18% of US couples who utilized assisted reproductive technology were affected by tubal infertility (Macaluso et al. 2008). Using health services data published for an English health district (Hull et al. 1985), Wiesenfeld and Cates estimated that one in six couples would seek infertility treatment from a specialist during their lives with tubal damage accounting for the infertility in 14% of infertile couples (Wiesendfeld and Cates 2008). In a Danish study, approximately 20% of infertility was attributed to tubal damage (Schmidt et al. 1995).

Determining what proportion of tubal infertility is attributable to *C. trachomatis* infection is difficult. A recent review of 15 cross-sectional and case–control studies provides the percent of tubal-factor infertility cases and nontubal-factor infertility controls, respectively, that had chlamydial antibody (Wiesenfeld and Cates 2008). These percents yield odds ratios of 5–93 (authors calculations). A recent Netherlands study utilized a serologic test that was species specific (den Hartog et al. 2004). The percent test positive for the cases and controls were 54% and 8%, respectively (odds ratio 14). These estimates might overstate the role of *C. trachomatis* if the serologic tests for *C. trachomatis* are less sensitive among controls than cases and if *C. trachomatis* infection is a marker for other causal infections, such as *N. gonorrhoeae* or *Mycoplasma genitalium*.

Determining the frequency of ectopic pregnancy has become difficult due to the increasing proportion of cases that are treated as outpatients. Recently, 1–3% of pregnancies were reported to be ectopic (Bakken 2008; Farquhar 2005). Wiesenfeld and Cates reviewed 12 case–control studies of ectopic pregnancy and *C. trachomatis* infection (Wiesenfeld and Cates 2008). The odds ratios for ectopic pregnancy following *C. trachomatis* infection, based on *C. trachomatis* serologic tests, are slightly lower than for infertility with point estimates ranging from 2 to 24. The caveats described above for infertility regarding these associations also apply to ectopic pregnancy.

Chronic pelvic pain is also an important sequela of *C. trachomatis* tubal infection because of the impact on the quality of life and the costs associated with diagnostic procedures and treatment (Haggerty et al. 2003). Although chronic pelvic pain is common, affecting 15% of women in the USA (Mathias et al. 1996), studies have not been conducted to assess the role of prior *C. trachomatis* infection.

20.3 Determinants of the Epidemiology of *C. trachomatis* Infection

Transmission of communicable infections through populations depends on a set of key variables: risk of transmission during contact between infected and susceptible individuals; time course of infections, including onset of symptoms; and rates and patterns of contacts, in this case, sexual contacts (Garnett 2002). Dynamic transmission models that are being used to evaluate chlamydial interventions (described subsequently) depend upon having estimates for these key model parameters.

20.3.1 Risk of an Initial C. trachomatis Infection

The risk of chlamydial infection following a single sexual exposure has not been estimated directly. Instead, Kretzschmar et al. (2001) utilized results of a study of the concordance of chlamydial infection between heterosexual partners attending an STD clinic (Quinn et al. 1996). The percents that were *C. trachomatis* test positive among female and male partners of test-positive index patients were approximately 70%. Treating transmission during individual exposures as independent binomial probability events, Kretzschmar et al. (2001) derived a per-contact probability of infection of 0.108 by assuming a mean of 10 exposures per casual partnership. Regan et al. (2008) similarly derived a transmission risk per exposure range of 0.0165–0.17 by assuming a range of exposures per partnership. However, such an approach may not provide an accurate estimate if, among concordantly positive partners, presumed source partners are actually "spread" partners. Turner et al. (2006a) arrived at a transmission probability per sex act of 0.0375 by fitting a simulation model to sexual behavior and prevalence information obtained from surveys and the literature.

20.3.2 Symptoms and Time Course of *C. trachomatis* Genital Infection

Given the 36–72 hour replication cycle of *Chlamydia*, a few days to 2–3 weeks is required for *C. trachomatis* infection to become established at which time an individual is presumed to be infectious. In the absence of a screening program, the infection would be expected to persist until (1) symptoms develop and the infected individual obtains curative treatment; (2) the individual is referred for curative treatment because an infected sex partner develops symptoms; or (3) the infection is resolved by an immune response. Determining the proportional distribution of incident *C. trachomatis* infections among these categories and the duration of infection within each is critical to modeling *C. trachomatis* infection in populations and to designing community interventions. However, such determinations are very problematic, since it is difficult to determine the time of onset of most infections and it is not ethically feasible to follow untreated individuals.

An early dynamic transmission model of *C. trachomatis* infection assumed that 75% of infected males and 30% of infected females develop symptoms (Kretzschmar et al. 1996). Subsequent studies have resulted in markedly reduced values for males. Korenromp et al. (2002) modeled the probability of developing symptoms, the probability of treatment, the point prevalence of symptoms, and the duration of infection. They fit their model to values for these variables obtained from the literature, survey data from Rakai District, Uganda, and expert opinion. They estimated that 6 and 11% of infected females and males, respectively, develop symptoms. Farley et al. (2003) conducted a retrospective cohort study in the United States by enrolling men and women who presented to potential chlamydia screening sites for reasons unrelated to chlamydial infection. Using a combination of history of symptoms during the prior year, medical chart review, and current prevalence of infection, they estimated that only 11% of males and 29% of females that became infected during the year developed symptoms and 85 and 80%, respectively, of these sought care and were treated.

In addition to the proportion asymptomatic, the duration of infection among those without symptoms importantly affects the effectiveness of screening. A number of studies have investigated the proportion of individuals with chlamydial infection who were still infected at a return visit for treatment. For a set of such studies, Korenromp et al. (2002) assumed that the rate of resolution of infection is constant and independent of the past duration of infection and, by applying an exponential distribution, calculated the total mean duration of infection for each study from the proportion still infected at the follow-up and the mean days of follow-up. The authors pooled the results for each gender, reporting an estimated mean duration of infection of 132 days for males and 499 days for females.

Clearly, considerable uncertainty exists regarding the proportion of incident chlamydial infections that result in symptoms and the duration of untreated infections. Nevertheless, these estimates suggest that only a small minority of infected individuals seek curative health care and, in the absence of treatment, infection persists for a few months in males and for over a year in females. The frequency with which infections are ended due to treatment secondary to onset of symptoms in an infected sex partner is unknown.

20.3.3 Time Course of Complicated C. trachomatis Genital Infection

A few studies provide some insight regarding risk of clinically evident PID following acquisition of chlamydia. Two early studies involved clinical trials in which 20 women with *N. gonorrhoeae* infection (Stamm et al. 1984) and 15 female partners of men with nongonococcal urethritis (Paavonen et al. 1980) were determined to have *C. trachomatis* infection but did not receive effective treatment for that organism. At follow-up, 30 and 20%, respectively, of the women had clinically evident PID compared with 2% and none of controls that received antibiotics active against *C. trachomatis*.

Subsequent studies, which involved follow-up of untreated women who tested positive for *C. trachomatis* infection, have reported lower rates of clinically evident PID. In these studies, 2%, 3.6%, and none of infected women developed evidence of PID during intervals without treatment of up to 60 days (Geisler et al. 2008), for 90 days (Rahm et al. 1986), and for 1 year (Morre et al. 2002), respectively. The reasons for the disparity in these rates of clinically evident PID during follow-up of women with chlamydial infection are unclear.

The classical cohort study of 1,309 Swedish women followed after treatment for laparoscopically confirmed PID is the principal source of estimates of the risk of sequelae following treated PID (Westrom et al. 1992). The authors reported a confirmed tubal infertility rate of 10.8% among treated PID cases compared with none among controls. Ectopic pregnancy occurred in 9.1% of the women treated for PID compared with 1.4% of controls. Chronic abdominal pain developed in 18.1% of a subsample of PID cases and 5% of controls (Westrom 1975).

The case–control studies described earlier in this chapter suggest that a substantial proportion of PID that progresses to sequelae is subclinical. The risk of sequelae following untreated chlamydial infection in the absence of clinically evident PID is unknown.

20.3.4 Formation and Dissolution of Sexual Partnerships

STI are transmitted through sexual partner networks embedded in and connecting communities. Network theory together with infectious disease modeling has been used extensively in recent years to better understand how these complicated and dynamic networks affect the frequency and distribution of STI, including chlamydial infection (Doherty et al. 2005; Garnett 2008; Morris et al. 2008). Important aspects of sexual partnering include the rate of formation and dissolution of sexual partnerships, the extent to which individuals form sexual partnerships with individuals of similar chlamydial risk status (assortative mixing), and the extent to which sexual partnerships overlap (concurrency).

Age is a strong risk factor for STI in general and especially for chlamydial infection. This is particularly true in developed countries where first sexual partnerships occur during the mid-to-late teens or early twenties, but marriage is delayed (Berman and Ellen 2008; Wellings et al. 2006). Median age at marriage/cohabitation is later for men than women (Wellings et al. 2006). Compared with older persons, a higher proportion of the sexually active in younger age groups report multiple or new partners (Johnson et al. 2001; Kretzschmar et al. 1996; Kretzschmar et al. 2001; Low et al. 2006; Mosher et al. 2005; Regan et al. 2008), have primary monogamous partnerships of shorter duration (Laumann 1994; Low et al. 2007; Turner et al. 2006a; Turner et al. 2006b), and are more likely to enter a new partnership, i.e., a concurrent partnership, while continuing a current relationship (Johnson et al. 2001; Kelley et al. 2003). Sexual partnering by age is strongly assortative, further contributing to the relative concentration of chlamydial infections among teens and young adults; males, however, tend to be slightly older than their female partners (Laumann 1994; Low et al. 2007; Morris et al. 2008; Regan et al. 2008; Turner et al. 2006a; Turner et al. 2006b). Increased susceptibility to chlamydial infection due to cervical ectopy in adolescent girls and relative lack of any immunity may add to their increased risk. The fact that *C. trachomatis* infections, unlike HIV or herpes simplex virus type 2, do not persist and accumulate with increasing age also serves to concentrate transmission within the teen and young adult age groups (Morris et al. 2008).

Sexual network differences also contribute to race-ethnicity disparities in prevalence of STIs, including chlamydial infections. National population surveys in Britain and the USA indicate differences by race ethnicity in numbers of partners, especially for males (Fenton et al. 2005; Mosher et al. 2005). Analyses of results from an earlier US survey, conducted in 1992, demonstrated strong assortative mixing by black and white races (Laumann and Yoosik 1999). Assortative mixing by race was greater for blacks than whites and, in part, explains the racial disparities in STDs; in addition, mixing between risk groups was more random among blacks than whites, which facilitates STD transmission through a population and also contributes to the observed racial disparities. These differences in mixing patterns reinforce the effects of differences in number of sex partners and other STI risk differences, e.g., health-care utilization, on race-ethnicity disparities.

20.4 Public Health Interventions

The four essential interventions related to STD prevention are clinical, screening, partner management, and individual and community behavioral services. Clinical services for individuals with symptomatic chlamydial infections are important, but most infections are asymptomatic. Consequently, identification and treatment of asymptomatic infections have been the focus of chlamydia prevention efforts. Screening appropriate populations for chlamydia and providing effective treatment reduce transmission – accomplishing primary prevention – by shortening duration of infection. Partner notification serves the same objective. In addition, both approaches can also serve secondary prevention objectives, by treating infected individuals, especially women, and preventing the development of complications, such as PID. The chlamydia-specific aspects of these activities are discussed below in some detail. Few aspects of individual or community level behavioral interventions are specific to chlamydia and are not addressed in this chapter.

20.4.1 Dynamic Models of Early Diagnosis and Treatment

Dynamic models that simulate heterosexual transmission of chlamydial infection through virtual communities have been used to evaluate early diagnosis and treatment interventions (Andersen et al. 2006; Brunham et al. 2006; de Vries et al. 2008; Fisman et al. 2008; Gift et al. 2008; Kretzschmar et al. 1996; Kretzschmar et al. 2001; Low et al. 2007; Regan et al. 2008; Turner et al. 2006a; Turner et al. 2006b). These models are based on the proximate determinants of transmission: rates of sexual contact; risk of transmission given contact between infected and susceptible sex partners; and the duration of infection (Garnett 2002). More realistic models involve greater complexity, subdividing groups of infected and susceptible males and females into subgroups, based on combinations of age and risky sexual behavior. Mixing matrices are applied to generate assortative sexual mixing between combinations of age and sexual behavior subgroups. The dynamic models are generally run under baseline conditions until chlamydial prevalence stabilizes at equilibrium. An intervention is then introduced and the model continued for sufficient time to capture the effect of the intervention on chlamydia prevalence.

The simplest of the dynamic models are deterministic compartmental models, which do not consider events at the individual level (Brunham et al. 2005; de Vries et al. 2006; de Vries et al. 2008; Fisman et al. 2008; Gift et al. 2008; Regan et al. 2008). These models consider only average rates of events (e.g., sexual contact and resolution of infection) that determine the flow of individuals between subgroups (Garnett 2002). Most *C. trachomatis* transmission models have been of the susceptible-infected-susceptible type, i.e., *C. trachomatis* infected individuals have been assumed to return immediately to a susceptible state upon resolution of their infection. Certain recent models have considered the impact of immunity by adding compartments for immune individuals (Brunmhan et al. 2005; Fisman et al. 2008; Regan et al. 2008).

A concern with deterministic compartmental *C. trachomatis* models has been their inability to take into account events within a given dyad – for example, that one member of a dually infected partnership may continue with that partnership following screening and treatment rather than selecting a new partner at random (Morris et al. 2008). The effect of screening may be nullified by reinfection if the partner is not referred and treated. Furthermore, the deterministic models do not adequately reflect the impact of concurrent relationships. To address these concerns, dynamic models have been developed that track individuals and sexual partnerships (Andersen et al. 2006; Kretzschmar et al. 1996; Kretzschmar et al. 2001; Low et al. 2007; Turner et al. 2006a; Turner et al. 2006b).

Parameter values for these models have been chosen by reviewing the literature and conducting local sexual behavior and chlamydial prevalence surveys. If initial model results deviate from the results of the surveys, the modelers have used their judgment to adjust, i.e., calibrate initial parameter values until the model generates results that reasonably fit survey results. As a consequence, some of the parameter values used in the published *C. trachomatis* dynamic modeling studies, e.g., probability of an infection becoming symptomatic and rate of resolution of infections differ substantially among studies even though the structure of the models and local survey results are similar.

Taken together, the modeling studies support a prediction that screening of females aged 15–24 would be an effective core component of a screening program intended to reduce prevalence in the population (Brunham et al. 2005; Fisman et al. 2008; Kretzschmar et al. 1996, 2001; Regan et al. 2008). Roughly a quarter to a third of that group must be screened annually to begin to have a substantial impact; the impact appears to accelerate with expanded screening and then the incremental gains decline as coverage exceeds a majority of the target population (Kretzschmar et al. 1996; 2001; Turner et al. 2006a; Turner et al. 2006b). The individual person models demonstrate the importance of partner notification (Andersen et al. 2006; Kretzschmar et al. 1996; Kretzschmar et al. 2001; Turner et al. 2006a; Turner et al. 2006b). The effect of partner notification interacts with screening, since partner notification cannot be initiated until the index individual's infection is detected. If screening coverage of women was high, increasing notification and treatment of male partners had a greater impact on prevalence among women than screening males (Kretzschmar et al. 2001). Some combination of partner notification and screening to detect and treat infected males contributed importantly to reducing prevalence when coverage of females aged 15–24, in particular, but also aged 15–29, was not high (Fisman et al. 2008; Turner et al. 2006a; Turner et al. 2006b).

An important exception to the findings of the dynamic transmission modeling studies described immediately above is the results of a study conducted to evaluate potential home-based screening in the UK (Low et al. 2007; Roberts et al. 2007). Although the structure and parameterization of the model used in this study appear to be similar to the individual-based models used in the foregoing studies, the reported impact of screening and partner notification on chlamydial prevalence was much lower.

20.4.2 Cost-Effectiveness of Early Diagnosis and Treatment

Appended to several of the chlamydia dynamic transmission models are economic models, which take chlamydial incidence, the probabilities of chlamydial complications and sequelae, and the costs of intervention activities and disease as inputs and provide estimates of the costs, the effectiveness, and the cost-effectiveness as outputs (Adams et al. 2007; Andersen et al. 2006; de Vries et al. 2008; de Vries et al. 2006; Gift et al. 2008; Roberts et al. 2007; Welte et al. 2000). Welte et al. (2000), in an early dynamic modeling cost-effectiveness study of chlamydia screening, found annual provider-based screening of females aged 15–24 to be cost saving, given a very high screening compliance rate, a moderately high partner treatment rate, and relatively high PID risk (0.25), PID hospitalization rate, and hospitalized PID treatment cost. In that study, the program was cost saving under a variety of univariate sensitivity analyses.

Recent *C. trachomatis* cost-effectiveness screening studies have utilized lower screening and partner notification rates based on the results of field studies, reduced the risk of PID associated with untreated infection in response to cohort studies of chlamydial infection, and reduced estimated costs associated with PID, to reflect that the vast majority of cases are managed without hospitalization. Certain studies have also added quality adjusted life years (QALYs) to major outcomes averted (MOAs) to provide an outcome measure that permits comparison of chlamydial interventions with interventions that target other diseases. Studies vary in whether they consider direct costs only (health systems perspective) or include indirect patient costs as well (societal perspective).

A study that simulated population-based *C. trachomatis* screening in Denmark by mailing of test specimens utilized a PID risk of 0.20. Program direct costs decreased steadily over the 10-year simulation, becoming negative in the 10th year (Andersen et al. 2006). The simulation study of provider-based opportunistic screening in the UK, described above (Turner et al. 2006a; Turner et al. 2006b) included a separately published cost-effectiveness component (Adams et al. 2007). The modelers considered only symptomatic PID and decided that a PID risk of 0.10 and hospitalization rate of 6.5% best matched UK PID study results (Simms et al. 2006) and service data. Screening females aged 16–24 or screening both genders aged 16–20 yielded direct costs per QALY gained compared with no screening of <£20,000. The incremental cost per QALY gained of adding screening of males aged 16–24 to screening of females aged 16–24 was relatively large, yielding direct costs per QALY gained compared with no screening in the £20,000–30,000 range. Overall, applying a UK standard of £20,000–30,000 per QALY gained, the authors considered chlamydia screening to be borderline cost-effective.

Cost-effectiveness dynamic modeling studies that have assessed adding male screening to female screening in schools (Fisman et al. 2008) or adding male screening in high prevalence venues to standard screening of females aged 15–24 years (Gift et al. 2008) yielded very satisfactory cost per QALY gained (Fisman et al. 2008). In general, sensitivity analyses conducted in dynamic modeling cost-effectiveness studies demonstrate low cost-effectiveness as PID rates drop toward 0.01 or as interventions are extended to older age groups (Andersen et al. 2006; Roberts et al. 2007).

20.4.3 Public Health Screening and Partner Treatment Programs

Following is a brief summary of efforts that North American and northern European countries have made to establish national chlamydia screening and partner notification programs.

20.4.3.1 Screening

In 1993, the US Centers for Disease Control and Prevention published "Recommendations for the prevention and management of *Chlamydia trachomatis* infections" (Centers for Disease Control and Prevention 1993). Screening was recommended for all sexually active women less than 20 years of age and for older women who met either (ages 20–24) or both (ages >24) of the additional criteria – inconsistent use of barrier contraception, or new or more than one sex partner during the last 3 months. The Recommendations were justified in part by a pilot project implementing chlamydia screening among attendees in 136 family planning clinics in four states in the northwestern United States. Prevalence decreased from 10.9% in 1988 to 6.8% in the last quarter of 1990 (Britton et al. 1992). Chlamydia screening was also motivated by the apparent success of a gonorrhea prevention program; following a tripling of US gonorrhea rates, rates peaked and then declined impressively subsequent to 1975, just 3 years after nationwide gonorrhea control efforts were implemented (Wasserheit and Aral 1996).

In 2001 the US Preventive Services Task Force recommended chlamydia screening for women <25 years of age (Nelson and Helfand 2001). The Task Force was strongly motivated by a randomized controlled trial that demonstrated a 56% reduction in incidence of PID by screening women selected by a set of risk factors (Scholes et al. 1996). The Task Force did not find convincing evidence that population prevalence rates were decreased as a result of screening. It also pointed out a lack of evidence concerning effectiveness of screening men for chlamydia.

In 1996, the Canadian Task Force on the Periodic Health Examination recommended annual screening of high-risk groups: sexually active women less than 25 years of age; men or women with new or multiple sexual partners during the preceding year; and women who use nonbarrier contraceptive methods (Davies and Wang 1996). Sweden began a program in 1982 to identify asymptomatic infection, and in 1988 passed legislation requiring clinicians to provide free chlamydia testing (Low 2007). However, beyond making free testing available, there is, in fact, no national program in the country; chlamydia control is locally organized, with intensity varying by geographic location (Low 2004).

In England, the National Chlamydia Screening Programme was launched in 2002, with phased implementation (Fenton and Ward 2004). The National Chlamydia Screening Programme targets men and women under 25 years of age and utilizes an opportunistic approach, as does the USA and Canada. An opportunistic screening approach, with screening taking place in health-care settings, rather than a registry-based approach with household screening, was adopted, because the latter was shown to be associated with substantially lower prevalences (Fenton and Ward 2004). The Netherlands, however, is implementing a pilot chlamydia screening project that does in fact utilize a systematic registry-based approach with invitations for testing sent by post (Op de Coul et al. 2007).

One basis for questioning the effectiveness of screening is that countries engaged in chlamydia screening have been experiencing increasing rates of reported chlamydia cases (Fine et al. 2008; Rekart and Brunham 2008; Velicko et al. 2007). However, the modeling studies described previously indicate that achieving decreases in chlamydia prevalence is dependent upon adequate screening coverage. The ability of countries that have implemented screening programs to monitor coverage independently of chlamydia infection rates varies greatly and has contributed to substantial confusion in assessing the effectiveness of these programs.

The UK appears to have the ability to monitor opportunistic screening rates. Unfortunately, the program target to screen 15% of the 15–24 year old population between April 1, 2007 and March 31, 2008 (National Chlamydia Screening Programme 2008) appeared to be aspirational; data suggest that the target was not achieved (White 2008). An analysis of services and outcomes in Uppsala, Sweden, found that, among females who were 15–24 years old between 1984 and 1989, during a follow-up that was up to 10 years, 70.7% were tested for chlamydia at least one time; of those ever tested, almost half (47.8%) were tested only once (Low et al. 2006). An analysis in Sweden evaluating the increases in rates of genital chlamydia that occurred over 10 years nationally reported that approximately 10% of 15–49 year olds were tested for *C trachomatis* in 2006, and that fewer were tested in previous years (Velicko et al. 2007).

Similarly in North America, although there are reports that rates of chlamydia in British Columbia have increased, there is little information about screening coverage; Low has estimated that annual coverage is unlikely to be over 10–20% (Low 2008). In the USA, which may be experiencing a modest decline in chlamydia burden (Datta et al. 2008), opportunistic screening coverage has been monitored in a group of commercial and Medicaid health plans. The chlamydia screening rate among sexually active female enrollees aged 16–25 years increased from 25.3% in 2000 to 41.6% in 2007, but is now leveling off (Douglas 2008).

20.4.3.2 Partner Notification

Efforts to treat partners of individuals diagnosed with chlamydia are justified for at least two reasons. First, it allows exposed or infected individuals to obtain prompt treatment, hopefully preventing possible sequelae. Second, partner treatment reduces ongoing transmission. The potential effectiveness of such an approach is related to the probability of infection in the exposed partners. Studies have documented a high concordance of infection (68%) in sexual partners (Quinn et al. 1996).

There are several recent excellent reviews of partner notification (Centers for Disease Control and Prevention 2008a; Hogben 2007; Hogben et al. 2007; Trelle et al. 2007). Partner notification has either involved public health professionals notifying partners (provider referral) or required the patient to notify partners (patient- or self-referral) (Hogben et al. 2007). Although the labor-intense provider referral approach is not typically utilized for chlamydia cases in the USA, there is some evidence that the approach is cost-effective (Katz et al. 1988). Evaluations among individuals with chlamydia, gonorrhea, trichomoniasis, or syndromic STDs have found that partner-delivered therapy or another form of expedited partner treatment (EPT, approaches that do not require an intervening clinical encounter with the partner) were associated with a greater number of partners being treated (Golden et al. 2005; Kissinger et al. 2005) and a reduced risk of reinfection with gonorrhea or chlamydia, when compared with simple patient referral methods. Similarly, there is evidence that providing infected patients an informative booklet in addition to relying on the simple patient referral method also increases the number of partners that receive treatment (Kissinger et al. 2006). Recently, the Internet has been utilized for partner notification. However, Internet notification has been evaluated primarily for exposure to syphilis (Hogben 2007).

Policies and approaches to partner notification differ by country. In Europe, only in Sweden and Norway is partner notification compulsory (not surprisingly, it is estimated that in Sweden 76–99% of partners exposed to chlamydia are tested and/or treated) (Arthur et al. 2005). In the USA, laws vary by state. Certain states have laws requiring practitioners to warn persons they know to be at risk for infection with a communicable disease, an STD, or HIV because of exposure to their patients. Many other states have laws permitting but not requiring practitioners to warn persons that they are at risk (i.e., privilege to warn) (Centers for Disease Control and Prevention 2008a). Also, in the USA, partner notification efforts undertaken by health department personnel are closely related to the etiologic agent; in one study, partner notification interviews were conducted with 89% of syphilis, 17% of gonorrhea, and 12% of chlamydia cases (Golden et al. 2003).

In the USA, because of differences in laws or pharmacy regulations, EPT is legally permissible in some states, prohibited in others, and potentially allowable elsewhere (Hodge et al. 2008). In the UK, partner-delivered therapy is clearly not consistent with Good Medical Practice guidance from the General Medical Council. Although there is support for the practice among those in the genitourinary medicine community (Coyne et al. 2007), such support is clearly not universal (Markos 2008).

20.5 Monitoring Impact of Public Health Interventions

Chlamydial interventions described in the previous section began in Sweden in the early 1980s and somewhat later in the USA. Although evaluations were provided that convinced authorities to launch prevention efforts, adequately monitoring the impact of such efforts on chlamydia prevalence and chlamydia-related sequelae has been challenging.

20.5.1 Tracking Prevalence of C. trachomatis Infection

Case report data, expressed as cases per population (typically 100,000), have not proven useful in tracking changes in chlamydia burden, since increased case rates represent expanded efforts at detecting asymptomatic infection rather than disease trends. In the USA, the rate of reported chlamydia has increased every year in all regions (Centers for Disease Control and Prevention 2008b). Furthermore, since screening has been performed primarily among females, the rate of reported infection has appeared substantially greater among females than among males (Centers for Disease Control and Prevention 2008b; Hiltunen-Back et al. 2003; Klovstad and Aavitsland 2009), although prevalence by gender, when measured by a population survey, is actually rather comparable (Datta et al. 2007).

Monitoring chlamydia test positivity is another approach to track chlamydia burden. In the United States, such an approach provides positivity data in all 50 states, stratified by clinic type (i.e., family planning clinics, prenatal care clinics, STD clinics) (Centers for Disease Control and Prevention 2009). Such data have been useful for evaluating screening strategies (La Montagne et al. 2004), and for targeting resources to sites and populations with higher disease burden (Gorgos et al. 2008). Median state-specific positivity among 15–24 year old women tested in family planning clinics has increased steadily from 5.2% in 2000 to 6.9% in 2007 (Centers for Disease Control and Prevention 2008b). However, annual analyses may not include the same individual clinics consistently, and screening criteria employed by the clinics may change over time. Because of such factors, and also because clinic populations themselves may change, some authors have pointed out the marked bias that may be associated with such assessments (Miller 2008). Similarly, in Norway, the proportion of tests for chlamydia that were positive increased from 4.1% in 1993 to 7.7% in 2006. However, the extent to which this represents a true increase in disease burden is not clear, since the case definition had changed, there was increased use of NAATs, and perhaps increased testing among high-risk groups (Klovstad and Aavitsland 2009).

A more methodologically appropriate way to track chlamydia would be to assess prevalence in a defined population, accessed in a consistent fashion. In the United States, the National Health and Nutrition Examination Survey (NHANES) allows tracking of chlamydia in just such a manner. Analysis of data from 1999 to 2006 has provided strong evidence that chlamydia burden has not been increasing, and may actually be decreasing; the overall prevalence of *C. trachomatis* among 14–39 year olds was: 1999–2000, 2.6% (95%, CI 2.0–3.5%); 2001–2002, 1.8%, (1.3–2.6%); 2003–2004, 2.1% (1.5–2.9%); and 2005–2006, 1.4% (0.9–1.9%). Furthermore, statistically significant decreases were seen among females 14–19 years of age, a group targeted for screening (Datta et al. 2008). In addition, in the USA, prevalence has been tracked among National Job Program entrants, economically disadvantaged young people 16–24 years of age, who have met consistent criteria for participation. From 1990 to 1997, chlamydia prevalence among female entrants decreased from 14.9 to 10.0% (Mertz et al. 2001); a more modest decline was seen from 1998 to 2004, 11.7–10.3% (Joesof and Mosure 2006).

The UK is one of the few other countries that have population-based prevalence data on chlamydia. The 2000 National Survey of Sexual Attitudes and Lifestyles (NATSAL 2000) found that *C trachomatis* prevalence was 2.2% (95%, CI 1.5–3.2%) among men and 1.5% (95%, CI 1.11–2.14%) among women; prevalence was greater among young males and females (Fenton et al. 2001). The results of the next evaluation, planned for 2010, will be of great interest, since the National Chlamydia Screening Program was implemented in England in 2002 (Fenton and Ward 2004).

20.5.2 Tracking Complications and Sequelae

20.5.2.1 Pelvic Inflammatory Disease

The diagnosis of PID is clinical and correlation with salpingitis is imperfect; salpingitis was identified in 65 and 46% of PID cases in two studies utilizing specific diagnostic criteria (Chaparro et al. 1978; Jacobson and Westrom 1969). Doxanakis (STI 2008) found in the same clinical setting great clinician variability in the frequency of PID diagnosis (Doxanakis et al. 2008). Furthermore, the criteria recommended in the US Centers for Disease Control and Prevention STD Treatment Guidelines for identifying cases that warrant PID treatment became increasingly sensitive and less specific in the last three versions (Centers for Disease Control and Prevention 1998, 2002, 2006).

These challenges not withstanding, rates of PID in several countries have been decreasing. In Sweden, rates of PID hospitalizations were stable or increased from the 1970s to the early 1980s. Subsequently, from 1987 to 1997, rates fell sharply; during that time endemic *N. gonorrhoeae* was nearly eliminated, and cases of PID were increasingly managed in outpatient settings (Kamwendo et al. 1998). Similarly, during that same time, community rates of PID fell sharply in Lund, Sweden (Westrom et al. 1992). In the United States, where approximately 91% of

PID cases are managed in ambulatory settings (Sutton et al. 2005), rates of hospitalization fell by 68% between 1985 and 2001 and ambulatory visits for PID decreased by 47–68%, depending on the data source utilized (Sutton et al. 2005).

These declines in PID are encouraging. Nevertheless, additional research is clearly needed to identify a reliable surveillance definition that is not so affected by clinician subjectivity and that accurately identifies chlamydia-associated cases.

20.5.2.2 Ectopic Pregnancy

Assessing trends in chlamydia-associated outcomes of ectopic pregnancy or infertility is no easier or more certain. Regardless, incidence of ectopic pregnancy increased substantially in a number of nations, including the USA, during the 1970s and 1980s (Centers for Disease Control and Prevention 1995; Coste et al. 1994; Makinen et al. 1998). More recently, declines in rates of ectopic pregnancy have been noted in some places, but not others (Coste et al. 2004). Sweden experienced a 21% decrease among women ≥25 years from 1990–1994 to 1997 (Kamwendo et al. 2000). An ecologic evaluation from 1985 to 1995 in a county in Sweden (Egger et al. 1998) found that falling rates of chlamydia were associated with declines in ectopic pregnancy. However, such an association was not found in Australia, where between 1992 and 2001 hospitalizations for ectopic pregnancy remained constant, while case reports of chlamydia increased fourfold (Chen et al. 2005). Evaluations in the United States have only monitored hospitalizations, which is an increasingly less relevant approach since most ectopic pregnancies are managed as outpatients (Zane et al. 2002).

20.5.2.3 Infertility

Tracking the prevalence of chlamydia-related infertility is also problematic. In fact, some have questioned the estimates of the contribution chlamydial infection makes to overall infertility, highlighting the limitations of the supporting evidence (Wallace et al. 2008). Registry data from some Scandinavian countries have allowed evaluations linking chlamydia case reports or test results with birth and care records, but the results have not been very helpful, since it is not clear how infertility rates following *treated chlamydial infections* relate to chlamydia control activities.

Data available from women in the USA, who have received infertility services, provide some additional information about infertility trends and tubal factor infertility. In 2006, 18% of couples utilizing assisted reproductive technology (ART) to conceive had tubal factor infertility (Macaluso et al. 2008) compared with 33% in 1996 (Macaluso, personal communication). Although such findings suggest that the prevalence of tubal factor infertility is decreasing – consistent with chlamydia control efforts – other factors may well be responsible.

20.6 Challenges

The discipline of epidemiology and the closely related discipline of public health are at an important juncture with respect to understanding and addressing the burden of *C. trachomatis* infection in populations. The distribution of *C. trachomatis* infections is well understood. Accurate, effective, and inexpensive tests and antibiotics are available to detect and treat these infections. The effectiveness of these tools to reduce progression to PID by proactive screening of women, as demonstrated in randomized controlled trials (RCTs) (Scholes et al. 1996), has motivated certain authoritative groups and governments to recommend and institute national screening programs. In parallel, advances in infectious disease epidemiology and simulation modeling have provided powerful tools to better understand the dynamics of *C. trachomatis* transmission through populations and the effects of interventions. With important exceptions, the results of studies that have utilized these tools have encouraged public health workers to expect that the primary prevention benefits of *C. trachomatis* screening programs are a cost-effective extension of the secondary prevention benefits demonstrated by the RCTs.

A number of serious challenges need to be addressed to ensure continuation of the foregoing progress. A particularly pressing challenge is to develop diagnostic methods and population-based surveillance systems to track PID and its sequelae. A second critical challenge is to improve our ability to monitor screening coverage and success rates in notifying sex partners of individuals treated for chlamydial infection. This challenge is especially great in countries such as the USA with highly heterogeneous health-care delivery systems and limited population level information concerning individuals. At least as urgent is the need to develop field evaluations that incorporate the improved measures of burden and intensity of interventions.

The large literature on the immunology of *C. trachomatis* infection, developed largely with a focus on vaccine development, was beyond the scope of this chapter. The transmission modeling studies reviewed in this chapter assumed rapid loss of any immunity following chlamydial infection. However, concerns have been raised about an increase in transmission due to a reduction in herd immunity and an increased reinfection rate following screening (Brunham et al. 2005). This chapter includes a brief mention of dynamic transmission models of chlamydial infection that demonstrate the possibility of such an effect (Brunham et al. 2005). Thus, a final challenge is to integrate the work on vaccine development, the epidemiology of *C. trachomatis* infections, and early diagnosis and treatment interventions.

References

Adams EJ, Turner KM, Edmunds WJ (2007) The cost effectiveness of opportunistic chlamydia screening in England. Sex Transm Infect 83:267–274

Andersen B, Gundgaard J, Kretzschmar M, Olsen J, Welte R, Oster-Gaard L (2006) Prediction of costs, effectiveness, and disease control of a population-based program using home sampling for diagnosis of urogenital *Chlamydia trachomatis* Infections. Sex Transm Dis 33: 407–415

Arthur G, Lowndes CM, Blackham J, Fenton KA (2005) Divergent approaches to partner notification for sexually transmitted infections across the European Union. Sex Transm Dis 32:734–741

Bakken IJ (2008) *Chlamydia trachomatis* and ectopic pregnancy: recent epidemiological findings. Curr Opin Infect Dis 21:77–82

Berman SM, Ellen JM (2008) Adolescents and STDs, including HIV infection. In: Holmes KK, Sparling PF, Stamm WE, Piot P, Wasserheit JN, Corey L, Cohen MS, Watts DH (eds) Sexually Transmitted Diseases. McGraw-Hill, New York, pp 165–185

Britton TF, DeLisle S, Fine D (1992) STDs and family planning clinics: a regional program for Chlamydia control that works. Am J Gynecol Health 6:80–87

Brunham RC, Pourbohloul B, Mak S, White R, Rekart ML (2005) The unexpected impact of a *Chlamydia trachomatis* infection control program on susceptibility to reinfection. J Infect Dis 192:1836–1844

Centers for Disease Control and Prevention (1993) Recommendations for the prevention and management of *Chlamydia trachomatis* infections, 1993. MMWR Recomm Rep 42:1–39

Centers for Disease Control and Prevention (1995) Ectopic pregnancy – United States, 1990–1992. MMWR Morb Mortal Wkly Rep 44:46–48

Centers for Disease Control and Prevention (1998) Guidelines for treatment of sexually transmitted diseases 1998. MMWR Recomm Rep 47:1–111

Centers for Disease Control and Prevention (2002) Sexually transmitted diseases treatment guidelines 2002. MMWR Recomm Rep 51:1–78

Centers for Disease Control and Prevention (2006) Sexually transmitted diseases treatment guidelines, 2006. MMWR Recomm Rep 55:1–94

Centers for Disease Control and Prevention (2008a) Recommendations for partner services programs for HIV infection, syphilis, gonorrhea, and chlamydial infection. MMWR Recomm Rep 57:1–83

Centers for Disease Control and Prevention (2008b) Sexually transmitted disease surveillance, 2007. Atlanta, GA, U.S. Department of Health and Human Services

Centers for Disease Control and Prevention (2009) Sexually transmitted disease surveillance 2007 supplement, chlamydia prevalence monitoring project annual report 2007. Atlanta, GA, U.S. Department of Health and Human Services

Chaparro MV, Ghosh S, Nashed A, Poliak A (1978) Laparoscopy for the confirmation and prognostic evaluation of pelvic inflammatory disease. Int J Gynaecol Obstet 15:307–309

Chen MY, Fairley CK, Donovan B (2005) Discordance between trends in chlamydia notifications and hospital admission rates for chlamydia related diseases in New South Wales, Australia. Sex Transm Infect 81:318–322

Coste J, Bouyer J, Ughetto S, Gerbaud L, Fernandez H, Pouly JL, Job-Spira N (2004) Ectopic pregnancy is again on the increase. Recent trends in the incidence of ectopic pregnancies in France (1992–2002). Hum Reprod 19:2014–2018

Coste J, Job-Spira N , ublet-Cuvelier B , Germain E , Glowaczower E , Fernandez H , Pouly JL (1994) Incidence of ectopic pregnancy. First results of a population-based register in France. Hum Reprod 9:742–745

Coyne KM, Cohen CE, Smith NA, Mandalia S, Barton S (2007) Patient-delivered partner medication in the UK: an unlawful but popular choice. Int J STD AIDS 18:829–831

Datta SD, Sternberg M, Johnson RE, Berman S, Papp JR, McQuillan G, Weinstock H (2007) Gonorrhea and chlamydia in the United States among persons 14 to 39 years of age, 1999 to 2002. Ann Intern Med 147:89–96

Datta, S. D., Sternberg, M., Satterwhite, C. L., Johnson, R., Papp, J., McQuillan, G., Berman, S.,, Weinstock, H (2008) Trends in chlamydia population prevalence in the US, 1999-2006. Results from the National Health and Nutrition Examination Survey (NHANES). Annual Meeting, Infectious Diseases Society of America, Washington DC

Davies HD, Wang EE (1996) Periodic health examination, 1996 update: 2. Screening for chlamydial infections. Canadian Task Force on the Periodic Health Examination. CMAJ 154:1631–1644 de Vries R, van Bergen JE, de Jong-van den Berg LT, Postma MJ, PILOT-CT Study Group (2008) Cost-utility of repeated screening for *Chlamydia trachomatis*. Value Health 11: 272–274

de Vries R, van Bergen JE, de Jong-van den Berg LT, Postma MJ, PILOT-CT Study Group (2006) Systematic screening for *Chlamydia trachomatis:* estimating cost-effectiveness using dynamic modeling and Dutch data. Value Health 9:1–11

den Hartog JE, Land JA, Stassen FR, Slobbe-van Drunen ME, Kessels AG, Bruggeman CA (2004) The role of chlamydia genus-specific and species-specific IgG antibody testing in predicting tubal disease in subfertile women. Hum Reprod 19:1380–1384

Doherty IA, Padian NS, Marlow C, Aral SO (2005) Determinants and consequences of sexual networks as they affect the spread of sexually transmitted infections. J Infect Dis 191 (suppl 1):S42–S54

Douglas JM (2008) Dear colleague: Announcing new national chlamydia screening coordinator. Division of STD Prevention, Centers for Disease Control and Prevention. Available at http://www.cdc.gov/std/general/dcl-3-31-2008-chlam-coord.pdf Accessed April 11, 2009

Doxanakis A, Hayes RD, Chen MY, Gurrin LC, Hocking J, Bradshaw CS, Williams H, Fairley CK (2008) Missing pelvic inflammatory disease? Substantial differences in the rate at which doctors diagnose PID. Sex Transm Infect 84:518–523

Egger M, Low N, Smith GD, Lindblom B, Herrmann B (1998) Screening for chlamydial infections and the risk of ectopic pregnancy in a county in Sweden: ecological analysis. Brit Med J 316:1776–1780

Farley TA, Cohen DA, Elkins W (2003) Asymptomatic sexually transmitted diseases: The case for screening. Prev Med 36:502–509

Farquhar CM (2005) Ectopic pregnancy. Lancet 366:583–591

Fenton KA, Korovessis C, Johnson AM, McCadden A, McManus S, Wellings K, Mercer CH, Carder C, Copas AJ, Nanchahal K, Macdowall W, Ridgway G, Field J, Erens B (2001) Sexual behaviour in Britain: reported sexually transmitted infections and prevalent genital *Chlamydia trachomatis* infection. Lancet 358:1851–1854

Fenton KA, Mercer CH, McManus S, Erens B, Wellings K, Macdowall W, Byron CL, Copas AJ, Nanchahal K, Field J, Johnson AM (2005) Ethnic variations in sexual behaviour in Great Britain and risk of sexually transmitted infections: a probability survey. Lancet 365: 1246–1255

Fenton KA, Ward H (2004) National chlamydia screening programme in England: making progress. Sex Transm Infect 80:331–333

Fine D, Dicker L, Mosure D, Berman S (2008) Increasing chlamydia positivity in women screened in family planning clinics: do we know why? Sex Transm Dis 35:47–52

Fisman DN, Spain CV, Salmon ME, Goldberg M (2008) The Philadelphia high-school STD screening program: Key insights from dynamic transmission modeling. Sex Transm Dis 35:S61–S65

Garnett GP (2002) An introduction to mathematical models in sexually transmitted disease epidemiology. Sex Transm Infect 78:7–12

Garnett GP (2008) The transmission dynamics of sexually transmitted infections. In: Holmes KK, Sparling PF, Stamm WE, Piot P, Wasserheit JN, Corey L, Cohen MS, Watts DH (eds) Sexually Transmitted Diseases. Ch. 3. McGraw-Hill, New York

Geisler WM, Wang C, Morrison SG, Black CM, Bandea CI, Hook EW, III (2008) The natural history of untreated *Chlamydia trachomatis* infection in the interval between screening and returning for treatment. Sex Transm Dis 35:119–123

Gift TL, Gaydos CA, Kent CK, Marrazzo JM, Rietmeijer CA, Schillinger JA, Dunne EF (2008) The program cost and cost-effectiveness of screening men for *Chlamydia* to prevent pelvic inflammatory disease in women. Sex Transm Dis 35:S66–S75

Golden MR, Hogben M, Handsfield HH, St Lawrence JS, Potterat JJ, Holmes KK (2003) Partner notification for HIV and STD in the United States: low coverage for gonorrhea, chlamydial infection, and HIV. Sex Transm Dis 30:490–496

Golden MR, Whittington WL, Handsfield HH, Hughes JP, Stamm WE, Hogben M, Clark A, Malinski C, Helmers JR, Thomas KK, Holmes KK (2005) Effect of expedited treatment of sex partners on recurrent or persistent gonorrhea or chlamydial infection. N Engl J Med 352:676–685

Gorgos L, Fine D, Marrazzo J (2008) Chlamydia positivity in American Indian/Alaska Native women screened in family planning clinics, 1997–2004. Sex Transm Dis 35:753–757

Haggerty CL, Schulz R, Ness RB (2003) Lower quality of life among women with chronic pelvic pain after pelvic inflammatory disease. Obstet Gynecol 102:934–939

Hiltunen-Back E, Haikala O, Kautiainen H, Ruutu P, Paavonen J, Reunala T (2003) Nationwide increase of *Chlamydia trachomatis* infection in Finland: highest rise among adolescent women and men. Sex Transm Dis 30:737–741

Hodge JG, Jr., Pulver A, Hogben M, Bhattacharya D, Brown EF (2008) Expedited partner therapy for sexually transmitted diseases: assessing the legal environment. Am J Public Health 98: 238–243

Hogben M (2007) Partner notification for sexually transmitted diseases. Clin Infect Dis 44 Suppl 3:S160–S174

Hogben M, Brewer DD, Golden MR (2007) Partner notification and management intervention. In: Aral SO, Douglas JM, Lipshutz JA (eds) Behavioral Interventions for Prevention and Control of Sexually Transmitted Diseases. Ch. 7. Springer, New York, 170–189

Hull MG, Glazener CM, Kelly NJ, Conway DI, Foster PA, Hinton RA, Colson C, Lambert PA, Watt EM, Desai KM (1985) Population study of causes, treatment and outcome of infertility. Br Med J 291:1693–1697

Jacobson L, Westrom L (1969) Objectivized diagnosis of acute pelvic inflammatory disease. Diagnostic and prognostic value of routine laparoscopy. Am J Obstet Gynecol 105:1088–1098

Joesoef MR, Mosure DJ (2006) Prevalence trends in chlamydial infections among young women entering the national job training program, 1998–2004. Sex Transm Dis 33:571–575

Johnson AM, Mercer CH, Erens B, Copas AJ, McManus S, Wellings K, Fenton KA, Korovessis C, Macdowall W, Nanchahal K, Purdon S, Field J (2001) Sexual behaviour in Britain: partnerships, practices, and HIV risk behaviours. Lancet 358:1835–1842

Kamwendo F, Forslin L, Bodin L, Danielsson D (1998) Programmes to reduce pelvic inflammatory disease—the Swedish experience. Lancet 351 Suppl 3:25–28

Kamwendo F, Forslin L, Bodin L, Danielsson D (2000) Epidemiology of ectopic pregnancy during a 28 year period and the role of pelvic inflammatory disease. Sex Transm Infect 76:28–32

Katz BP, Danos CS, Quinn TS, Caine V, Jones RB (1988) Efficiency and cost-effectiveness of field follow-up for patients with *Chlamydia trachomatis* infection in a sexually transmitted diseases clinic. Sex Transm Dis 15:11–16

Kelley SS, Borawski EA, Flocke SA, Keen KJ (2003) The role of sequential and concurrent sexual relationships in the risk of sexually transmitted diseases among adolescents. J Adolesc Health 32:296–305

Kissinger P, Mohammed H, Richardson-Alston G, Leichliter JS, Taylor SN, Martin DH, Farley TA (2005) Patient-delivered partner treatment for male urethritis: a randomized, controlled trial. Clin Infect Dis 41:623–629

Kissinger P, Schmidt N, Mohammed H, Leichliter JS, Gift TL, Meadors B, Sanders C, Farley TA (2006) Patient-delivered partner treatment for *Trichomonas vaginalis* infection: a randomized controlled trial. Sex Transm Dis 33:445–450

Klovstad H, Aavitsland P (2009) *Chlamydia trachomatis* infections in Norway, 1986 to 2006, surveillance data. Sex Transm Dis 36:17–21

Korenromp EL, Sudaryo MK, de Vlas SJ, Gray RH, Sewankambo NK, Serwadda D, Wawer MJ, Habbema JD (2002) What proportion of episodes of gonorrhoea and chlamydia becomes symptomatic? Int J STD AIDS 13:91–101

Kretzschmar M, van Duynhoven YT, Severijnen AJ (1996) Modeling prevention strategies for gonorrhea and chlamydia using stochastic network simulations. Am J Epidemiol 144: 306–317

Kretzschmar M, Welte R, van den HA, Postma MJ (2001) Comparative model-based analysis of screening programs for *Chlamydia trachomatis* infections. Am J Epidemiol 153:90–101

La Montagne DS, Patrick LE, Fine DN, Marrazzo JM (2004) Re-evaluating selective screening criteria for chlamydial infection among women in the U S Pacific Northwest. Sex Transm Dis 31:283–289

Laumann EO (1994) The social organization of sexuality: Sexual practices in the United States. University of Chicago Press, Chicago, IL

Laumann EO, Yoosik Y (1999) Racial/ethnic group differences in the prevalence of sexually transmitted diseases in the United States: A network explanation. Sex Transm Dis 26: 250–261

Low, N(2004) Current status of chlamydia screening in Europe. Eurosurveillance 8(41), 1–4

Low N (2007) Screening programmes for chlamydial infection: when will we ever learn? Brit Med J 334:725–728

Low N (2008) Caution: chlamydia surveillance data ahead. Sex Transm Infect 84:80–81

Low N, Egger M, Sterne JA, Harbord RM, Ibrahim F, Lindblom B, Herrmann B (2006) Incidence of severe reproductive tract complications associated with diagnosed genital chlamydial infection: the Uppsala Women's Cohort Study. Sex Transm Infect 82:212–218

Low N, McCarthy A, Macleod J, Salisbury C, Campbell R, Roberts TE, Horner P, Skidmore S, Sterne JA, Sanford E, Ibrahim F, Holloway A, Patel R, Barton PM, Robinson SM, Mills N, Graham A, Herring A, Caul EO, Davey SG, Hobbs FD, Ross JD, Egger M (2007) Epidemiological, social, diagnostic and economic evaluation of population screening for genital chlamydial infection. Health Technol Assess 11:iii-xii, 1

Macaluso M, Wright-Schnapp TJ, Chandra A, Johnson R, Satterwhite CL, Pulver A, Berman SM, Wang RY, Farr SL, Pollack LA (2008) A public health focus on infertility prevention, detection, and management. Fertil Steril

Makinen J, Rantala M, Vanha-Kamppa O (1998) A link between the epidemic of ectopic pregnancy and the "baby-boom" cohort. Am J Epidemiol 148:369–374

Markos A (2008) Patient-delivered partner medication: the antagonism of clinical standards and good medical practice. Int J STD AIDS 19:283–284

Mathias SD, Kuppermann M, Liberman RF, Lipschutz RC, Steege JF (1996) Chronic pelvic pain: prevalence, health-related quality of life, and economic correlates. Obstet Gynecol 87: 321–327

Mertz KJ, Ransom RL, St Louis ME, Groseclose SL, Hadgu A, Levine WC, Hayman C (2001) Prevalence of genital chlamydial infection in young women entering a national job training program, 1990–1997. Am J Public Health 91:1287–1290

Miller WC (2008) Epidemiology of chlamydial infection: are we losing ground? Sex Transm Infect 84:82–86

Miller WC, Ford CA, Morris M, Handcock MS, Schmitz JL, Hobbs MM, Cohen MS, Harris KM, Udry JR (2004) Prevalence of chlamydial and gonococcal infections among young adults in the United States. JAMA 291:2229–2236

Morre SA, van den Brule AJ, Rozendaal L, Boeke AJ, Voorhorst FJ, de Blok S, Meijer CJ (2002) The natural course of asymptomatic *Chlamydia trachomatis* infections: 45% clearance and no development of clinical PID after one-year follow-up. Int J STD AIDS 13:Suppl-8

Morris M, Goodreau S, Moody J (2008) Sexual networks, concurrency, and STD/HIV. In: Holmes KK, Sparling PF, Stamm WE, Piot P, Wasserheit JN, Corey L, Cohen MS, Watts DH (eds) Sexually Transmitted Diseases. Ch. 7. McGraw-Hill, New York

Mosher WD, Chandra A, Jones J (2005) Sexual behavior and selected health measures: Men and women 15–44 years of age, United States, 2002. Advance data from vital and health statistics; no 362. National Center for Health Statistics, Hyattsville, MD

National Chlamydia Screening Programme (2008) NCSP: Five years. Annual report of the National Chlamydia Screening Programme in England 2007/08. Health Protection Agency, London.

Nelson HD, Helfand M (2001) Screening for chlamydial infection. Am J Prev Med 20(suppl 3): 95–107

Ness RB, Soper DE, Holley RL, Peipert J, Randall H, Sweet RL, Sondheimer SJ, Hendrix SL, Amortegui A, Trucco G, Songer T, Lave JR, Hillier SL, Bass DC, Kelsey SF (2002) Effectiveness of inpatient and outpatient treatment strategies for women with pelvic inflammatory disease: results from the Pelvic Inflammatory Disease Evaluation and Clinical Health (PEACH) Randomized Trial. Am J Obstet Gynecol 186:929–937

Op de Coul E , van den Broek IVF, Kretzschmar M (2007) Planned evaluation of an internet-based chlamydia screening implementation in the Netherlands. 17th ISSTDR 10th IUSTI World Congress, 393

Paavonen J, Kousa M, Saikku P, Vartiainen E, Kanerva L, Laussus A (1980) Treatment of nongonococcal urethritis with trimethoprim-sulphadiazine and with placebo: A double-blind partner-controlled study. Br J Vener Dis 56:101–104

Paavonen J, Westrom L, Eschenbach D (2008) Pelvic Inflammatory Disease. In: Holmes KK, Sparling PF, Stamm WE, Piot P, Wasserheit JN, Corey L, Cohen MS, Watts DH (eds) Sexually Transmitted Diseases. Ch. 56. McGraw-Hill, New York, 1017–1050

Quinn TC, Gaydos C, Shepherd M, Bobo L, Hook EW, III, Viscidi R, Rompalo A (1996) Epidemiologic and microbiologic correlates of *Chlamydia trachomatis* infection in sexual partnerships. JAMA 276:1737–1742

Rahm VA, Belsheim J, Gleerup A, Gnarpe H, Rosen G (1986) Asymptomatic carriage of *Chlamydia trachomatis*: a study of 109 girls. Eur J STD AIDS 3:91–94

Regan DG, Wilson DP, Hocking JS (2008) Coverage is the key for effective screening of *Chlamydia trachomatis* in Australia. J Infect Dis 198:349–358

Rekart ML, Brunham RC (2008) Epidemiology of chlamydial infection: are we losing ground? Sex Transm Infect 84:87–91

Roberts TE, Robinson S, Barton PM, Bryan S, McCarthy A, Macleod J, Egger M, Low N (2007) Cost effectiveness of home based population screening for *Chlamydia trachomatis* in the UK: economic evaluation of chlamydia screening studies (ClaSS) project. Brit Med J 335:291

Schachter J, Stephens RS (2008) Biology of *Chlamydia trachomatis*. In: Holmes KK, Sparling PF, Stamm WE, Piot P, Wasserheit JN, Corey L, Cohen MS, Watts DH (eds) Sexually Transmitted Diseases. Ch. 31. McGraw-Hill, New York,

Schmidt L, Munster K, Helm P (1995) Infertility and the seeking of infertility treatment in a representative population. Br J Obstet Gynaecol 102:978–984

Scholes D, Stergachis A, Heidrich FE, Andrilla H, Holmes KK, Stamm WE (1996) Prevention of pelvic inflammatory disease by screening for cervical chlamydial infection. N Engl J Med 334:1362–1366

Simms I, Stephenson JM, Mallinson H, Peeling RW, Thomas K, Gokhale R, Rogers PA, Hay P, Oakeshott P, Hopwood J, Birley H, Hernon M (2006) Risk factors associated with pelvic inflammatory disease. Sex Transm Infect 82:452–457

Simms I, Warburton F, Westrom L (2003) Diagnosis of pelvic inflammatory disease: time for a rethink. Sex Transm Infect 79:491–494

Stamm WE (2008) *Lymphogranuloma venereum*. In: Holmes KK, Sparling PF, Stamm WE, Piot P, Wasserheit JN, Corey L, Cohen MS, Watts DH (eds) Sexually Transmitted Diseases. McGraw-Hill, New York

Stamm WE, Guinan ME, Johnson C (1984) Effect of treatment regimens for Neisseria gonorrhoeae on simultaneous infection with *Chlamydia trachomatis*. N Engl J Med 310:545–549

Stephen EH, Chandra A (2006) Declining estimates of infertility in the United States: 1982–2002. Fertil Steril 86:516–523

Sutton MY, Sternberg M, Zaidi A, St Louis ME, Markowitz LE (2005) Trends in pelvic inflammatory disease hospital discharges and ambulatory visits, United States, 1985–2001. Sex Transm Dis 32:778–784

Trelle S, Shang A, Nartey L, Cassell JA, Low N (2007) Improved effectiveness of partner notification for patients with sexually transmitted infections: systematic review. Brit Med J 334:354

Turner KM, Adams EJ, Gay N, Ghani AC, Mercer C, Edmunds WJ (2006a) Developing a realistic sexual network model of chlamydia transmission in Britain. Theor Biol Med Model 3:3

Turner KM, Adams EJ, LaMontagne DS, Emmett L, Baster K, Edmunds WJ (2006b) Modelling the effectiveness of chlamydia screening in England. Sex Transm Infect 82:496–502

van Bergen J, Gotz HM, Richardus JH, Hoebe CJ, Broer J, Coenen AJ, PILOT CT study group (2005) Prevalence of urogenital *Chlamydia trachomatis* increases significantly with level of urbanisation and suggests targeted screening approaches: results from the first national population based study in the Netherlands. Sex Transm Infect

Velicko I, Kuhlmann-Berenzon S, Blaxhult A (2007) Reasons for the sharp increase of genital chlamydia infections reported in the first months of 2007 in Sweden. Euro Surveill 12:E5–E6

Wallace LA, Scoular A, Hart G, Reid M, Wilson P, Goldberg DJ (2008) What is the excess risk of infertility in women after genital chlamydia infection? A systematic review of the evidence. Sex Transm Infect 84:171–175

Wasserheit JN, Aral SO (1996) The dynamic topology of sexually transmitted disease epidemics: implications for prevention strategies. J Infect Dis 174 Suppl 2:S201–S213

Wellings K, Collumbien M, Slaymaker E, Singh S, Hodges Z, Patel D, Bajos N (2006) Sexual behaviour in context: a global perspective. Lancet 368:1706–1728

Welte R, Kretzschmar M, Leidl R, van den Hoek A, Jager JC, Postma MJ (2000) Cost-effectiveness of screening programs for *Chlamydia trachomatis*: a population-based dynamic approach. Sex Transm Dis 27:518–529

Westrom L (1975) Effect of acute pelvic inflammatory disease on fertility. Am J Obstet Gynecol 121:707–713

Westrom L, Joesoef R, Reynolds G, Hadgu A, Thompson SE (1992) Pelvic inflammatory disease and fertility: A cohort study of 1,844 women with laparoscopically verified disease and 657 women with normal laparoscopy. Sex Transm Dis 19:185–192

White, C (2008) Government to press trusts to meet screening targets for chlamydia. Brit Med J 336:299

Wiesenfeld HC, Cates W, Jr. (2008) Sexually transmitted diseases and infertility. In: Holmes KK, Sparling PF, Stamm WE, Piot P, Wasserheit JN, Corey L, Cohen MS, Watts DH (eds) Sexually Transmitted Diseases. Ch. 99. McGraw-Hill, New York, 1493–1510

Zane SB, Kieke BA, Jr., Kendrick JS, Bruce C (2002) Surveillance in a time of changing health care practices: estimating ectopic pregnancy incidence in the United States. Matern Child Health J 6:227–23

Chapter 21
Vector-Borne Transmission: Malaria, Dengue, and Yellow Fever

Tomas Jelinek

21.1 Malaria

At least 2 billion people live in malarious areas (Snow et al. 2005). The disease primarily affects poor populations in tropical and subtropical areas, where the temperature and rainfall are most suitable for the development of the malaria-causing *Plasmodium* parasites in *Anopheles* mosquitoes. This limited geographic distribution is no necessity: malaria once occurred widely in temperate areas, including Western Europe and the USA. The infection receded with economic development and public health measures. It was finally eliminated in the USA between 1947 and 1951 through a campaign that included household spraying of the insecticide dichloro-diphenyl-trichloroethane (DDT) . WHO launched the Global Malaria Eradication Program 1955 (WHO 1999). The planning depended on two key tools: chloroquine for treatment and prevention and DDT for vector control. Implementation of the program had substantial impact in some areas, particularly areas with relatively low transmission rates, such as India and Sri Lanka. Despite these successes, lost political will, the emergence of chloroquine-resistant *Plasmodium* parasites, and of DDT-resistant *Anopheles* mosquitoes led to a failure of the campaign. The global eradication of malaria was officially abandoned as a goal in 1972 (Greenwood et al. 2008). Since the Global Malaria Eradication Program ended, the burden of malaria increased substantially in many parts of the world. The resurgence of malaria was sometimes dramatic, including epidemics in Sri Lanka in 1968–1969 and in Madagascar in 1987–1988. However, economic development, improved health infrastructure, and continued anti-vector measures led to a continued decline of transmission in some countries (e.g., Thailand). Recently, good prospects for malaria elimination in some defined epidemiological settings have been emerging (Tanner and de Savigny 2008). This new momentum is supported by the recent demonstration of a dramatic reduction in malaria transmission, morbidity, and mortality in several countries in Africa (Greenwood et al. 2008;

T. Jelinek (✉)
Berlin Center for Travel and Tropical Medicine, Jägerstrasse 67–69, 10117 Berlin, Germany
e-mail: jelinek@bctropen.de

A. Krämer et al. (eds.), *Modern Infectious Disease Epidemiology*, Statistics for Biology and Health, DOI 10.1007/978-0-387-93835-6_21,

Tanner and de Savigny 2008), owing to the implementation of effective malaria control measures, such as insecticide-treated bednets (ITNs) , indoor residual spraying (IRS), and artemisinin-based combination therapies (ACTs).

Currently a mixed epidemiological picture is emerging. While malaria transmission is spreading to higher altitudes, probably due to improved climate conditions for the vector, highly endemic areas are reporting a clear decline of cases (Greenwood et al. 2008). A good example for this unclear situation is the Gambia. In a retrospective study on the malaria indices of this country, a clear decrease was evident. From 2003 to 2007, at four sites with complete slide examination records, the proportions of malaria-positive slides decreased by 50–82%. During the same period, the proportions of malaria admissions fell by 27–74% in three sites, while proportions of deaths attributed to malaria in two hospitals decreased by 90–100% (Ceesay et al. 2008). On the other hand, in November 2008, a significant cluster of *falciparum* malaria imported by tourists from the Gambia to Europe and an accompanying increase of local cases indicated a local resurgence of the disease (Promed 2008).

21.1.1 The Parasite and Its Life Cycle

Plasmodium falciparum is the most virulent among the four *Plasmodium* species that cause malaria in humans. It is also distinguished by the particular pathophysiology it causes, in particular through its ability to bind to endothelium during the blood stage of the infection and to sequester in organs, including the brain. This causes the vast majority of deaths from malaria. *Plasmodium vivax* is a far less deadly parasite but highly disabling; it is common in tropical areas outside Africa. The ability of *P. vivax* and also the very similar *Plasmodium ovale* to remain dormant for months as hypnozoites in the liver makes infection with these parasites difficult to eradicate. The fourth plasmodial species that is pathogenic for humans, *Plasmodium malariae*, does not form hypnozoites, but it can persist for decades as an asymptomatic blood stage infection. The *Plasmodium* life cycle leads to numerous transitions and stages of the parasite, all necessitating a specific immune response during this particular part of the cycle. Following inoculation by an *Anopheles* mosquito into the human dermis, motile sporozoites access blood vessels in the skin, are transported to the liver, and then transit through macrophages and hepatocytes to initiate liver stage infection. Subsequently, each sporozoite yields tens of thousands of merozoites. After an incubation period of 1–4 weeks, infected hepatocytes rupture and release merozoites. The clinical disease begins. The merozoites invade erythrocytes. They develop further and multiply within these cells while digesting the hemoglobin. Asexual blood stage parasites produce 8–20 new merozoites every 36–48 h (or 72 h for *P. malariae*), causing parasite numbers to rise rapidly to levels as high as 10^{13} per host. The asexual stages are pathogenic, and infected individuals can present with diverse sequelae affecting different organ systems. The blood stages of infection also include gametocytes (male and female sexual forms) that await ingestion by mosquitoes before developing further. Sexual stage parasites are nonpathogenic but are transmissible to the *Anopheles* vector, where they recombine and generate genetically distinct sporozoites. The mosquito becomes infectious to its next blood meal donor 1–2 weeks after ingesting gametocytes, a time frame that is influenced by the external temperature. Development of *P. vivax* within the mosquito can occur at a lower environmental temperature than that required for the development of *P. falciparum*, explaining the preponderance of *P. vivax* infections outside tropical and subtropical regions.

21.1.2 Course of Disease and Diagnosis

Uncomplicated malaria usually presents with fever and nonspecific symptoms, such as vomiting and/or diarrhea while severe malaria caused by *P. falciparum* is characterized by multiorgan damage, including renal failure. The clinical picture is different in children, who present with prostration, respiratory distress, severe anemia, and cerebral malaria. Additional complications, such as hypoglycemia and acidosis, can occur. The determinants of severe malaria in an individual case are not fully understood. Genetic factors are important (Kwiatkowski 2005). Also, both the age of the patient and the intensity of transmission in the community influence the susceptibility to complicated malaria (Reyburn et al. 2005). Cerebral malaria is a more common presentation of severe malaria where transmission intensity is low, whereas severe anemia predominates where transmission intensity is high. Malaria can interact with other infectious diseases to modify the susceptibility and/or severity of either disease. Solid evidence now indicates that infection with HIV increases the risk of uncomplicated and severe malaria (Korenromp et al. 2005). Conversely, malaria causes a transitory increase in viral load, and this could promote HIV transmission. An important percentage of patients with severe malaria have associated bacteremia, and these patients show increased mortality (Berkley et al. 1999). Microscopy of thin and thick blood films remains the central tool for diagnosis. However, laboratory diagnosis has now become possible through the development of rapid diagnostic tests (Moody 2002). Following initial problems with sensitivity after their introduction, the immunochromatographic tests have become quite reliable.

21.1.3 Global Distribution and Surveillance

Considerable progress has been made in defining the global distribution of malaria and its burden. Since the clinical diagnosis of malaria is imprecise, estimates of the burden of malaria that rely upon clinical data without laboratory support are unreliable. Improved regional and global estimates of the malaria burden have used accurate data collected at selected areas with well-defined geographical, entomological, and population characteristics. Results are then extrapolated to other areas with similar characteristics and known populations. Studies of this kind suggest that malaria directly causes just under 1 million deaths and at least 500 million clinical cases each year (Snow et al. 2005; Greenwood et al. 2008; Rowe et al. 2006). Furthermore, malaria in pregnancy contributes to a substantial number of maternal deaths as well as infant deaths resulting from low birth weight. However, overall data are still hard to collect. Most malaria-endemic countries, particularly those in sub-Saharan Africa, have weak health information systems and civil registries. Since the consequences of a malaria infection vary, many indicators are used to measure the impact of an intervention. Malaria-specific mortality is very difficult to document because most deaths from malaria occur at home. Data collection on malaria morbidity requires either the use of health facilities as sentinel sites or regularly conducted community-based surveys.

Most important factors that determine the epidemiology of malaria:

- Presence of *Anopheles* mosquitoes and humans: There is no real animal reservoir for the four plasmodial species that cause disease in humans, nor does epidemiologically relevant transmission outside of mosquitoes occur. One of the most indices of malaria transmission intensity is the vectorial capacity, the number of infectious bites that would arise from all bites on a single infected human on a single day (Garret-Jones 1964).
- Climatic factors are a key determinant: Rainfall creates water collections where *Anopheles* can breed. Such breeding sites may dry up prematurely in the absence of further rainfall, or conversely they can be flushed and destroyed by excessive rains. Once adult mosquitoes have emerged, ambient temperature, humidity, and rains will determine their chances of survival. To transmit malaria successfully, female *Anopheles* must survive long enough after they have become infected through a blood meal on an infected human. The parasite development inside the mosquito lasts 9–21 days at 25°C. Warmer ambient temperatures shorten the duration of the extrinsic cycle, thus increasing the chances of transmission. Conversely, below a minimum ambient temperature of 15°C for *P. vivax* and of 20°C for *P. falciparum*, malaria cannot be transmitted. Current trends of global warming may increase the geographic range of malaria and may be responsible for future malaria epidemics.
- Behavior of *Anopheles* mosquitoes: Not all *Anopheles* species transmit malaria parasites. In addition, *Anopheles* species differ in selected behavior traits, with important consequences on their abilities as malaria vectors. In some species the females are anthropophilic, in other they are zoophilic. Some species prefer to bite indoors (endophagic), while others prefer outdoor biting (exophagic). All other factors being equal, the anthropophilic, endophagic species will have more frequent contacts with humans and will thus be more effective malaria vectors. Those *Anopheles* that are able to transmit the infection show distinct variations in their breeding habits. For example, *Anopheles gambiae*, the main mosquito host in Africa, prefers to breed in open, savanna-like country. In contrast, the *Anopheles* species of Southeast Asia that transmit malaria are predominantly forest breeders. Thus, malaria decreased significantly in these areas when forests were cut down. Next to all *Anopheles* species prefer fresh, unpolluted water for their breeding sites. This

is developing into a major handicap in important parts of the world since access to clean water is decreasing with the spread of human urban and in particular slum habitation.

• Behavior and biologic characteristics of humans: Genetic and acquired characteristics and behavioral traits can influence an individual's malaria risk and, on a larger scale, the intensity of transmission in a population. For example, the heterozygotic form of sickle cell anemia protects against development of severe malaria.

• Characteristics of the malaria parasite: Occurrence of particular plasmodial species, infection with several strains of the same species and drug resistance influence the impact of malaria on human populations. For example, *P. falciparum* (and to a lesser extent *P. vivax*) have developed strains that are resistant to several antimalarial drugs. Such strains are not uniformly distributed. Constant monitoring of the susceptibility of these two parasite species to drugs used locally is critical to ensure effective treatment and successful control efforts.

As malaria numbers continue to decline in highly endemic areas, patterns of infection and disease will change. An increasing proportion of cases will occur in older children and adults, leading to an increased risk of local outbreaks. The latter will be especially likely to occur if control measures are allowed to lapse in the face of a decreasing burden of infection. Extensive and continuous surveillance will be required to monitor changes and to define optimal and cost-effective strategies for managing the situation. The most effective control programs are those that apply a combination of tools with particular emphasis on mosquito control. Interventions are insufficient to meet the ambitious goal of global eradication. All programs have to be monitored for the efficacy of their interventions since one day they will be lost to a changing parasite or mosquito.

21.2 Dengue Fever

Dengue fever has become acknowledged as one of the world's major emerging infectious diseases. In fact, the infection is by now correctly seen as a global pandemic with recorded prevalence in over 101 countries (WHO 2008b, c). Dengue infection is caused by one of the four serologically distinct dengue virus serotypes (DENV-1, DENV-2, DENV-3, DENV-4) of the family Flaviviridae. Each one is leading to life-long immunity to this homologous serotype, but only to a short period of cross-reactive heterotypic immunity. This cross-protection is thought to last 2–12 months (Kliks et al. 1988).

Dengue viruses are usually transmitted by bites of an infected mosquito vector, mainly *Aedes aegypti*. For transmission to occur, the female *Aedes* mosquito must bite an infected human during the viremic phase of the illness which generally lasts 4–5 days but may last up to 12 days (McBride and Bielefeldt-Ohmann 2000). The incubation period in humans ranges from 3 to 12 days, most common between 5 and 7 days. *Aedes* mosquitoes are efficient vectors and their global distribution goes hand in hand with that of the dengue viruses. *Aedes* are highly susceptible to dengue viruses and they feed preferentially and frequently on human blood, the only important reservoir besides mosquitoes themselves. In particular *A. aegypti* is a highly domesticated mosquito and breeds in man-made containers such as pots, tin cans, and tyres. It mainly bites during the day or early evening, and most biting occurs out of doors in urban areas. Dengue viruses are transovarially transmitted in some *Aedes* mosquitoes (McBride and Bielefeldt-Ohmann 2000). It has been shown that dengue viruses in mosquitoes cause an infection of the nervous system, consecutively leading to prolonged feeding periods with a higher likelihood to be interrupted by the host, which increases the chance that this infected mosquito will probe or feed on additional hosts.

These facts impact the clinical and epidemiological role of dengue: first, because of the short incubation period a high proportion of infected persons will suffer from disease within a short time after infection. For example, travelers being infected in endemic countries will fall ill during their stay abroad. Most of them will not seek medical care in the country of sojourn or when returning to their home country, and the disease will be underreported by far in both national surveillance systems. Second, dengue is a disease which occurs mainly, but not exclusively, in urbanized areas. These areas nowadays are globally much closely connected to each other. Overcrowding, urbanization, poverty, insufficient water storage systems, and insufficient vector control are major causes for the dramatic resurgence of dengue disease (Lifson 1996). With increasing international air travel, new and potentially more virulent viral strains can be introduced to other areas infested with *Aedes* species. Therefore, travelers not only play a role as a potential victim of infection but also as an important transmission vessel in the global distribution of the viruses.

21.2.1 The Disease and Its Symptoms

Dengue virus infection may be asymptomatic or may lead to undifferentiated febrile illness (viral syndrome), dengue fever (DF), or dengue hemorrhagic fever (DHF) with or without shock, depending largely on age and immunological conditions (Jelinek et al. 2002).

In DF, the severity of the clinical features increases with age of the patient (Rigau-Perez et al. 1998). Therefore, classical dengue fever is primarily a disease of older children and adults, characterized by a sudden onset of fever, headache, joint or muscle pain, rash, leukopenia, and thrombocytopenia. Mild hemorrhagic manifestations, such as epistaxis, petechiae, gingival bleeding, and menorrhagia, are accepted as a rare part of the clinical picture of DF. The disease is self-limited, and in classical dengue fever usually no deaths occur. In a study performed in Swedish patients with DF after return from travel, 21 out of 74 had hemorrhagic manifestations but none presented as DHF.

In contrast, dengue hemorrhagic fever (DHF) is primarily a disease in children under 15 years in hyperendemic areas where two or more virus serotypes are circulating simultaneously, but it might also occur in adults. The early clinical features of DHF are indistinguishable from DF (Halstead 1989). Even though the severity of hemorrhage in DHF tends to be greater than in DF and severe gastrointestinal bleeding may sometimes occur, dengue hemorrhagic fever is somewhat inaptly named, because its central clinical and pathogenetical lesion is not bleeding. The major pathophysiological change that determines the severity of disease in DHF and differentiates it from DF is the leakage of plasma which results into hemoconcentration (manifested as a rise in hematocrit), pleural or other effusions, or hypoalbuminemia or hypoproteinemia. This feature typically occurs simultaneously with a drop in platelet count at the time of defervescence, 2–9 days after the onset of symptoms, and may progress to hypovolemic shock (DSS) and death. Within the European Network on Imported Infectious Disease Surveillance (www.tropnet.eu), 2.7% of all dengue cases (n=483) were reported as DHF (Jelinek et al. 2002). In recent years, there have been an increase in the number of reports on dengue infections with unusual manifestations, mainly with cerebral and hepatic involvement.

21.2.2 Pathogenesis: Current Knowledge and Opinions

The pathogenesis of dengue is not fully understood. There are currently several concepts that try to explain why dengue viruses lead to DHF in some individuals and not in others. The major pathophysiological change, however, that determines the severity of DHF and differentiates it from DF is the acute increased vascular permeability which results in plasma leakage, leading to hypovolemia and shock. Other hallmarks are hemorrhagic diathesis and complement activation.

The observations that classical dengue fever without complications occur in non-indigenous foreigners while DHF occurs in indigenous children, and that most aspects of the disease become prominent only after several days of illness when fever and viremia remit, support an immunological explanation. Fundamental to the immunological events in DHF is the existence in nature of four antigenically related but distinct dengue serotypes that parenterally enter human hosts: Prior infection with a dengue virus of one serotype confers only transient immunity to infections with heterologous serotypes, but does give rise to antibodies broadly cross-reactive with virions of all four serotypes. Several prospective studies demonstrated that the presence of circulating dengue antibodies, acquired actively by prior infection or passively by heterotypic maternal dengue IgG antibodies in infants, is an important risk factor for the development of severe manifestations of infections (Thein et al. 1997).

It has been well documented that higher viral burden is associated with more severe disease. According to the immune enhancement theory cross-reactive non-neutralizing antibodies facilitate virus entry and replication in Fc receptor-bearing cells leading to higher viral loads. These activate precursor cross-reactive memory T cells and lead to the release of chemical mediators that cause plasma leakage.

In infants it has been shown that maternal dengue antibodies are important in the development of DHF. These antibodies have a dual role: in the first 6 months of life maternal dengue neutralizing antibodies protect infants from dengue infection;

at 7–8 months the neutralizing activity decreases below the protective level and antibody-dependent enhancement activity rises to peak levels causing a period of greatest risk to acquire DHF/DSS. Beyond this critical 2-month period, further IgG degradation results in a decrease of infection-enhancing antibodies. The observation of transient heterotypic immunity followed by a period of highest risk 7–8 months after acquiring dengue antibodies would explain why DHF is rare in travelers. One other recently established explanation for higher viral loads is that cross-reactive T cells (CD8+) activated by original antigenic sin may have lower affinity and be less effective at clearing a secondary infection with dengue viruses.

However, even primary dengue infection can in rare occasions also be associated with fatal dengue hemorrhagic disease and shock. Therefore, the virus itself might play an important role in disease severity. Dengue virus structural differences were shown to correlate with pathogenesis and epidemiological studies showed strong evidence that there are significant differences in disease severity between secondary infections of American and Asian origin (White 1999). Alternatively, there might be differences in the ability of pre-existing dengue antibodies to neutralize or enhance specific viral strains (subtypes). If virus virulence plays an important role in the pathogenesis of dengue, and more virulent strains are widespread, this will also have an effect on dengue morbidity and mortality in travelers.

Since antibodies play a role in enhancing or preventing infection while cellular immunity limits viral infected cells, some of these processes might be under genetic control. Several studies revealed both protective and pathogenic roles in disease severity for specific HLA class genetic variations (Halstead 2002). There is also some epidemiological evidence that there must be genes in blacks that play a major role in restricting severity of dengue infection. Genetic variations might also be an explanation why DHF is rare in Caucasian travelers.

21.2.3 Epidemiology

Dengue is endemic in most tropical parts of the world. Worldwide, 3.5 billion people live in dengue endemic areas. The incidence of epidemic and endemic dengue has increased substantially (Fig. 21.1). This increased epidemic activity, which is caused by all four virus serotypes, is associated with the geographical expansion of both, the mosquito vectors and the viruses, the development of hyperendemicity (the co-circulation of multiple virus serotypes in an area), and the emergence of dengue hemorrhagic fever (DHF) . Hyperendemicity is the most constant factor associated with the evolution of epidemic DHF in a geographical area (Gubler 1997). Today, DF/DHF has emerged as the most important arboviral disease of humans, with an estimated 50–100 million cases of dengue fever and several hundred thousand cases of DHF occurring each year, depending on epidemic activity (Gibbons and Vaughn 2002). DHF is a leading cause of hospitalization and death especially among children in Southeast Asian countries where epidemics first occurred in the 1950s. Epidemic DHF spread out to the South Pacific islands in the 1970s, and reached the American region in the 1980s and 1990s (Pinheiro and Nelson 1997). Of major

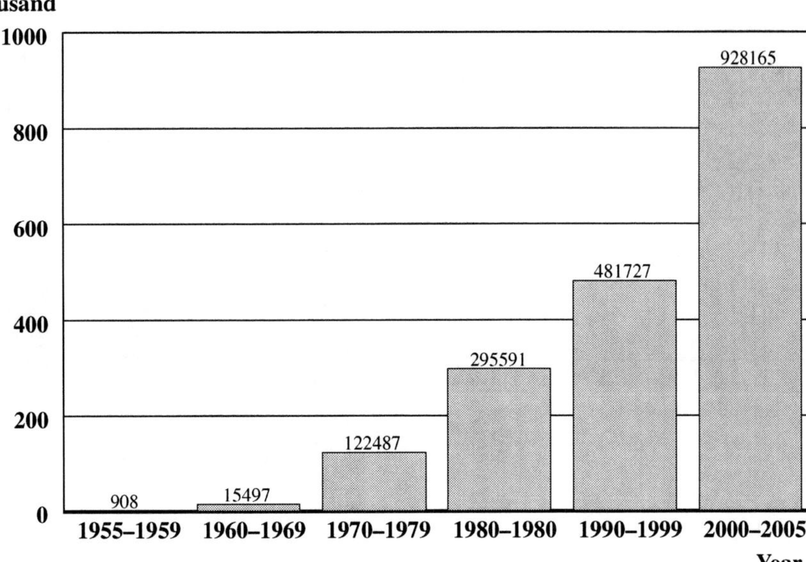

Fig. 21.1 Number of reported cases of dengue per decade, 1950–2005 (Moody 2002; Gibbons and Vaughn 2002)

concern is the potential area of dengue transmission due to the spread of its vectors: such areas include sizeable parts of the USA and Europe. In such a manner, the introduction of dengue fever by returning travelers as yet unafflicted by the disease poses a very real threat to public health systems of the western world, as has already been demonstrated with the introduction of dengue into Australia (Queensland), and the USA (Hawaii and Mississippi) (WHO 2008b,c). One of the largest dengue fever epidemics known in history, with approximately 1 million cases and 1000 deaths, occurred in Greece during 1927–1928. At that time, the vector was the later locally eradicated *A. aegypti*. In this context, the recent introduction of *Aedes albopictus* to Europe, notably Italy, France, and Albania, might serve as a warning of things to come (Romi 2001). In most disease-endemic areas dengue transmission has a definite seasonality, but the reasons for the seasonal patterns are not fully understood. However, studies on the vector showed that the larval index per house increased during the wet season due to a higher proportion of colonized containers at each house, as well as increased number of available containers.

21.3 Yellow Fever

Yellow fever is caused by a flavi virus. The disease is transmitted by infected mosquitoes, in particular *A. aegypti*. The clinical spectrum of yellow fever shows a wide spectrum, ranging from mild symptoms of acute viral infection to severe

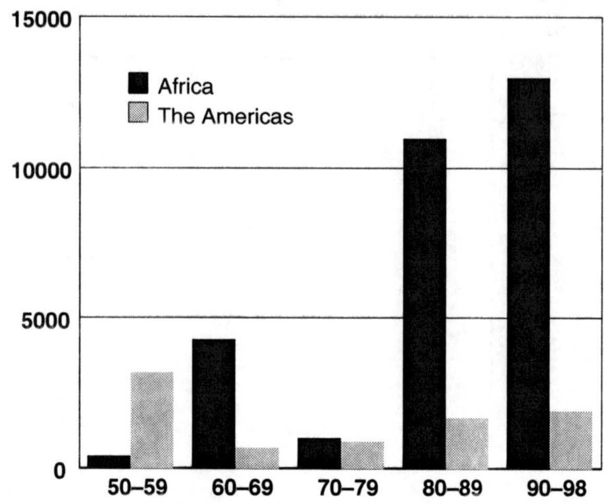

Fig. 21.2 Number of reported cases of yellow fever per decade, 1950–1998 (Gibbons and Vaughn 2002)

disease and death (WHO 2000; Monath 2001). Jaundice caused by hepatitis, kidney failure, and hemorrhagic signs dominate the picture of severe disease; hence the name yellow fever. Case fatality rates during outbreaks tend to be in the range of 15–50%. The disease has caused large epidemics in Africa and the Americas in the past and can be recognized from historic texts stretching back at least 400 years. Following a long period of comparatively low case numbers during the last century, case reports have been increasing for two decades, and yellow fever is now again a serious threat to public health (Fig. 21.2) (WHO 2000; WHO 2005). Yellow fever is one of the diseases that are reportable under the International Health Regulations (IHR) . Reporting began in 1948. Countries are required to report cases and deaths to WHO within 24 h of being notified. As with other diseases under the IHR, it is estimated that only a small fraction of true cases are reported to WHO (1–10%). However, it is also assumed that large outbreaks have not been missed due to the public disturbances they cause.

Important reasons for the re-emergence of yellow fever are an increased presence of vector mosquitoes and the lapse of yellow fever immunization programs in endemic areas (Monath 2001). Although a very effective and safe live-attenuated vaccine is available, large unvaccinated populations are now living at risk of the disease. Another important factor is the increasing urbanization in many developing countries. Since the vector is anthropophilic and breeds in abundance in slum areas, the potential for explosive urban outbreaks is constantly increasing.

Non-human primates in tropical areas of Africa and the Americas and several *Aedes* spp. form a reservoir for the virus. Thus, eradication of the disease is currently impossible. Close contacts of humans to forested areas and infestation of human habitations by vector mosquitoes form the ground for epidemics. In Africa, 33 countries with a population of 468 million are currently at risk. These inhabit an area ranging from 15°N to 10°S of the equator. In the Americas, yellow fever is endemic in ten countries and several Caribbean islands. It has recently been spreading south and reached Argentina and Paraguay. It remains unclear why yellow fever is confined to areas in Africa and the Americas, even though the vectors do occur in Asia and are spreading freely into Europe, Central America, and North America (Barros and Boecken 1996). One explanation is the occurrence of dengue in areas free of yellow fever, but this theory no longer holds since dengue has spread rapidly to most tropical and subtropical countries.

Three types of transmission: A variety of species of *Aedes* and *Haemagogus* mosquitoes transmit the yellow fever virus, the latter in South America only. These vectors exhibit domestic, semi-domestic, or wild habits but they are, in general, anthropophilic and day-active. There are three potential transmission cycles of yellow fever: sylvatic, intermediate, and urban.

Sylvatic (or jungle) yellow fever: Monkeys in tropical rainforests are infected by wild mosquitoes. The infected monkeys do not necessarily fall sick and pass the virus to the next mosquito that feeds on them. Thus, a disease reservoir is formed. The infected mosquitoes may bite humans that enter the forest, resulting in sporadic cases of yellow fever. The majority of cases occur in people visiting the forest for their livelihood, e.g., loggers, hunters, but this may also affect visitors to national parks. Occasionally, and increasingly so in the last years, the virus is transported by the infected individual into human dwellings, transmitted to semi-domestic or domestic mosquitoes, and spreads to other persons.

Intermediate yellow fever: Small epidemics can occur in humid or semi-humid areas at the forest fringes. This has been observed particularly in Africa. These village outbreaks behave differently from urban epidemics: usually several villages are affected at the same time, but fewer patients are reported. Semi-domestic mosquitoes in the vicinity infect both monkeys and humans. These areas are classified as "zones of emergence" (WHO 2000), with an increased contact between animal reservoir and humans that may lead to disease. This type of outbreak can easily shift into a more urban epidemic if the virus is carried into a suitable environment.

Urban yellow fever: This type of transmission has a potential for large outbreaks. It occurs when the virus is carried into an urban setting with a high density of human population (frequently slums) that is infested by suitable domestic vectors. In particular *A. aegypti* is a very effective slum breeder. Here the disease is carried by mosquitoes from person to person, no animal reservoir is involved. Outbreaks of this type tend to spread rapidly from single sources and have the potential for many cases.

The potential for large urban epidemics is increasing in many parts of the world. Urbanization and intense mosquito infestation of human settlements go hand in hand in increasing the possibilities of outbreaks. In particular the density of *A. aegypti* has expanded dramatically in rural and urban areas over the last 30 years. The mosquito has re-infested regions where it was previously eradicated and has reached new areas, too. Therefore, areas with *Aedes* populations have to be considered as risk for yellow fever outbreaks, even if the disease has not occurred there yet. This holds for Europe, the Caribbean, Central America, and North America, since these areas had yellow fever outbreaks in the past, but also for Asia, which has been free of the disease as far as historical records go.

Prevention: The availability of a highly effective and comparatively safe, life-attenuated, single shot vaccine is a great advantage in yellow fever control. Immunity occurs in 95% of vaccines within 1 week. Immunization lasts officially for 10 years with actual protection being much longer, in a considerably amount of vaccinees life-long. Next to mosquito control measures, increasing the vaccine coverage in populations at risk is the most effective measure in preventing outbreaks. Thus immunization with yellow fever vaccine should be part of the routine vaccination campaigns in endemic areas, preferably with administration at the same time as measles vaccine. The vaccine can also be used in mass vaccination campaigns at the beginning of an outbreak in order to block the spread of disease. As this is far less effective than preventive childhood vaccination, the latter is vastly preferable. Current examples of mass vaccination campaigns include those initiated by PAHO and national authorities after the re-introduction of yellow fever in Paraguay (WHO 2008b,c). Another campaign initiated in 2008 was the mass vaccination in 37 districts of Burkina Faso, following deaths by yellow fever (WHO 2008a).

References

Barros MLB, Boecken G (1996) Jungle yellow fever in the central Amazon. Lancet 348:969–970

Berkley J, Mwarumba S, Bramham K, Lowe B, Marsh K (1999) Bacteraemia complicating severe malaria in children. Trans R Soc Trop Med Hyg 93:283–286

Ceesay SJ, Casals-Pascual C, Erskine J, Anya SE, Duah NO, Fulford AJ, Sesay SS, Abubakar I, Dunyo S, Sey O, Palmer A, Fofana M, Corrah T, Bojang KA, Whittle HC, Greenwood BM, Conway DJ (2008) Changes in malaria indices between 1999 and 2007 in The Gambia: a retrospective analysis. Lancet 372:1545–1554

Garret-Jones C (1964) Prognosis for interruption of malaria transmission through assessment of the mosquito's vectorial capacity. Nature 204:1173–1175

Gibbons RV, Vaughn DW (2002) Dengue: an escalating problem. BMJ 324: 1563–1566

Greenwood BM, Fidock DA, Kyle DE, Kappe SH, Alonso PL, Collins FH, Duffy PE (2008) Malaria: progress, perils, and prospects for eradication.J Clin Invest 118(4):1266–1276

Gubler DJ (1997) Epidemic dengue/dengue hemorrhagic fever: A global public health problem in the 21st century. In: World Health Organization, the South-East Asia and Western Pacific Region. Dengue Bulletin – Vol. 21. New Delhi: WHO; pp. 1–13

Halstead SB (1989) Antibody, macrophages, dengue virus infection, shock, and hemorrhage: a pathogenetic cascade. Rev Infect Dis 11: S830–S839

Halstead SB (2002) Dengue Curr Opin Infect Dis 15: 471–476

Jelinek T, Mühlberger N, Harms G et al (2002) Epidemiology and clinical features of imported dengue fever in Europe: Sentinel surveillance data from TropNetEurop. Clin Infect Dis 35: 1047–1052

Kliks SC, Nimmanitya S, Nisalak A, Burke DS (1988) Evidence that maternal dengue antibodies are important in the development of dengue hemorrhagic fever in infants. Am J Trop Med Hyg 38: 411–419

Korenromp EL et al. (2005) Malaria attributable to the HIV-1 epidemic, sub-Saharan Africa. Emerg Infect Dis 11:1410–1419

Kwiatkowski DP (2005) How malaria has affected the human genome and what human genetics can teach us about malaria. Am J Hum Genet 77:171–192

Lifson A (1996) Mosquitos, models, and dengue. Lancet 347: 1201–1202

McBride WJ, Bielefeldt-Ohmann H (2000) Dengue viral infections; pathogenesis and epidemiology. Microbes infect 2000; 2: 1041–1050

Monath TP (2001) Yellow fever: an update. The Lancet Infect Dis 1:11–20

Moody A (2002) Rapid diagnostic tests for malaria parasites. Clin Microbiol Rev 15:66–78

Pinheiro F, Nelson M (1997) Re-emergence of dengue and emergence of dengue haemorrhagic fever in the Americas. In: World Health Organization, the South-East Asia and Western Pacific Region. Dengue Bulletin – Vol. 21. New Delhi: WHO; pp. 16–23

Promed post (2008) Malaria, Europa and US, from Gambia. http://www.promedmail.org /pls/otn/f?p=2400:1001:2917102731875827::NO::F2400_P1001_BACK_PAGE,F2400_P1001_PUB_MAIL_ID:1000,74978

Reyburn H et al. (2005) Association of transmission intensity and age with clinical manifestations and case fatality of severe Plasmodium falciparum malaria. JAMA 293:1461–1470

Rigau-Perez J, Clark G, Gubler D et al. (1998) Dengue and dengue haemorrhagic fever. Lancet 352: 971–977

Romi R (2001) Aedes albopictus in Italy: an underestimated health problem. Ann Inst Super Sanita 37: 241–247

Rowe AK et al. (2006) The burden of malaria mortality among African children in the year 2000. Int J Epidemiol 35:691–704

Snow RW, Guerra CA, Noor AM, Myint HY, Hay SI (2005) The global distribution of clinical episodes of Plasmodium falciparum malaria. Nature 434:214–217

Tanner M, de Savigny D (2008) Malaria eradication back on the table. Bull. World Health Organ 86, 82

Thein S, Aung MM, Shwe TN et al (1997) Risk factors in dengue shock syndrome. Am J Trop Med Hyg 56: 566–572

White NJ (1999) Variation in virulence of dengue virus. Lancet 23: 1401–1402

WHO (1999) Making a difference. The World Health Report. Health Millions 25:3–5

WHO (2000) Report on Global Surveillance of Epidemic-prone Infectious Diseases, World Health Organization 2000, WHO/CDS/CSR/ISR/2000.1; www.who.int/emc ; last accessed 30 June 2008

WHO (2005) International Health Regulations. Geneva: World Health Organization, 1–60. http://www.who.int/csr/ihr/en /

WHO (2008a) Epidemic and Pandemic Alert and Response. Yellow Fever in Burkina Faso. http://www.who.int/csr/don/2008_11_03/en/index.html

WHO (2008b) DengueNet http://www.who.int/globalatlas/default.asp; accessed 30 June 2008

WHO (2008c) Epidemic and Pandemic Alert and Response. Yellow Fever in Paraguay. http://www.who.int/csr/don/2008_02_20a/en/index.html

Chapter 22
Nosocomial Transmission: Methicillin-Resistant *Staphylococcus aureus* (MRSA)

M.J.M. Bonten and M.C.J. Bootsma

22.1 Introduction

Nosocomial, or hospital-acquired, infections are an important cause of morbidity and mortality in health-care settings. Within hospitals, we find a gathering of patients with a weakened immune system, who receive all kinds of treatment that may even further weaken host defense mechanisms and that may break natural barriers against pathogens by surgery or by inserting intravascular lines. In such circumstances, even microorganisms that are generally considered harmless may cause fulminate infections. Such potentially pathogenic microorganisms are ubiquitous in health-care settings. They are continuously introduced by patients being admitted and can also be transmitted between patients. The latter is facilitated by the frequent contacts between health-care workers and patients, creating many opportunities for cross-transmission. Finally, because of the frequent use of antimicrobial agents, there is a selective advantage for pathogens resistant to these agents, and, hence, reported prevalence rates of antimicrobial resistant pathogens, which are more difficult to treat, are usually high in these settings.

Apart from these factors, there are several other factors, which clearly distinguish nosocomial infections from other infections.

- The concept of colonization. Typically, infections with nosocomial pathogens are preceded by colonization (i.e., the presence of the microorganism at a body site without signs of infection) with the same pathogen. Since only a fraction of colonized patients will develop overt infection, dynamics of nosocomial pathogens are mainly determined by patients being colonized instead of infected. It is estimated that the ratio between colonized and infected patients is at least 10:1.
- Population size. The typical size of hospital units is small (5–20 beds) and, therefore, natural fluctuations in the prevalence of colonization are high. These

M.J.M. Bonten (✉)
Department of Medical Microbiology and the Julius Center for Health Sciences and Primary Care; University Medical Center Utrecht, Utrecht, The Netherlands
e-mail: mbonten@umcutrecht.nl

A. Krämer et al. (eds.), *Modern Infectious Disease Epidemiology*, Statistics for Biology and Health, DOI 10.1007/978-0-387-93835-6_22,

fluctuations, together with dependency between colonized patients due to transmission, complicate the analysis of preventive interventions.

- Patient dynamics. The length of stay of patients in hospitals (or in certain units) is short (days), which leads to a high turnover of patients.
- Readmission of patients. Many patient categories, e.g., haemodialysis patients, are frequently readmitted. If colonization persists after discharge (which holds for most nosocomial pathogens), there will be frequent re-introductions of pathogens.
- External interactions. Units (and hospitals) are not isolated and will be in contact, through transfer of patients, with other units (or hospitals).

22.2 The Burden of Disease

An abundance of data demonstrates the high prevalence of hospital-acquired infections. In the United States these infections now rank among the leading causes of death, with conservative estimates of 260,000 years of life lost each year from premature deaths directly related to nosocomial bloodstream infections alone. Such infections lead to billions of dollars of expenditures and to an unquantified diminution of the quality of life for thousands of patients each year (Wenzel 2003). Actual estimated figures are 1.7 million individuals in the United States acquiring a nosocomial infection, yielding 100,000 deaths (Klevens et al. 2007a) and an additional $6.5 billion in health-care expenditures (Stone et al. 2005). Within hospitals, *Staphylococcus aureus* is the most frequent cause of opportunistic infections and the proportion of these infections caused by MRSA has increased rapidly in most developed countries in the last decade. More than 18,000 deaths were estimated to have occurred among patients with invasive MRSA infections in the United States during 2005, and most of these infections had been acquired in health-care settings (Klevens et al. 2007b).

22.2.1 Staphylococcus aureus and MRSA

S. aureus is a bacterium colonizing many healthy persons. The predilection site for colonization is the anterior nares. For unknown reasons, about 25% of healthy people are always found to be colonized and another 25% appear to be resistant to nasal colonization with *S. aureus*. The remaining proportion is intermittently colonized. In the hospital, *S. aureus* is the most important bacterial cause of hospital-acquired infections, such as postoperative wound infections and pneumonia. In most cases, these infections are caused by the bacteria that could initially be detected in the nose of the patient.

At the time that penicillin was introduced for clinical use, in the 1940 s, all *S. aureus* isolates were susceptible to penicillin. However, within 5 years almost all isolates causing infections in hospitalized patients had become resistant to penicillin, due to the bacterial production of enzymes that destroy penicillin (beta-lactamases). In the 1950 s a new class of penicillin antibiotics was developed that was resistant to these beta-lactamases, the first being methicillin. Within several years, though, methicillin-resistant *S. aureus* (MRSA) isolates were described as well. Now resistance did not result from production of beta-lactamases, but from a new protein in the bacterial cell wall that prevents the interaction of the antibiotic with the bacterium. As a result, MRSA are resistant to all beta-lactam antibiotics.

During the 1980s, MRSA became an important cause of nosocomial infections in virtually all developed countries. In this chapter, we focus on the transmission dynamics and modelling of MRSA in hospital settings. For simplicity we call these strains hospital-acquired MRSA (HA-MRSA). Recently, we have seen a rapid emergence of infections caused by MRSA strains in the community, especially in the United States, as well as among animals in Europe with secondary spread to professional caretakers. From an epidemiological point of view, these so-called community-acquired MRSA (CA-MRSA) have different characteristics. The modelling as described in this chapter, therefore, does not automatically apply to CA-MRSA.

22.2.2 Transmission Routes

Within a health-care setting, several different bacterial transmission routes can be distinguished:

- Airborne transmission. This occurs through aerosols after coughing or sneezing. This route is relevant for respiratory viral diseases such as influenza and severe acute respiratory syndrome (SARS) but it seems to be of little relevance for antibiotic-resistant bacteria such as HA-MRSA.
- Environmental contamination. Although this may occur for MRSA, its role in the epidemiology of nosocomial MRSA is unclear. There are reported outbreaks due to contaminated surfaces or equipment, but in most instances, the contribution of contamination to the transmission dynamics is unknown. Moreover, there are no studies demonstrating that a single intervention reducing environmental contamination as a sole measure reduces acquisition with MRSA by patients (Dancer 2008).
- Direct transmission. This can occur when a health-care worker is persistently colonized with MRSA and acts as a constant source for non-colonized patients. Such occasions have been documented for MRSA, but these are considered to occur only sporadically.
- Indirect transmission, usually through temporarily contaminated hands of health-care workers. This transmission route, usually considered most important for HA-MRSA, will be discussed in detail below.

22.2.3 Indirect Transmission of MRSA

Health-care workers (more specifically their hands) are considered important in the nosocomial transmission of HA-MRSA. In this respect, health-care workers act as vectors and they spread pathogens after direct contact with a colonized patient followed by a contact with an uncolonized patient (Grundmann et al. 2002). The dynamics of this process mimics the dynamics of malaria, with health-care workers acting as mosquitoes, and is described in the Ross–MacDonald model (Ross 1911; MacDonald 1957) (Figure from Austin et al. 1999). This model was, more or less simultaneously, applied to describe the epidemiology of nosocomial pathogens by Cooper et al.(1999) and Bonten et al. (2001), and later by Grundmann et al.(2002).

In this theoretical framework, patients can be admitted and discharged and on admission patients are either uncolonized or colonized. Uncolonized patients can only acquire colonization after a contact with a contaminated health-care worker. Health-care workers can become contaminated after contact with a colonized patient. With adequate hand disinfection, a contaminated health-care worker may clear contamination, and become uncontamined again. From this model, it becomes immediately clear that improved hand hygiene (through either more frequent or more effective cleaning) will reduce the number of contacts between contaminated health-care workers and uncolonized patients, and, hence, reduce the spread of HA-MRSA. This underscores the prominent role that improved hand hygiene campaigns nowadays have in many hospitals worldwide.

Another possibility to reduce the number of contacts between colonized patients and uncontaminated health-care workers as well as between uncolonized patients and contaminated health-care workers is cohorting. The level of cohorting can be quantified as the likelihood that a next health-care worker's contact will be with the same patient. In the extreme case (cohorting level is 1) each health-care worker contacts only a single patient and colonization cannot be transmitted from one patient to another. The level cohorting has been determined in intensive care units in the United States, the United Kingdom and the Netherlands, and was approximately 70% in all (Grundmann et al. 2002; Nijssen et al. 2005; Bonten unpublished data). The importance of a high level of cohorting underscores the need of adequate staffing levels. In general, the number of contacts needed by patients depends on the severity of their disease, and should be seen as a given parameter that is difficult to change (without compromising the quality of patient care). A reduction in the number of staff, with a similar need of patient contacts, may well reduce the level of cohorting as nurses need to assist more frequently in the care of different patients. On top of that, the increased working load for nurses may also reduce the frequency (and appropriateness) of hand hygiene, which will even more facilitate transmission.

The likelihood that a health-care worker acquires contamination with HA-MRSA on his/her hands depends on the fraction of patients in the unit being colonized. This parameter has been termed colonization pressure (Bonten et al. 1998). Even when compliance of hand disinfection is far from optimal (in both frequency and efficiency), the rate at which the hands of health-care workers become decolonized is much higher than the rate at which the colonization pressure is changing, i.e. health-care workers will successfully clear contamination several times per shift. This is confirmed by studies where, even for high colonization pressure, contamination on the hands of health-care workers was only seen infrequently (Grundmann et al. 2002). The risk of an uncolonized patient acquiring colonization depends on the prevalence of hand contamination of health-care workers. However, due to the high decolonization rate of health-care workers, the probability that the hands of a given health-care worker are contaminated at a certain time is proportional to the colonization pressure, i.e., a doubling in the colonization pressures doubles the probability that the hands of a given health-care worker are contaminated. Therefore, from a mathematical point of view, the risk for an uncolonized patient of acquiring colonization can be described by the colonization pressure and health-care workers need not be modelled explicitly. In other words, the dynamics with health-care workers will resemble a situation without health-care workers where patients have direct contacts with each other. The frequency of such 'direct contacts' between patients depends of course on the frequency of contact between health-care workers and patients and on the efficacy of hand disinfection.

Environmental contamination is not part of the theoretical framework depicted in Fig. 22.1. If a colonized patient contaminates his or her direct inanimate environment (bed, washbasin, or air due to sneezing) and this contamination is only short-lived (for instance, because the environment is successfully cleaned after patient discharge) we can consider the inanimate environment as part of the patient. Contamination of a health-care worker then still fulfills the assumptions of indirect "patient-to-patient" transmission. However, if environmental contamination persists longer, the risk of an uncolonized patient to acquire colonization no longer depends on the actual number of colonized patients in the unit. In such a scenario, indirect "patient-to-patient" is no longer an accurate description of the transmission dynamics.

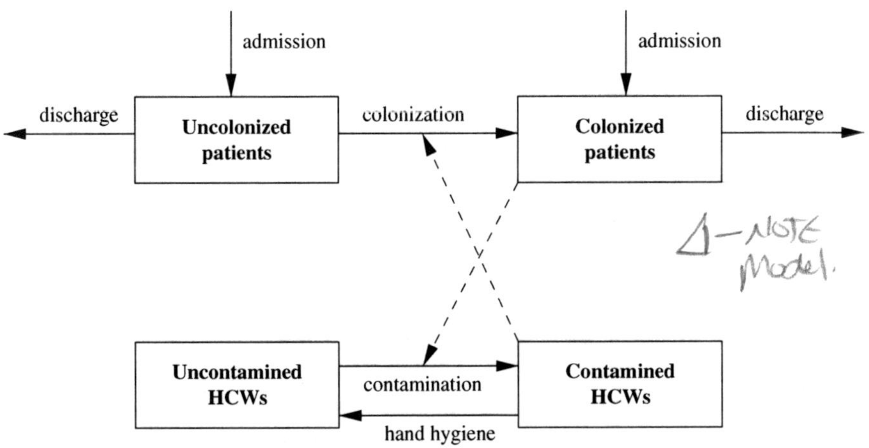

Fig. 22.1 Model of the transmission dynamics of HA-MRSA

This distinction between transmission routes that do (patient dependent), and that do not depend (patient independent), on the colonization pressure is extremely important. Examples of patient-independent transmission routes are transmission due to persistently colonized health-care workers, colonized (or contaminated) visitors, and persistent contamination of the inanimate environment. Naturally, efficacy of intervention measures will differ for both scenarios, but even more importantly, differences in dynamics become obvious in statistical analysis. If patient dependency is relevant, dynamics become nonlinear and standard statistical tests that are usually applied (e.g., chi square tests or student t-tests) for intervention studies are no longer appropriate (Nijssen et al. 2006). Therefore, distinction between both transmission routes, and determination of their relative contribution, is necessary when interpreting epidemiologic data and evaluations of interventions. Genotyping to determine events of cross-transmission and mathematical methods (Bootsma et al. 2007; Cooper 2007; Cooper and Lipsitch 2004; Drovandi and Pettitt 2008; Forrester and Pettitt 2005; McBryde et al. 2004; McBryde et al. 2007; Mikolajczyk et al. 2007; Pelupessy et al. 2002) are available to distinguish between the two.

For clarity, the models described in this chapter focus on nosocomial pathogens for which colonization pressure is relevant, as is the case for HA-MRSA and vancomycin-resistant enterococci (VRE).

22.2.4 Intervention Strategies

The aims of intervention strategies for HA-MRSA are to reduce the number of infections with MRSA, by reducing the prevalence of HA-MRSA carriage. Intervention strategies can be divided into those which work for many pathogens simultaneously and pathogen-specific strategies. General strategies generally include improvement of hygiene measures, such as hand hygiene (hand washing with an alcohol-based rub instead of water and soap), usage of gloves and gowns, better environmental cleaning, and cohorting of health-care workers.

Pathogen-specific intervention measures typically aim to physically separate colonized and uncolonized patients, by treating colonized patients in isolation rooms, single bed rooms, or by cohorting these patients (Cooper et al. 2003). Although such a separation in theory should be effective in reducing spread of pathogens, several clinical studies failed to confirm this (Cepeda et al. 2005; Cooper et al. 2003).

Detection of carriage is an important aspect for the success of such an intervention strategy. The simplest way is to use bacteriological cultures that have been obtained for clinical reasons. However, as could be assumed from the high colonization–infection ratio, most colonized patients will not develop infections and may, therefore, not be subjected to clinical testing. This problem can be overcome by active screening, either of all patients or of a high-risk population. Active screening means obtaining cultures to detect certain pathogens even in the absence of clinical suspicion of infection. Such strategies could include weekly surveillance of all patients, screening on admission of all patients, of those with a history of colonization or other risk factors for colonization. The faster colonized patients are isolated, the more effective this measure will be. Therefore, the best time to screen suspected carriers is directly after admission (Robotham et al. 2006). One should also realize that there is a diagnostic delay between obtaining the culture sample and the microbiological result, during which colonized patients would not be treated in isolation. For HA-MRSA, conventional microbiological techniques have a diagnostic delay of up to 5 days for patients not carrying HA-MRSA. Recent advances in diagnostic techniques have reduced this diagnostic delay to several hours, although these tests still have delay of about 1 day in routine daily practice (Harbarth et al. 2006). Preventive isolation of patients at high risk for colonization until culture results have excluded such carriage (or documented it) could be used to minimize the likelihood of transmission during the period of unrecognized carriage. However, if there is a trade-off between accuracy and rapidness of a test, the effect of rapid tests depends on the screening strategy (Bootsma et al. 2006; Raboud et al. 2005).

22.3 Mathematical Models for the Dynamics of Hospital-Associated MRSA

In the last decade, a considerable number of mathematical models to describe the spread of nosocomial pathogens have been published (Austin et al. 1999; Boldin 2007; Bonten et al. 2001; Bootsma et al. 2006; Cooper et al. 1999; Cooper et al. 2004; D'Agata et al. 2005; Grundmann et al. 2002; Lipsitch et al. 2000; McBryde et al. 2007; Robotham et al. 2006; Robothamet al. 2007; Sébille and Valleron 1997; Sébille et al. 1997; Smith et al. 2004; Smith et al. 2005). With these models investigators aimed to highlight key aspects of pathogen dynamics, as well as to predict the effect of intervention measures.

For models that want to go beyond qualitative relationships between parameters, two model ingredients are essential. The first one is that the model should be stochastic because hospital units are small with large fluctuations in prevalence (Bootsma et al. 2006; Cooper et al. 1999; Cooper et al. 2004; Raboud et al. 2005; Sébille and Valleron 1997; Sébille et al. 1997). The second is that readmission of discharged patients should be taken into account. The average number of secondary cases per primary case per admission if all other patients are uncolonized (the R_A-value) (Cooper et al. 2004) is typically below 1. This implies that after the first introduction of HA-MRSA in a hospital, there may be a small outbreak, but it is unlikely that there is a major epidemic shortly afterwards in which a substantial fraction of the hospitalized patients is involved. However, a patient who was colonized at the time of hospital discharge can still be colonized when readmitted. So, although the spreading capacity of HA-MRSA per admission is insufficient to generate an epidemic, the readmission loop (or feedback loop) ensures that the average total number of secondary cases per primary case per infectious period, i.e. the R_0-value, is above 1 (Bootsma et al. 2006; Cooper et al. 2004; Robotham et al. 2007).

Almost all models assume that the probability of an uncolonized patient acquiring colonization is proportional to the colonization pressure. As mentioned earlier, this mass action assumption is correct when health-care workers are vectors of transmission, and as long as contamination of their hands is short-lived. However, although mass action may be a reasonable assumption for the dynamics within a single ward, it is not a good description of the pathogen dynamics in a hospital with multiple wards. In general, most health-care workers are confined to a single ward, and some, e.g., physicians, move between wards. The compartmental structure of a hospital has several consequences for the dynamics. First, depletion of susceptible patients occurs much more rapidly in a small unit, which may reduce the growth of an epidemic. Second, when outbreaks occur within a single unit, intervention measures can be restricted to the affected unit, although such a local outbreak may exceed the local capacity to deal, e.g. because no isolation beds are available, with possible subsequent spread to other wards.

Another feature of the models is that all uncolonized patients are assumed to be equally susceptible and all colonized individuals to be equally infectious. The main reason for this assumption is simplicity and incorporation of heterogeneity in susceptibility and infectivity is challenging. Factors that influence susceptibility are known from clinical trials, the factors that increase infectivity, however, are less known. More importantly, correlations between infectivity, susceptibility, readmission rates, and decolonization rates are hardly known. However, variation in susceptibility and infectivity typically leads to smaller outbreaks (Kuulasma 1982) and a model with equal susceptibility and infectivity can therefore be seen as a worst-case scenario.

22.3.1 Insights Derived From Mathematical Models of Hospital-Associated MRSA

Here, we briefly describe the most salient observations in some models addressing the nosocomial epidemiology of HA-MRSA. Of note is that all models stress the importance of hand hygiene and cohorting, but these were not specifically investigated in any of the models (only by considering changes in the transmission parameter).

Grundmann and coworkers fitted observational data of MRSA colonization in an intensive care unit during a 1-year period to the previously described model of vector-borne indirect transmission (Grundmann et al. 2002). During the study period there were two outbreaks, and these were linked to temporal shortage of nursing staff. For most periods of the year the calculated R_A-value of MRSA was <1, but this increased to values just above 1 at the time of outbreaks. Overall, it was estimated that the R_A-value of MRSA (in the absence of any control measures) was close to 12 and that infection control measures as used had reduced this value to <1 for most of the time.

Several researchers have explicitly addressed the relation between antibiotic consumption and selection of resistant strains (Bergstrom et al. 2004; Boldin 2007; Bonten et al. 2001; D'Agata et al. 2005; Lipsitch et al. 2000; Stewart et al. 1998), and all demonstrate a direct relation between the amount of antibiotic consumption and the prevalence of antibiotic-resistant strains. However, all models assume that there is a fitness cost of resistance. This implies that, in the absence of the selective pressure of antibiotics, susceptible bacteria will have a growth advantage over the resistant ones and that in time carriage with resistant strains will disappear. Although this concept has been assumed for decades, there is increasing evidence that this paradigm of a fitness cost due to resistance is not always correct. In the absence of fitness costs of resistance, prevalence levels of resistant strains will not decline or decline much slower after withdrawing the selective pressure of antibiotics.

Cooper et al. (2004) used a Markovian stochastic simulation model to mimic the dynamics of MRSA both in the hospital as well as in the catchment population outside the hospital. They were the first to stress the importance of readmission of patients still colonized with MRSA for the nosocomial dynamics of MRSA. Especially, patients with frequent hospital admissions are of pivotal importance. Cooper et al. also demonstrated that when infection prevention resources (here the number of isolation beds) are insufficient to control an outbreak, the efficacy of such measures decreases rapidly. Finally, they nicely demonstrated the importance of stochastic effects. With the same parameters, MRSA could be controlled (even without extensive control measures) for years, but catastrophic failure resulting in high endemic prevalence levels might occur as well. Their findings advocate the use of infection preventions strategies before a pathogen becomes a major problem.

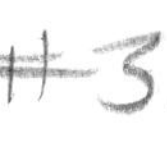

In another study, a more "game-theory like" approach was used (Smith et al. 2004; Smith et al. 2005). In order to preserve or reach a low nosocomial prevalence rate of MRSA carriage or infection, it would be optimal if all hospitals implemented intervention measures. However, for an individual hospital, it may be cost-effective not to implement these costly measures, as long as the other hospitals do (the so-called tragedy of the commons). In return, the efficacy (and thus cost-efficacy) will be lower for the hospitals with implemented measures. This exemplifies the need and the economic benefits of coordinated actions for controlling the spread of nosocomial pathogens, such as MRSA. In the extreme, the outcomes of this model would even justify legal enforcement to comply with such measures.

We have also used a Markovian stochastic simulation model to investigate the dynamics of MRSA in hospitals and their catchment population, as well as the effects of different intervention measures hereon (Bootsma et al. 2006). The main difference with the Cooper model (Cooper et al. 2004) is the much more detailed modelling of the transmission dynamics within the hospital. This includes a compartmentalized structure due to wards, two different types of wards (with regard to transmission and patient flow), the presence of health-care workers persistently carrying MRSA (and being a continuous source for patients) as well as health-care workers temporarily contaminated with MRSA and acting as vectors for MRSA transmission. This more detailed modelling structure mimics reality more closely and allows for the evaluation of the contribution of the individual components of the so-called Search and Destroy policy. This policy consists of a set of infection prevention measures and is thought to be responsible for the low prevalence of MRSA among nosocomial *S. aureus* infections in Scandinavian countries and the Netherlands. The "Search and Destroy" policy aims at treating MRSA carriers in single rooms with barrier precautions. On admission, high-risk patients are screened for MRSA carriage and preventively isolated until documented absence of such carriage. When MRSA is unexpectedly found in a patient who is not treated in isolation, all patients and health-care workers in the same ward or that otherwise might have had contact with the index case are screened for carriage. Finally, eradication of MRSA (in those identified as infected or colonized) through nasal application of mupirocin (in combination with chlorhexidine body washing) is attempted after hospitalization.

First we analyzed how the cumulative use of these measures will benefit control of MRSA in a low-endemic setting. Isolation of MRSA carriers that are detected by clinical cultures alone will not be sufficient to control MRSA in the long term, even if isolation is 100% effective. However, it might take many years before the nosocomial prevalence of carriage will start to increase. With isolation we mean all measures that limit the transmission of MRSA to another patient. The highest likelihood to achieve this will be reached when such a patient is placed in a single room, with limited exposure to health-care workers that adhere maximally to barrier precautions. This may not be feasible in many circumstances, though, and therefore, we have used different efficacy levels for isolation in our model. In a low-endemic setting, addition of either admission screening and preventive isolation of high-risk patients or active search for carriage among contact patients in case of an unexpected case to isolation of carriers seems sufficient to control MRSA. Yet, in the analytical model perfect performance of these combined measures would only be sufficient to control a pathogen with an R value of 1.4–1.5. Considering that such measures will never be executed perfectly, application of both screening interventions (on admission and after detection of an index patient) simultaneously is much safer. In the combined approach, the R value that could be controlled successfully increased to 2.2. In such a scenario, active decolonization after hospital discharge would only add little to its effectiveness.

Second, we analyzed how a modified Search and Destroy approach would perform in a setting with a high prevalence of MRSA carriage in the hospital. Considering the problems of realizing perfect isolation in such setting, for instance, because of shortage of isolation facilities, two strategies were evaluated. In the first scenario, three measures were implemented (isolation of all documented carriers; screening of high-risk patients on admission with preemptive isolation; screening of contact patients when an index patient was identified). Because of anticipated problems in achieving appropriate isolation in the beginning (when prevalence of carriage is high) we assumed that efficacy of colonization would be 50% in the first 5 years and would then increase to 80% thereafter. From Fig. 22.2, it is obvious

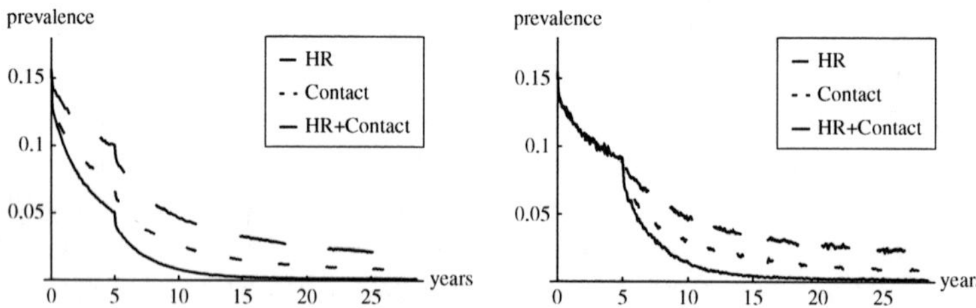

Fig. 22.2 Mean nosocomial prevalence in 1000 simulations. *Left*: The isolation efficacy is 50% during the first 5 years and 80% thereafter for three intervention scenarios. Admission screening of high-risk patients (HR), Screening of contact patients (contact) and a combination of both. *Right*: The first 5 years only documented carriers are isolated with an efficacy of 80%. After 5 years, additional interventions are implemented.

that the combined approach of all three measures is more effective than the other combinations. In the second scenario, all efforts were placed on achieving good isolation (80% efficacy) of documented carriers in the first 5 years, with the addition of screening high-risk patients and contacting patients after this period (while maintaining 80% efficacy of isolation). Again, the combined approach of all three measures was most efficient. This scenario analysis can also be used to determine the burden of infection prevention for the hospital, expressed as the number of isolation beds needed. This is represented by the area under the curves. Accepting the assumptions made, there were marked differences in the number of isolation beds needed, which might be helpful in choosing the most cost-effective strategy.

Finally, the effects of rapid screening methods for MRSA were compared to conventional microbiological culture methods. Conventional microbiological methods have a diagnostic delay of up to 5 days for excluding MRSA carriage and of several days (up to 3) for detecting MRSA. This diagnostic delay can be reduced, in theory, to several hours, although a turn-around-time of about 1 day has been realized in clinical trials (Harbarth et al. 2006). Rapid diagnostic tests can prevent unnecessary isolation days when using preventive isolation. When not using preventive isolation, rapid diagnostic tests can reduce the duration of non-isolation of colonized patients. Therefore, in theory, rapid diagnostic tests must be beneficial for controlling MRSA if these tests have equally good sensitivity and specificity as the conventional microbiological culture methods. Yet, rapid tests will be more expensive and these additional costs must be balanced against these benefits.

Several interesting scenarios arise if the test characteristics of the rapid test are different from those of conventional microbiological tests. Occurrence of false negative results (sensitivity <100%) will prevent colonized patients from being isolated, which may increase transmission (and nosocomial prevalence) and will, thus, determine whether the use of rapid test reduces the nosocomial prevalence. As prevalence may grow only slowly, rapid tests may initially seem beneficial, but may ultimately increase the number of patient days in isolation. However, our model predicts that rapid tests will reduce the number of isolation days required in high-endemic settings, even if test characteristics are not optimal.

Going back to the two proposed scenarios for gradually increasing MRSA control in high-endemicity settings, we have evaluated to what extent the use of rapid diagnostic tests can reduce the number of isolation beds needed. Depending on the turn-around-time of test results and their specificity this number could be reduced by as much as 47%, which might make such control strategies feasible, even in high-endemicity settings.

References

Austin DJ, Bonten MJM, Weinstein RA et al. (1999) Vancomycin-resistant enterococci in intensive-care hospital settings: Transmission dynamics, persistence, and the impact of infection control programs. Proc Natl Acad Sci USA 96:6908–6913

Bergstrom CT, Lo M, Lipsitch M (2004) Ecological theory suggests that antimicrobial cycling will not reduce antimicrobial resistance in hospitals. Proc Natl Acad Sci USA 101:13285–13290

Boldin B (2007) Relative effects of barrier precautions and topical antibiotics on nosocomial bacterial transmission: results of multi-compartment models. Bull Math Biol 69:2227–2248

Bonten MJM, Slaughter S, Ambergen AW et al. (1998) The role of "colonization pressure" in the spread of vancomycin-resistant enterococci. An important infection control variable. Arch Intern Med 158:1127–1132

Bonten MJM, Austin DJ, Lipsitch M (2001) Understanding the spread of antibiotic resistant pathogens in hospitals: mathematical models as tools for control. Clin Infect Dis 33: 1739–1746

Bootsma MCJ, Diekmann O, Bonten MJM (2006) Controlling methicillin-resistant *Staphylococcus aureus*: Quantifying the effects of interventions and rapid diagnostic testing. Proc Natl Acad Sci USA 103:5620–5625

Bootsma MCJ, Bonten MJM, Nijssen S et al. (2007) An algorithm to estimate the importance of bacterial acquisition routes in hospital settings. Am J Epidemiol 166:841–851

Cepeda JA, Whitehouse T, Cooper B et al. (2005) Isolation of patients in single rooms or cohorts to reduce spread of MRSA in intensive-care units: prospective two-centre study. Lancet 365: 295–304

Cooper BS (2007) Confronting models with data. J Hosp Infect 65(S2):88–92

Cooper BS, Lipsitch M (2004) The analysis of hospital infection data using hidden Markov models. Biostatistics 5:223–237

Cooper BS, Medley GF, Scott GM (1999) Preliminary analysis of the transmission dynamics of nosocomial infections: stochastic and management effects. J Hosp Infect 43:131–147

Cooper BS, Stone SP, Kibbler CC et al. (2003) Systematic review of isolation policies in the hospital management of methicillin-resistant *Staphylococcus aureus*: a review of the literature with epidemiological and economic modelling. Health Technol Assessment 7:1–194

Cooper BS, Medley GF, Stone SP et al. (2004) Methicillin-resistant *Staphylococcus aureus* in hospitals and the community: Stealth dynamics and control catastrophes. Proc Natl Acad Sci USA 101:10223–10228

D'Agata EM, Horn MA, Webb GF (2005) A mathematical model quantifying the impact of antibiotic exposure and other interventions on the endemic prevalence of vancomycin-resistant enterococci. J Infect Dis 192:2004–2011

Dancer SJ (2008) Importance of the environment in methicillin-resistant *Staphylococcus aureus* acquisition: the case for hospital cleaning. Lancet Infec Dis 8:101–113

Drovandi CC, Pettitt AN (2008) Multivariate Markov process models for the transmission of methicillin-resistant *Staphylococcus aureus* in a hospital ward. Biometrics. doi: 10.1111/j.1541–0420. 2007. 00933.x

Forrester M, Pettitt AN (2005) Use of stochastic epidemic modeling to quantify transmission rates of colonization with methicillin-resistant *Staphylococcus aureus* in an intensive care unit. Infect Control Hosp Epidemiol 26:598–606

Grundmann H, Hori S, Winter B et al. (2002) Risk factors for the transmission of methicillin-resistant *Staphylococcus* aureus in an adult intensive care unit: fitting a model to the data. J Infect Dis 185:481–488

Harbarth S, Masuet-Aumatell C, Schrenzel J et al. (2006) Evaluation of rapid screening and preemptive contact isolation for detecting and controlling methicillin-resistant *Staphylococcus aureus* in critical care: an interventional cohort study. Crit Care 10:R25

Klevens RM, Edwards JR, Richards CL Jr et al. (2007a) Estimating health care-associated infections and deaths in U.S. hospitals, 2002. Public Health Rep. 122:160–166

Klevens RM, Morrison MA, Nadle J et al. (2007b) Invasive methicillin-resistant *Staphylococcus aureus* infections in the United States. J Am Med Assoc 298:1763–1771

Kuulasma K (1982) The spatial general epidemic and locally dependent random graphs. J Appl Prob 19:745–758

Lipsitch M, Bergstrom CT, Levin BR (2000) The epidemiology of antibiotic resistance in hospitals: Paradoxes and prescriptions. Proc Natl Acad Sci USA 97:1938–1943

MacDonald G (1957) The epidemiology and control of malaria. Oxford University Press, London

McBryde ES, Bradley LC, Whitby M et al. (2004) An investigation of contact transmission of methicillin-resistant *Staphylococcus aureus*. J Hosp Infect 58:104–108

McBryde ES, Pettitt AN, McEwain DLS (2007) A stochastic mathematical model of methicillin resistant *Staphylococcus aureus* transmission in an intensive care unit: Predicting the impact of interventions. J Theor Biol 245:470–481

Mikolajczyk RT, Sagel U, Bornemann R et al. (2007) A statistical method for estimating the proportion of cases resulting from cross-transmission of multi-resistant pathogens in an intensive care unit. J Hosp Infect 65:149–55

Nijssen S, Bonten MJM, Weinstein RA (2005) Are active microbiological surveillance and subsequent isolation needed to prevent the spread of methicillin-resistant Staphylococcus aureus? Clin Infect Dis 40:405–409

Nijssen S, Bootsma MCJ, Bonten,MJM (2006) Potential confounding in evaluating infection control interventions in hospital settings: changing antibiotic prescription. Clin Infect Dis 43:616–623

Pelupessy I, Bonten MJM, Diekmann O (2002) How to assess the relative importance of different colonization routes of pathogens within hospital settings. Proc Natl Acad Sci USA 99: 5601–5605

Raboud J, Saskin R, Simor A et al. (2005) Modeling transmission of methicillin-resistant *Staphylococcus aureus* among patients admitted to a hospital. Infect Control Hosp Epidemiol 26:607–615

Robotham JV, Jenkins DR, Medley GF (2006) Screening strategies in surveillance and control of methicillin-resistant *Staphylococcus aureus* (MRSA). Epidemiol Infect 13:1–15

Robotham JV, Scarff CA, Jenkins DR et al. (2007) Meticillin-resistant *Staphylococcus aureus* (MRSA) in hospitals and the community: model predictions based on the UK situation. J Hosp Infect 65(S2):93–99

Ross R (1911) The prevention of malaria (2nd edition). Murray, London

Sébille V, Valleron A-J (1997) A computer simulation model for the spread of nosocomial infections caused by multidrug-resistant pathogens. Comput Biomed Res 30:307–322

Sébille V, Cheuret S, Valleron A-J (1997) Modeling the spread of resistant nosocomial pathogens in an intensive-care unit. Infect Control Hosp Epidemiol 18:84–92

Smith DL, Dushoff J, Perencevich E et al. (2004) Persistent colonization and the spread of antibiotic resistance in nosocomial pathogens: resistance is a regional problem. Proc Natl Acad Sci USA 101:3709–3714

Smith DL, Levin SA, Laxminarayan R (2005) Strategic interactions in multi-institutional epidemics of antibiotic resistance. Proc Natl Acad Sci USA 102:3153–3158

Stewart FM, Antia R , Levin BR et al. (1998) The population genetics of antibiotic resistance. II: Analytic theory for sustained populations of bacteria in a community of hosts. Theor Popul Biol 53:152–165

Stone PW, Hedblom EC, Murphy DM et al. (2005) The economic impact of infection control: Making the business case for increased infection control resources. Am J Infect Control 2005 33:542–547

Wenzel RP (2003) Prevention and Control of Nosocomial Infections, 4th edition, Lippincott Williams & Wilkins, Chicago

Chapter 23
Infectious Diseases and Cancer: HPV

Helen Trottier and Eduardo L. Franco

23.1 Introduction

Many types of cancer are etiologically linked to infections. Historically, it has been a challenge to prove the causal link between an infectious agent and a given type of cancer; different sets of causal criteria have been applied according to the methodological approach used to study the putative association (Franco et al. 2004). Yet, epidemiologic and molecular evidence to date unequivocally demonstrate causal links between viruses, bacteria, and protozoan and metazoan parasites, and many forms of cancer. The main infectious agents that are known to cause cancer in humans are the human papillomavirus (HPV), hepatitis B and C viruses, Epstein–Barr virus (EBV), human T cell lymphotropic virus I, human immunodeficiency virus (HIV), human herpes virus 8 (HHV-8), *Helicobacter pylori*, Schistosomes, and liver flukes (genus *Opistorchis*). Altogether, it has been estimated that these agents cause 17.8% of incident cancers worldwide (12.1%, 5.6%, and 0.1% for viral, bacterial, and parasitic infections, respectively) including as much as 5.2% for HPV alone (Parkin 2006).

HPV infection is recognized today as the necessary causal factor of all cervical cancer cases in the world and of a substantial proportion of many other anogenital neoplasms. HPV has also been implicated in the genesis of several other cancers, such as head and neck cancer, non-melanoma skin malignancies and other cancers. In this chapter, we provide an overview of the types of cancer in which HPV infection has been etiologically implicated or is suspected to play a causal role.

H. Trottier (✉)
Division of Cancer Epidemiology, Departments of Oncology and Epidemiology and Biostatistics, McGill University, Montreal, Canada
e-mail: helen.trottier@mcgill.ca

A. Krämer et al. (eds.), *Modern Infectious Disease Epidemiology*,
Statistics for Biology and Health, DOI 10.1007/978-0-387-93835-6_23,

23.2 HPV Biology

23.2.1 HPV Structure

HPVs belong to the Papillomaviridae family. They have a double-stranded circular DNA genome of around 8,000 base pairs (5 million MW) with six early genes (E1, E2, E4–E7) and two late genes (L1 and L2, the capsid proteins) that are all located on the same circular DNA structure (Fig. 23.1). Over 100 HPV genotypes have been identified based on the isolation of complete genomes (de Villiers et al. 2004) and have a similar genomic organization. The L1 protein is highly conserved among all HPV types and is thus used for taxonomical purposes. A new HPV isolate is recognized as a new genotype (type for short) if the complete genome has been cloned and the nucleotide sequence of the L1 gene differs by more than 10% from the type with which it has greatest homology in DNA sequence. Differences of less than 10% but more than 2% characterize a new subtype, and of less than 2% they define a new molecular variant. Viral DNA is detectable as free-form episomes in the nucleus of the infected cell and/or as integrated sequences into the host chromosomes. In general, HPV-associated cancer arises from the integration of the viral genome into a host cell chromosome which causes disruption of cellular genes and overexpression of viral oncogenes, although there is some evidence that integration may not be a requirement for cell transformation and neoplastic development (Cullen et al. 1991; Pirami et al. 1997).

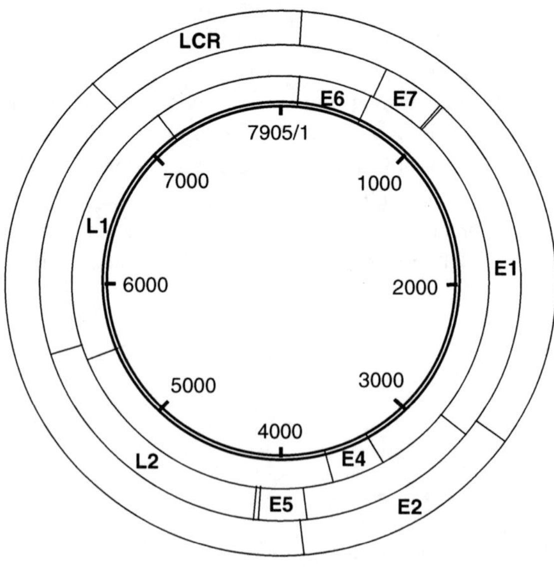

Fig. 23.1 The Papillomavirus genome

23.2.2 Classification of HPVs and Carcinogenicity

The more than 100 HPV types that have been catalogued so far (De Villiers et al. 2004) are classified according to their tissue tropism (mucosal or cutaneous) and oncogenic potential. Table 23.1 shows the general properties of HPVs in terms of tissue tropism, carcinogenic potential, and associated diseases. About 40 types infect the epithelial lining of the anogenital tract and other mucosal areas of the body. Infection with low-oncogenic risk HPVs (LR-HPV), such as HPV-6 and 11, can cause benign lesions of the anogenital areas known as *Condylomata acuminata* (genital warts), as well as a large proportion of low-grade squamous intraepithelial lesions (LSIL) of the cervix. LR-HPV infections are responsible for substantial morbidity and incur high costs associated with the treatment of clinically relevant lesions. Perinatal transmission of HPV is also possible and can cause in rare instances recurrent respiratory papillomatosis in infants and young children (Amstrong et al. 2000). Among the mucosal HPVs, some 13–18 types have been

Table 23.1 Classification of HPV genotypes and diseases associated with them. Adapted from: de Villiers et al. (2004)

Genus	Tissue tropism	HPV types		Diseases
Alpha	Mucosal and cutaneous	High-oncogenic risk:	16,18,31,33,35,39, 45,51,52,56,58,59, 66,68,73,82	Intraepithelial neoplasia/cervical, other anogenital cancers and head and neck cancer
		Low-oncogenic risk	6,11,42,44,51,53, 83	Condylomata acuminata/intraepithelial neoplasia /mucosal lesions
			32,42	Benign lesion (oral or genital)
			3,10,28,29,78	Cause more frequently cutaneous than mucosal lesions
			61,72,81,83,84,62, 86,87,89	Benign mucosal lesion
			2, 27, 57	Common skin warts
			13,26,30,34,54,71, 74,53,67,69,70,85, 90,PcPV	Mucosal lesion
			7,40,43,91	Mucosal and cutaneous lesions
Beta	Cutaneous	5,8,9,12,14,15,17,19,20,21,22, 23,25,36,37,38,47,80 49,75,76		Commonly associated with epidermodysplasia verruciformis (mostly benign lesion)
Gamma	Cutaneous	4,48,50,60,65		Cutaneous lesion
Mu	Cutaneous	1		Plantar wart
Nu	Cutaneous	63		Plantar wart

identified as probable or definite high-oncogenic risk (HR-HPV) according to their frequency of association with cervical cancer and other anogenital cancers. Since the 1990s, several classifications have been made according to the research development (reviewed in Trottier and Franco 2006). The latest classification published by the World Health Organization's International Agency for Research on Cancer (IARC) referred HPV-16, 18, 31, 33, 35, 39, 45, 51, 52, 55, 56, 58, 66 as HR-HPVs (IARC 2007). This new classification included also HPV type 6 and 11 as possibly carcinogenic.

Many HPV types can also infect the dry skin, causing verrucous lesions, more commonly known as warts. In addition to the above-mentioned carcinogenic types that belong to the alpha genus, the IARC (2007) has classified HPV-5 and 8 (genus beta) as carcinogenic. Epidermodysplasia verruciformis (EV) can occur among hosts with genetic defects in their ability to control the cutaneous proliferation of HPVs. HPV infections in EV patients are more likely to undergo malignant transformation than other warty lesions in normal individuals, although oncogenic transformation of an epithelial HPV infection is very rare.

23.3 HPV and Human Cancer

Extensive research in the last 20 years has contributed to today's recognition of HPV infection as the main etiologic agent of cervical cancer and other anogenital neoplasms, and a leading cause of death from cancer worldwide. It is now widely accepted that HR-HPV infections are a necessary, but not sufficient, cause of virtually all cases of cervical cancer worldwide and are a likely cause of a substantial proportion of other anogenital, upper aero-digestive tract, and non-melanoma skin cancers. HPV has also been suspected to play a role in several other human tumors.

23.3.1 Cervical Cancer

Cervical cancer is the second most common malignant neoplasm affecting women worldwide, after breast cancer. In 2002, 4,93,000 new cases were diagnosed in the world from which 83% occurred in developing countries (Ferlay et al. 2004; Pisani et al. 1999). This translates into a high mortality rate with an estimated 1,90,000 deaths from cervical cancer worldwide every year, with over 75% of them in developing countries, where mortality from this disease is the highest among deaths caused by neoplasms (Pisani et al. 1999). The highest-risk areas for cervical cancer are in Southern and Eastern Africa, Melanesia, the Caribbean, and Central and South America, with average incidence rates well above 30 per 1,00,000 women per year (Parkin et al. 2005). In the United States there are approximately 12,800 new cases of invasive cervical cancer and 4,600 deaths due to this disease each year (Ries et al. 2000). Overall annual cervical cancer prevention and treatment costs in the United States were estimated at $3.4 billion, with expenditures for routine screening of $2.1 billion, impact of false-positive Papanicolaou test results at $300 million, management and treatment of CIN 1 of $150 million, CIN 2/3 of $450 million, and invasive cancer of $350 million (Insinga et al. 2004; 2004).

23.3.1.1 Causal Role of HPV in Cervical Cancer

Cervical cancer was early hypothesized as related to sexual activity; since nuns did not develop this neoplasm whereas prostitutes had an increased risk. Moreover, sexual behavior variables were recognized as key risk factors, such as age at first sexual coitus, number of sexual partners, etc. (Harris et al. 1980; Brock et al. 1989; Cuzick et al. 1990; Parazzini et al. 1992; Munoz et al. 1993; De vet et al. 1994; Kjellberg et al. 1999). Over the years, many sexually transmitted microbes such as herpes simplex virus (HSV-2), syphylis, gonorrhea, or either *Chlamydia trachomatis* have been suspected as etiologic agents of cervical cancer. However, with the international multidisciplinary effort that began more than 25 years ago, there was a gradual realization that not only most cervical carcinomas harbored HPV DNA but also that cervical HPV infection was common in women without cervical abnormalities, with prevalences in the 10–40% range (Franco et al. 1991).

Many investigations examined the nature of the relationship between HPV and cervical cancer. In addition to the Hill's criteria (strength of the association, consistency, biologic gradient, temporality, coherence, biologic plausibility, experimental evidence, etc.), sets of other useful guidelines for causal attributions involving infectious agents have been proposed (Evans 1976; Evans et al. 1990; Fredricks et al. 1998). These causal criteria take into account the knowledge about the timing, specificity, and level of immune response against putative viruses, or the advances in nucleic acid detection methodology as used in modern molecular epidemiologic investigations (Franco et al. 2004). All those criteria help establishing that infection with HR-HPV types is the central causal factor in cervical cancer (Bosch et al. 2002; Franco et al. 1999; IARC 1995; Schiffman and Brinton 1995; Schiffman and Kjaer 2003; Herrero 1996; Holly 1996; Walboomers and Meijerr 1997; Walboomers et al. 1999; Clifford et al. 2003; Muñoz et al. 2003). The relative risk for the relation between HPV and cervical cancer is the strongest ever observed between an etiologic agent and a human cancer. For example, the relative risk between tobacco and lung cancer is estimated between 7 and 15 (IARC 1986), whereas the relative risk between HPV-16 and squamous cell cervical cancer estimated from the pool of IARC case–control studies is 435 (Muñoz et al. 2003). Although only a small proportion of HPV-infected women develop cervical cancer, it is now well known that virtually 100% of cervical cancers are caused by HR-HPV (Walboomers et al. 1999). The association is supported by strong epidemiological evidence and the detection of HPV DNA in up to 99.7% of cervical cancers from all geographic areas (Schiffman et al. 1993; Bosch et al. 1995; Walboomers et al. 1999; Munoz et al. 2003). HPV-16 is the

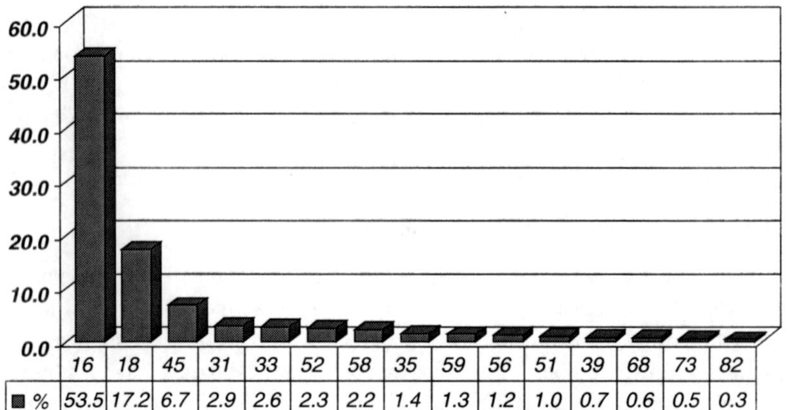

	16	18	45	31	33	52	58	35	59	56	51	39	68	73	82
■ %	53.5	17.2	6.7	2.9	2.6	2.3	2.2	1.4	1.3	1.2	1.0	0.7	0.6	0.5	0.3

Fig. 23.2 Distribution of type-specific HPV in cervical tumor specimens. Adapted from: Munoz et al., IJC 2004

most prevalent type causing approximately 54% of cervical cancers worldwide, followed by HPV-18 which is associated with approximately 17% of cervical cancers (Fig. 23.2). In combination, HPV types 16 and 18 are the most important in terms of the attributable risk they pose causing altogether about 70–75% of all cervical cancers (Muñoz et al. 2004). The remaining tumors have been shown to contain DNA from other HR types such as HPV-45, HPV-31, and HPV-33 (Clifford et al. 2003).

23.3.1.2 Natural History of Cervical Cancer

The natural history of cervical cancer is represented by acquisition of HPV, development of a persistent HPV infection with HR types, and cervical neoplastic development (Fig. 23.3). Cervical neoplastic development is a slow process of disruption of the normal maturation of the transformation zone epithelium of the uterine cervix near its squamo-columnar junction (Franco and Ferenczy 2002). This process of abnormal changes is initially limited to the cervical epithelium. These preinvasive lesions known as dysplasia or as squamous intraepithelial lesion (SIL) can be discovered through cytological examination using the Papanicolaou technique and confirmed by colposcopic examination and biopsy as cervical intraepithelial neoplasia (CIN). They are invariably asymptomatic and if left untreated, the low-grade lesions may eventually extend to the full thickness of the cervical epithelium (cervical carcinoma in situ (CIS)) and traverse the lining formed by the basement membrane to become invasive. This process may take a decade or longer but will eventually occur in a substantial proportion of CIS patients.

Although HPV infection is the central cause of cervical cancer, only a small percentage of women who are infected go on to develop cervical cancer or its precursors. In fact, HPV alone is not a sufficient cause and much work has been devoted to determining why certain HPV-positive women develop cervical cancer while

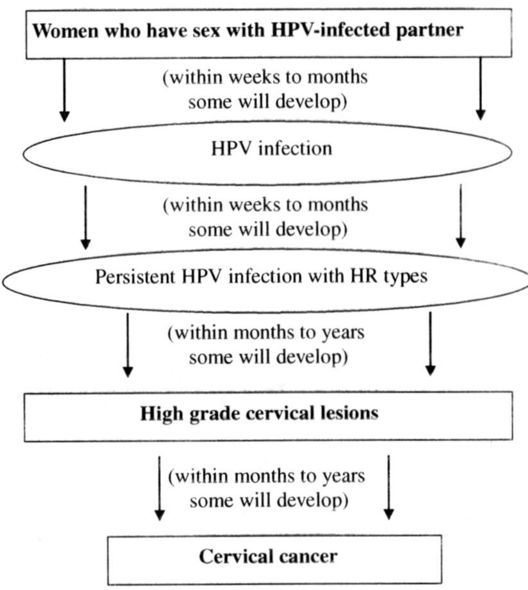

Fig. 23.3 Cervical cancer carcinogenesis. Source: Franco and Ferenczy 2002

others do not. The multifactorial model of cervical cancer etiology shows an interplay of various cofactors in the relation between persistent HPV, the main etiologic agent, and cervical cancer (Spence et al. 2005). Smoking, high parity, long-term use of oral contraceptive, coinfections, and immunosuppression have been found to increase risk of cervical cancer (Spence et al. 2005; Richardson et al. 2003; Winer et al. 2003; Koutsky 1997; Moscicki et al. 2001; Sellors et al. 2003; Baseman and Koutsky, 2005; Giuliano et al. 2002; Rousseau et al. 2000; Aral and Holmes 1999; Kahn et al. 2002; Manhart and Koutsky 2002; Stone et al. 1999). Results about condom are inconsistent; the majority showing that condom is not protective while other have shown that consistent condom use by their partners appears to reduce the risk of cervical lesions (Manhart and Koutsky 2002; Winer et al. 2006). Others factors such as genetic polymorphisms in the human leukocyte antigen (HLA) system, p53 polymorphism, nutrition, insulin-like growth factors (IGFs), and viral factors (molecular variants of HPV-16 and 18 and high viral load) have been associated with cervical cancer (Schaffer et al. 2007; Wang and Hildesheim 2003; Maciag et al. 2002; Garcia-Closas et al. 2005; Giuliano et al. 2003; Sichero et al. 2007; Schlecht et al. 2003).

23.3.2 Other Anogenital Cancers

HPV has also been implicated in the development of malignancies of other anogenital sites including anus, vagina, vulva, and penis. Unlike the situation for cervical cancer, in which 100% of cancers are caused by HPV, cancers of other anogenital

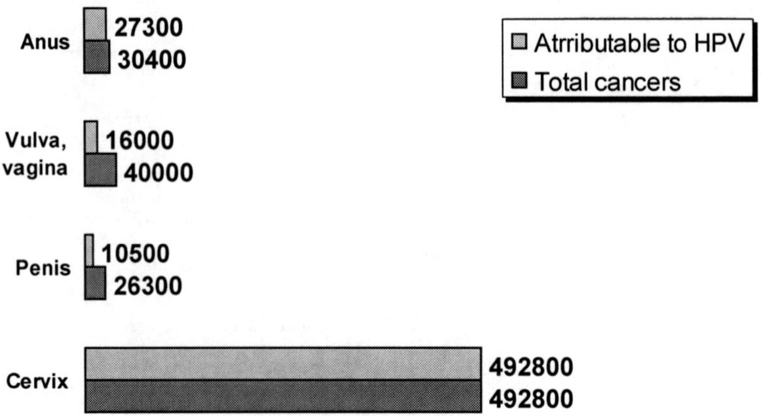

Fig. 23.4 Total number of annual incident cancers in the world and total attributable to HPV. Adapted from Parkin 2006

sites show lower risk attributions for HPV. It is estimated that 85–95% of anal cancers, 60–65% of vaginal cancers, 20–50% of vulvar cancers, and 40–50% of penile cancers are attributed to HPV (Fig. 23.4) (Parkin 2006).

23.3.2.1 Anal Cancer

Anal cancer is relatively rare although there has been a considerable increase in the incidence over the last 25 years among both men (160%) and women (78%) (Melbye et al. 1994; Frisch et al. 1993; Johnson et al. 2004). This increase was especially pronounced among homosexual men, particularly those who are HIV positive. Such subpopulations as homosexuals, HIV-positive persons, transplant recipients, and women with cervical squamous intraepithelial lesions are at a higher risk than the general population (Palefsky 2000a; Ryan et al. 2000).

Historically, anal cancer was believed to develop as a result of chronic irritation resulting from benign conditions (e.g., hemorrhoids, fissures) and was also associated with inflammatory bowel disease (Ryan et al. 2000). These factors notwithstanding, a substantial proportion of anal cancer are unequivocally linked to HPV (Welton et al. 2004). The proportion of anal cancers due to HPV is around 90% (Palefsky et al. 1991; Frisch et al. 1997; Daling et al. 2004). Similar to cervical cancer, HPVs 16 and 18 are the most common types present in anal carcinoma specimens. The model of anal cancer pathogenesis is very similar to that of cervical cancer: HPV infection is associated with the development of precursor lesions (SILs), which can be low grade (LSIL) or high grade (HSIL) and progression of anal SIL to invasive anal cancer is influenced by other cofactors. In men, homosexual behavior is the strongest risk factor for anal cancer (Daling et al. 1987). Immunosuppression is also an important risk factor. The incidence of anal cancer in men who have sex with men (MSM) is doubled with HIV positivity (Palefsky et al.

2000b). In heterosexual men, syphilis, lifetime number of sexual partners, being unmarried, anogenital warts, anal fissures, or hemorrhoids are risk factors (Holly et al. 1989; Frisch et al. 1997). In women, anogenital warts, cervical squamous intraepithelial lesions, C. *trachomatis* and HSV-2 infections, gonorrhea, hemorrhoids, anal intercourse, lifetime number of sexual partners, partners with history of venereal disease, smoking, and anal fissures are risk factors for anal cancer (Daling et al. 1987; Holly et al. 1989; Frisch et al. 1997).

23.3.2.2 Vaginal Cancer

Cancer of the vagina is extremely rare with an average incidence rate of approximately 1 case per 1,00,000 women per year worldwide (Parkin et al. 1997). In the United States, little more than 2,000 new cases occurred and 800 died from vaginal cancer in 2006 (Ries et al. 2006). HPV seems to play a central role in the causal pathway, being found in the majority of cases (Daling et al. 2002; Ikenberg et al. 1990). HPV DNA is detected in 64–91% of vaginal cancers and 82–100% of their precursor lesions (vaginal intraepithelial lesions of grade 3) and HPV-16 appear to be the most prevalent type (Munoz et al. 2006). The model of vaginal cancer pathogenesis is very similar to that of cervical cancer and is highly associated with sexual behaviors (Daling et al. 2002). In addition, women with primary vaginal carcinoma are more likely to have been previously diagnosed with an anogenital tumor, particularly of the cervix (Daling et al. 2002).

23.3.2.3 Vulvar Cancer

Invasive squamous cell carcinoma of the vulva is relatively rare; it accounts for slightly less than 5% of all female tract malignancies but the incidence of vulvar cancer has increased over the past 30 years, especially in younger women (Judson et al. 2006). In the United States, it was estimated that there were 3,740 new cases and 880 deaths from vulvar cancer in 2006 (Ries et al. 2006). Approximately 60% of vulvar cancers contain HPV DNA. HPV-16 is the most frequently observed type in these tumors (Hampl et al. 2006; IARC 2007). However, there seems to be two distinct risk factor profiles for vulvar cancer that are age dependent (Fig. 23.5). Keratinizing squamous cell carcinomas mostly affect older women and are rarely associated with HPV infection (less than 10%). On the other hand, warty or basaloid carcinomas are more often diagnosed in young women and constitute a HPV-related subgroup of tumors (60–90% are positive for HPV) (Al-Ghamdi et al. 2002; Munoz et al. 2006). These HPV-positive tumors have seem to have become more frequent in recent decades (Hørding et al. 1994) and tend to have the same risk profile as other anogenital cancers, i.e., association with high-risk sexual behaviors.

23.3.2.4 Penile Cancer

Squamous cell carcinoma (SCC) of the penis is a relatively rare disease in developed countries in Europe and North America, where incidence rates vary between 0.3 and

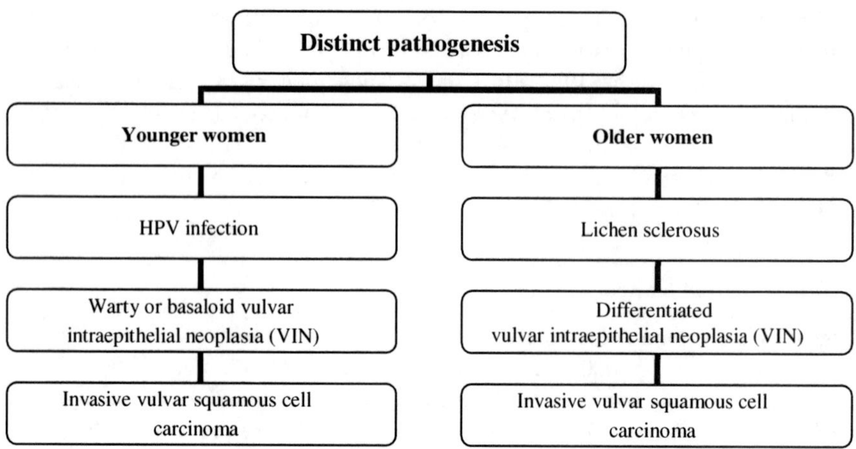

Fig. 23.5 Pathogenesis of vulvar invasive squamous cell carcinoma in young versus old women

1 cases per 1,00,000 men-years. Incidence is higher in parts of Africa (Uganda), Asia, and South America (Brazil and Colombia) where it may reach four cases per 1,00,000 men-years (Parkin et al. 2002; Malek et al. 1993). The etiology of penile cancer also appears to be multifactorial, with a history of smoking, phymosis, poor hygiene, history of genital warts, large number of lifetime sexual partners, and lack of circumcision during childhood being commonly associated with this neoplasm (Dillner et al. 2000; Heideman et al. 2007; Rubin et al. 2001; Maden et al. 1993; Hellberg et al. 1987). Interestingly, wives of men who have been diagnosed with penile cancer are at higher risk of cervical neoplasia (Spence et al. 2005). The exact etiologic mechanisms that lead to the development of penile cancer are largely unknown although HPV has been associated with this neoplasm (Parkin 2006). Similarly to vulvar cancer, basaloid or warty penile carcinomas show the highest HPV prevalence (up to 100%) (Cubilla et al. 2000; Cubilla et al. 1998; Rubin et al. 2001). Keratinizing penile SCCs, which represent more than 95% of penile cancer diagnosed in Europe and the United States generally showed a lower HPV prevalence (approximately 30–40%) (Heideman et al. 2007; Ferreux et al. 2003; Rubin et al. 2001). HPV-16 is also the most prevalent type detected in HPV-related penile cancer (Rubin et al. 2001; Maden et al. 1993; Heideman et al. 2007).

23.3.3 Head and Neck Cancer

In 2000, head and neck cancer (cancers of the oral cavity, pharynx, and larynx) was ranked as the eighth leading cause of cancer death worldwide with an average incidence rate of 8.8 and 5.1 per 1,00,000 males and females per year, respectively (Shibuya et al. 2002). There is an extensive variation in head and neck squamous cell carcinoma (HNSCC) incidence by both sex and geographic region (Parkin et al. 2002). In North America, the incidence rates are 5.0 and 2.6 per 1,00,000 males and females per year, respectively; whereas in Europe the equivalent rates are 8.6 and 2.7, respectively (Shibuya et al. 2002). However, the results of many studies suggest that head and neck cancer, particularly oral tongue cancer, is increasing in young adults internationally (Macfarlane et al. 1992; Shiboski et al. 2000; Schantz and Yu 2002).

The main risk factors are tobacco and alcohol but it has been proposed that HPV also play a role in a subset of head and neck squamous cell carcinomas. The association is strongest in the oropharynx, particularly in the tonsil (Klussmann et al. 2003a; Venuti et al. 2004; Tran et al. 2007; Dahlstrand et al. 2004; Gillison 2004; Klussmann et al. 2003b; El-Mofty and Lu 2003; Klussmann et al. 2001; Mork et al. 2001; D'Souza et al. 2007). Sexual activity (high numbers of sexual partners, younger age of first sexual intercourse, the practice of oral sex, and a history of genital warts) has been associated with an increased risk of oropharyngeal cancer (Kreimer et al. 2004; Garrote et al. 2001; Maden et al. 1992). Also, husbands of women who had cervical cancer are more likely to have tonsillar and other upper aerodigestive cancers (Hemminki et al. 2000).

Evidence supports the idea that HNSCC is a multifactorial disease with at least two distinct pathogenesis models, one model implicating smoking and alcohol consumption, and the other driven by HPV (Ragin et al. 2007). The overall prevalence of HPV in head and neck cancer is 26% (Kreimer et al. 2005). For oropharyngeal, oral, and laryngeal SCCs considered separately, the prevalence of HPV is 36, 23, and 24%, respectively (Kreimer et al. 2005). Higher proportions are seen for tonsillar carcinomas, where 51% are found to be HPV DNA positive (Syrjanen 2005). HPV-16 and HPV-18 are the most prevalent types detected in HNSCC (Munoz et al. 2006) whereas HPV-6 and 11 are strongly associated with the development of respiratory papillomas (Kashima et al. 1992; Silverberg et al. 2003).

23.3.4 Non-melanoma Skin Cancer

Non-melanoma skin cancer (NMSC), which includes squamous cell carcinoma (SCC) and basal cell carcinoma (BCC) have also been linked to HPV. However, the types implicated among these types of cancers are different than the types implicated in the anogenital and head and neck cancer. The HPV family includes many cutaneous types (the most important clinically being EV-associated HPVs) which are involved, particularly HPV-5 and HPV-8, in the development of NMSC. About 30–50% of NMSC of immunocompetent individuals contain HPV DNA and this proportion increases to up to 90% among immunosuppressed organ transplant recipients (Pfister 2003; Munoz et al. 2006). It is clear that UV light is the primary etiological agent in NMSC, but it is now becoming clear that HPV may act as co-carcinogen with UV radiation or immunosuppression (Munoz et al. 2006).

23.3.5 Squamous Cell Carcinoma of the Conjunctiva

Squamous cell carcinoma of the conjunctiva is a rare tumor of the eye (Gichuhi and Irlam 2007; McKelvie et al. 2002). However, in Africa it is becoming more common, more aggressive, and more likely to affect young persons (Ateenyi-Agaba 1995). This pattern seems to be related to the coexistence of the HIV/AIDS pandemic, high HPV exposure, and solar radiation in the region. So far the causes of the disease are not adequately understood. There have been a number of investigations that have studied the impact of several factors, including solar exposure (Newton 1996) and HPV. The presence of HPV is strongly correlated with the occurrence of conjunctival papilloma (Sjo et al. 2007) and HPV has been detected in 35–100% of SCC of the conjunctiva (McDonnell et al. 1992; Tabrizi et al. 1997; Scott et al. 2002; Moubayed et al. 2004; Ateenyi-Agaba et al. 2004; Nakamura et al. 1997). However, since some studies failed to detect HPV in SCC of conjunctiva (Eng et al. 2002; Palazzi et al. 2000), the IARC has concluded that there is limited evidence for the carcinogenicity of HPV in this ocular site (IARC 2007).

23.4 Other Cancers in Which HPV Is Suspected to Play a Causal Role

It has been proposed that HPV may also play a role in the development of a whole range of other epithelial cancers such as malignancies of the bladder and urethra (Chrisofos et al. 2004; Youshya et al. 2005), lung (Chen et al. 2004; Giuliani et al. 2007; Coissard et al. 2005), retina (Orjuela et al. 2000; Palazzi et al. 2003), breast (de Villiers et al. 2005; Damin et al. 2004), prostate (Dennis and Dawson, 2002; Sutcliffe et al. 2007), colon (Lee et al. 2001; Pérez et al. 2005), ovary, and endometrium (Atalay et al. 2007; Konidaris et al. 2007). However, the role of the HPV in these cancers is still subject of considerable debate, as a strong proof of a causal relation is still lacking for each of them. Simply showing that HPV DNA is present in a lesion is not sufficient to demonstrate causality; contamination is a possible factor when testing specimens from these cancers. These cancers have usually more than one etiologic factor and even if it is eventually shown that HPV may be causally implicated it would probably not explain a large proportion of cases. Carefully performed molecular epidemiologic studies (using PCR as a more sensitive HPV detection method) with appropriate control groups and meticulous avoidance of sample contamination is needed to obtain unequivocal evidence for causal associations between HPV and these cancers.

23.5 Clinical Implications, HPV DNA Testing, and HPV Vaccines

HR-HPV has been definitely recognized as the main causal factor for cervical cancer. The recognition of this etiologic relationship has an enormous impact on prevention research and policy. This has led to the development of two new exciting fronts for cervical cancer prevention: HPV DNA testing for screening and HPV vaccination. Recent research on the safety and efficacy of two prophylactic vaccines against HPV has shown nearly 100% efficacy in preventing persistent infections and development of cervical precancerous lesions caused by the vaccine-targeted HPV types (Harper et al. 2004; Harper et al. 2006; Villa et al. 2006). An important caveat is that the vaccines are prophylactic only and not therapeutic. They are efficacious only in women without evidence of genital HPV DNA at the time of vaccination. The first one to be licensed, Gardasil^{TM} (Merck Inc.) is a quadrivalent vaccine and protects against HPV types 6, 11 (the two types that cause most anogenital warts), 16, and 18 (the two main HPV types that together cause about 75% of all cervical cancers). A bivalent Cervarix^{TM} (GlaxoSmithKline Inc.) has also been licensed in many countries; it protects against HPVs 16 and 18. A small degree of cross-protection against other HR-HPVs may also be expected (Harper et al. 2006). HPV vaccines are certainly among the most prominent public health achievements of the decade and can serve a central role in the prevention of cervical cancer. High vaccine coverage, sustained over many decades, with a long duration of vaccine-conferred protection would have a great impact on type-specific cancer incidence. Testing for HPV DNA has also shown great promise as a screening tool with much greater sensitivity but slightly lower specificity than Pap cytology (Mayrand et al. 2007). In combination with vaccination, HPV testing has the potential to improve the overall effectiveness of cervical cancer screening, thus allowing for increased testing intervals, which would lower program costs with acceptable safety.

23.6 Conclusions

HPV is the most common sexually transmitted viral infection and has been unequivocally considered as a human carcinogen. Progress has been grounded on the recognition that HPV infection is the central, necessary cause of many neoplastic diseases. This virus is the main causal factor of all cervical cancer cases in the world and of a substantial proportion of many other anogenital neoplasms (vagina, vulva, anus, and penis). To date, it has also been etiologically linked to a non-negligible proportion of head and neck cancer (oral cavity, pharynx, and larynx) and non-melanoma skin cancer. A causal role for HPV in other malignancies such as the conjunctiva, bladder, urethra, lung, retina, breast, prostate, colon, ovarian or endometrium, is yet to be credibly established. Properly designed and conducted molecular epidemiologic studies will be necessary to provide conclusive evidence for an association between HPV and these cancers. What is clear, however, is that vaccination against HPV-16/18 can serve a central role in the prevention of cervical cancer and of a substantial proportion of anogenital, and head and neck cancers. HPV vaccination is among the most important public health achievement of this decade.

Acknowledgments Cervical cancer research activities in the Division of Cancer Epidemiology at McGill University have been funded by an endowment from the Cancer Research Society and multiple grants from the Canadian Institutes of Health Research (CIHR), National Cancer Institute of Canada (NCIC), and US National Institutes of Health. The authors have also received salary awards from the CIHR (Distinguished Scientist to ELF), Fonds de la recherche en santé du Quebec (Chercheur National to ELF) and chercheur-boursier to HT. Supplemental unconditional financial support to the work of the division has been provided by Merck Frosst.

References

Al-Ghamdi A, Freedman D, Miller D, Poh C, Rosin M, Zhang L, Gilks CB (2002) Vulvar squamous cell carcinoma in young women: a clinicopathologic study of 21 cases. Gynecol Oncol; 84(1):94–101

Aral SO, Holmes KK (1999) Social and behavioural determinants of epidemiology of STDs: industrialized and developing countries. .. In: Holmes KK, Mardh P, Sparling PF, et al. eds. Sexually transmitted diseases. 3rd ed. New York, NY: McGraw-Hill; 39–76

Armstrong LR, Preston EJ, Reichert M, Phillips DL, Nisenbaum R, Todd NW, Jacobs IN, Inglis AF, Manning SC, Reeves WC (2000) Incidence and prevalence of recurrent respiratory papillomatosis among children in Atlanta and Seattle. Clin Infect Dis; 31(1):107–9

Atalay F, Taskiran C, Taner MZ, Pak I, Or M, Tuncer S (2007) Detection of human papillomavirus DNA and genotyping in patients with epithelial ovarian carcinoma. J Obstet Gynaecol Res; 33(6):823–828

Ateenyi-Agaba C (1995) Conjunctival squamous-cell carcinoma associated with HIV infection in Kampala, Uganda. Lancet; 345(8951):695–6

Ateenyi-Agaba C, Weiderpass E, Smet A, Dong W, Dai M, Kahwa B, Wabinga H, Katongole-Mbidde E, Franceschi S, Tommasino M (2004) Epidermodysplasia verruciformis human papillomavirus types and carcinoma of the conjunctiva: a pilot study. Br J Cancer; 90(9):1777–9

Baseman JG, Koutsky LA (2005) The epidemiology of human papillomavirus infections. J Clin Virol 2005 ; 32(suppl 1):S16–24.

Bosch FX, Manos MM, Muñoz N, Sherman M, Jansen AM, Peto J, Schiffman MH, Moreno V, Kurman R, Shah KV (1995) Prevalence of human papillomavirus in cervical cancer: a worldwide perspective. International biological study on cervical cancer (IBSCC) Study Group. J Natl Cancer Inst; 87(11): 796–802.

Bosch FX, Lorincz A, Munoz N, Meijer CJ, Shah KV (2002) The causal relation between human papillomavirus and cervical cancer. J Clin Pathol; 55(4):244–65

Brock KE, MacLennan R, Brinton LA, Melnick JL, Adam E, Mock PA, Berry G (1989) Smoking and infectious agents and risk of in situ cervical cancer in Sydney, Australia. Cancer Res; 49(17):4925–8

Chen YC, Chen JH, Richard K, Chen PY, Christiani DC (2004) Lung adenocarcinoma and human papillomavirus infection. Cancer; 15: 1428–36

Chrisofos M, Skolarikos A, Lazaris A, Bogris S, Deliveliotis Ch (2004) HPV 16/18-associated condyloma acuminatum of the urinary bladder: first international report and review of literature. Int J STD AIDS;15(12):836–8

Clifford GM, Smith JS, Plummer M, Munoz N, Franceschi S (2003) Human papillomavirus types in invasive cervical cancer worldwide: a meta-analysis. Br J Cancer; 88:63–73

Coissard CJ, Besson G, Polette MC, Monteau M, Birembaut PL, Clavel CE (2005) Prevalence of human papillomaviruses in lung carcinomas: a study of 218 cases. Mod Pathol; 18(12):1606–9

Cubilla AL, Reuter VE, Gregoire L et al. (1998) Basaloid squamous cell carcinoma: A distinctive human papilloma virus-related penile neoplasm—A report of 20 cases. Am J Surg Pathol 22:755–61

Cubilla AL, Velazques EF, Reuter VE et al. (2000) Warty (condylomatous) squamous cell carcinoma of the penis: A report of 11 cases and proposed classification of 'verruciform' penile tumors. Am J Surg Pathol 24:505–12

Cullen AP, Reid R, Camption M. Lorincz AT (1991) Analysis of the physical state of different human papillomavirus DNAs in intraepithelial and invasive cervical neoplasm. J Virol; 65(2):606–12

Cuzick J, Singer A, De Stavola BL, Chomet J (1990) Case-control study of risk factors for cervical intraepithelial neoplasia in young women. Eur J Cancer; 26(6):684–90

Dahlstrand H, Dahlgren L, Lindquist D et al. (2004) Presence of human papillomavirus in tonsillar cancer is a favourable prognostic factor for clinical outcome. Anticancer Res; 24:1829–35

Daling JR, Madeleine MM, Johnson LG, Schwartz SM, Shera KA, Wurscher MA, Carter JJ, Porter PL, Galloway DA, McDougall JK (2004) Human papillomavirus, smoking, and sexual practices in the etiology of anal cancer. Cancer 15;101(2):270–80

Daling JR, Madeleine MM, Schwartz SM, Shera KA, Carter JJ, McKnight B, Porter PL, Galloway DA, McDougall JK, Tamimi H (2002) A population-based study of squamous cell vaginal cancer: HPV and cofactors. Gynecol Oncol; 84(2):263–70

Daling JR, Weiss NS, Hislop TG, Maden C, Coates RJ, Sherman KJ, Ashley RL, Beagrie M, Ryan JA, Corey L (1987) Sexual practices, sexually transmitted diseases, and the incidence of anal cancer. N Engl J Med 15; 317(16):973–7

Damin AP, Karam R, Zettler CG, Caleffi M, Alexandre CO (2004) Evidence for an association of human papillomavirus and breast carcinomas. Breast Cancer Res Treat; 84:131–7

D'Souza G, Kreimer AR, Viscidi R, Pawlita M, Fakhry C, Koch WM, Westra WH, Gillison ML (2007) Case-control study of human papillomavirus and oropharyngeal cancer. N Engl J Med.10; 356(19):1944–56

de Vet HC, Sturmans F (1994) Risk factors for cervical dysplasia: implications for prevention. Public Health;108(4):241–9

de Villiers EM, Sandstrom RE, zur Hausen H, Buck CE (2005) Presence of papillomavirus sequences in condylomatous lesions of the mamillae and in invasive carcinoma of the breast. Breast Cancer Res; 7:R1–11

de Villiers EM, Fauquet C, Broker TR, Bernard HU, zur Hausen H (2004) Classification of papillomaviruses. Virology; 324(1):17–27

Dennis LK, Dawson DV (2002) Meta-analysis of measures of sexual activity and prostate cancer. Epidemiology; 13:72–9

Dillner J, von Krogh G, Horenblas S, Meijer CJ (2000) Etiology of squamous cell carcinoma of the penis. Scand J Urol Nephrol Suppl; (205):189–93

El-Mofty SK, Lu DW (2003) Prevalence of human papillomavirus type 16 DNA in squamous cell carcinoma of the palatine tonsil, and not the oral cavity, in young patients: a distinct clinicopathologic and molecular disease entity. Am J Surg Pathol; 27:1463–70

Eng HL, Lin TM, Chen SY, Wu SM, Chen WJ (2002) Failure to detect human papillomavirus DNA in malignant epithelial neoplasms of conjunctiva by polymerase chain reaction.Am J Clin Pathol; 117(3):429–36

Evans AS (1976) Causation and disease: the Henle-Koch postulates revisited. Yale J Biol Med; 49(2):175–95

Evans AS, Mueller NE (1990) Viruses and cancer. Causal associations. Ann Epidemiol; 1(1):71–92

Ferlay J, Bray F, Pisani P, Parkin DM (2004) GLOBOCAN 2002: Cancer Incidence, Mortality and Prevalence Worldwide. IARC CancerBase No. 5, version 2.0. IARC Press, Lyon

Ferreux E, Lont AP, Horenblas S, et al. (2003) Evidence for at least three alternative mechanisms targeting the p16INK4A/cyclin D/Rb pathway in penile carcinoma, one of which is mediated by high-risk human papillomavirus. J Pathol 201:109–18

Franco EL (1991) Viral etiology of cervical cancer: a critique of the evidence. Rev Infect Dis; 13(6):1195–206

Franco EL, Correa P, Santella RM, Wu X, Goodman SN, Petersen GM (2004) Role and limitations of epidemiology in establishing a causal association. Semin Cancer Biol; 14(6):413–26

Franco EL, Ferenczy A (2002) Part III, site-specific precancerous conditions: Cervix. In: EL Franco, TE Rohan eds. Cancer Precursors: Epidemiology, Detection, and Prevention. New York, NY: Springer- Verlag; 249–86

Franco EL, Rohan TE, Villa LL (1999) Epidemiologic evidence and human papillomavirus infection as a necessary cause of cervical cancer. J Natl Cancer Inst; 91: 506–11

Fredricks DN, Relman DA (1998) Infectious agents and the etiology of chronic idiopathic diseases. Curr Clin Top Infect Dis; 18:180–200

Frisch M, Glimelius B, van den Brule AJ, Wohlfahrt J, Meijer CJ, Walboomers JM, Goldman S, Svensson C, Adami HO, Melbye M (1997) Sexually transmitted infection as a cause of anal cancer. N Engl J Med; 337(19):1350–8

Frisch M, Melbye M, Moller H (1993) Trends in incidence of anal cancer in Denmark. BMJ; 306:41922

Garcia-Closas R, Castellsague X, Bosch X, Gonzalez CA (2005) The role of diet and nutrition in cervical carcinogenesis: A review of recent evidence. Int J Cancer; 117:629–37

Garrote LF, Herrero R, Reyes RM, Vaccarella S, Anta JL, Ferbeye L, Muñoz N, Franceschi S (2001) Risk factors for cancer of the oral cavity and oro-pharynx in Cuba. Br J Cancer; 85: 46–54

Gichuhi S, Irlam JJ. Interventions for squamous cell carcinoma of the conjunctiva in HIV-infected individuals (2007) Cochrane Database Syst Rev; (2):CD005643

Gillison ML (2004) Human papillomavirus-associated head and neck cancer is a distinct epidemiologic, clinical, and molecular entity. Semin Oncol; 31:744–54

Giuliano AR, Papenfuss M, Abrahamsen M, Inserra P (2002) Differences in factors associated with oncogenic and nononcogenic human papillomavirus infection at the United States–Mexico border. Cancer Epidemiol Biomarkers Prev; 11(9):930–4

Giuliani L, Favalli C, Syrjanen K, Ciotti M (2007) Human papillomavirus infections in lung cancer. Detection of E6 and E7 transcripts and review of the literature. Anticancer Res.; 27(4C): 2697–704

Giuliano AR, Siegel EM, Roe DJ, Ferreira S, Baggio ML, Galan L, Duarte-Franco E, Villa LL, Rohan TE, Marshall JR, Franco EL (2003) Dietary intake and risk of persistent human papillomavirus (HPV) infection: the Ludwig-McGill HPV Natural History study. J Infect Dis; 188:1508–16

Hampl M, Sarajuuri H, Wentzensen N, Bender HG, Kueppers V (2006) Effect of human papillomavirus vaccines on vulvar, vaginal, and anal intraepithelial lesions and vulvar cancer. Obstet Gynecol; 108(6):1361–8

Harper DM, Franco EL, Wheeler C, Ferris DG, Jenkins D, Schuind A et al. (2004) Efficacy of a bivalent L1 virus-like particle vaccine in prevention of infection with human papillomavirus types 16 and 18 in young women: a randomised controlled trial. Lancet; 364(9447): 1757–65

Harper DM, Franco EL, Wheeler CM et al. (2006) Sustained efficacy up to 4.5 years of a bivalent L1virus-like particle vaccine against human papillomavirus types 16 and 18: follow-up from a randomized control trial. Lancet; 367:1247–55

Harris RW, Brinton LA, Cowdell RH, Skegg DC, Smith PG, Vessey MP, Doll R (1980) Characteristics of women with dysplasia or carcinoma in situ of the cervix uteri. Br J Cancer; 42(3):359–69

Heideman DA, Waterboer T, Pawlita M, Delis-van Diemen P, Nindl I, Leijte JA, Bonfrer JM, Horenblas S, Meijer CJ, Snijders PJ (2007) Human papillomavirus-16 is the predominant type etiologically involved in penile squamous cell carcinoma. J Clin Oncol; 25(29):4550–6

Hellberg D, Valentin J, Eklund T, Nilsson S (1987) Penile cancer: is there an epidemiological role for smoking and sexual behaviour? Br Med J (Clin Res Ed).; 295(6609):1306–8

Hemminki K, Dong C, Frisch M (2000) Tonsillar and other upper aerodigestive tract cancer among cervical cancer patient and their husbands. Eur J Cancer Prev; 9: 433–7

Herrero R (1996) Epidemiology of cervical cancer. J Natl Cancer Inst Monogr; 21: 1–6

Holly EA (1996) Cervical intraepithelial neoplasia, cervical cancer, and HPV. Annu Rev Public Health; 17: 69–84

Holly EA, Whittemore AS, Aston DA, Ahn DK, Nickoloff BJ, Kristiansen JJ (1989) Anal cancer incidence: genital warts, anal fissure or fistula, hemorrhoids, and smoking. J Natl Cancer Inst; 81(22):1726–31

Hørding U, Junge J, Daugaard S, Lundvall F, Poulsen H, Bock JE (1994) Vulvar squamous cell carcinoma and papillomaviruses: indications for two different etiologies. Gynecol Oncol; 52(2):241–6

Ikenberg H, Runge M, Goppinger A, Pfleiderer A (1990) Human papillomavirus DNA in invasive carcinoma of the vagina. Obstet Gynecol; 76:432–8

International Agency for Research on Cancer (IARC) (1986) Tobacco smoking. Lyon, France: IARC. IARC monographs on the evaluation of carcinogenic risk of chemical to human. Vol. 38

International Agency for Research on Cancer (IARC) (1995) Human papillomaviruses. Lyon, France: IARC. IARC monographs on the evaluation of carcinogenic risks to humans. Vol. 64

International Agency for Research on Cancer (IARC) (2007) Human Papillomaviruses. Lyon, France: IARC. IARC monographs on the evaluation of carcinogenic risks to humans.,: International Agency for Research on Cancer, vol. 90

Insinga RP, Glass AG, Rush BB (2004) The health care costs of cervical human papillomavirus–related disease. Am J Obstet Gynecol. l; 191(1):114–20

Insinga RP, Glass AG, Rush BB (2004) Pap screening in a U.S. health plan. Cancer Epidemiol Biomarkers Prev; 13(3):355–60

Johnson LG, Madeleine MM, Newcomer LM, Schwartz SM, Daling JR (2004) Anal cancer incidence and survival: the SEER experience, 1973-2000. Cancer; 101: 281–288

Judson PL, Habermann EB, Baxter NN, Durham SB, Virnig BA (2006) Trends in the incidence of invasive and in situ vulvar carcinoma. Obstet Gynecol; 107(5):1018–22

Kahn JA, Rosenthal SL, Succop PA, Ho GY, Burk RD (2002) Mediators of the association between age of first sexual intercourse and subsequent human papillomavirus infection. Pediatrics; 109(1):E5

Kashima HK, Shah F, Lyles A, et al.(1992) A comparison of risk factors in juvenile-onset and adult-onset recurrent respiratory papillomatosis. Laryngoscope; 102:9–13

Kjellberg L, Wang Z, Wiklund F, Edlund K, Angstrom T, Lenner P, Sjoberg I, Hallmans G, Wallin KL, Sapp M, Schiller J, Wadell G, Mahlck CG, Dillner J (1999) Sexual behaviour and papillomavirus exposure in cervical intraepithelial neoplasia: a population-based case-control study. J Gen Virol; 80(Pt 2):391–8

Klussmann JP, Gultekin E, Weissenborn SJ, et al. (2003a) Expression of p16 protein identifies a distinct entity of tonsillar carcinomas associated with human papillomavirus. AmJ Pathol; 162:747–53

Klussmann JP, Weissenborn SJ, Wieland U, et al. (2003b) Human papillomavirus-positive tonsillar carcinomas: a different tumor entity? Med Microbiol Immunol (Berl);192:129–32

Klussmann JP, Weissenborn SJ, Wieland U, Dries V, Kolligs J, Jungehuelsing M, Eckel HE, Dienes HP, Pfister HJ, Fuchs PG (2001) Prevalence, distribution, and viral load of human papillomavirus 16 DNA in tonsillar carcinomas. Cancer ; 92:2875–84.

Konidaris S, Kouskouni EE, Panoskaltsis T, Kreatsas G, Patsouris ES, Sarivalassis A, Nonni A, Lazaris AC (2007) Human papillomavirus infection in malignant and benign gynaecological conditions: a study in Greek women. Health Care Women Int; 28(2):182–91

Koutsky L (1997) Epidemiology of genital human papillomavirus infection. Am J Med; 102(5A):3–8

Kreimer AR, Alberg AJ, Daniel R, Gravitt PE, Viscidi R, Garrett ES, Shah KV, Gillison ML (2004) Oral human papillomavirus infection in adults is associated with sexual behavior and HIV serostatus. J Infect Dis; 189: 686–98

Kreimer AR, Clifford GM, Boyle P, Franceschi S (2005) Human papillomavirus types in head and neck SCCs worldwide: a systematic review. Cancer Epidemiol Biomarkers Prev; 14:467–75

Lee YM, Leu SY, Chiang H, Chiang H, Fung CP, Liu WT (2001) Human papillomavirus type 18 in colorectal cancer. J Microbiol Immunol Infect; 34: 87–91

Maciag PC, Schlecht NF, Souza PS, Rohan TE, Franco EL, Villa LL (2002) Polymorphisms of the human leukocyte antigen DRB1 and DQB1 genes and the natural history of human papillomavirus infection. J Infect Dis; 186: 164–72

Macfarlane GJ, Boyle P, Scully C (1992) Oral cancer in Scotland: changing incidence and mortality. BMJ; 305:1121–3

Madeleine MM, Daling JR, Carter JJ, Wipf GC, Schwartz SM, McKnight B, Kurman RJ, Beckmann AM, Hagensee ME, Galloway DA (1997) Cofactors with human papillomavirus in a population-based study of vulvar cancer. J Natl Cancer Inst; 89:1516–23

Maden C, Beckmann AM, Thomas DB, McKnight B, Sherman KJ, Ashley RL, Corey L, Daling JR (1992) Human papillomaviruses, herpes simplex viruses, and the risk of oral cancer inmen. AmJ Epidemiol; 135:1093–102

Maden C, Sherman KJ, Beckmann AM, Hislop TG, Teh CZ, Ashley RL, Daling JR (1993) History of circumcision, medical conditions, and sexual activity and risk of penile cancer. J Natl Cancer Inst; 85(1):19–24

Malek RS, Goellner JR, Smith TF, Espy MJ, Cupp MR (1993) Human papillomavirus infection and intraepithelial, in situ, and invasive carcinoma of penis. Urology; 42(2):159–70

Manhart LE, Koutsky LA (2002) Do condoms prevent genital HPV infection, external genital warts, or cervical neoplasia? A meta-analysis. Sex Transm Dis; 29: 725–35

Mayrand MH, Duarte-Franco E, Rodrigues I, Walter SD, Hanley J, Ferenczy A, Ratnam S, Coutlée F, Franco EL (2007) Canadian Cervical Cancer Screening Trial Study Group. Human papillomavirus DNA versus Papanicolaou screening tests for cervical cancer. N Engl J Med; 357(16):1579–88

McDonnell JM, McDonnell PJ, Sun YY (1992) Human papillomavirus DNA in tissues and ocular surface swabs of patients with conjunctival epithelial neoplasia. Invest Ophthalmol Vis Sci;33(1):184–9

McKelvie PA, Daniell M, McNab A, Loughnan M, Santamaria JD (2002) Squamous cell carcinoma of the conjunctiva: a series of 26 cases. Br J Ophthalmol; 86(2):168–73

Melbye M, Rabkin C, Frisch M, Biggar RJ (1994) Changing patterns of anal cancer incidence in the United States, 19401989. Am J Epidemiol; 139:77280

Mork J, Lie AK, Glattre E, Hallmans G, Jellum E, Koskela P, Møller B, Pukkala E, Schiller JT, Youngman L, Lehtinen M, Dillner J (2001) Human papillomavirus infection as a risk factor for squamous-cell carcinoma of the head and neck. N Engl J Med; 344:1125–31

Moscicki AB, Hills N, Shiboski S, Powell K, Jay N, Hanson E, Miller S, Clayton L, Farhat S, Broering J, Darragh T, Palefsky J (2001) Risks for incident human papillomavirus infection and low-grade squamous intraepithelial lesion development in young females. JAMA; 285: 2995–3002

Moubayed P, Mwakyoma H, Schneider DT (2004) High frequency of human papillomavirus 6/11, 16, and 18 infections in precancerous lesions and squamous cell carcinoma of the conjunctiva in subtropical Tanzania. Am J Clin Pathol; 122(6):938–43

Munoz N, Bosch FX, Castellsague X, Diaz M, de Sanjose S, Hammouda D, Shah KV, Meijer CJ (2004) Against which human papillomavirus types shall we vaccinate and screen? The international perspective. Int J Cancer; 111(2):278–85

Munoz N, Bosch FX, de Sanjose S, Herrero R, Castellsague X, Shah KV, Snijders PJ, Meijer CJ (2003) Epidemiologic classification of human papillomavirus types associated with cervical cancer. N Engl J Med; 348(6):518–27

Muñoz N, Castellsagué X, de González AB, Gissmann L (2006) Chapter 1: HPV in the etiology of human cancer. Vaccine. 2006 Aug 21; 24S3:S1–10

Nakamura Y, Mashima Y, Kameyama K, Mukai M, Oguchi Y (1997) Detection of human papillomavirus infection in squamous tumours of the conjunctiva and lacrimal sac by immunohistochemistry, in situ hybridisation, and polymerase chain reaction. Br J Ophthalmol; 81(4):308–13

Newton R (1996) A review of the aetiology of squamous cell carcinoma of the conjunctiva. Br J Cancer; 74(10):1511–3

Orjuela M, Castaneda VP, Ridaura C, Lecona E, Leal C, Abramson DH, Orlow I, Gerald W, Cordon-Cardo C (2000) Presence of human papilloma virus in tumor tissue from children with retinoblastoma: an alternative mechanism for tumor development. Clin Cancer Res; 6(10):4010–6

Palazzi MA, Erwenne CM, Villa LL (2000) Detection of human papillomavirus in epithelial lesions of the conjunctiva. Sao Paulo Med J; 118(5):125–30

Palazzi MA, Yunes JA, Cardinalli IA, Stangenhaus GP, Brandalise SR, Ferreira SA, Sobrinho JS, Villa LL (2003) Detection of oncogenic human papillomavirus in sporadic retinoblastoma. Acta Ophthalmol Scand; 81(4):396–8

Palefsky JM (2000b) Anal squamous intraepithelial lesions in human immunodeficiency virus-positive men and women. Semin Oncol.; 27(4):471–9

Palefsky JM (2000a) Human papilloma virus related tumors. AIDS; 14(Suppl 3):S18995

Palefsky JM, Holly EA, Gonzales J, Berline J, Ahn DK, Greenspan JS (1991) Detection of human papillomavirus DNA in anal intraepithelial neoplasia and anal cancer. Cancer Res; 51(3): 1014–9

Parazzini F, La Vecchia C, Negri E, Fedele L, Franceschi S, Gallotta L (1992) Risk factors for cervical intraepithelial neoplasia. Cancer; 69(9):2276–82

Parkin DM (2006) The global health burden of infection-associated cancers in the year 2002. Int J Cancer; 118(12):3030–44.

Parkin DM, Bray F, Ferlay J, Pisani P (2005) Global cancer statistics, 2002. CA Cancer J Clin; 55(2):74–108

Parkin DM, Whelan SL, Ferlay J, et al. (2002) Cancer Incidence in Five Continents. Lyon, France, IARC Scientific Publication 155

Parkin DM, Whelan S, Ferlay J, Raymond LE, Young J (1997) Cancer incidence in five continents, Vol. VII. Lyon: International Agency for Research on Cancer, IARC Scientific Publications No. 143

Pirami L, Giache V, Becciolini A (1997) Analysis of HPV 16, 18, 31, and 35 DNA in pre-invasive and invasive lesions of the uterine cervix 1997. J Clin Pathol; 50(7):600–4

Pisani P, Parkin DM, Bray F, Ferlay J (1999) Estimates of the worldwide mortality from 25 cancers in 1990. Int J Cancer; 83:18–29

Pérez LO, Abba MC, Laguens RM, Golijow CD (2005) Analysis of adenocarcinoma of the colon and rectum: detection of human papillomavirus (HPV) DNA by polymerase chain reaction. Colorectal Dis; 7(5):492–5

Pfister H (2003) Chapter 8: Human papillomavirus and skin cancer. J Natl Cancer Inst Monogr; 31:52–6

Ragin CC, Modugno F, Gollin SM (2007) The epidemiology and risk factors of head and neck cancer: a focus on human papillomavirus. J Dent Res; 86(2):104–14

Ryan DP, Compton CC, Mayer RJ (2000) Carcinoma of the anal canal. N Engl J Med; 342: 792– 800

Richardson H, Kelsall G, Tellier P, Voyer H, Abrahamowicz M, Ferenczy A, Coutlée F, Franco EL (2003) The natural history of type-specific human papillomavirus infections in female university students. Cancer Epidemiol Biomarkers Prev;12:485–90

Ries LAG, Eisner MP, Kosary CL, Hankey BF, Miller BA, Clegg L, Edwards BK eds. (2000) SEER Cancer Statistics Review, 1973–1997, National Cancer Institute. Bethesda, MD

Ries LAG, Harkins D, Krapcho M, Mariotto A, Miller BA, Feuer EJ, et al. eds.(2006) SEER Cancer Statistics Review, 1975-2003. Bethesda (MD): National Cancer Institute. Available at: http://seer.cancer.gov/csr/1975_2003

Rousseau MC, Franco EL, Villa LL, Sobrinho JP, Termini L, Prado JM, Rohan TE (2000) A cumulative case-control study of risk factor profiles for oncogenic and nononcogenic cervical human papillomavirus infections. Cancer Epidemiol Biomarkers Prev; 9:469–76

Rubin MA, Kleter B, Zhou M, Ayala G, Cubilla AL, Quint WG, Pirog EC (2001) Detection and typing of human papillomavirus DNA in penile carcinoma: evidence for multiple independent pathways of penile carcinogenesis. Am J Pathol; 159(4):1211–8

Schaffer A, Koushik A, Trottier H, Duarte-Franco E, Mansour N, Arseneau J, Provencher D, Gilbert L, Gotlieb W, Ferenczy A, Coutlée F, Pollak MN, Franco EL (2007) Insulin-like growth factor-I and risk of high-grade cervical intraepithelial neoplasia. Cancer Epidemiol Biomarkers Prev; 16(4):716–22

Schantz SP, Yu GP (2002) Head and neck cancer incidence trends in young Americans, 1973–1997, with a special analysis for tongue cancer.Arch Otolaryngol Head Neck Surg; 128(3):268–74

Schiffman MH, Bauer HM, Hoover RN, Glass AG, Cadell DM, Rush BB, Scott DR, Sherman ME, Kurman RJ, Wacholder S, et al. (1993) Epidemiologic evidence showing that human papillomavirus infection causes most cervical intraepithelial neoplasia. J Natl Cancer Inst; 85(12): 958–64

Schiffman MH, Brinton LA (1995) The epidemiology of cervical carcinogenesis. Cancer; 76 (10 Suppl): 1888–901

Schiffman M, Castle PE (2003b) Human papillomavirus: epidemiology and public health. Arch Pathol Lab Med; 127(8):930–4

Schiffman M, Kjaer SK (2003) Chapter 2: Natural history of anogenital human papillomavirus infection and neoplasia. J Natl Cancer Inst Monogr; (31):14–9

Schlecht NF, Trevisan A, Duarte-Franco E, et al. (2003) Viral load as a predictor of the risk of cervical intraepithelial neoplasia. Int J Cancer; 103:519–24

Scott IU, Karp CL, Nuovo GJ (2002) Human papillomavirus 16 and 18 expression in conjunctival intraepithelial neoplasia. Ophthalmology; 109(3):542–7

Sellors JW, Karwalajtys TL, Kaczorowski J, Mahony JB, Lytwyn A, Chong S, Sparrow J, Lorincz A (2003) Survey of HPV in Ontario Women Group. Incidence, clearance and predictors of human papillomavirus infection in women. CMAJ;168:421–5

Shibuya K, Mathers CD, Boschi-Pinto C, Lopez AD, Murray CJ (2002) Global and regional estimates of cancer mortality and incidence by site: II. Results for the global burden of disease 2000. BMC Cancer; 2(1):37

Shiboski CH, Shiboski SC, Silverman SJ (2000) Trends in oral cancer rates in the United States, 1973–1996. Community Dent Oral Epidemiol; 28:249–56

Sichero L, Ferreira S, Trottier H, Duarte-Franco E, Ferenczy A, Franco EL, Villa LL (2007) High grade cervical lesions are caused preferentially by non-European variants of HPVs 16 and 18. Int J Cancer; 120(8):1763–8

Silverberg MJ, Thorsen P, Lindeberg H, Grant LA, Shah KV (2003) Condyloma in pregnancy is strongly predictive of juvenile-onset recurrent respiratory papillomatosis. Obstet Gynecol; 101:645–52

Sjö NC, von Buchwald C, Cassonnet P, Norrild B, Prause JU, Vinding T, Heegaard S (2007) Human papillomavirus in normal conjunctival tissue and in conjunctival papilloma: types and frequencies in a large series. Br J Ophthalmol; 91(8):1014–5

Spence AR, Franco EL, Ferenczy A (2005) The role of human papillomavirus in cancer. Am J Cancer; 4(1):49–64

Stone KM, Timyan J, Thomas EL (1999) Barrier methods for the prevention of sexually transmitted diseases. In: Holmes KK, Mardh P, Sparling PF, et al. eds.. Sexually Transmitted Diseases. 3rd ed. New York, NY: McGraw- Hill:1307–21

Sutcliffe S, Giovannucci E, Gaydos CA, Viscidi RP, Jenkins FJ, Zenilman JM, Jacobson LP, De Marzo AM, Willett WC, Platz EA (2007) Plasma antibodies against Chlamydia trachomatis, human papillomavirus, and human herpesvirus type 8 in relation to prostate cancer: a prospective study. Cancer Epidemiol Biomarkers Prev; 16(8):1573–80

Syrjanen S (2005) Human papillomavirus (HPV) in head and neck cancer. J Clin Virol; 32 Suppl 1:S59–66

Tabrizi SN, McCurrach FE, Drewe RH, Borg AJ, Garland SM, Taylor HR (1997) Human papillomavirus in corneal and conjunctival carcinoma. Aust N Z J Ophthalmol; 25(3):211–5

Tran N, Rose BR, O'Brien CJ (2007) Role of human papillomavirus in the etiology of head and neck cancer. Head Neck; 29(1):64–70

Trottier H, Franco EL (2006) The epidemiology of genital human papillomavirus infection. Vaccine; 24 Suppl 1:S1–15

Venuti A, Badaracco G, Rizzo C, Mafera B, Rahimi S, Vigili M (2004) Presence of HPV in head and neck tumours: high prevalence in tonsillar localization. J Exp Clin Cancer Res; 23: 561–6

Villa LL, Ault KA, Giuliano AR, Costa RL, Petta CA, Andrade RP, Brown DR, Ferenczy A, Harper DM, Koutsky LA, Kurman RJ, Lehtinen M, Malm C, Olsson SE, Ronnett BM, Skjeldestad FE, Steinwall M, Stoler MH, Wheeler CM, Taddeo FJ, Yu J, Lupinacci L, Railkar R, Marchese R, Esser MT, Bryan J, Jansen KU, Sings HL, Tamms GM, Saah AJ, Barr E (2006) Immunologic responses following administration of a vaccine targeting human papillomavirus types 6, 11, 16, and 18. Vaccine; 24:5571–83

Walboomers JM, Jacobs MV, Manos MM, Bosch FX, Kummer JA, Shah KV, Snijders PJ, Peto J, Meijer CJ, Munoz N (1999) Human papillomavirus is a necessary cause of invasive cervical cancer worldwide. J Pathol; 189: 12–9

Walboomers JM, Meijer CJ (1997) Do HPV-negative cervical carcinomas exist? J Pathol; 181: 253–4

Wang SS, Hildesheim A (2003) Chapter 5: Viral and host factors in human papillomavirus persistence and progression. J Natl Cancer Inst Monogr; (31):35–40

Welton ML, Sharkey FE, Kahlenberg MS (2004) The etiology and epidemiology of anal cancer. Surg Oncol Clin N Am; 13:263–75

Winer RL, Lee SK, Hughes JP, Adam DE, Kiviat NB, Koutsky LA (2003) Genital human papillomavirus infection: incidence and risk factors in a cohort of female university students. Am J Epidemiol; 157(3):218–26

Winer RL, Hughes JP, Feng Q et al. (2006) Condom use and the risk of genital human papillomavirus infection in young women. N Engl J Med; 354:2645–54

Youshya S, Purdie K, Breuer J, Proby C, Sheaf MT, Oliver RT, Baithun S (2005) Does human papillomavirus play a role in the development of bladder transitional cell carcinoma? A comparison of PCR and immunohistochemical analysis. J Clin Pathol; 58(2):207–10

Index

A. Krämer et al. (eds.), *Modern Infectious Disease Epidemiology*, Statistics for Biology and Health, DOI 10.1007/978-0-387-93835-6,

P

CPSIA information can be obtained at www.ICGtesting.com
Printed in the USA
LVOW06*0928190715

446791LV00003B/35/P